Massimo Rossi

Orthodontics in Clinical Practice

Published in the UK by:-

Anshan Ltd
6 Newlands Road
Tunbridge Wells
Kent. TN4 9AT

Tel: +44 (0) 1892 557767
Fax: +44 (0) 1892 530358

e-mail: info@anshan.co.uk
web site: www.anshan.co.uk

ISBN: 978 1 848290 73 0

British Library Cataloguing in Publication Data

A catalogue record for this book is available from the British Library.

Copy Editor: Catherine Lain
Copy Editor: Andrew White
Cover Design: Emma Randall
Typeset by: KerryPress Ltd

Printed and bound in India by Replika Press Pvt. Ltd.

Author

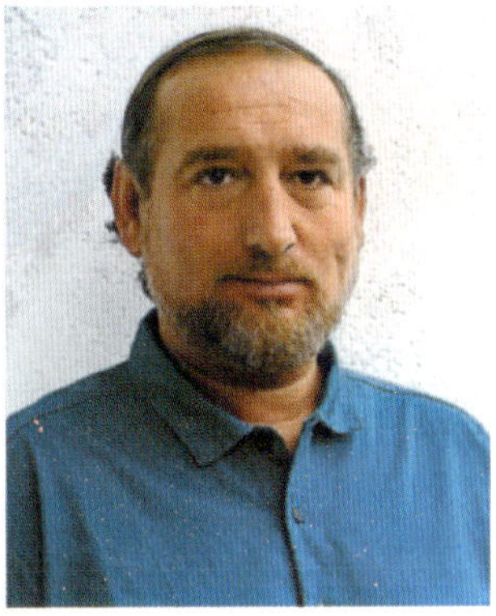

Massimo Rossi.

Born in Arona, northern Italy, on 27th April, 1953. Graduated in Medicine and Surgery cum laude in 1977 at the University of Pavia. He graduated again in 1979, also cum laude, with a Diploma of Specialization in Clinical Stomatological Odontoiatrics from the University of Milan, and followed this in 1982 with a specialization in Orthognathodontics under the guidance of Prof. Ennio Gianni. He continues to live and work in Arona.

dedicated to all those who supported me during the creation of this book and who continue to support me.

μοι νυνὶ γέγονεν ἐκ τοῦ διαλόγου μηδὲν εἰδέναι
As for me, all I know is that I know nothing

Socrates

Acknowledgements

I would like to thank my colleagues and friends who have made contributions to the production of this work.

I also thank Leone Orthodontics and Implantology S.p.A - Florence and Wisil Latoor SRL dental laboratory - Milan

Table of Contents

All the images in this book are available for viewing on the Anshan website www.anshan.co.uk Go to Orthodontics in Clinical Practice and click on View Illustrations.

CHAPTER 1 General Introduction

- Embryology 2
- Craniofacial Growth 3
- Ossification 5
- Stomatognathic Growth 6
- Growth Forecast 8
- Diagnosis and Treatment Plan 8
- Examination of the Patient and Family 9
- *Dental Plaster Models* 12
- *Orthopantomography* 12
- *Lateral Cephalogram* 12
- Importance of Radiological Examinations 13
- *Importance of Clinical Observation Combined with Radiological Analysis* 15
- Data Provided by Radiology and by Modelling 16
- *Changes from Deciduous to Permanent Occlusions* 16
- *Relationship between Teeth and the Dental Arch* 17
- *With or without Extractions* 18
- Classification of Malocclusions 19
- Cephalometric Analysis 19
- *Lateral Cephalogram* 19
- Postero-Anterior X-Ray 23
- Orthodontics and Aesthetics 24
- *Clinical Evaluation* 24
- *Mixed Evaluation* 25
- *Discussion* 26
- *Conclusion* 26
- Biomechanics 26
- *Teeth Displacement* 27
- Dental Movement 29
- *Tipping-Uprighting* 29
- *Torque* 29
- Anchorage 31
- *Orthodontic wires* 32
- *Stainless Steel Wires* 32
- *Cobalt-Chromium Wires* 32

Table of Contents

- *Beta-Titanium Wires* 32
- *Multi-Stranded Wires* 32
- *Nickel-Titanium (NiTi) Wires* 32
- *Traditional NiTi* 32
- Why an Orthodontic Treatment? 33
- *When to begin a Treatment?* 34
- Prevention in Orthodontics 35
- Myofunctional Exercises 36
- *Tongue* 36
- *Orofacial Musculature Exercises* 36
- Removable or Fixed Appliances? 37
- Fixed Techniques in Orthodontics 38
- *Edgewise* 38
- *Tweed* 38
- *Begg* 39
- *Phase 1, 2, 3* 39
- *Andrews Straight Wire* 39
- *Alexander* 41
- *Segmented Arch* 42
- *Bioprogressive* 42
- *Common Considerations about Brackets* 44
- *Anterior Teeth* 44
- *Posterior Teeth* 44
- *"Best" Technical System* 45
- *Self Ligating Low Friction* 46
- Aesthetic Techniques 47
- *Lingual Orthodontics* 48
- *Clear Aligners* 48
- Elastics 48

CHAPTER 2 Class I

- Class I 54
- Expansion in Orthodontics 54
- *Maxilla* 55
- Types of Expansion 57
- *Rapid Expansion* 57
- *Slow Expansion* 58
- *Ultra-Slow Expansion* 59
- *Until What Age is it Possible to Perform Maxillary Expansion?* 60

Table of Contents

- *Expansion to Gain Space* 60
- Mandible 60
- *Transverse Expansion* 60
- *To Extract or not to Extract?* 61
- *Dental Arch Limits* 61
- *Who is Right?* 62
- Naturally Beyond the Limits:Bialveolar Protrusions 66
- How to Gain Space Distally (Molar Distalization) 70
- *Kloehn Headgear* 70
- Distalization of Upper Molars with Non-Compliance Appliances 71
- *Are We Always Talking about Non-Compliance Appliances?* 71
- *Conclusions* 71
- *Lip Bumper* 75
- *Palatal Bar* 77
- *Stripping* 77
- *Conclusions* 78
- Extractions:Which Teeth to Extract? 90
- *Third Molars* 80
- *First Molars* 80
- *Second Molars* 80
- *Conclusions* 87
- *Sectional Treatments* 93

CHAPTER 3 Class II

- Class II 98
- Treatment 98
- *Functional Appliances* 99
- *Andresen Activator* 100
- *Frankel* 103
- *Functional Plate of Cervera* 105
- *Bimler* 105
- *Bionator* 105
- *Kinetor* 107
- *Sander's Appliances* 107
- *Twin Block* 109
- *RV1-RV2* 109
- *Herbst Appliance* 111
- *Headgears* 114

Table of Contents

- *Orthodontic Use* 116
- *Orthopedic Use (with forces greater than 300g)* 118
- *Headgears Combined with Activators* 118
- *Centres of Resistance* 118
- *Can Headgears be Dangerous?* 123
- Orthodontic Fixed Appliances in Conservative Treatment of Class II 124
- *Class II: One Phase or Two Phase Treatment?* 125
- *Conclusions* 125
- *Class II Treatment at the End of Growth (Adult Patients)* 126
- *Class II Division 1* 126
- *When is it Better to Avoid Extraction of the Upper Premolars?* 126
- *When can only Two Upper Premolars be Extracted?* 126
- *When do Four Upper Premolars Need to be Extracted?* 127
- *What are the Limits of Lower Incisor Proclination?* 127
- *How Many Millimetres can a "Gnathological Skid" Be?* 127
- Four Extraction Treatments in Class II Malocclusions 132
- Class II Treatments with Two Extractions 137
- Treatment of a Class II with Two Upper First Molar Extractions 138
- *Cases with Two Unusual Extractions* 139

CHAPTER 4 Class III

- Description and Etiology 144
- *Maxilla* 144
- *Mandible* 145
- *Treatment* 145
- *Functional Appliances* 145
- *Chin Cup* 148
- *Protraction Facemask* 148
- *At the End of Growth* 156
- *Treatment with Fixed Appliances* 157
- *Discussion* 157
- *Conclusions* 158

CHAPTER 5 Issues Common to the Three Classes

- Serial Extractions 160
- Dental Anomalies (Supernumerary and Agenesis) 163
- Problems (and Mistakes) in Orthodontics 164

Table of Contents

- Vertical Dimension 166
- Increased Vertical Dimension 166
- *Treatment* 167
- *Class II* 167
- *Class I* 167
- *Class I - Class II* 167
- *Treating the Problems of Dysfunction* 167
- *Conclusions* 168
- Decreased Vertical Dimension 173
- *Treatment* 173
- Retainers 177
- Diastemas 178
- *Canine Displacement* 180
- *Treatment* 182
- *Iatrogenic Displacement* 187
- *Root Resorption* 188
- *What are the Limits of Treatment on Impacted Canines?* 188
- *Other Teeth Displacement* 191
- *Transpositions* 192

CHAPTER 6 MultiDisciplinary Treatments: the Relationship between Orthodontics and Other Disciplines

- Orthodontics and Periodontology 196
- *How Can Teeth with Periodontal Problems be Moved?* 197
- *Intrusion* 197
- *Extrusion* 197
- *Gingival Recessions* 197
- Orthodontics and Prosthesis 205
- *Incisors* 206
- *The Cases of Two Brothers* 208
- *Canines* 210
- *Molars and Premolars* 211
- *Molar Uprighting* 213
- *A-B Modalities* 214
- *Second Lower Right Molar Uprighting* 215
- *More Cases to illustrate the Ortho-Prosthesis Relationship* 216
- Orthodontics-Implantology 220
- *What Can Implantology Do for Orthodontics?* 220

Table of Contents

- *What Implantology Can Do for Orthodontics* 223
- Surgical Management of MiniScrew Insertion and Removal: a Step by Step Approach 224
- *Preparation Phase (Steps 1-6)* 225
- *Soft Tissue Phase (Steps 7-15)* 227
- *Cortical Bone Phase (Step 16)* 230
- *Trabecular Bone Insertion Phase (Step 17)* 231
- *Final Positioning Phase (Steps 18-24)* 233
- *Surgical Management for the Removal of Mini-Implants* 234
- *Example of MiniScrew Application* 236
- Orthodontics and the Temperomandibular Joint (TMJ) 238
- *Relationship between Orthodontics and Gnathology* 238
- *Temperomandibular Joint Disorders* 238
- *Relationship between the TMJ and Orthodontics* 239
- *Transverse Evaluation* 241
- *Vertical Evaluation* 242
- *Treatment* 246
- *Conclusions* 246
- *Interdisciplinary Cases* 246

CHAPTER 7 Orthognathic Surgery

- Orthognathic Surgery 254
- *Treatment* 257,263

Chapter I:

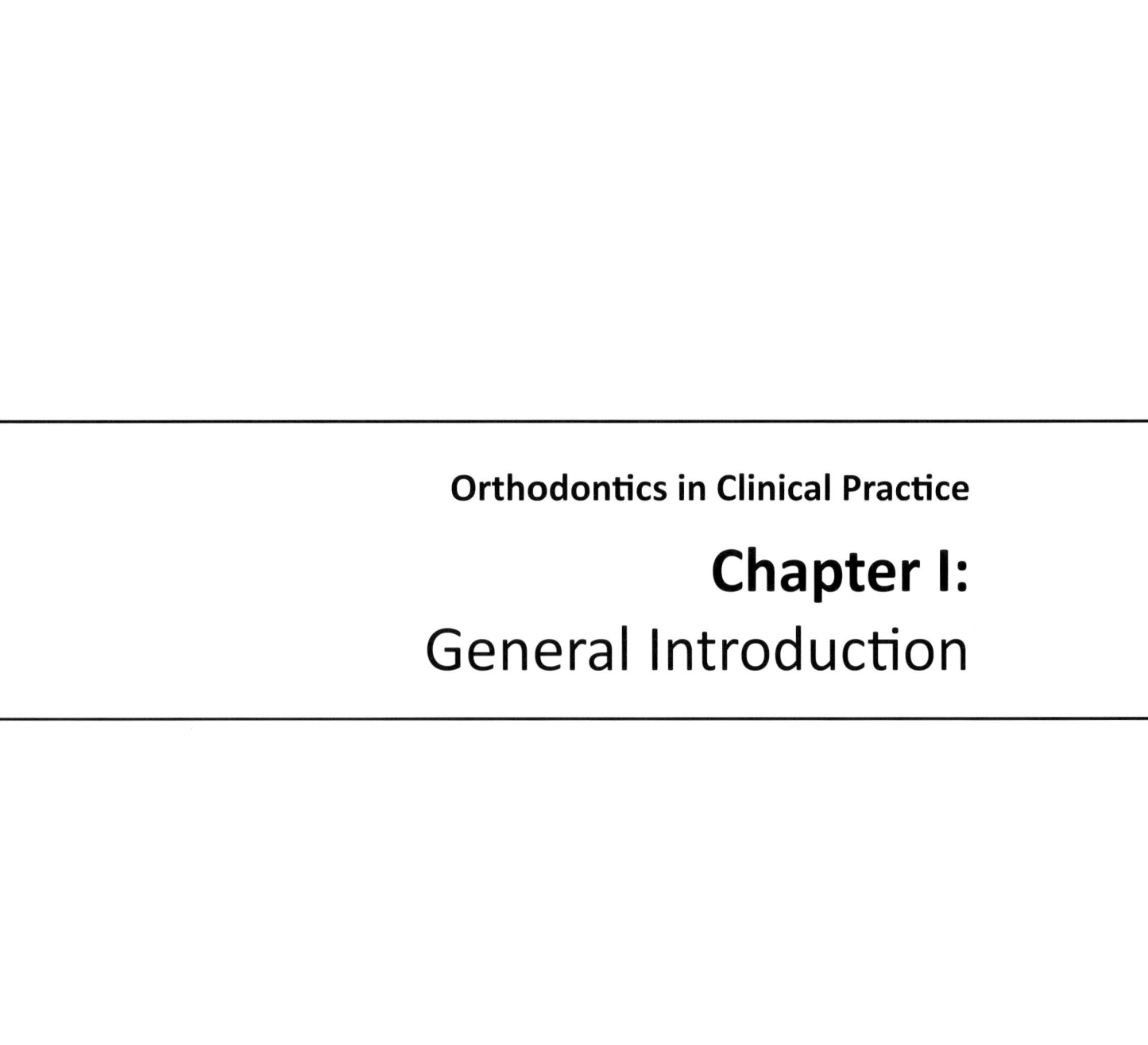

General Introduction

EMBRYOLOGY

It is useful for the clinician to consider craniofacial embryology so that they can understand the nature of malocclusion and otherwise inexplicable symptoms. After ovum fertilization and its embedding in the endometrium fetal organogenesis begins. It ends at the third month of gestation. This is the period of maximum vulnerability of the fetus. Pathogenic factors can have catastrophic consequences and result in a miscarriage or malformations of considerable gravity.

Organs are shaped and defined between 4 and 6 months. Then between 7 and 9 months fetal growth and maturation occur.

The skull can be divided into two parts: the neurocranium that protects the brain and the viscerocranium, from which the skeleton of the face forms.

The base of the skull or condrocranium is common to both parts.

The skeletal structure of the face (Fig. 1-1) is formed around the stomodeum, which is a single cavity at first that is later divided into the nasal part (top) and in the buccal part (bottom). The stomodeum is bordered on top by the fronto - nasal process, laterally by the maxillary processes with the nasal processes, above and on the bottom by the mandibular processes.

At the bottom of the stomodeum is the fusion of the ectoderm and the entoderm of the intestinal cephalic portion, with the formation of the oral lamina or bucco - pharyngeal membrane.

After its re-absorption around the third week the oral cavity appears, still communicating with the nasal cavity. The maxillary processes (from the first branchial arch) are close to the midline and join the medial and lateral nasal processes.

In this way the palatal septum that separates the oral cavity from the nasal one is formed. The latter is divided into two nasal cavities with the union of the medial nasal processes.

Branchial arches, pouches, grooves are beneath the stomodeum.

An orthodontist should be aware that the **first** branchial arch differs on both sides in a dorsal section (maxillary processes) and a ventral section (mandibular processes).

From the union of the maxillary processes on the sides with the fronto - nasal process in the middle position the maxilla is formed, together with the contours of the mouth and nasal region.

From the mandibular processes the following parts derive:

- the jaw, which is formed around the Meckel cartilage whose resorption leads to the forming of the incus and the malleus
- the lower lip with the body of the tongue and the front of the alveolar processes

1-1

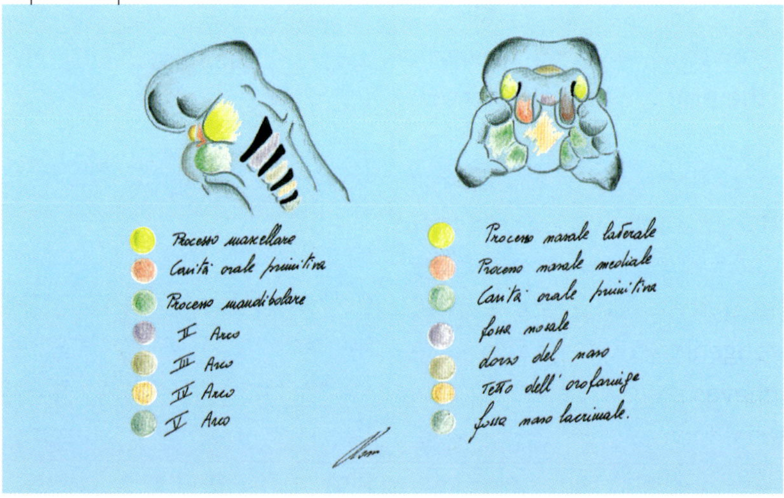

Fig. 1-1
Human embryo: branchial arches, pouches, grooves.

- the muscles of mastication (masseter, pterygoid, anterior belly of digastric) with the tensor tympani and tensor veli palatini muscles
- the wings of the sphenoid with the temporal bone and maxillary margin of the orbits
- part of the ear (concha, tragus, helix).

From the **second** branchial arch the following parts form:

- the remaining portion of the ear
- the stirrup
- the facial muscles (mimic muscles) with the facial nerve (VII), in addition to the posterior belly of the digastric, the stylohyoid and the stapedius

The **third** arch forms the body of the hyoid bone and the posterior part of the tongue. The annexed nerve is the glossopharyngeal.

The **fourth** and **fifth** branchial arches form the thyroid cartilage, laryngeal muscles and back muscles of the neck (sternocleidomastoid and trapezius). The vagus nerve is attached.

Thus it is clear that disturbances during fetal growth can lead to clinical outcomes that are very interesting for an orthodontist.

One in particular is Treacher Collins syndrome, where there is hypertelorism, ear malformations, facial hypoplasia; the first and second branchial arch syndrome with ear malformations is associated with malocclusion, facial asymmetry and mandibular hypoplasia.

An alteration in the fusion between the nasal process and maxillary processes results in a median cleft condition:

- cleft lip
- cleft palate
- cleft lip and palate.

These clinical situations differ from others that may also affect the orthodontist such as examples of craniosynostosis. Among these the most common is Crouzon syndrome where at birth sagittal and coronal sutures are obliterated, while the front suture and the anterior fontanelle fuse together soon after birth.

Achondroplasia should also not be forgotten where the lack of facial growth is due to the absence of cartilage growth centres. However, there can be Class III intermaxillary relationships in both cases although with different mechanisms.

CRANIOFACIAL GROWTH

Crucial to an orthodontist is the knowledge of craniofacial growth and development of the stomatognathic system.

For a long time it was thought that the activity of the sutures was responsible for craniofacial growth. Koski and Enlow[139] showed that the primary input in increasing new bone and its displacement is not sutural, for example like the epiphyseal cartilages. Moreover, they suggested that developing soft tissues move the sutures away and the space they create is filled with their osteogenic activities. Therefore the suture behaves passively and not having the potential for independent growth, adapts to its surroundings.

According to Koski[142] the only centre of growth would be the cartilage of the nasal septum. If it is removed early the antero-posterior facial growth is compromised.

Moss[178] looked at the genetic component of growth, the functional aspect, and formulated the theory of the "functional matrix". This represents the set of structures and soft tissues in relation to certain functions. In other words, the functional matrix is composed of relatively independent skeletal parts, functionally coordinated, whose components are related to the main functions of sight, breathing, swallowing, phonation.

For example, the orbit depends on sight and that is its function. Consequently, vision and bone develop with the eye.
The maxilla is in contact with the orbit. An orbital enucleation can cause morphological changes of bone segments among the functional matrix and also possible alterations of the maxilla.
Another example of a functional matrix is the skull development together with the growth of the brain. The brain mass reaches 90% of its volume at around 12 years or so.
And thus the stomatognathic system develops following its skeletal components by adapting to the functional matrix.
The mandible is not a single structure but is instead a set of relatively independent components. The alveolar bone depends on the teeth, the angle and the coronoid apophysis of the muscles. The condyle develops independently from the body. The pterygium-maxillary apophysis , in contact with the palatine apophysis, has its upper portion connected to the respiratory function while the lower portion relates to the digestive function. Its position, as well as its growth, is therefore affected by the function.
However, as underlined by Enlow[82] the growth of the face does not depend only on the suture ossification, but also on a modelling ossification process, which is

1-2

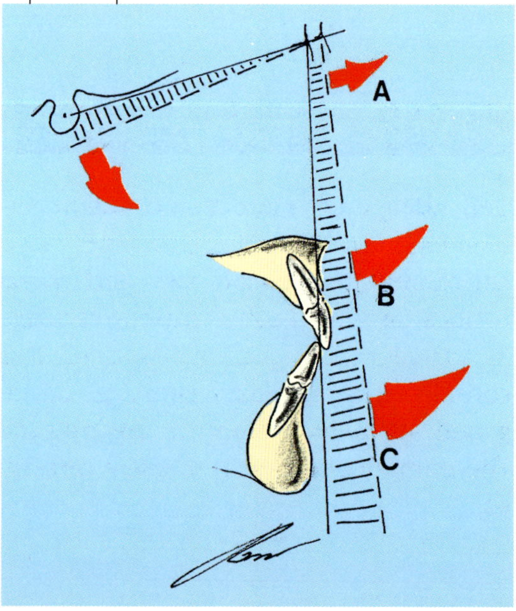

Fig. 1-2
In normal growth the jaws move downward and forward with a counterclockwise rotation. To keep a well-balanced relationship among the facial structures, the sagittal advancement is different at various sites. Sassouni says that if the growth amount corresponds to 1 at the nasal – frontal suture (A), it will be twice more at the anterior nasal spine (B) and 3 times more at pogonion (C).

theoretically independent although coordinated. It is a continuous remodelling, which occurs simultaneously from one end to the other, involving each part of the facial skeleton and maintaining constant proportions and forms.
Particularly interesting for orthodontists is the fact that in **normal growth, the maxilla and the mandible move downward and forward with a counterclockwise rotation**.
The mandible is affected by a measurably higher development than the maxilla in order to maintain a constant relationship between the two.
This is the image that is commonly obtained by superimposing many cephalometric tracings of the same person at different times of growth along the line SN (S is the centre of the sella turcica, N is the nasal-frontal suture).
Although it offers some validity in viewing the complex changes that occur, it is a simplified conception of the development that actually happens (Fig. 1-2). As mentioned above, size increases, remodelling and displacement determines bone changes.
Thus we can say that in effect the mandible does not grow down and forwards, because although it increases in size, its remodelling is essentially posteriorly and upward, even though it displaces downwards.
Similarly the mandible ramus is repositioned posteriorly and increases its width because the parallel processes of bone apposition, which take effect on the back surface, are greater than the resorption occurring on the anterior surface (Fig. 1-5). In other words, part of the ramus is transformed into the posterior part of the body. This determines the mandibular arch lengthening needed for teeth eruption.
These examples show how important it is for an orthodontist to understand craniofacial growth. As a matter of fact, only by knowing the physiology it is possible to understand and treat the pathology.

1-3

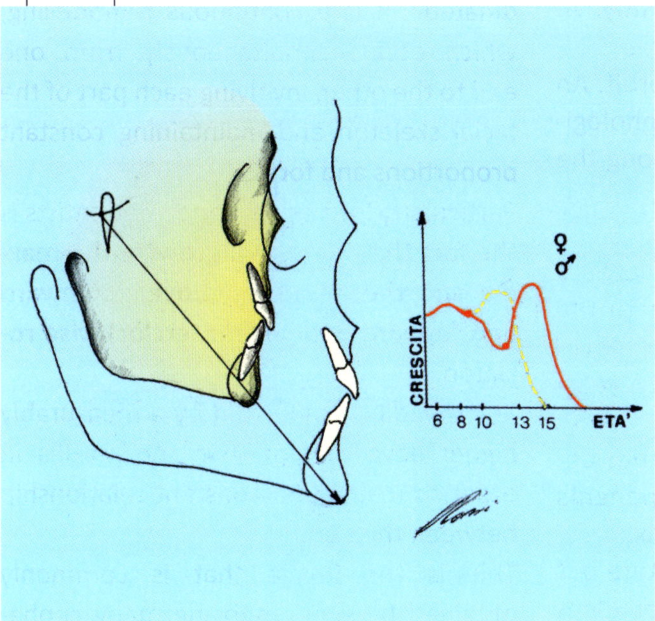

1-4

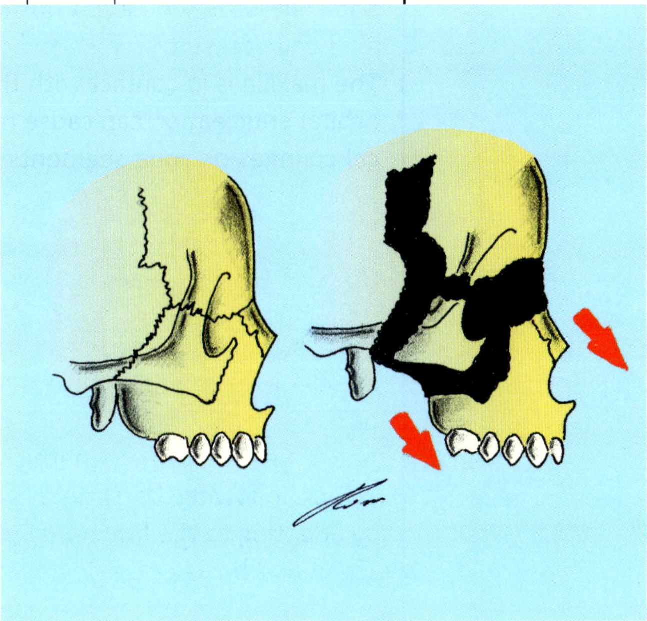

1-5

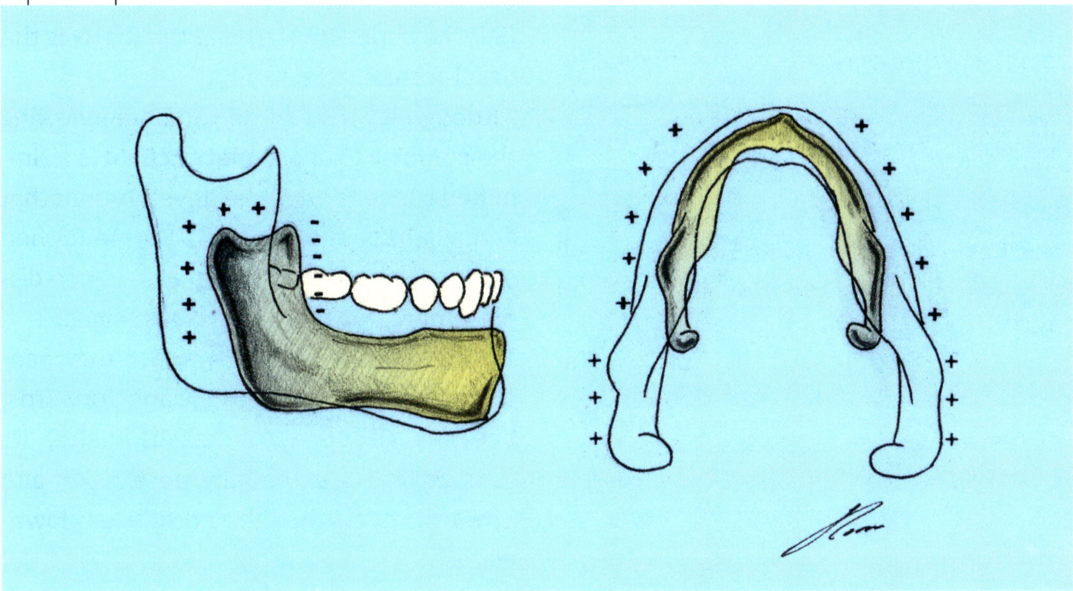

Fig. 1-3
Cranio-facial growth is normally directed downward and forward with counterclockwise rotation of the jaws. There are two growth spurts, age and sex related.

Fig. 1-4
The expansion of the cranial structures as a consequence of functional stimuli determines the displacement of the jaws.

Fig. 1-5
Bone increase and remodelling: (+) indicates apposition, (-) indicates resorption.

OSSIFICATION

The ossification process can be intramembranous or cartilaginous. The first is given by the periosteum from the outside and by endosteum from the inside.

These two components produce a fibrous bone that develops from connective but non-calcified tissue elements and a lamellar bone where there needs to be a pre-existing mineralized structure. The latter can involve a cartilage which is then replaced by bone.

Depending on the direction of the mineralization process, this last process is called pericondral ossification and enchondral ossification. The most interesting cartilage in orthodontics is the condilar one. It is considered a secondary cartilage, phylogenetically derived from the periosteum. The primary ones are epiphyseal cartilages.

STOMATOGNATHIC GROWTH

Stomatognathic growth occurs parallel to the rest of the skeletal structure.

It is important for the clinician to know the bone age (which does not necessarily coincide with the chronological age) because many researchers have demonstrated that the success of an orthopaedic treatment is related to the maturation period of the jaws.[106, 188, 196]

It may therefore be useful to examine an X-ray of the wrist which allows a definition of the stage of growth (carpal index). The carpal bones present are the hamate, the capitate, the triquetrum, the lunate and the trapezoid.

Children of both sexes have an initial growth spurt between 6 and 8 years. It usually coincides with the eruption of permanent incisors (Fig. 1-3 earlier).

There follows a period of slow growth until about 10 years in females and 12 years in males when the trapezium and the scaphoid appear.

With the appearance of the pisiform and sesamoid bones there is a resumption of growth that reaches a new peak in puberty. This period offers the best growth response from 10½ years up to 12 ½ in the female, and 12 ½ years up to about 15 years in the male (Fig. 1-3 earlier).

In the female around 13 years of bone age, the onset of menarche indicates the near-term development.

After the pubertal peak, growth decreases. In females it lasts until about 15 years while in the male up to 18. In the meantime there is complete ossification of the phalangeal and metacarpal bones and finally those of the ulna and the radio. (Fig 1-6)

After puberty the response to an orthopaedic treatment is poor.

Some of the details worth remembering are:

- the skull at the age of 5 is nearly the size of the adult (90% approximately), with areas of growth at the level of the sella turcica, basion, nasion and spheno-occipital synchondrosis
- the cranial vault at birth is characterized by the presence of the fontanelles (bregmatica, lamboidea, pteriche, asterisk) that become sutures by the eighteenth month, except for the bregmatica which closes between 2 and 3 years
- the anterior cranial fossa, with its growth, influences the nose and the maxilla

1-6

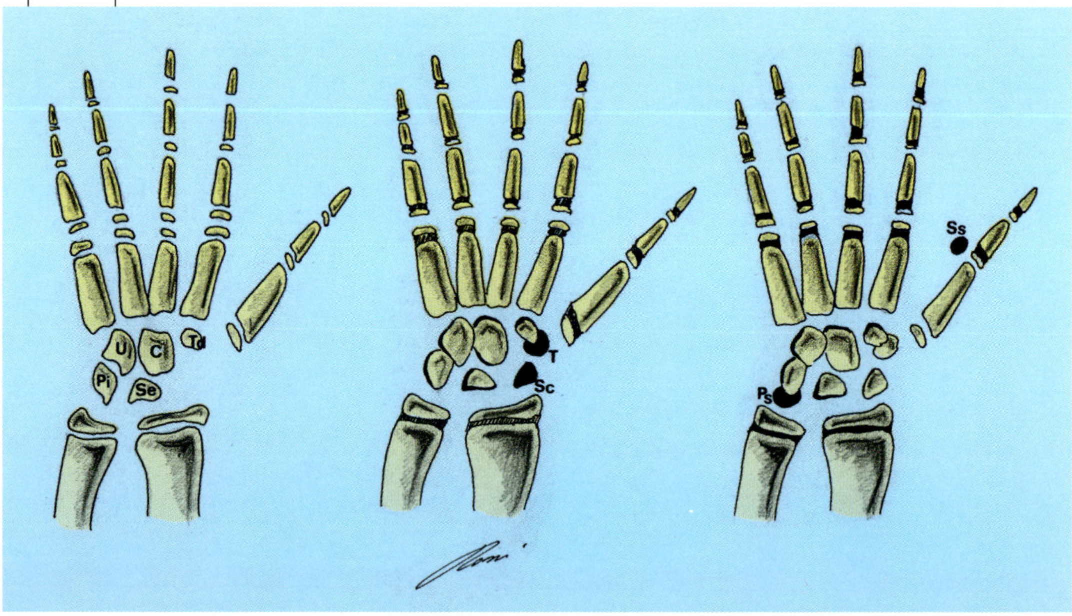

Fig. 1-6 Periods of carpal ossification.

- maxillary retrusion or protrusion may result from an imbalanced growth of the anterior cranial fossa
- the jaws can also be influenced by middle cranial fossa activity where the brain mass expansion activates the growth of the spheno-occipital synchondrosis
- the growth of the posterior cranial fossa follows the middle one (Fig. 1-7).

The upper jaw and the nose (up to about 4 years) are influenced by the ethmoid bone, then by the nasal septum cartilage (up to 8 years approximately). Thus, the maxillary tubers area becomes the fastest growing location.

Functional stimulations are important in determining functional development and shape of the palate, while the role of the incisor-canine suture is controversial in promoting the advancement of the premaxilla.

The median palatine suture is a fibrous sinartrosis until about 15 years when it begins to obliterate, becoming a synostosis at about 25 years of age.

Giannì[106] indicates growth for this suture of 1 mm per year until the age of 5, followed by an increase of 0.25 mm a year until puberty.

After puberty there is a residual growth of 1.5 mm.

Regarding the mandible, the condylar cartilage is an area of primary growth, activated by functional stimulations.

Mandibular development is also due to the periosteal activity while the enlargement of the oropharynx induces a downwards and forwards translation movement.

For a long time the growth of the mandible has been identified with the condyle.

Experimentally it has also been observed that despite the removal at a young age of both condyles, the mandibular structure had a normal form, position and size.

The epiphyseal cartilage of long bones increases both in vitro and in vivo if placed in other anatomic sites.

Following these observations, other experiments showed the intracerebral graft of condylar cartilage to reveal a possible capacity of autonomous growth. The results showed little or no potential, unlike the cartilage of the nasal septum and cartilages (synchondrosis) of the skull base.

Therefore, at present the condyle is mainly considered a structure that fits the relationship between lower jaw and skull base.

1-7

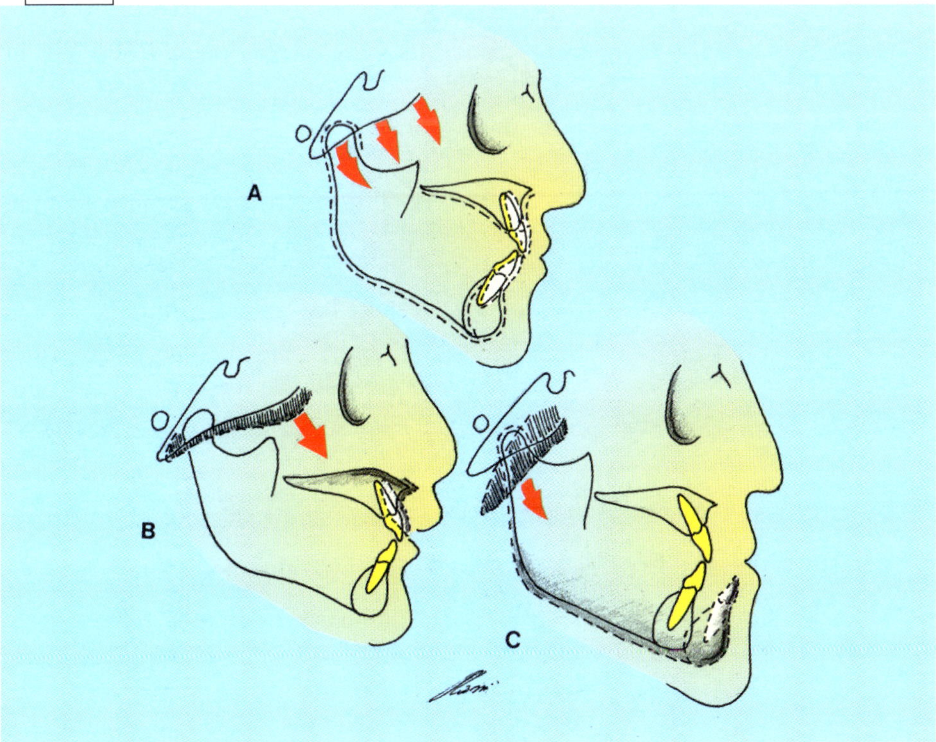

Fig. 1-7
Possible influence of the cranial base on the growth of the jaws.

a) Class 1. Secondary movements: harmonic growth of the jaws. Alteration of secondary displacements

b) Class II

c) Class III

GROWTH FORECAST

Predicting with certainty the growth of a patient would certainly seem to be useful for an orthodontist. However, unfortunately there are mixed opinions on the subject.
In fact, the many factors that influence growth make it difficult to predict, even though Bjork and other researchers have established that in 90% of cases there is a tendency of counter clockwise growth.[27]
Do not forget that what works for some can be worth very little when the clinician must make a difficult decision. To say that an analysis is reliable in 80% of cases means for an orthodontist that in 20 cases out of 100 he can make a mistake and this is certainly not a good prospect.
Things get complicated if you try to assess the growth of subjects orthodontically treated given the additional variables introduced by the latter (mode of application of devices, effectiveness of the devices, patient cooperation, time to start of treatment, etc.).
Sheldon Baumrind author of some interesting research and comments on the subject, outlines the limits of forecasting methods and suggests a cautious assessment. Baumrind and his collaborators[17] conducted a study where a sample of selected lateral cephalograms was presented to five very experienced orthodontists. They were informed that some of those cases would have a mandibular clockwise growth. Then, with a growth forecast, they were invited to detect which ones were those cases.
A consensus was not achieved.
Conclusion: you cannot trust anyone!

DIAGNOSIS AND TREATMENT PLAN

Once the complexity of the matter has been understood, it is clear that the orthodontist should not formulate a diagnosis and set up a treatment plan based solely on an examination of dental casts (Fig 1-8),which often happens.
The examination of dental models is important, but must be accompanied by X-ray examinations: panoramic radiograph, lateral cephalogram, postero-anterior cephalogram, hand-wrist X-ray (Figs. 1-9, 1-10, 1-11, 1-12).
They allow the evaluation of the relationship among the bone bases, the inclination of the teeth on them, the asymmetries, the lingual posture, the upper airway, the cervical spine, the period of growth, etc. of the patient.
Everything must be integrated with a careful medical history that considers, among other things, the presence of "bad" habits: thumb sucking, tongue swallowing, lip sucking, etc.
Therefore, observation of the patient (and relatives to identify possible genetic influences, not only on the malocclusion, but also, for example the shape of the nose) is fundamental.
Never forget the evaluation, mainly clinical, of temporomandibular joints and of the periodontal conditions.
Finally do not forget that the formulation of a treatment plan requires a modern aesthetic evaluation of the patient. The photographic documentation of a case, including the face and profile of the patient, is an important element in orthodontic practice.

1-8

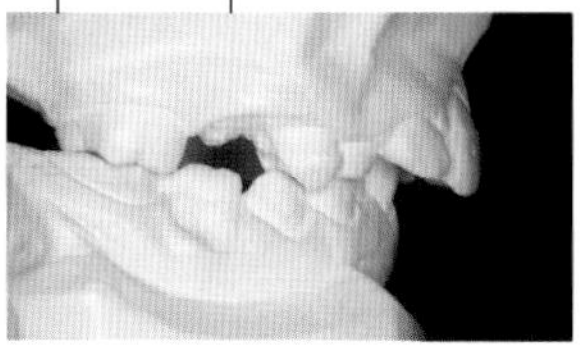

1-9

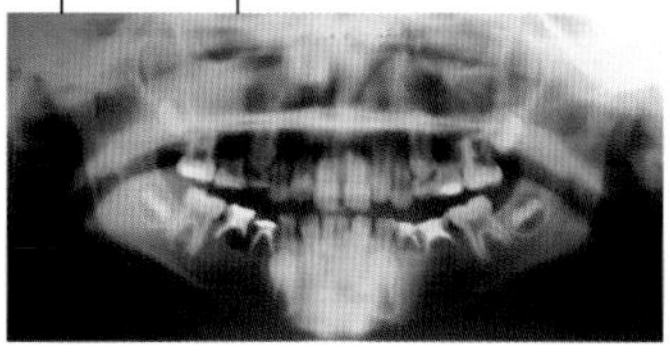

Fig. 1-8 Dental casts.

Fig. 1-9 Panoramic radiograph.

1-10

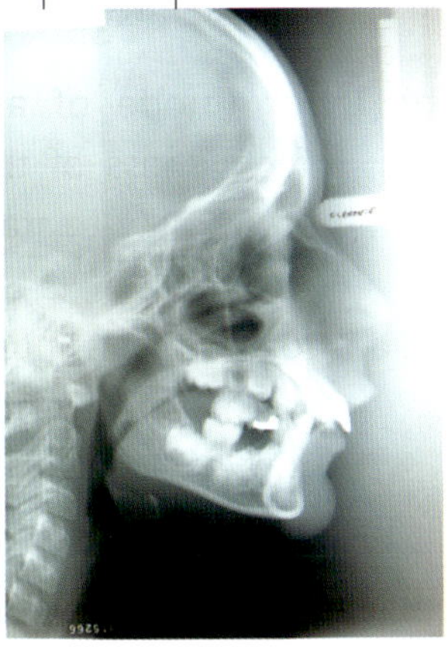

1-11

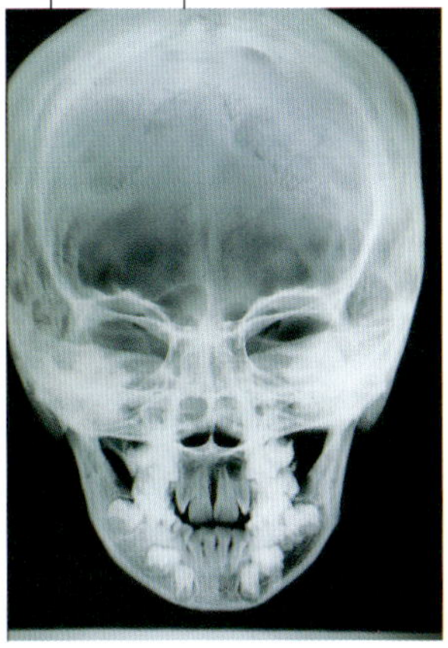

1-12

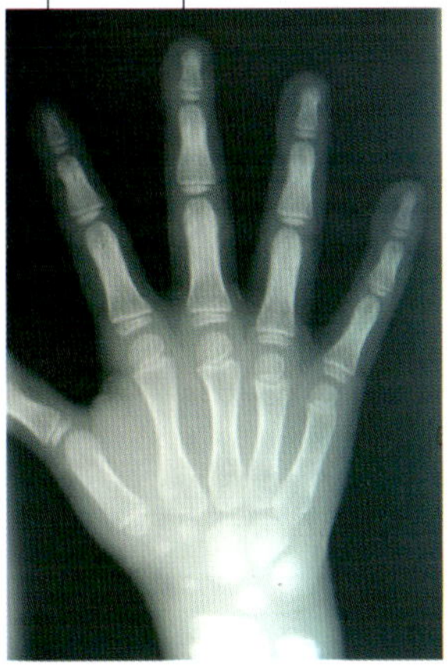

Fig. 1-10
Lateral cephalogram.

ig. 1-11
Postero-anterior cephalogram.

Fig. 1 -12
Hand-wrist X-ray.

EXAMINATION OF THE PATIENT AND FAMILY

FAMILY

Facial examination

- The shape of the nose (excluding traumatic outcomes) may be important for the choice of the therapeutic strategy. It is under genetic control.
- Profile: it is important to assess the trend of growth influenced by heredity.

Stomatognathic examination

- It can be helpful in assessing the genetic influence of malocclusion.

PATIENT

Facial examination

- Local diseases.
- Asymmetry conditions (Fig. 1-15).
- Nasopharyngeal disorders which disturb normal nasal breathing (tonsils, adenoids, etc.), trauma, angiomas, tumors etc. can cause malocclusions.

General diseases

- Endocrine disorders can cause abnormalities of jaw growth, alterations of teeth eruption, etc..
- Chromosomal abnormalities (Franceschetti syndrome, cleido-cranial dysostosis, trisomy 21, labial-palatal cleft, ectodermal dysplasia, etc.).
- Allergies (because they can lead to breathing alterations, among other things).

Include in the facial examination the record of the facial biotype.

Mesofacial

- There is a perfect harmony according to the more widespread standard among the transverse and vertical diameters. Muscles tend to be normotonic.
- Probable mandibular growth: **ideal** with rotation around an hypothetical incisal fulcrum.

Brachifacial (Fig. 1-13)

- Prevalence of transverse diameters.
- Muscles tend to be hypertonic.
- Probable mandibular growth: clockwise-rotation with hypothetical premolar fulcrum

Dolicofacial (Fig. 1-14)

- Prevalence of vertical diameters.
- Muscles tend to be hypotonic.
- Probable mandibular growth: counterclockwise rotation with hypothetical molar fulcrum.

1-13

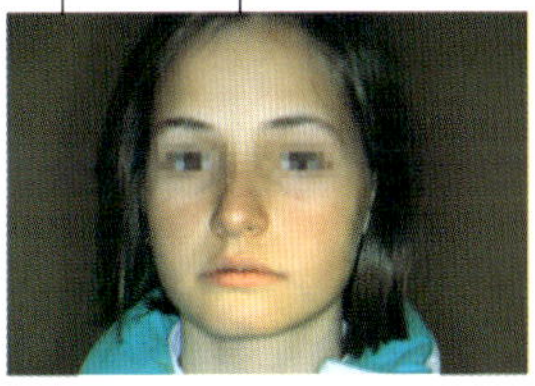

1-14

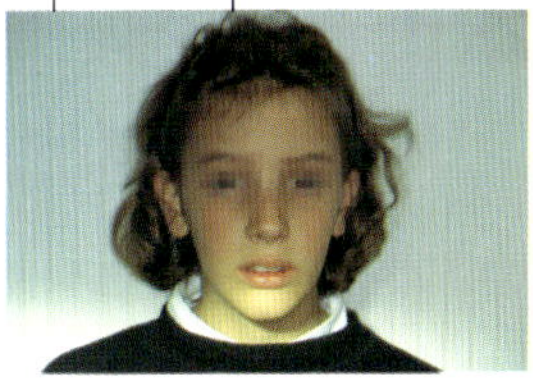

Fig. 1-13
Brachi

Fig. 1-14
Dolico

This assessment is important because it may indicate the growth trend which is, statistically, most likely. It also suggests which shape to give the dental arch, no small consideration when planning the course of treatment.

Essentially asymmetry assessment!

In women the menarche is also known for its correlation to the growth of a person.

Add any postural defects, not to mention observation of the nose.

Deviations of the septum may explain irregularities in the maxillary growth. A different shape and size can suggest different orthodontic treatment strategies such as extractions or non-extractions.

Of course, when there is a bad nose, it is better to change its shape with a rhinoplasty (Figs. 1-16 to 1-19).

Stomatognathic assessment

- Decay, fillings and root treatments.
- Periodontal examination: plaque, calculus, gum recession.
- TMJ (temporomandibular joint) evaluation – jaw clicking, aching.
- Dental class evaluation.
- Centric relation or dual bite (see figs 23 &24.)
- Overjet and overbite.
- Cross-bite.
- Scissor-bite.
- Teeth malposition.
- Diastemas.
- Supernumerary teeth.
- Frenula, (especially if the frenulum is tectolabial)
- Anodontia.
- Oral muscle tone.
- Swallowing.
- Oral respiration.
- Bad habits.

1-15

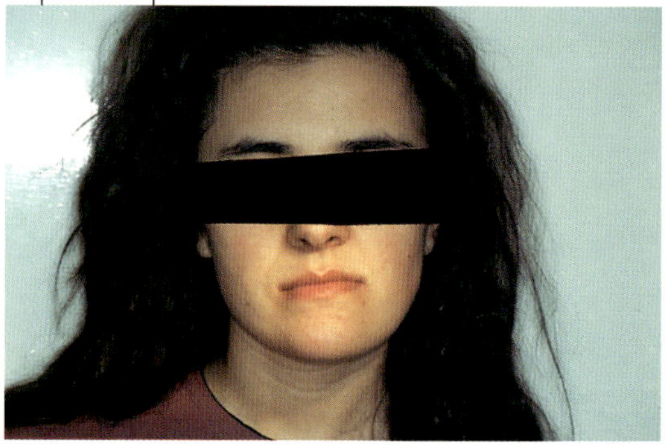

Fig. 1 -15
Facial asymmetry with mandibular lateral displacement.

1-16

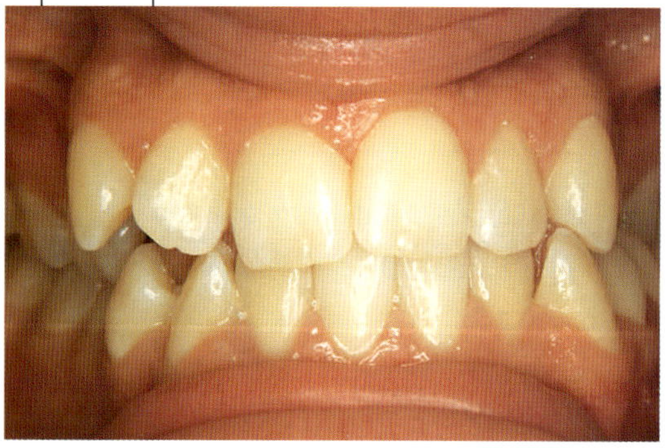

1-17

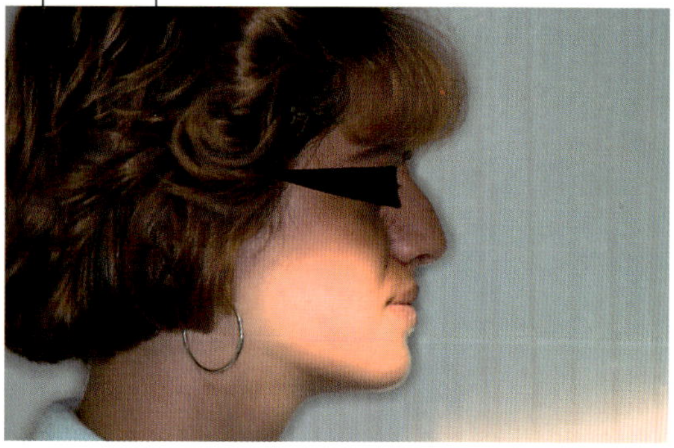

Fig. 1-16 /17
Occlusion before the orthodontic treatment and rhinoplasty.

1-18

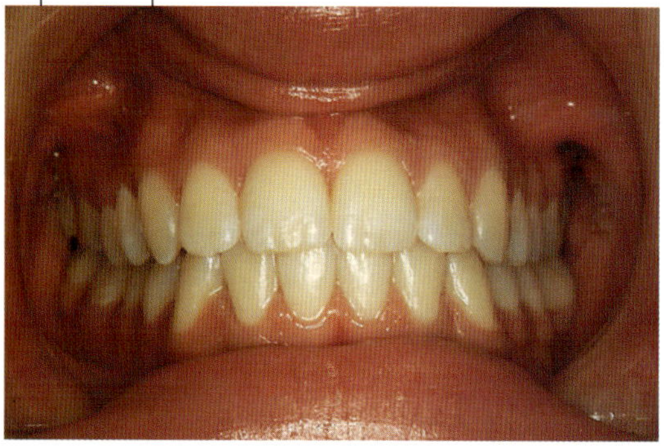

1-19

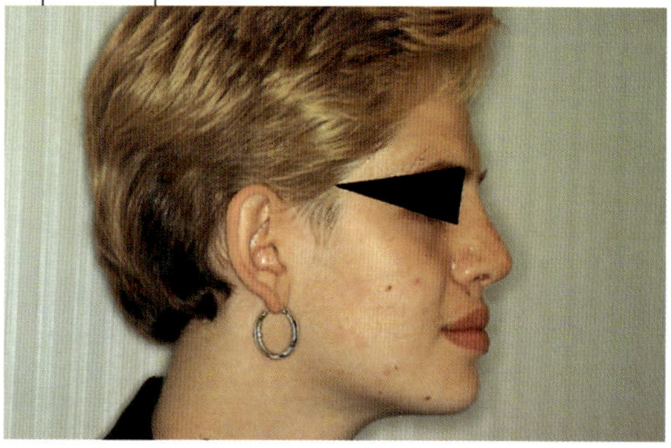

Fig.1-18 /19
Occlusion after the orthodontic treatment followed by rhinoplasty.

A malocclusion depends on both inherited genetic and functional factors. An orthodontist cannot have any influence on the genetics but he can improve the function. Therefore, remember:

A) Muscular tone

Teeth position is determined by a balance between opposite muscle forces.

The tongue pushes the teeth out while the peri-oral musculature (lips, cheeks etc.) pushes the teeth in. An improper balance corresponds to a malocclusion.

For example, when there is a tongue prevalence the incisors tend to be proclined.

The contrary happens with lip musculature hyperactivity.

Tongue dysfunctions like infantile swallowing can cause dental open bites.

B) Oral respiration

In these cases the tongue is positioned down and during swallowing there is no physiological pressure on the palatal surface. As a consequence, in many cases the upper dental arch has a narrow transverse dimension which causes a posterior crossbite. This situation can also cause mandible clockwise growth.

C) Habits

Thumb sucking and lip biting are examples of the most common habits which can cause a malocclusion. Also chewing a pencil or smoking a pipe in adulthood.

Examples of Bad Habits

1-20

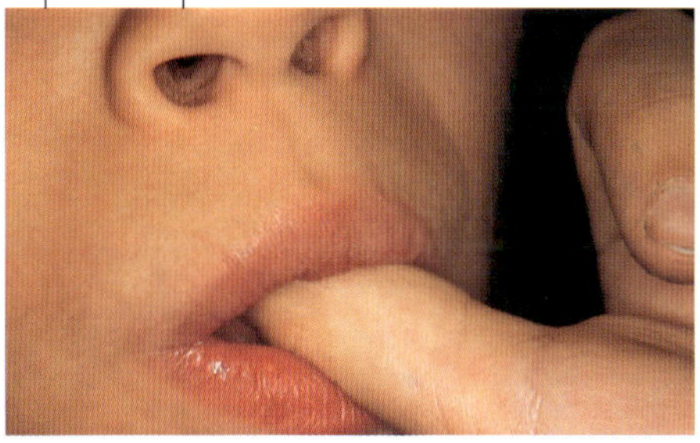

Fig. 1-20
Thumb sucking.

1-21

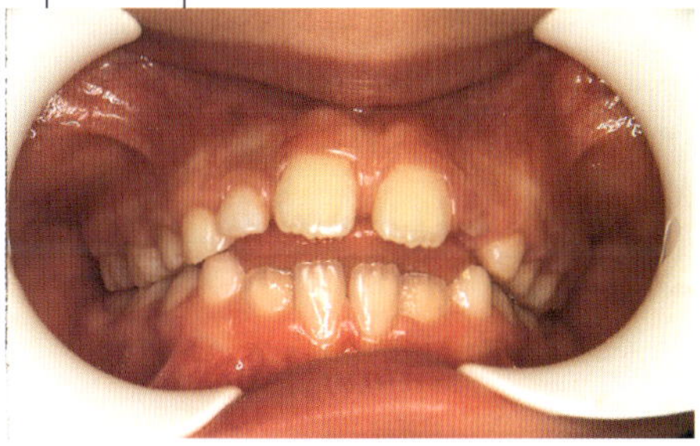

Fig. 1-21
Infantile swallowing.

1-22

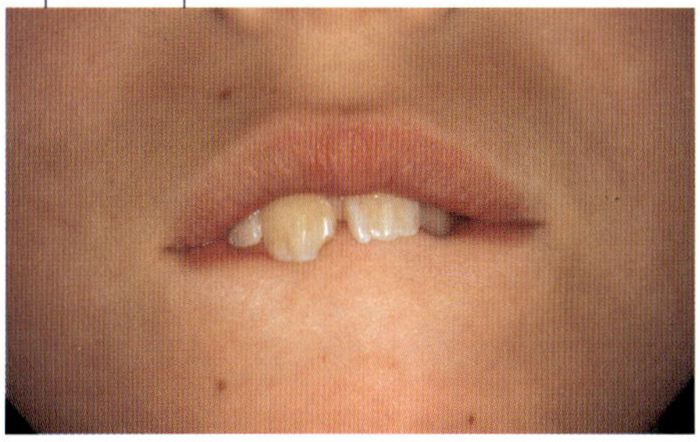

Fig. 1-22
Lip biting.

Dual bite. The same mouth:

1-23

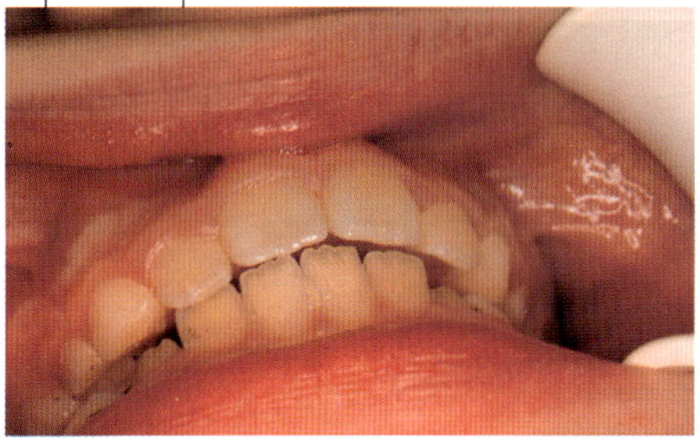

Fig. 1-23
Habitual occlusion compared to

1-24

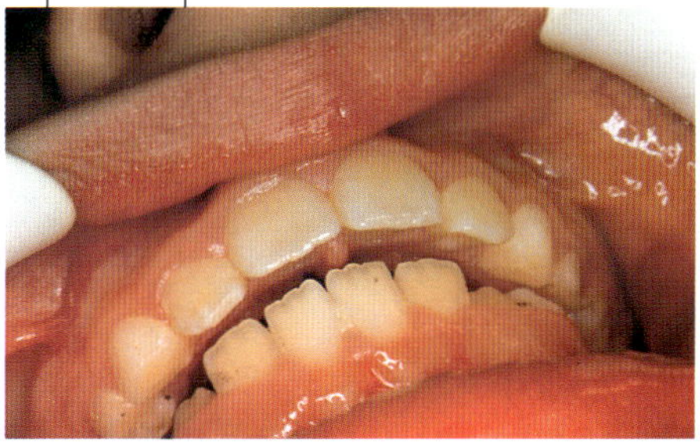

Fig. 1-24
the occlusion with condyles in centric relation.

DENTAL PLASTER MODELS

Plaster models are essential for the study of malocclusions and setting the treatment plan.
They are also used to assess the changes that occur during an orthodontic treatment.
There must be clearly visible anatomical details:

- Teeth (of course).
- Frenula.
- Gingiva.
- Maxillary tuberosity.
- Lower retromolar space.
- Alveolar – lingual solcus.

The height of each model should be about 3.5 cm. If well executed the model allows the occlusion to be easily found. Personally I think it is important that the clinician seeks the occlusion by "feeling" the correct gearing of the teeth.
With the most current assessment of what I call "static", the following should be noted:

- number and shape of the teeth in the arch
- dental class
- median-line at the palatal mid-line

It is also possible to obtain parameters from various sources - Pont, Bolton, Peck, etc..
A "static" evaluation highlights a situation without asking the reasons that led to it, while in a "dynamic" evaluation the clinician tries to reconstruct the sequence that led to that type of occlusion. For example, a reduced extraction space can be recorded as such, or it can be perceived as the mesial movement of the distal elements coinciding with the collapse of the hemi-arch. Another example would be a vestibularised lateral incisor. Why is it like that? How can a permanent canine be in a pre-eruptive phase?

ORTHOPANTOMOGRAPHY

It is a fundamental exam which allows us to:

- assess caries
- count the dental elements (and the extra non-developed elements)
- assess the presence of obstacles in tooth eruption
- assess abnormalities of eruption
- assess the temporomandibular joint
- detect deviations of the nasal septum
- view the mandibular shape anomalies.

LATERAL CEPHALOGRAM

Essential for cephalometric tracing but also useful for:

- assessment of impacted teeth (especially canines and incisors)
- estimation of impacted wisdom teeth
- evaluation of airway obstructions
- evaluation of the position of the hyoid bone
- visualization of the cervical spine.

1-25

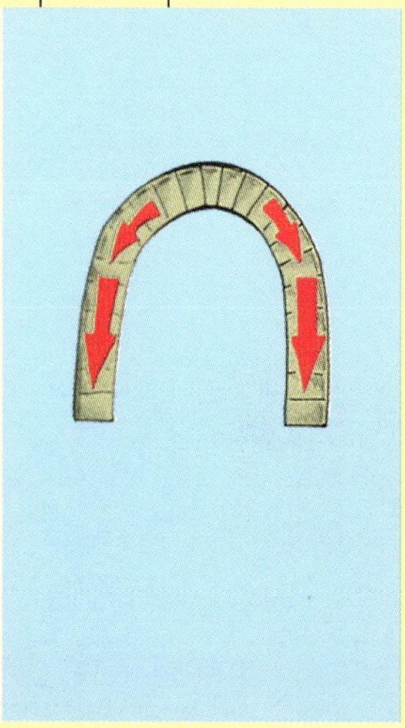

An architectural arch is capable of supporting surprisingly high load because the centripetal forces weighing down on individual sections are counterbalanced by the opposite reactive forces which maintain the equilibrium. In a dental arch the situation is analogous – the centripetal forces (perioral musculature) are more tolerable than the centrifugal forces (from the tongue). One must also bear in mind that when the perioral musculature is stronger distally rather than mesially, then it is the larger teeth (molars) which offer the most resistance. They themselves are contained within thick cortical bone at the front of the upper branch of the mandible. In addition to that, when chewing the forces involved tend to discharge mesially. For these reasons teeth incline and "open up" more easily.

Fig. 1-25
The principle of the architectural arch applied to orthodontics.

THE IMPORTANCE OF RADIOLOGICAL EXAMINATIONS

Modern orthodontics cannot ignore a careful assessment of radiological documentation, as shown by the following examples.

Fig. 1-26: An unscrupulous operator has put two brackets on the lower lateral incisors, probably to apply an elastic traction which brought them together, but without performing a preliminary radiological control.

After a panoramic radiograph though there is a surprise! (Fig. 1-27).

The patient, who already has the agenesis of upper left (25) and lower second (35 - 45) deciduous molars, has a transposition of the lower canines, The attempt to bring the lower lateral incisors closer includes the risk of harmful interference between the lower lateral incisors' roots and the teeth that have not yet erupted.

Once the brackets are removed nature proceeds intelligently to patch things up with the eruption of the canines in a better position. (Fig 1-28). It will not be a perfect arch, but it is better than the risk of losing other teeth besides the three that are already missing (Seven if we consider the absence of the wisdom teeth).

A radiological control over time is important, not only with a lateral cephalogram in order to evaluate the stomatognathic growth, but also with a panoramic radiograph.

Fig. 1-29A shows what we could define as a case of pseudo-agenesis. On the lower panoramic radiograph there is no evidence of the germ of the second lower left premolar. The germ appears on a panoramic radiograph performed the following year (Fig. 1-29B).

Another example of what we might call a radiological dynamic control is outlined below. In Fig 1-30 a panoramic radiograph performed on a young patient does not show any particular problems besides decay of the lower first molar. Over time an ankylosis of this molar is clear.

1-26

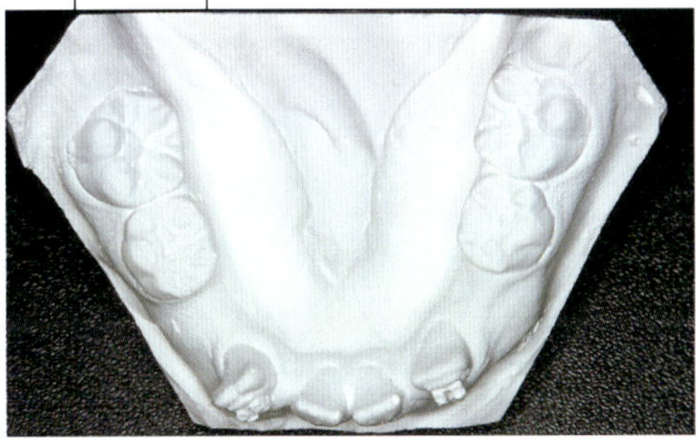

1-27

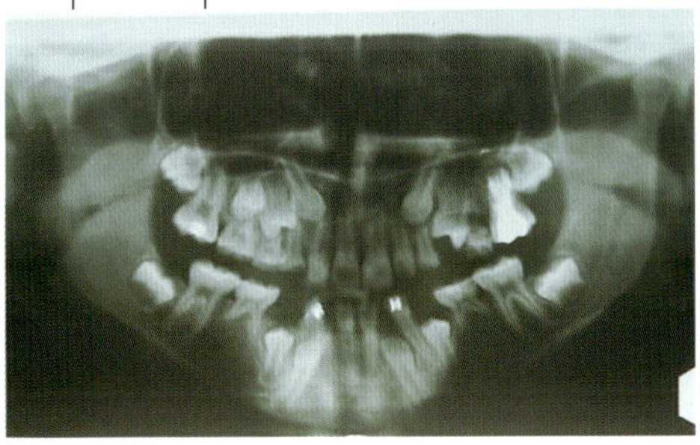

1-28

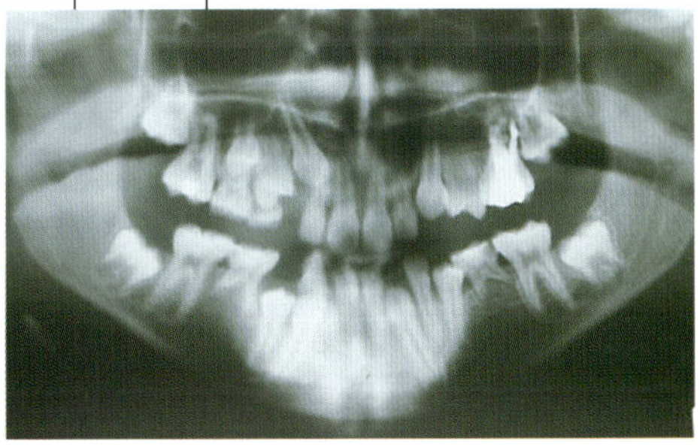

1-29A

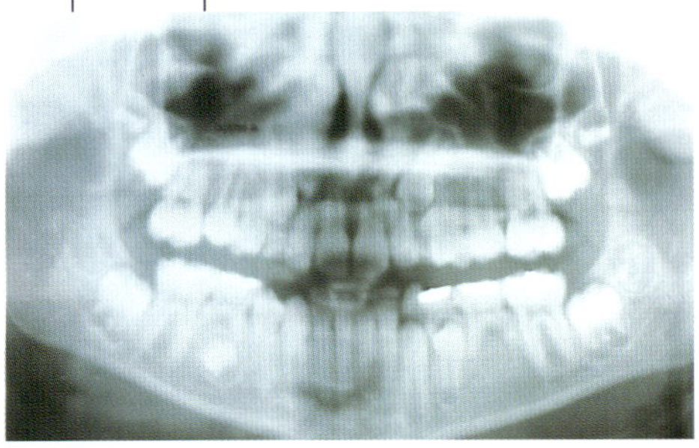

1-29B

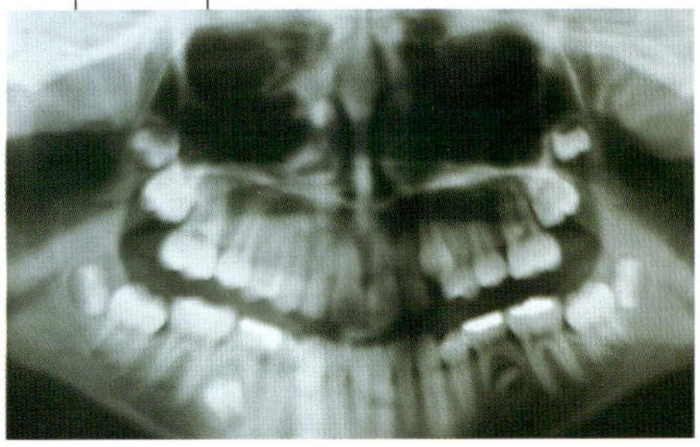

1-30

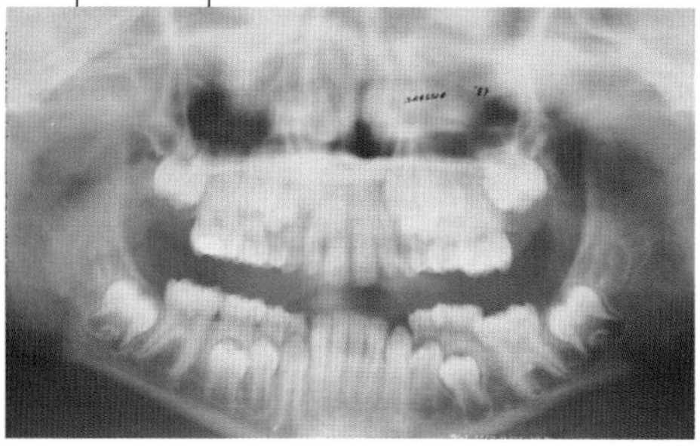

1-31

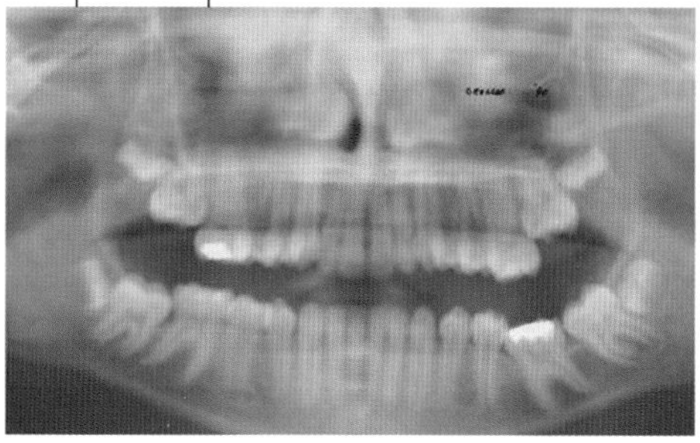

1-32

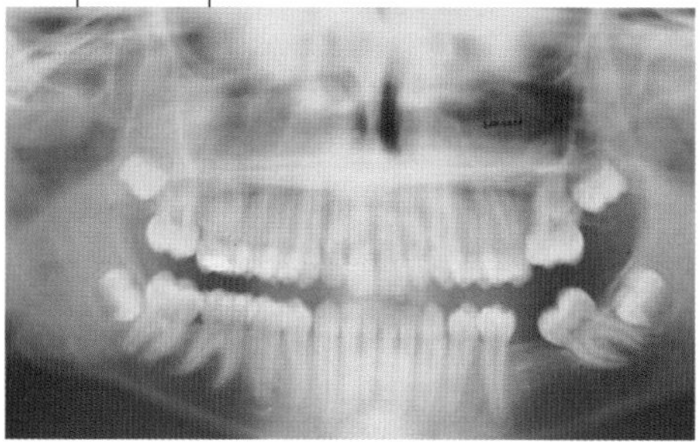

1-33

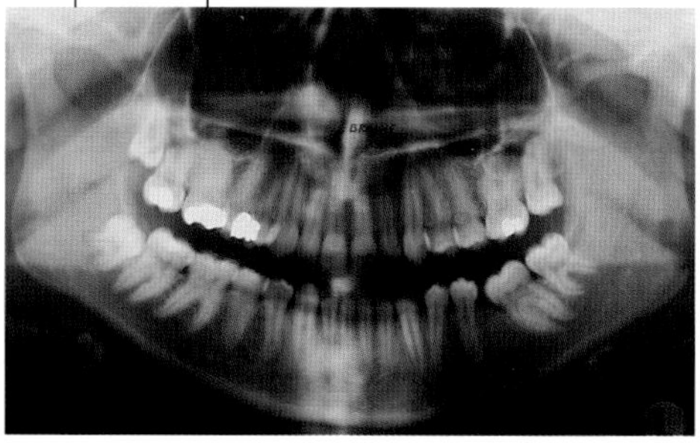

The pseudo-intrusion is accompanied by the upper first molar extrusion (Fig. 1-31). The parents are offered two types of treatment:

A) Orthodontic treatment with uncertain results.
B) Extraction of the first upper and lower molars with the hope of functional recovery of the eighths

The lower molar particularly would find little room under the first treatment, so the parents choose the second option (Fig. 1-32). We can see the evolution after five years (Fig. 1-33). All in all not a bad result. At this point, with a simple second left lower molar uprighting a very good occlusion can be obtained.

A panoramic radiograph may also be useful for a preliminary analysis of the temporomandibular joints.

In the case presented (Fig. 1-34), the panoramic radiograph indicates a different conformation of the two condyles on the bottom. This could explain a clinical situation characterized by joint disorders. A series of radiograms aimed at opening and closing the mouth allow a better definition of the difference between the two condyles. (observing the apparent hypertrophy of one condyle, while waiting for an arthroscopy, we assume the anterior displacement of a calcified disc.)

1-34

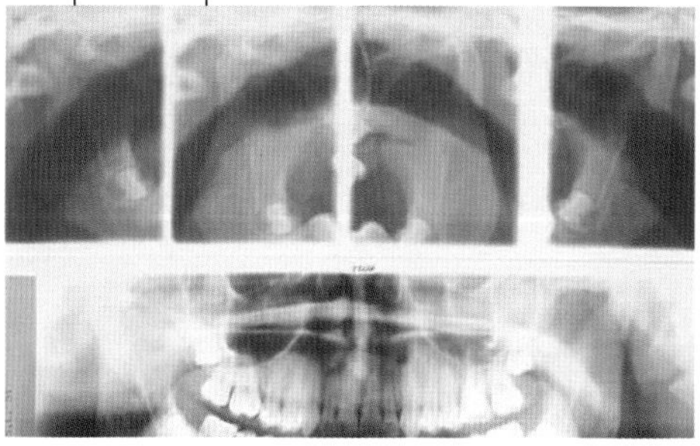

A panoramic radiograph is also useful for things that are more basic but often forgotten such as counting the teeth before they are clinically evident.

1-35

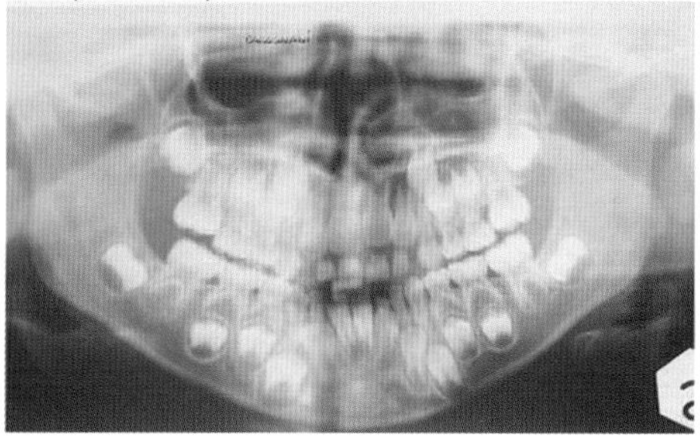

Fig. 1-35
In this case there are five lower incisors.

1-36

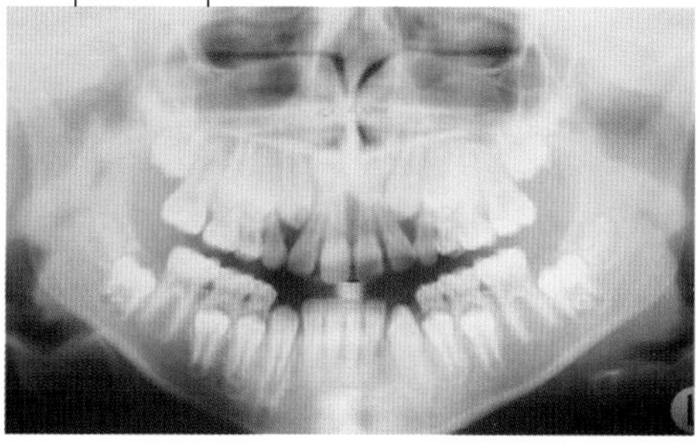

Fig. 1-36
Panoramic radiograph after the supernumerary incisor extraction.

THE IMPORTANCE OF CLINICAL OBSERVATION COMBINED WITH RADIOLOGICAL ANALYSIS

Although in the few examples seen so far the importance of radiological investigations is clear, it is fundamental not to ignore the clinical observation which is essential for a correct diagnosis. Consider the following case documented from Fig. 1-37 to Fig. 1-41.

The panoramic radiograph indicates the presence of supernumerary elements that prevent the eruption of upper right incisors (Fig. 1-37). It seems clear that the previous clinical observation has not been very careful. The operator should have suspected that something was wrong: the upper permanent incisors erupted only on one side (upper left), while they did not on the other side (Fig. 1-38).

After the extraction of deciduous and supernumerary teeth (Fig. 1-39), an orthodontic traction to extrude the incisors is applied (Fig. 1-40).

The situation, one year later (Fig. 1-41).

One more case points out the importance of a careful clinical analysis followed by X-rays.

The upper incisors of this young patient are badly positioned and the left central one is also rotated. (Fig. 1-42). Why? A panoramic radiograph is performed but sometimes, from a frontal viewpoint, it is not very clear. (Fig. 1-43) In this case, in combination with a lateral cephalogram, one can identify an extra tooth vertically positioned (Fig. 1-44/arrow).

After the supernumerary extraction it is possible to perform suitable orthodontic treatment. (Fig. 1-45).

1-37

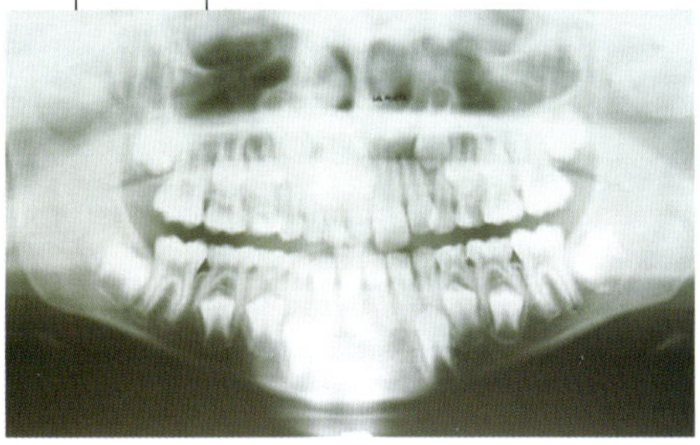

1-38

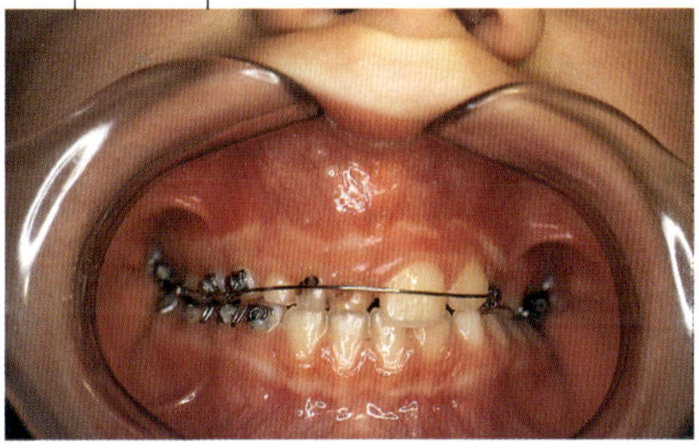

1-39

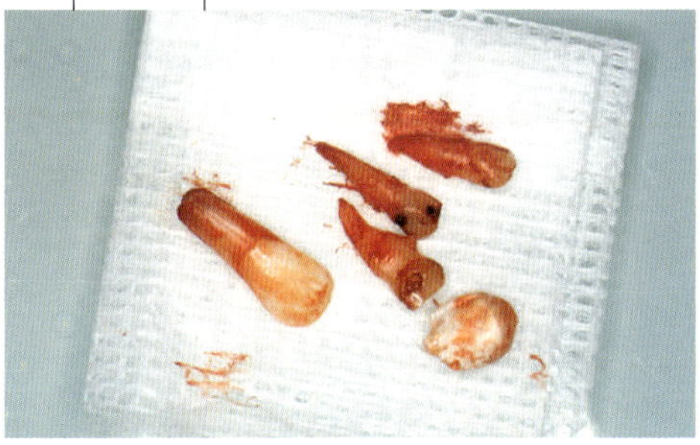

1-40

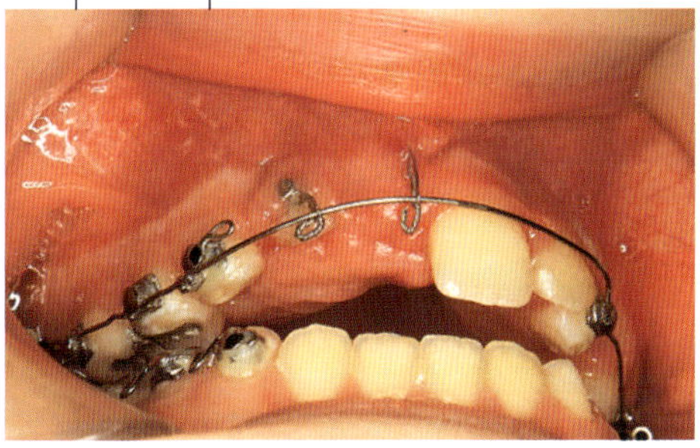

1-41

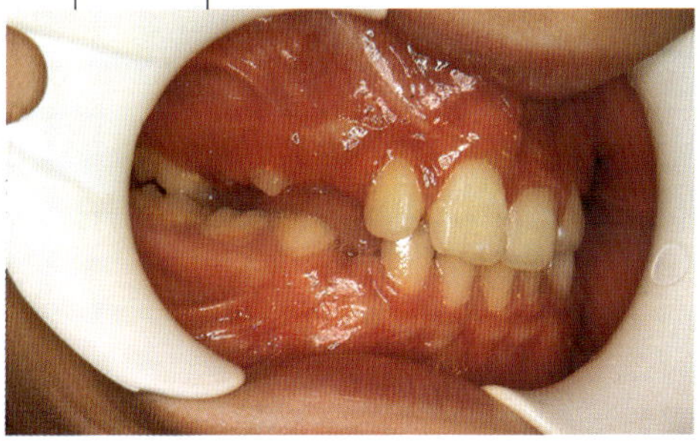

Fig. 1-37
Panoramic radiograph indicates presence of supernumerary elements

Fig. 1-38
An orthodontic fitting in place , ready for the traction of the upper right permanent incisors after the extractions of deciduous and supernumerary teeth

Fig. 1-39
Deciduous and supernumerary teeth removed

Fig.1-40
Orthodontic traction to extrude the incisors applied

Fig.1-41
One year after the removal of the fixed fitting. There follows a period of maintenance of the spaces and assistance of eruption with a removable fitting.

1-42

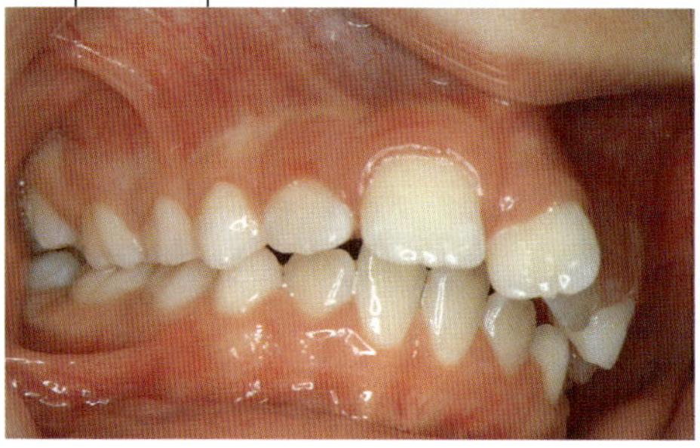

1-43

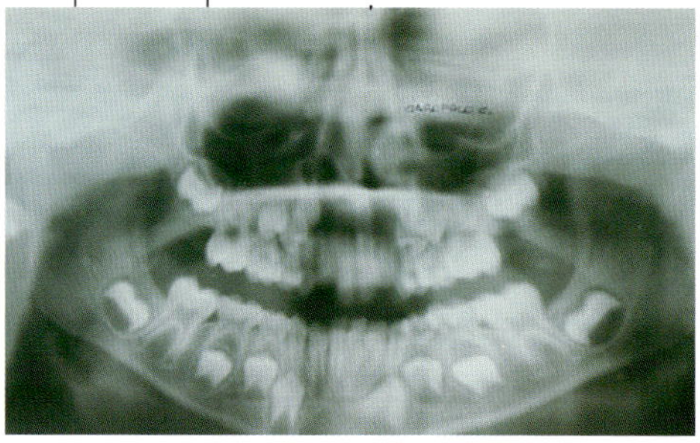

1-44

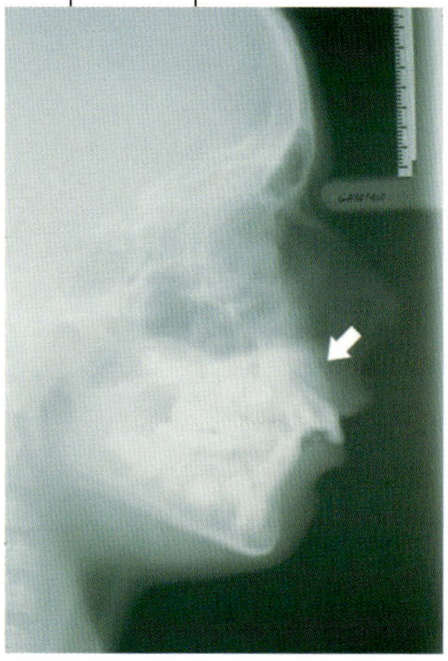

1-45

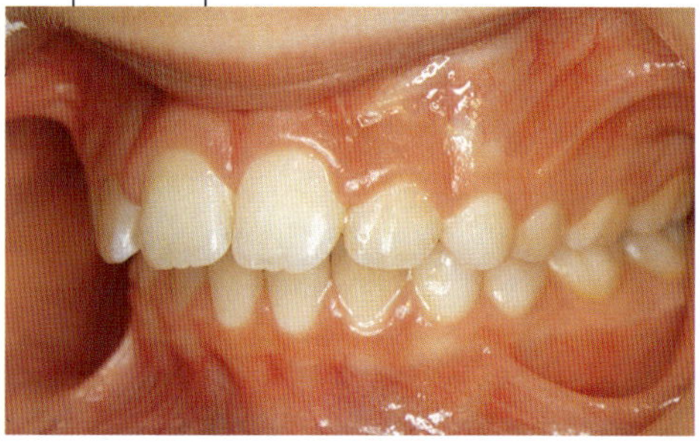

DATA PROVIDED BY RADIOLOGY AND BY MODELLING

CHANGES FROM DECIDUOUS TO PERMANENT OCCLUSIONS

Permanent teeth tend to erupt more externally than deciduous teeth, thus a small (2 mm) but useful space is available to resolve eventual crowding. Lee Way space according to Nance: the sum of the mesial - distal diameters of the 3 - 4 – 5 deciduous teeth is greater than the sum of the diameters of 3 - 4 - 5 permanent teeth by 3.4 mm (1.7 mm per side lower, 0.9mm per side upper), see Fig. 1-46.

Based on these data, if we have a well-spaced deciduous dentition, we will not have space problems in permanent dentition see Fig. 1-47.

However, if the teeth are "beautiful and united" as proud mothers sometimes note, we must expect a crowded permanent dentition.

The Relationship between Deciduous and Corresponding Elements not yet Erupted

1) **Method of Hixon and Oldfather (by Rx)**[122] to assess the size before their eruption of lower 3-4-5. Take an X-ray of 3-4-5 not yet erupted: they are likely to be as measured + 0.6 mm (maximum).
2) **Ballard and Wylie (by models)**[238] by measuring the mesial-distal diameters of the four lower incisors, refer to the table to obtain the probable size of the canine and two premolars.
3) **Tanaka - Johnston rule (by models)**[238] to estimate the size of premolars and canines not yet erupted:

$$\frac{\text{mesial-distal diameters sum of 31-32-41-42}}{2} + 10.5\text{ mm}$$

for lower canines and premolars

$$\frac{\text{mesial-distal diameters sum of 31-32-41-42}}{2} + 11\text{ mm}$$

for upper canines and premolars

4) **Moyer's tables**[173] for the prediction of permanent canines and premolars not yet erupted. Based on the sum of the mesio-distal diameter of the lower incisors, the tables indicate, to an approximation of 75%, the space occupied by canines and premolars (one quadrant) not yet erupted.

1-46

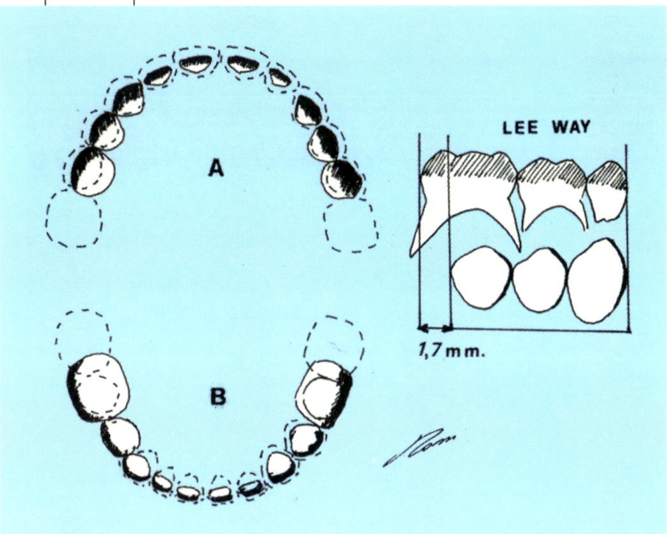

1-47

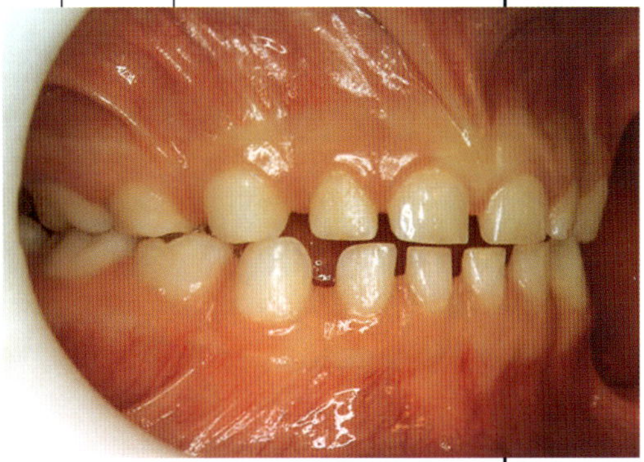

1-48

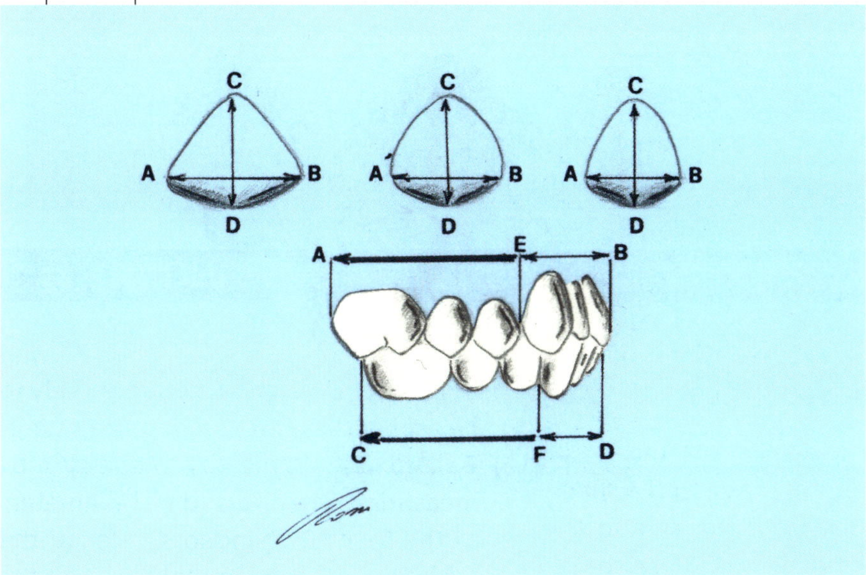

THE RELATIONSHIP BETWEEN TEETH AND THE DENTAL ARCH

1) **Peck and Peck Index (Fig. 1-48 top)**[195] Diameter ratio of mesial-distal and bucco-lingual of the lower incisors. According to the authors, it is acceptable that the first is greater than or at least equal to the second. The index can help with carrying out the procedure of reductive coronoplasty.
2) **Bolton Index (Fig. 1-48 bottom)**[31] The sum of the mesial-distal diameters of the six lower front teeth (distal 3 to distal 3) is approximately 77% (77.2%) of the sum of the same upper elements. The sum from distal 6 right to distal 6 left in the lower arch is about 91% (91.3%) of the corresponding distance in the upper arch. This analysis might lead us, for example, to decide whether or not we need to close the spaces in a dental arch with diastemas.

In orthodontics, one of the primary goals is firstly to place the treated teeth upright and secondly to obtain a Class I relationship. In a skeletal Class I, we may have a crowding condition (dento–alveolar discrepancy). In order to reposition the teeth with an orthodontic treatment, we need to measure on a model the space available and the space required. The reference to use is the mandibular arch.

A simple method is the following:

A) the sum of the mesial-distal diameters of the tooth is measured from 35 to 45, the lower deciduous molars, with a gauge or compass

B) the length of the arch is detected by modelling a flexible metal wire (brass) from the contact points between 36-35 and 46 to 45 passing through the cusps and the margin of the incisors (the most being centred on the crest) (Fig. 1-49 A).

The difference between the two measurements tells us how much space is needed in order to align the teeth according to the development of the arch.

Another convenient way is to measure the mesio-distal teeth dimension using the Brader arch form. To this value we add 2 to 4 mm to correct the curve of Spee if it is accentuated. How can you obtain the space you need?

WITH OR WITHOUT EXTRACTIONS

Without extractions:

- use of the Lee way space
- transverse expansion
- incisor proclination
- ditalization
- enamel interproximal removal (stripping).

If we are not in a skeletal Class I relationship we must consider an alignment as a change of inclination of the front teeth to create a "tooth compensation" of the jaws discrepancy.

Based on the values of ANB, the angle formed by the incisors with lines NA/NB and the distance between these lines and the incisal edge, Steiner indicates the following possibilities of compensation (Fig. 1-50).

With a similar concept, in a vertical assessment between bone bases there might be a possible dental compensation that provides, in subjects with *increased vertical dimension, more vertically positioned teeth* (Fig 1-51A). The same teeth are more labially inclined in subjects with a diminished vertical dimension (Fig. 1-51C). Picture 1-51B shows a normal vertical dimension; compare the incisor's relationship with the other ones.

1-49

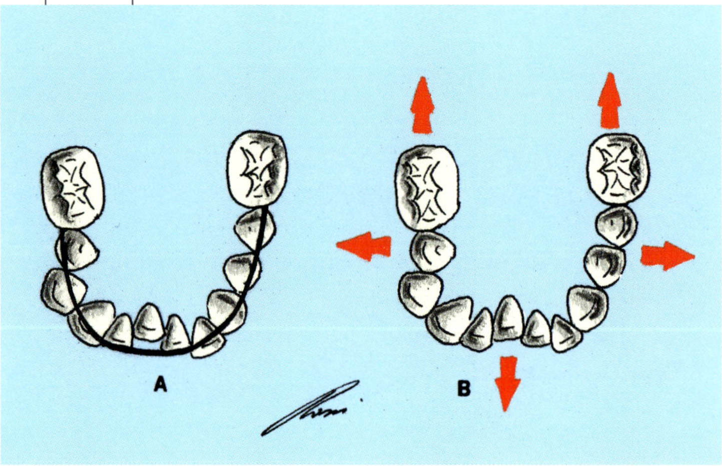

1-51

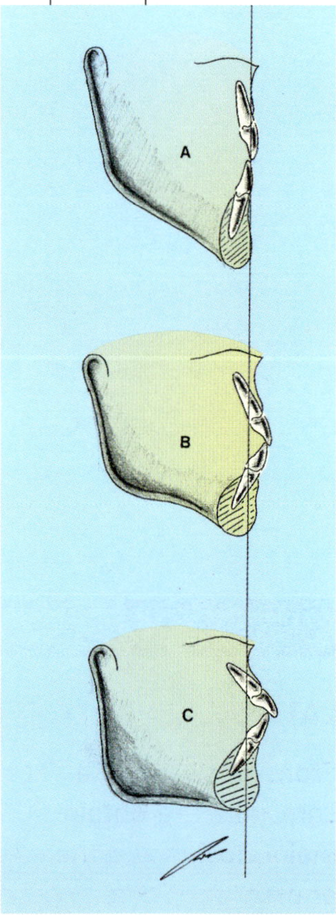

1-50

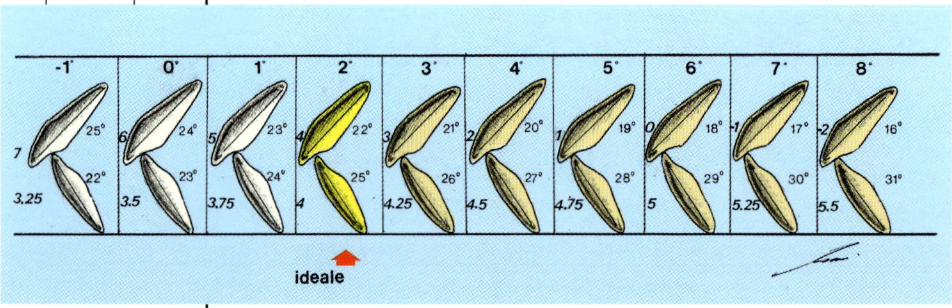

THE CLASSIFICATION OF MALOCCLUSIONS

The definitions of Class I, Class II, Class III are recurrent in orthodontics but what do they mean exactly? First of all we must distinguish dental aspects from skeletal ones. Edward Angle was the first to talk about dental classes, and his classification is still commonly used when referring to occlusion. As far as the sagittal jaws relationship various classifications have been proposed, one of the most famous (albeit with some limitations) considers the value of the ANB angle, as shown here.
As depicted in the diagram (Fig. 1-52: 1) in a Class I the jaws have a good sagittal skeletal relationship.
In a skeletal Class II (Fig. 1-52: 2) the upper jaw is too far ahead compared to the mandible (or the lower jaw is too far back, or both).
In a skeletal Class III (Fig. 1-52: 3) we have exactly the contrary.
The sagittal evaluation must be accompanied by a vertical one. Many classifications have been proposed by various authors. In this book I prefer to use the Ricketts analysis, expressed by dividing the biotypes in:

- Brachifacial (decreased vertical values)
- Mesofacial (normal vertical values)
- Dolicofacial (increased vertical values).

By increasing the verticality there is a clockwise rotation of the mandible which causes a Class II sagittal worsening. Decreasing the verticality, a Class II tends to improve.
The opposite happens in a Class III.
A dental class *does not always* imply a similar skeletal class (eg. dental class I -> skeletal class I), however, it is more likely to happen.
An ideal model to aspire to consists of a dental Class 1 in the context of a skeletal Class I.
With our therapeutic efforts we try to achieve an optimal occlusion and an harmonious relationship between the bone bases and their soft parts. Everything is done paying great attention to periodontal health, the temporomandibular joint and facial aesthetics. A correct classification requires cephalometric analysis.

1-52

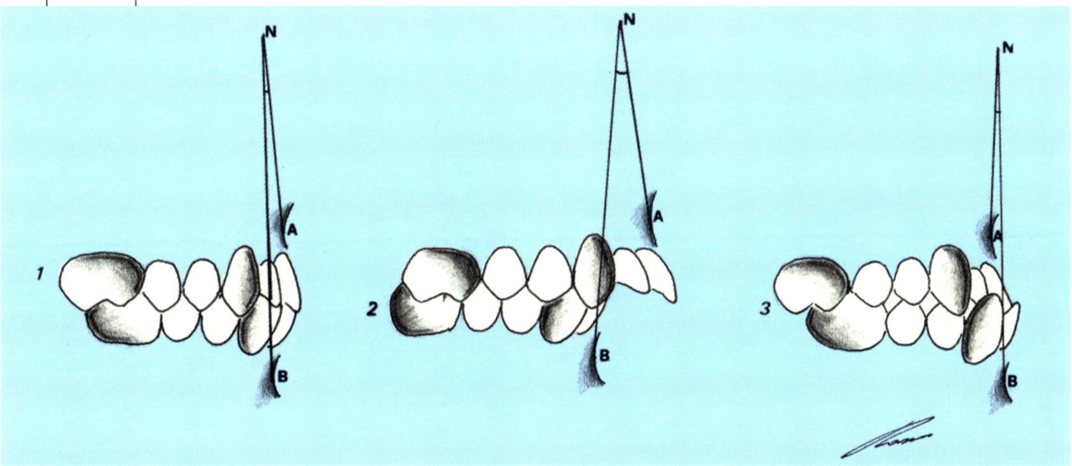

Fig. 1-52
Dental classification according to Angle and the relationship between the jaws at the angle ANB.

CEPHALOMETRIC ANALYSIS

LATERAL CEPHALOGRAM

From analysis of a lateral cephalogram, core data are obtained for the study of a malocclusion and the execution of a proper orthodontic treatment.

Technically, the X-ray film is placed at a distance of 1.50 m from the radiation source. If the anatomical contours of the left and right halves are not perfectly superimposed even when the examination is well executed (and this concerns especially the lower mandibular border) it is because the parties do not lie on the same plane. This leads to a different distance from the radiation's emission, and also some divergence of the rays.

From the lateral cephalometric radiographs, anatomical information is obtained (such as the size of the adenoids or the curvature of the cervical spine). Even more importantly, we are able to trace a lay out for a program for treatment.

The tracing is the basis of a series of linear and angular measurements which the clinician, noticing the differences when compared with the ideal values, can refer to.

1-53

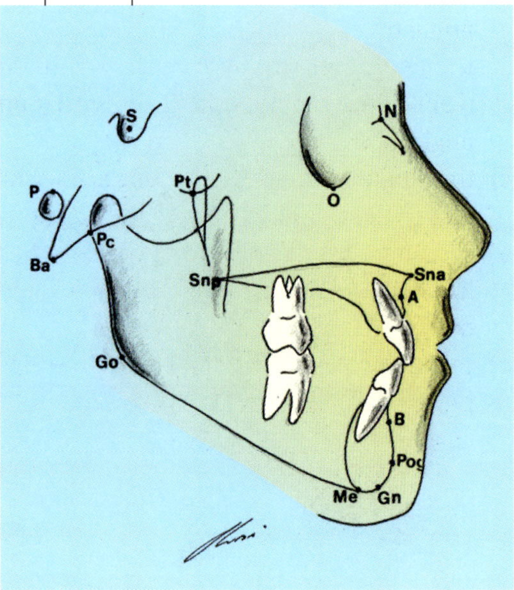

CEPHALOMETRIC POINTS OF A BASIC TRACING

FIG. 1-53

S	Sella:	*Midpoint of sella turcica.*
N	Nasion:	*Most anterior point on fronto-nasal suture.*
(Sna) ANS		*Anterior Nasal Spine*
(Snp) PNS		*Posterior Nasal Spine*
Go	Gonion:	*Where the bisector of the angle between the ramus plane and the mandibular plane meets the angle of the mandible.*
Gn	Gnathion:	*Where the bisector of the angle between the Nasion Pogonion line and the mandibular plane meets the mandibular symphysis.*
A	Point:	*Position of deepest concavity on anterior profile of the maxilla.*
B	Point:	*Position of deepest concavity on anterior profile of mandibular symphysis.*
Ba	Basion:	*The median point of the anterior margin of the foramen magnum.*
Pog	Pogonion:	*Most anterior point of chin symphysis.*
Me	Menton:	*Lowest point on the mandibular symphysis.*
O	Orbitale:	*Lowermost anterior point of the orbit.*
P	Porion:	*Highest point on bony external auditory meatus.*
Pc	Condylar point:	*Intersection of the posterior border of the condyle and the occipital bone (Gianni). Other authors indicate as **Ar** the same point.*
Pt	Pterygoid:	*Intersection of pterygomaxillary fissure and foramen rotunduum.*

1-54

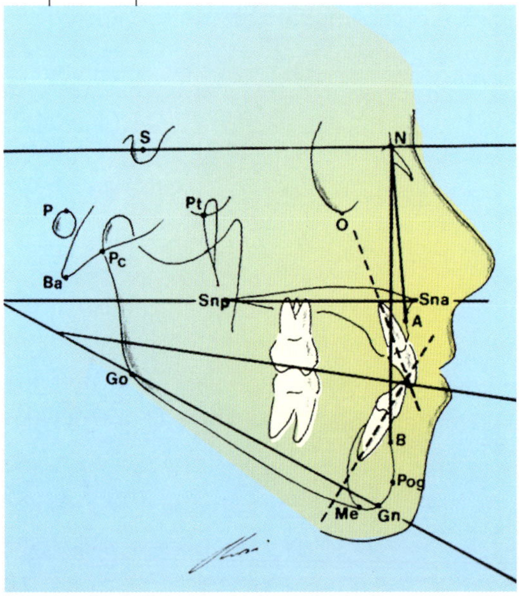

ANGLES AND PLANES

IDEAL VALUES AND VARIABLE

SNA	82° ± 2°
SNB	80° ± 2°
ANB	2° ± 2°
SN - GoGn	32° ± 5°
SN - (Sna) Ans I (Snp) Pns	10° ± 3°
SN - Occl	14° ± 3°
Occl - GoGn	14°
(Sna) Ans - (Snp) Pns - GoGn	25° ± 3°
1 NA	22°
1 NB	25°
1/1	131°
1 GoGn	93°

DATA EVALUATION

SNA and SNB angles greater or lesser than normal indicate whether the maxilla and mandible are anteriorly or posteriorly positioned, which may be due to a difference in jaw growth and size.

The ANB angle indicates the relative position of the maxilla to the mandible and allows the measurement of the extent of the jaw size/position discrepancy.

ANB 2 ± 2° = skeletal Class I

ANB > 4° = skeletal Class II

ANB < 0° = skeletal Class III

Evaluation is made possible by the angles between the following planes:

I) SN / Ans –Pns

The normal value is 10° ± 3° and indicates the inclination of the maxillary plane.

By applying traction you can change the inclination of the plane while, of course, you cannot change the values of SN.

2) SN / occlusal plane

The normal value is 14° ± 3°, considering the occlusal plane passing tangent to the cusp of the lower first molar and the midpoint between the edges of the upper and lower incisors.

This assessment does not consider, unlike others, the functional occlusal plane which is tangential to the cusps of the lower molars and premolars.

The occlusal plane can be changed with treatment.

3) SN / GoGn

The normal value is of 32 ± 5° and indicates the angle of the mandible compared to the skull base.

4) Ans-Pns / GoGn

It has an average value of 26° and represents the divergence between the maxillary bone bases.

The degree of divergence may be influenced by a direct treatment on bony parts or indirectly by changing the occlusal plane.

Under ideal conditions:

a) the upper incisor is placed 4 mm in front of the NA line and forms with it an angle of 22°
b) the lower incisor is placed 4 mm in front of the NB line and forms with it an angle of 25°
c) the angle formed by the upper incisor axis with lower incisor axis is of 131°
d) the angle between the axis of the lower incisor with the GoGn plane has a value of 93°
e) the angle between the axis of the upper incisor with the SN line is 103° ± 2°

ADVANCED TRACING

FROM JARABAK ANALYSIS[130]

ANGLES:

N-S-Pc	122° ± 5°	Saddle angle
S-Pc-Go	143° ± 6°	Articular angle
Pc-Go-Gn	120° ± 5°	Gonial angle
Pc- Go-N	50° ± 2°	Upper gonial angle
N-Go-Gn	70° ± 2°	Lower gonial angle

PLANES:

FROM RICKETTS'S ANALYSIS[211]

Pt-Gn	Facial axis (Ricketts). Corresponds to a normal growth direction. It forms with the Ba –N line an angle with 90° ± 3° as normal value.
A-Pog	Normal value: 1 ± 2 mm of distance from the edge of the lower incisor.
P – Or	Frankfurt plane.

An increased value of gonial angle and a straight mandibular canal are typical of a clockwise mandibular growth. This worsens in a sagittal Class II jaws relationship and even worse when the saddle and articular angles are also increased.

The McNamara line is also known as mini-VTO (visualization treatment objective). A simple line can, at a glance, show the sagittal jaws relationship.[165]

In a well-balanced profile:

1) In children the perpendicular from Nasion (N) to Frankfurt plane passes through the maxillary A point and is anterior to the chin (bone).
2) In an adult female the same line passes 1 mm behind the A point and it is still anterior to the chin (bone).
3) In an adult male the line passes 1 mm behind the A point but it is tangent to the chin (bone).

The distinction between basic and advanced tracing is not a rule. It simply represents what I usually do in my clinical practice where I add to the basic the advanced tracing with a more complex diagnosis.

1-55

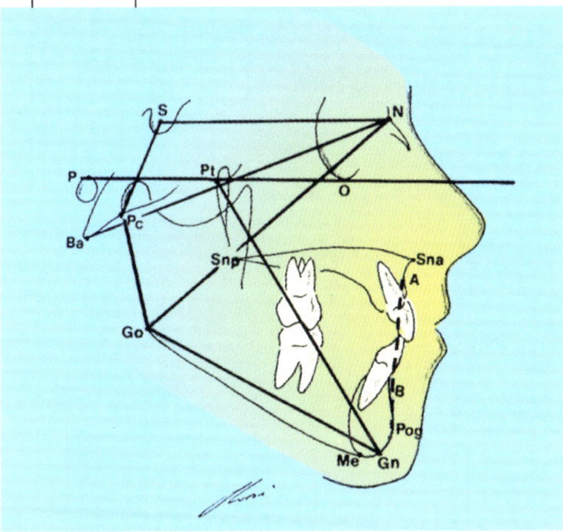

1-56

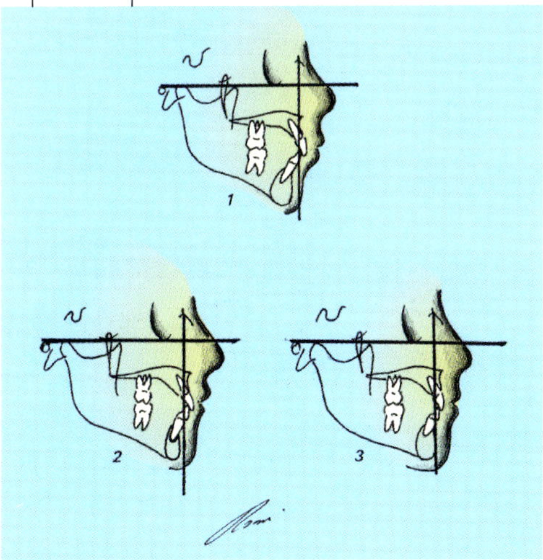

Fig. 1-56
McNamara Line.

VERTICAL EVALUATION

(according to Ricketts – Gugino)

PATIENTS:
A) 15%: Increased Verticality (Dolico facial)
B) 70%: Normal Verticality (Mesio facial)
C) 15%: Decreased Verticality (Brachi facial)

The arrows show an increasing difficulty with more extreme values.

If the verticality between the bone bases increases with a mandibular clockwise growth, a Class II worsens its sagittal jaws relationship. The opposite happens in a Class III.

SAGITTAL INTERMAXILLARY RELATIONSHIP (SLAVICECK)

N = Normal
P = Protruded
R = Retruded

1) Maxilla N / Mandible N:	27%
2) Maxilla N / Mandible R:	21%
3) Maxilla N / Mandible P:	4%
4) Maxilla P / Mandible N:	19%
5) Maxilla P / Mandible P:	11%
6) Maxilla P / Mandible R:	3%
7) Maxilla R / Mandible N:	3%
8) Maxilla R / Mandible P:	1%
9) Maxilla R / Mandible R:	11%

According to these data:

NN 27% + **PP** 11% + **RR** 11% = **49 %** of **Class I**
RN 21% + **PN** 19% + **PN** 3% = **43 %** of **Class II**
NP 4% + **RP** 1% + **RN** 3% = **8 %** of **Class III**

Do not forget the vertical aspect!

1-57

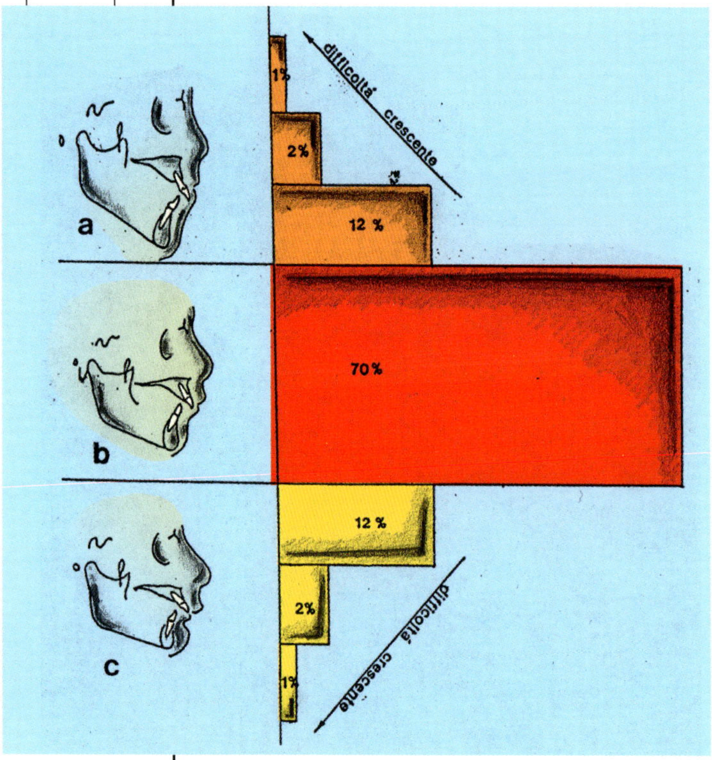

Ideal values have been derived and proposed by various authors having analysed large samples of subjects. Many tracings have been suggested. Personally I do not think that one tracing is better than another: if well used, they all give good directions.

What must be remembered is that each tracing, while having a global scope, may have some weaknesses. In some tracings it is difficult to find certain anatomical points while in others skeletal landmarks are more easily identifiable. If the data obtained is misinterpreted you can have contradictory information.

In tracings that use the ANB angle, the amplitude of the anterior skull base may cause apparently absurd values such as a value of ANB wider than 4° or below 0° in cases of evident occlusal harmony (Fig. 1-58 and 1-59).

It is therefore crucial to properly assess the various data by integrating the method you usually follow with other tracing analyses.

In cases where a deeper assessment is required, I integrate the data exposed with others, in particular that derived from the analysis of Jarabak and Ricketts (advanced tracing).

Finally, do not forget that as indicated by Giannì[106] (Fig. 1-60):

- from 6 to 12 years, the distance N-S increases l mm per year while the distance Go-Me increases 1.5/2 mm per year
- at 12 in both males and females the distance N-S should be the same as Me-Go. This ratio remains constant for the girls while for the boys it shifts in favour of the jaw. This assessment is important when we need to evaluate the size of the jaw.

The size of the posterior facial dimension IST-Go (lowest point of the sella turcica - gonion) is 62% of the anterior dimension SOR-Me (supraorbital point–menton). A decrease in this ratio indicates an increase in mandibular clockwise rotation. An increase indicates a counterclockwise rotation.

1-58

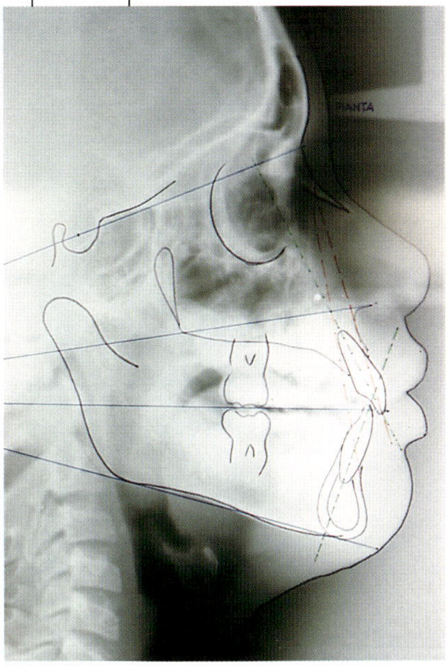

1-59

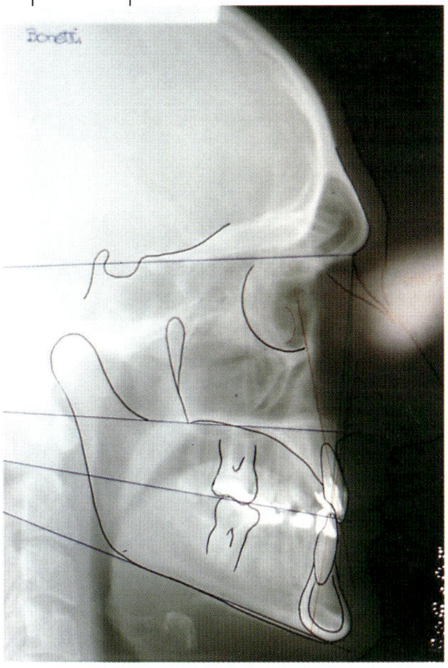

Fig. 1-58
ANB = 7°

Fig. 1-59
ANB = -0.3°

In tracings that use the ANB angle, the amplitude of the anterior skull base may cause apparently absurd values such as a value of ANB wider than 4° or below 0° in cases of evident occlusal harmony (Fig. 1-58 and 1-59).

POSTERO-ANTERIOR X-RAY

An X-ray of the skull in the posteroanterior projection is important for the analysis of craniofacial asymmetries, whose correction may be by orthopaedic, orthodontic or surgical means.
The lower jaw is a special case. Being mobile, its skeletal components may not be well centred either because of malposition or because it is structurally asymmetric. A gnathologic splint may be used to distinguish between these two possibilities and can lead to a mandible reallocation guided by jaw muscles and not forced by a deviant occlusion.
In order to evaluate the various structures on both the vertical and horizontal planes,

1-60

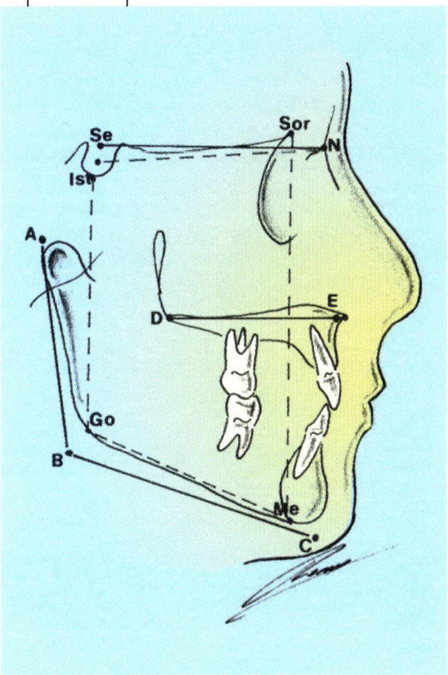

1-61

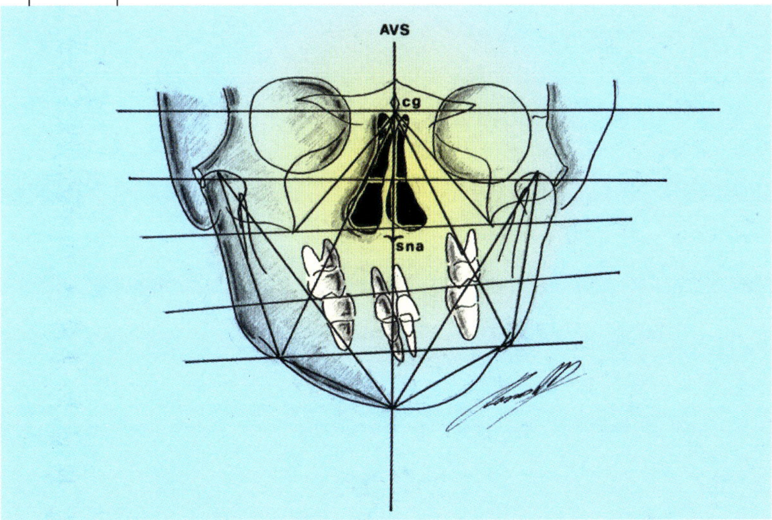

Fig. 1-61
Axes and planes of a posteroanterior tracing

lines or reference axes are essential. (Gianni proposes a vertical axis of symmetry passing through the highest point of the occipital foramen and perpendicular to the line joining the occipital condyles. Other authors, including DC Grummons, use another axis passing through the same CristaGalli apophysis and the anterior nasal spine.) Onto these axes, horizontal planes are traced passing through various anatomical points. Some of these such as the menton are more reliable than others, for example a frontozygomatic suture.
Taking teeth as references, mandibular canines are more reliable than mandibular molars.
The further addition of oblique lines makes these tracings more complete, allowing a linear and angular analysis of different situations.

ORTHODONTICS AND AESTHETICS

Since an orthodontic treatment is in many cases required in order to obtain a good smile, the concept of aesthetic research is implicit. Can the orthodontist limit this research to the teeth only? Evidently not. In the light of modern needs, he is definitely involved in the analysis of facial aesthetics; an analysis of the various parameters which have been proposed, aimed at defining the harmony between the parts.

CLINICAL EVALUATION

The face is divided into three parts (Fig. 1-62):

- Top third – from trichion (hairline) to the glabella
- Middle third – from glabella to subnasal point (between columella and philtrum)
- Bottom third – from the subnasal point to point under the chin (skin)

In a harmonic face these three parts are the same size.
From an evaluative point of view, the orthodontist is primarily interested in the presence of asymmetries although he does not ignore relevant details of the diagnosis and treatment plan, such as the flattening of the malar areas, which is indicative of a maxillary retrusion.

1-62

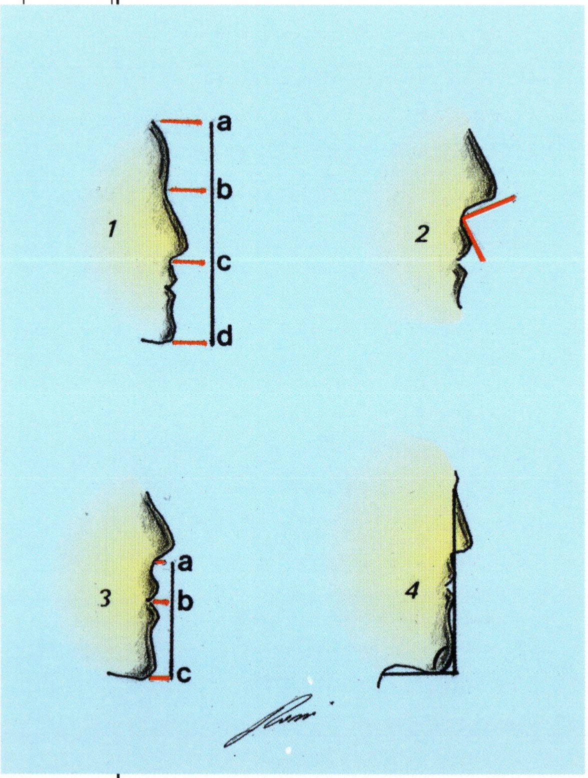

1-63

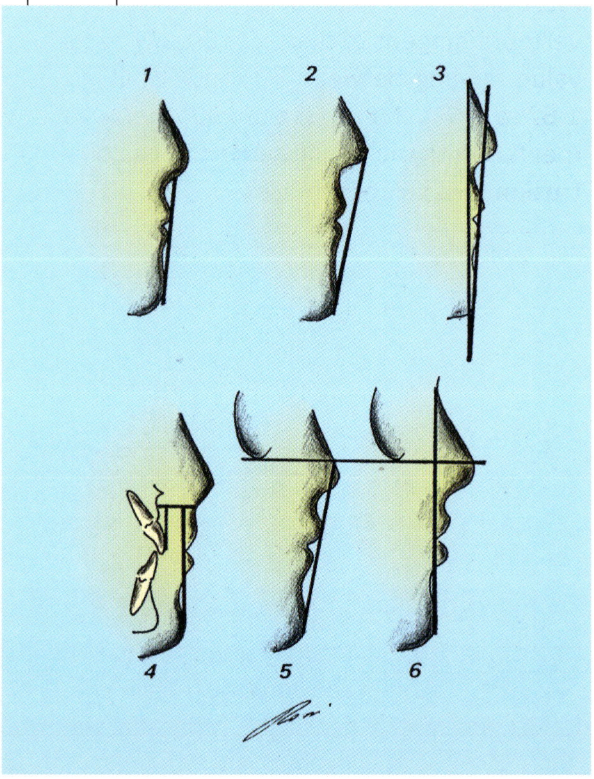

The upper third of the profile is characterized by the ratio between the forehead and the supraorbital rim. This ratio is variable and affected, for example, by the presence of orbital hypoplasia or by an exaggerated forehead.

In the middle third, the distance between the eyeball and the supraorbital margin is normally 8 to 15 mm. The angle of the nose-lip (formed by the tangent line to the upper lip with the line tangent to the columella) has a value between 90° and 110° (Fig. 1-62:2). Interventions on the maxilla can change its value, improving it if the angle is too oblique, or making the angle worse if the original value was normal. In a Class III with normal nasolabial angle, a mandibular retrusion will be preferable to maxillary advancement. Vice versa, if the nasolabial angle is increased it would be better to advance the maxilla.

The lower third is further divided into two parts: (a-b) from the subnasal point to the labial (stomion), and (b-c) from there to the chin (Figs. 1-62 and 1-63).

The optimum harmonic proportion is when a-b is half of b-c.

The angle chin-neck, formed by the straight line passing through the glabella tangent to the chin and with the line through the most prominent point of the third cervical vertebra tangent to the chin, usually has a value ranging between 90° and 95° (Figs. 1-62 to 1-64). If it is less than 90° there is a mental protrusion, while there is less protrusion if its value increases.

MIXED EVALUATION

Clinical – X-rays – Photography

- Under ideal conditions, in Steiner, the lips should be touching the line from the chin to the midpoint of the nose (Fig. 1-63: 1).[234]
- Ricketts defines the plane E that goes from the tip of the nose to the chin, stating that in a harmonic outline the lips are behind this by a few mm., with the upper lip in front of the lower one (Fig. 1-63: 2).[210]
- Holdaway indicates the angle formed between the NB line and the line tangent to the chin, passing through the outermost point of the upper lip. Its value is of 7°- 9° under ideal conditions (ANB: 2°). Larger values will have a protrusion of the soft parts of the lower third while lower values will have a retraction (Fig. 1-63: 3).[124]
- Bass suggests an analysis of the lower third of the chin correlated to the upper incisor. He divides into thirds the distance between point A and the subnasal point. The perpendiculars to the two division points are, in a harmonic subject, tangent to the outer edge of the upper incisor and to the chin (Fig. 1-63: 4).[12]
- Merrifield describes the Z angle between the Frankfurt plane and the line passing through the external border of the upper lip and the chin. In a balanced profile the ideal value is of 85° ± 5 ° (Fig. 63: 5).[170]
- For Gonzalez & Ulloa the perpendicular from the nasion to the Frankfurt plane

1-64

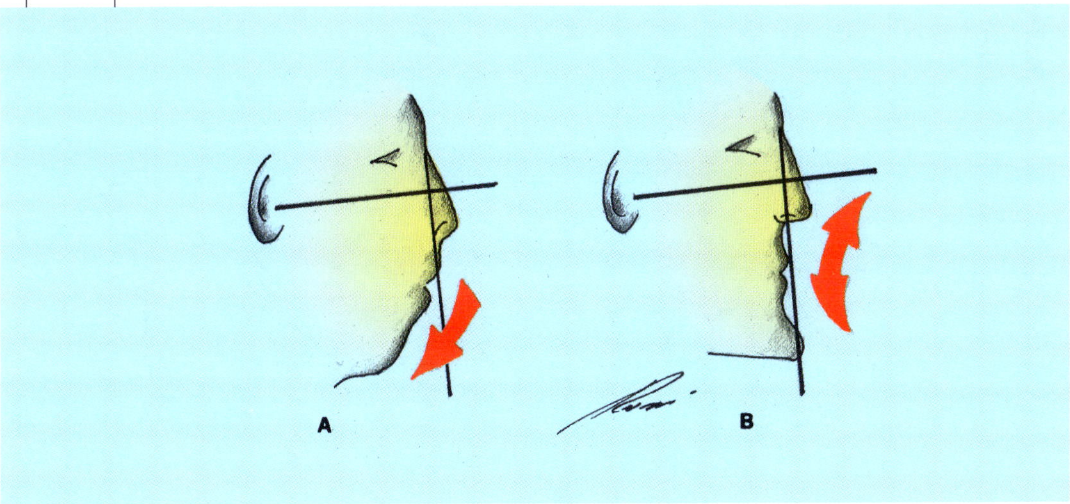

is tangent to the chin. (Fig. 1-63: 6)[108] McNamara suggests a similar assessment (mini VTO), indicating however a more retruse position of the chin in the female than in the male.[164]

We will have a *convex* profile (Fig. 1-64: A) if the chin is behind the perpendicular from point N to the plane of Frankfurt (for example in Class II with clockwise rotation of the mandible).

Conversely (Fig. 1-63: B), if the chin tends to approach or anteriorly exceed this perpendicular, we talk about a *concave* profile figure (for example in Class III).

DISCUSSION

There are many signs when it comes to defining facial harmony. Criticism affects every point of view.

- The position of the incisors in determining more or less pleasant lips was frequently pointed out. Several authors have shown different relationships between the lips and the posterior repositioning of the anterior teeth. 1.5-3 mm of incisal retraction, according to various opinions, corresponds to 1 mm of lip retraction. However, the thickness of the soft parts is highly variable. Therefore, if 1 mm for thin lips can be significant, it is much less for full lips.
- Aesthetic criteria are not absolute, especially over time. Just think of the ideal beauty of ancient Greece for example, and its comparision with that of the modern day. "What is beauty? A convention, a currency, whose value belongs only to a specific time and place." Ibsen (*Peer Gynt*)
- If the objective is aesthetic, people's opinion is what counts the most, even more than numbers, angles, etc... In a study involving women winning beauty contests, Riddle[213] observed that the public considered women with prominent teeth were more fascinating than those bestowed with normal teeth as measured by the cephalometric standards. Peck and Peck[194] reached a similar conclusion.
- As pointed out by Cox and Van der Linden[54] in their research, you can have a good aesthetic face even in the presence of a mild to moderate malocclusion.
- Do not forget that the concept of "beauty" is different in every part of the world.
- When a beautiful smile is considered synonymous of sexual attractiveness, keep in mind the differences among different cultures and historical periods.

Forty years ago, during the time of student protests, many women were extremely attracted to Woody Allen, who is not exactly the definition of beauty.

CONCLUSIONS

Aesthetic analyses suggested by various authors are useful in determining therapeutic choices, but their value is relative. Do not forget that among other things, aesthetic analysis is clearly influenced by the technique and philosophy of its proposers.

Therefore, once again, clinical sense remains the centre of an orthodontic treatment.

To conclude we should remember a quote from the Summa Theologica of St. Thomas Aquinas:

"Pulchra dicuntur quae visa placent" (beautiful are the things that please the eye).

BIOMECHANICS

Remember that according to the third law of Newton, every action has an equal and opposite reaction.

- Parallelogram of forces: two forces applied to a body with different directions produce a shift with an intensity and direction determined by the resultant vector (Fig. 1-65: A).
- Centre of rotation: the point around which a tooth rotates under the action of a force (Fig. 1-65: B).
- Centre of resistance: the point where a force causes bodily displacement. In a

1-65

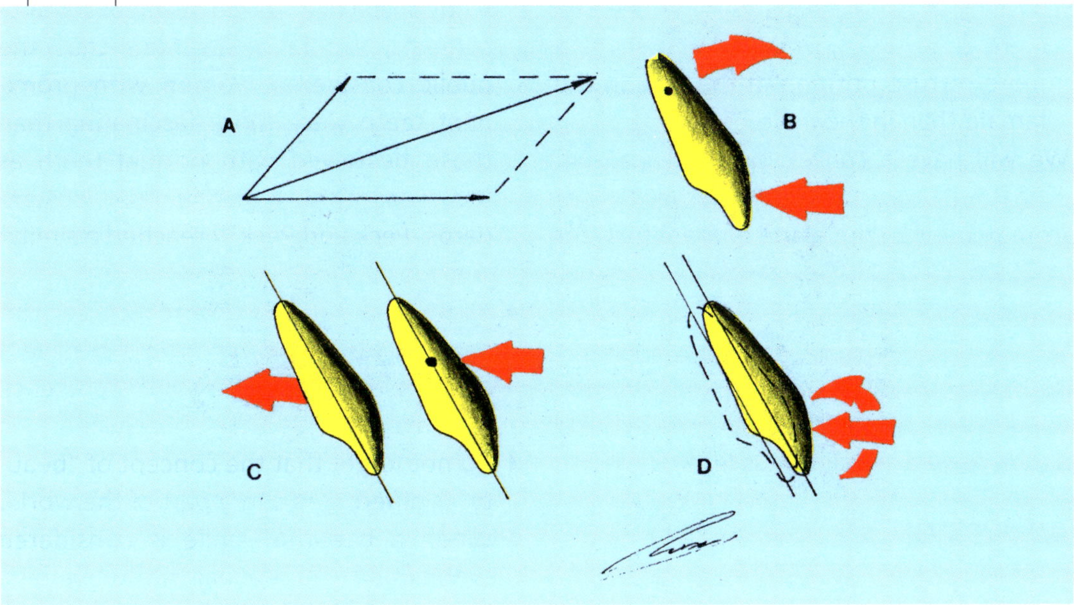

tooth with one root and healthy periodontium, it is located apically at 2/3 of the distance between the apex and the cementoenamel junction (Fig. 1-65: C).

In multirooted teeth the centre of resistance is in correspondence with the furcation.

In practice, since the centre of resistance is infrabony (Fig. 66: bottom), it is impossible to apply a force directly to it.

So, to obtain a bodily movement, we must apply a couple of forces (torque + linear force) (Fig. 1-65: D).

TEETH DISPLACEMENT

A force applied to a tooth results in areas where the periodontal ligament and the alveolar bone are subjected to pressure, and in areas that are subjected to tensile stress (Fig. 66: top).

In the first case occurs activation of osteoclasts and bone resorption: in the latter, osteoblasts by placing bone are activated. To have pressure only in the tooth displacement direction and to obtain a bodily movement, the force should be applied at the centre of resistance (Fig. 1=66: bottom) but this is impossible because the centre of resistance is infrabony. To obtain this movement it is necessary to apply a couple of forces.

For years orthodontists have discussed the definition of "optimal power", observing that in some cases (for example, in the presence of light forces) there is a balance between resorption and apposition that, using the expression of Fontenelle[92], "the tooth moves with the bone" like a turtle moves with the shell. In those cases the applied forces are beneficial. If they are excessive, as happens with heavy forces, the compression of the periodontal ligament against the wall of the alveolar determines an ischemia which induces necrosis

1-66

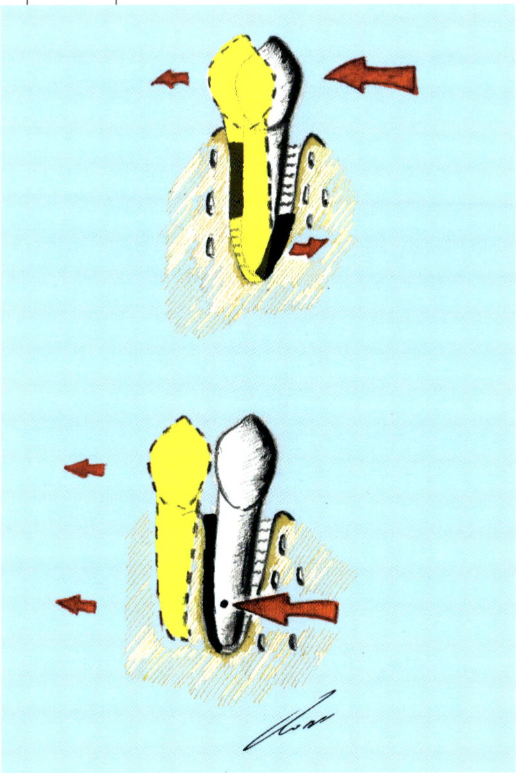

(hyalinization) of the lamina dura. Osteoclasts to remove the necrotic material are then activated, but the process takes time (about 15 days).

This explains the very common mistake of irrationally increasing the force applied in an attempt to move a dental element that seems unwilling to move. Such an action produces an opposite effect that could be called "mule" and can be particularly damaging in an adult patient. In other words, a heavy force induces a hyalinization resulting in an indirect bone resorption and a shift in the tooth "through the bone".

In clinical practice orthodontists usually consider "heavy" forces greater than 300g, but this is not a scientific evaluation. In fact, below this value the same force applied to a molar can be considered "light", while it would be "heavy" for a lower incisor. It is the root surface that makes the difference (Fig. 1-67).

We must also consider the type of movement. The forces necessary for a dental intrusion are much lighter than those needed for a dental displacement. A difference is seen in the technique used for obtaining a dental movement. For example, we can distalize a canine with a *"friction"* (Fig. 1-68: A) or with a *"no friction"* technique (Fig. 1-68: B).

In the first case the canine is distally displaced with the bracket slot sliding on the wire (friction). More anchorage and a force greater than in no-friction cases is needed. These examples have a relative value.

The orthodontic forces according to the application time can be divided into:

- continuous: usually fixed appliances where the applied force decreases with the tooth displacement. A relative exception is made using super elastic alloys.
- intermittent: usually removable appliances.

Remember that a dental displacement starts after four hours of force application time.[202]

1-67

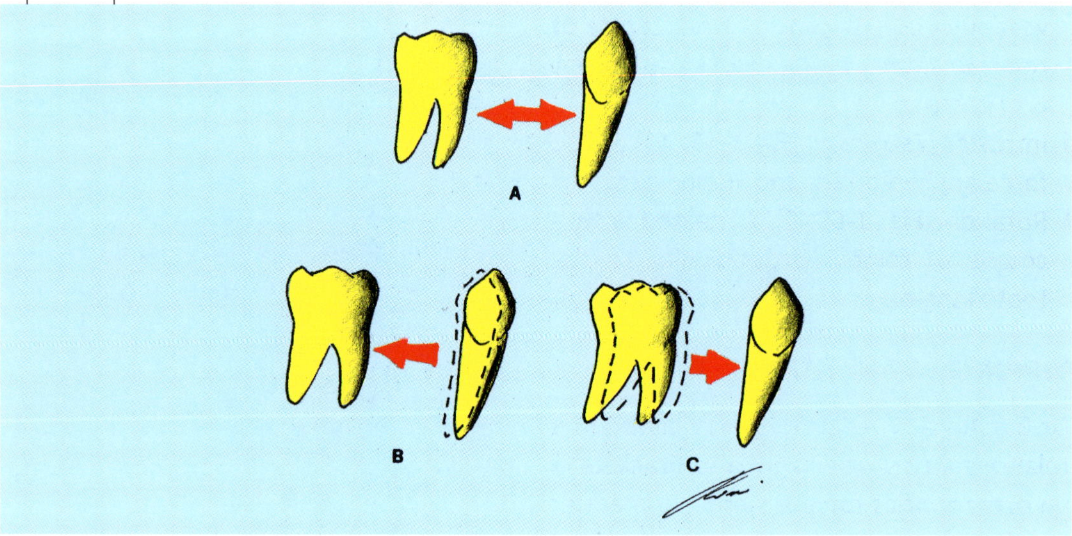

Fig. 1-67
Bodily retraction of a canine with a "friction" technique. A force is applied between molar and canine (A) If the force is lower than 150 g the teeth do not move. When the force is between 150 and 300 g there is a prevalence of canine displacement (B). With a force greater than 300 g there is a prevalence of molar movement (C).

1-68

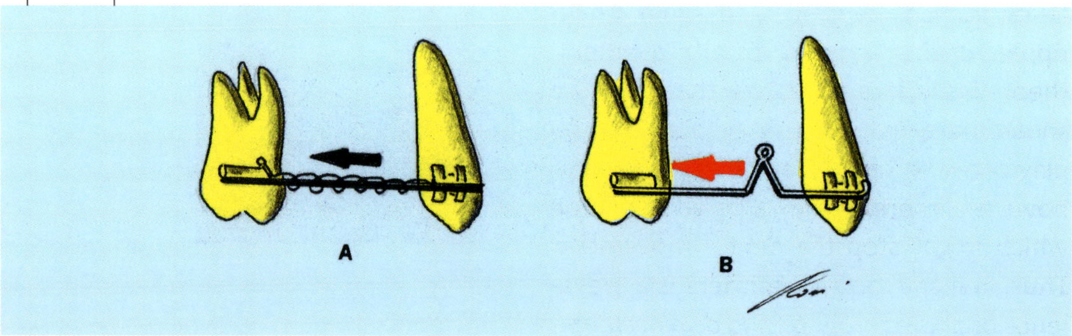

Fig. 1-68
Tooth distalization with: A friction mechanics. B no friction mechanics.

DENTAL MOVEMENT

According to Burstone's indications:[40]

- Non-controlled tipping (Fig. 1-69: A). A single force applied to the dental crown determines a dental buccal–palatal (or lingual) rotation around an intrabony centre of rotation (near the centre of resistance).
- Controlled tipping (Fig. 1-69: B). Tooth rotation around the root apex is obtained combining a single force (f) with a couple of forces (rotational moment M). **M** is clinically known as **torque**. M/f ratio is **5**/1.
- Bodily movement (Fig. 1-69: C). To have this movement a force must be theoretically applied to the centre of resistance which is intrabony. Therefore, a direct application is impossible. The desired result is possible with a combination of torque (M) and single force (f). M /f ratio **10**:1.
- Root torque (Fig. 69 D). To obtain a palatal (or lingual) root torque without vestibular crown proclination (centre of rotation: crown edge) a M/f ratio of **12**:1 is necessary.
- Intrusion/Estrusion (Fig 1-69: E). Single force applied on the tooth long axis.
- Rotation (Fig. 1-69: F). Obtained with a couple of forces perpendicular to the tooth long axis.

TIPPING – UPRIGHTING

Dr Burstone [40] explained very clearly the relationship between wire and brackets in an orthodontics force system. It is easier to obtain a dental crown displacement than a bodily displacement of the roots.

Using friction mechanics, to avoid dental tipping during a mesio/distal movement, theoretically it is necessary that the wire should have the same slot dimension (no play between the slot and wire). This way, however, there is an excessive friction which might stop the dental movement. Thus, in many techniques there is a prevalence of *tipping – uprighting displacement.*

Dental tipping causes a wire deformation. The wire elastic memory determines the uprighting. When the wire elastic memory is not enough it can be very useful to apply an "uprighting spring" which basically follows the M/f relationship (Fig. 1-70).

Bends determine different forces when the wire is inserted between two brackets with the same slot inclination (Fig. 1-70).

In a similar way different forces are produced by a straight arch wire and brackets with different slot inclinations (Fig. 1-71).

TORQUE

In order to have correct buccal (labial) / palatal or buccal (labial) / lingual teeth

1-69

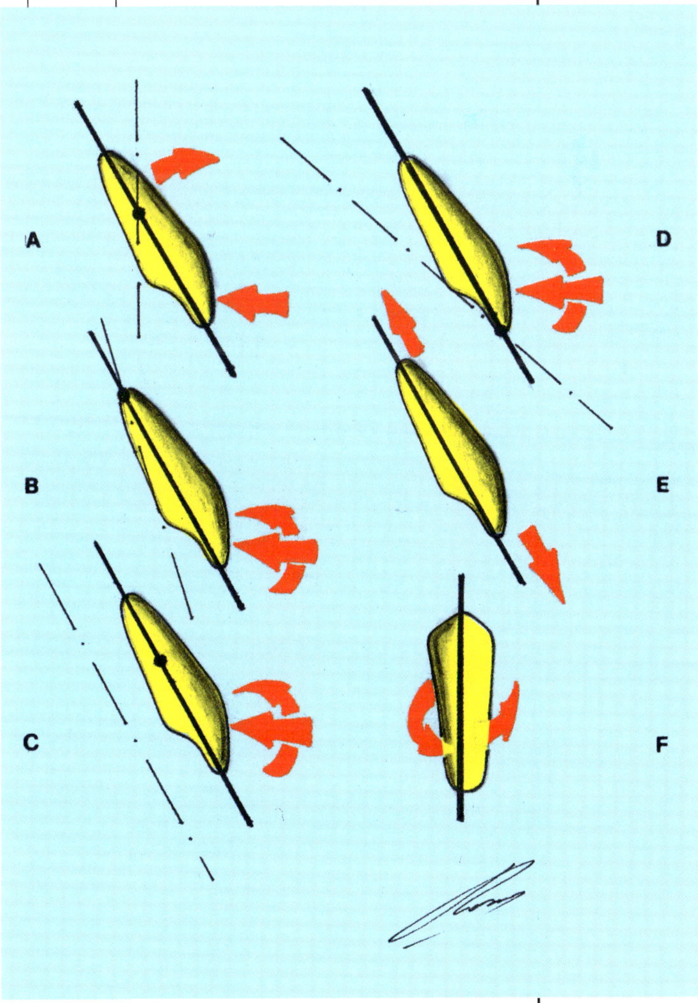

inclination the orthodontist must apply torque (a couple of forces) to the dental crown.

Dental torque is obtained using a rectangular wire. When the wire is inserted into the bracket slot it is deformed (rotated on its long axis) and causes friction between the wire edges and the bracket's slot walls. The reaction (springback) makes the teeth move (torque).

With pre-adjusted brackets there are various values of torque in their slots, otherwise the orthodontist himself must bend the wire to impose the torque value.

A buccal–labial crown inclination corresponds to a positive torque while a palatal / lingual inclination corresponds to a negative torque.

It is very important to remember that, as pointed out by Creekmore, *the interplay between wire and slot makes the difference.* With a 0.022" x 0.028" slot, using a 0.019" x 0.025" wire, there are 4.3° of torque more than when using a 0.018" x 0.025" wire. Using a 0.0215" x 0.025" there are 8° more. (T.D. Creekmore on torque (J Clin. Orthod 1979))

Fig. 1-70 V - bending wire
From left to right
A V bend is placed on a wire between two brackets with the same angulation.
When the apex of the V bend is placed halfway between the brackets, equal and opposite pairs of force are produced. As the V bend apex is moved off centre, different combinations of rotational moments and forces are created (arrows).
These schematic drawings show how, with different M/f relationships, it is possible to obtain different teeth movements: uprighting, extrusion, intrusion. They are also the rational basis for producing the desired force system and avoid unwanted teeth movements.

1-70

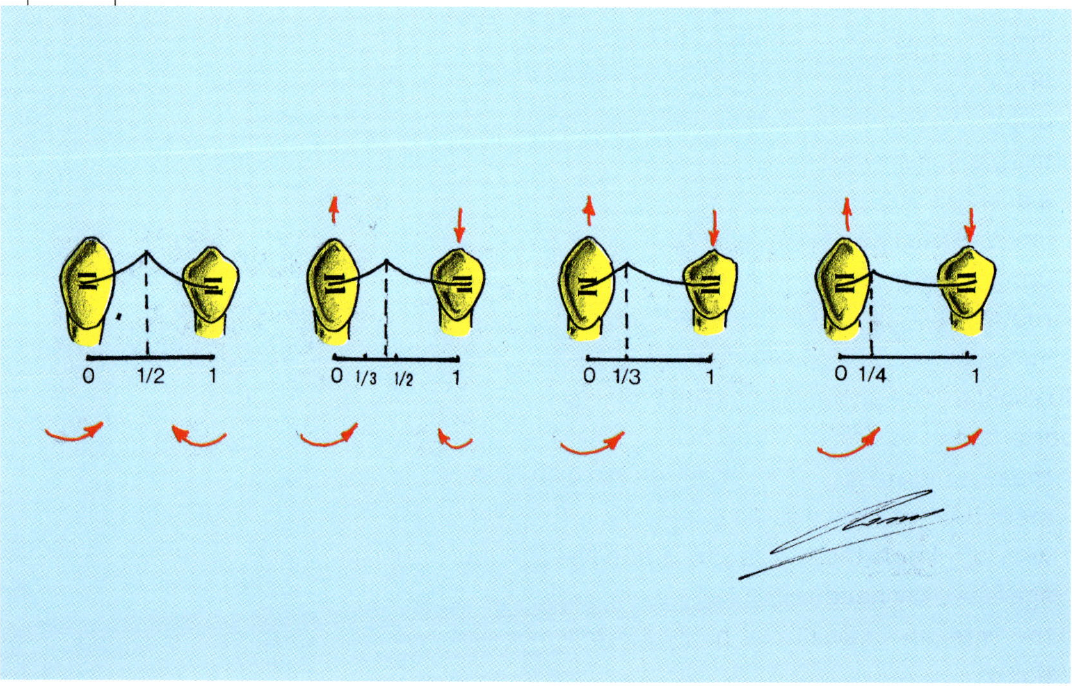

1-71

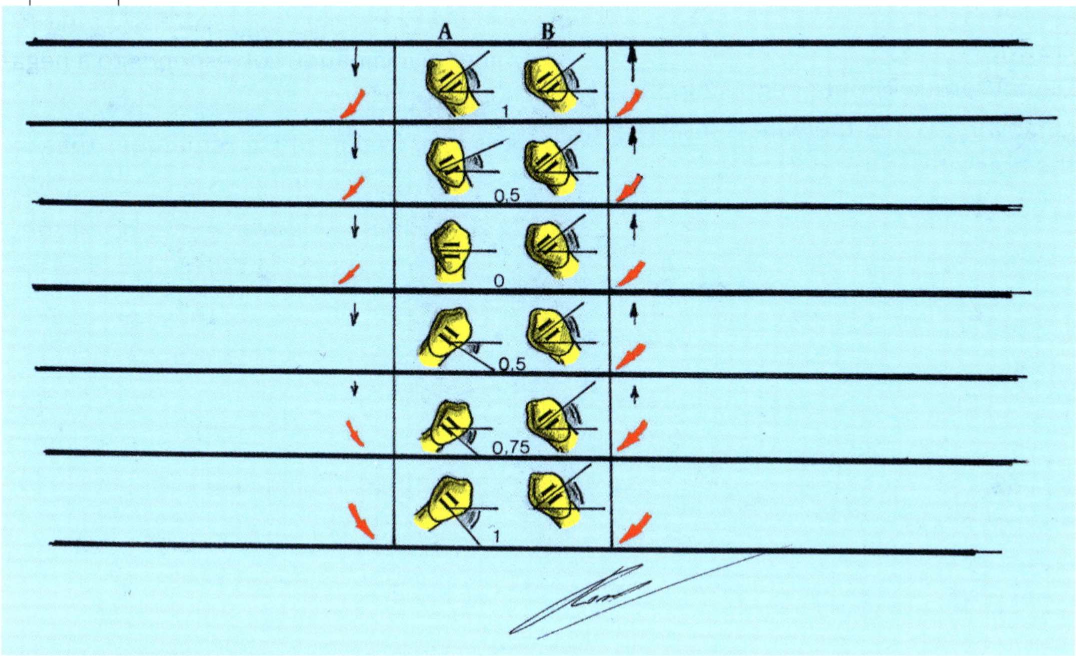

fig. 1-71 Burstone's Six Geometries
Using a straight wire, we obtain different linear forces and rotational moments (arrows) changing the position of the brackets. The concept is similar to the one explained above, but in this case there are no bends on the wire. Imagine a clockwise rotation of the left tooth (A) around the right (B). The slots between the brackets create different angles and six different geometries, to which correspond alternative forces.

ANCHORAGE

Imagine applying traction between two teeth with the same root surface. We see that -

A) They have a similar displacement – no anchorage.
B) Increasing the anchorage (left) there is a prevalence of right displacement - medium anchorage.
C) With maximum anchorage - only the tooth on the right moves.

We can increase the anchorage by:

- increasing the number of anchorage units
- using a headgear (upper)
- using a lip bumper (lower)
- a palatal bar
- inter-maxillary elastics
- uprighting springs
- root frictioning against cortical bone
- implants including mini-screws.

To evaluate the anchorage needed it is important to consider:

- the technique used for a tooth displacement (friction/no friction).
- with a friction technique more anchorage is usually needed.
- the wire/slot play (more play, less friction).
- the materials: stainless steel wires show less friction than TMA.
- ceramic brackets give more friction than stainless steel ones
- the *lowest friction is between stainless steel brackets and wires.*

1-72

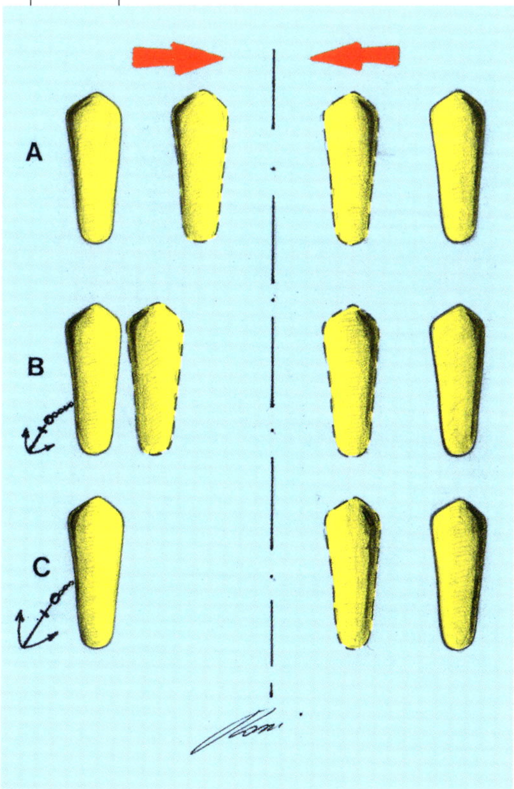

ORTHODONTIC WIRES

Before analysing the main characteristics of orthodontic wires it is useful to remember the basic vocabulary which accompanies the subject.

- Friction: usually present, in various mechanics, between the wire and slot.
- Springback: how far a wire can be deflected without permanent deformation.
- Stiffness: indicates the amount of force needed for a deflection.
- Formability: describes the amount and ability a wire can bend before being damaged.
- Resilience: the energy storing capacity of a wire without it being deformed.

Besides springs and elastics, orthodontic wires are the main "engine" of an orthodontic treatment. They are tied to the brackets and move the teeth. How does that happen?

When attached to the braces, wires temporarily lose their original shape but if they are not excessively deformed they return to their previous shape with a force that moves the teeth.

Thus, the wire should be springy, yet exert a gentle force. If it is too stiff and forced into the slots, it will be painful or detach the brackets when it is tied to them.

As teeth get straighter, stronger, stiffer and less elastic wires will be used. With such wires there is a greater control of the teeth movement.

Strength, springiness, stiffness etc. are influenced by the section (round, rectangular) and by the size of the arches. They are also influenced by the arch wire *materials*.

STAINLESS STEEL WIRES[147]

Stainless steel wires are widely used because of their formability, biocompatibility and environmental stability, stiffness, resilience and low cost. They can be welded or soldered to auxiliaries. To align the teeth in the first treatment phase they must be bent to create loops, otherwise they are too stiff. Therefore, they are mainly used *in the intermediate (for example, canine distalization with sliding mechanics) and in final treatment* phases.

COBALT-CHROMIUM WIRES[147]

Cobalt-chromium wires can be manipulated in a softened state when bends and loops are easily made.If subjected to heat treatment, these wires have properties similar to those of stainless steel. They are *mainly used in bioprogressive therapy.*

BETA–TITANIUM WIRES[38]

Beta-titanium wires have average stiffness, good formability, adequate springback and they can be welded to auxiliaries.

These wires serve as good intermediary wires between nickel-titanium and stainless steel.

They are mainly used in segmented arch treatments (Burstone) and they are also indicated in *patients who are allergic to nickel*.

MULTISTRANDED WIRES[147]

Thin stainless steel wires *braided or twisted together* have a low stiffness and high springback when compared to solid stainless steel wires. Therefore they can be *used to level and align the teeth at the beginning of treatment* even if nickel-titanium wires have practically taken their place.

NICKEL-TITANIUM (NI-TI) WIRES[39-133]

They represent a family of alloys with great elasticity, flexibility and shape memory.

Generally *these alloys are the best available wires for teeth levelling and alignment*.

TRADITIONAL NITI

NiTi alloy wires have been manufactured since 1972. They cannot be welded or soldered and only limited bending is possible. More friction in sliding mechanics, compared to stainless steel, is present. Among the positive aspects they offer are *high elasticity, springback and stored energy.*

Thermal NiTi are wires which are formed to the desired shape in a martensitic (a metallurgic) phase and, following the irregularities of the dental arch, are deformed

reaching an austenitic phase (another metallurgic phase). By increasing the temperature (to 37° in the mouth) these wires return to the original shape in the martensitic (memory) form.
The wires with an austenitic finish temperature less than 37° centigrade show some superelasticity.
The addition of copper allows the release of more constant forces. Compositional variations cause changes in the martensitic/austenitic start and finishing temperature. This is followed by different mechanical properties.
So we can have different forces at different temperatures. For example, there are some wires that are active with constant force at 27° centigrade for patients with an average pain tolerance and healthy periodontium, or some wires that are active at 35° centigrade developing low forces, suitable for patients with a low pain threshold and slightly compromised periodontium.
In the NiTi family, **copper NiTi** wires have a better springback, they are more resistant to permanent deformations and deliver more constant forces. Yet the **multistranding NiTi** wires introduced by Hanson are probably the ones that can profoundly reduce the forces imparted by arch wires. They have been commercially available since 1995 and apply the same mechanical principles of stainless steel multistranded wires.
The analysis of the load/deflection curve comparing the various wire materials is very important in order to understand their characteristics (Fig. 1-73).

1-73

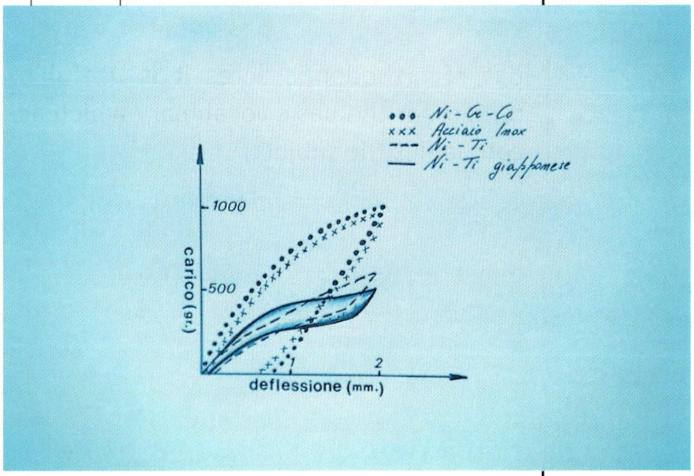

Fig. 1-73
Load-deflection diagram comparing: *Stainless steel (SS), Nickel cobalt chromium (Ni-Cr-Co), traditional NiTi, Japanese (superelastic) NiTi wires.*

SS and Ni-Cr-Co wires reach a similar deflection with a similar load. The same deflection is reached by NiTi wires with a lighter load.
When unloaded, SS and Ni-Cr-Co show significant and similar permanent deformation.
The NiTi wires show a very small amount of permanent deformation. *Clinically, the unloading corresponds to the force released to move the teeth.* In the NiTi group it is lighter than in SS and Ni-Cr-Co.
Another very important element is represented by the fact that with traditional NiTi wires the unloading curve is similar to the SS and NiCrCo one, while in Japanese (superelastic) wires it is flat (martensitic plateau). *Clinically it corresponds to a more constant released force to the teeth, considered by many to be more physiological.*
In other words, NiTi wires release light forces, but only superelastic wires do that in a more physiologically constant way.

WHY AN ORTHODONTIC TREATMENT?

We know that orthodontics can have functional and aesthetic aspects, but people demand an orthodontic treatment mainly for cosmetic improvement (Figs. 1-74 and 1-75).
It is very important to consider the positive psychological influence that an attractive smile can have. Many patients who had their malocclusions corrected have greater self-esteem than their friends whose malocclusions were not corrected. Self –esteem could mean more success in school, love, business etc..
Is there a pill that can lead to the same results?
Putting together functional and aesthetical aspects, I think that the goal of a modern orthodontic treatment is a Class I dental/

1-74

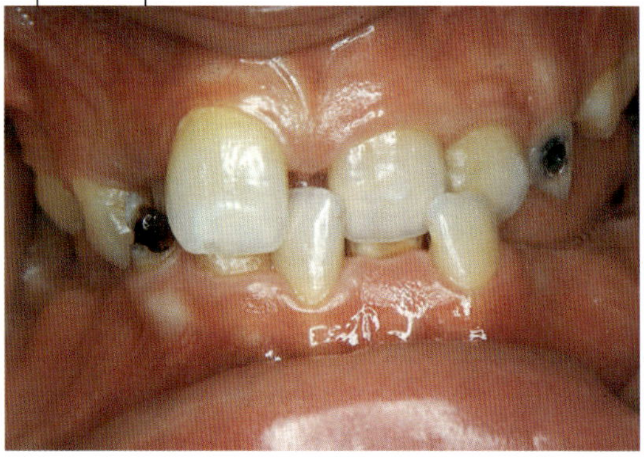

1-75

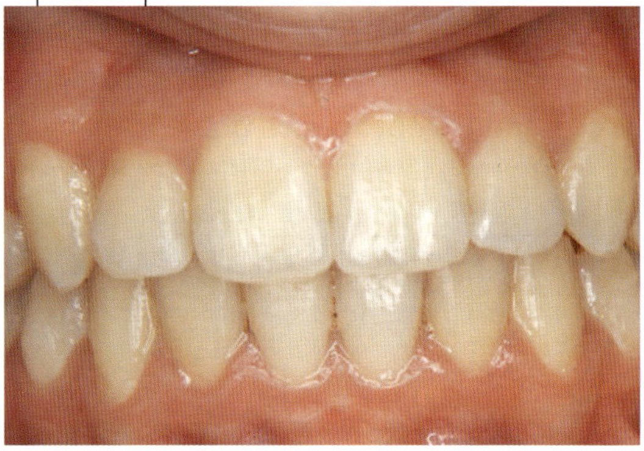

Figs. 1-74 & 1-75 Why should we opt for an orthodontic treatment? The best answer comes from the comparison between these two pictures. The smile on the right is much more attractive than the one on the left.

skeletal relationship with a healthy periodontium/TMJ, a correct overjet/overbite, and an optimal facial aesthetic.

A lot of attention is paid to the front teeth where the *overjet* and the *overbite* occupy a central position. The overjet is the distance between the upper and the lower incisors.

From a sagittal point of view, when the upper incisors have a correct inclination, they are just in front of the lower ones. From a vertical point of view, the upper incisors partially cover the lower ones touching them lightly.

When this relationship is excessive, beyond the upper incisors' cingulum, we speak of a dental deep bite. If there is a vertical space, we speak of a dental open bite.

WHEN TO BEGIN A TREATMENT?

The main distinction lies between *orthodontic* and *functional-orthopedic* treatments. In the first instance, it is possible to move teeth at all ages but there are cases when it is better to correct them as soon as possible. Cross bites are a classic example. Minor corrections can be done using removable appliances but fixed ones offer better teeth displacement control.

Fixed braces are usually more accepted in younger patients than in adults. There is a prevalence of orthodontic treatments in young patients where, for example, there are more opportunities for non-extraction cases.

Functional-orthopedic treatments do not obviously concern adults. They begin early, mostly using removable appliances. Skeletal Class III relationships are a typical example. It is better to perform an orthopedic treatment during a growth spurt.

1-76

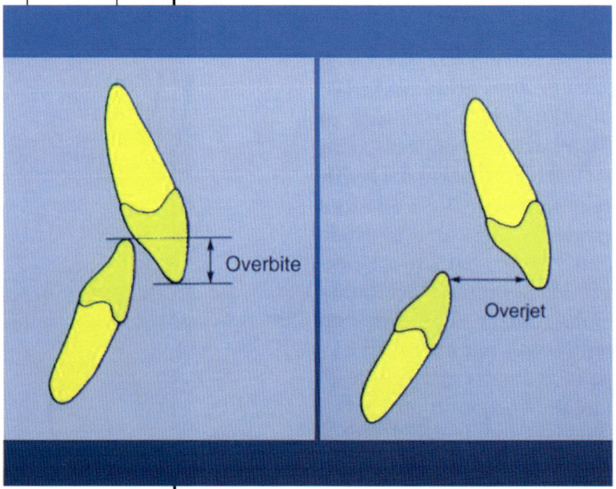

1-77

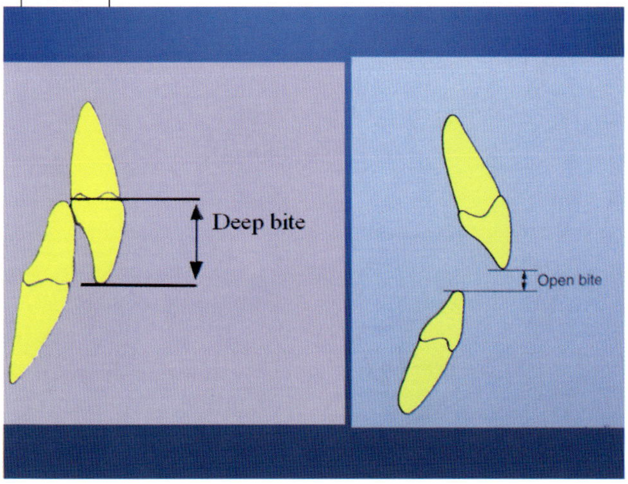

PREVENTION IN ORTHODONTICS

Malocclusions are caused by coexisting genetic and functional factors. We cannot influence genetics but we can prevent many negative situations. See for example (Figs. 1-78 to 1-80):

Fig. 1-78
A) care of deciduous teeth
B) space recovery
C) space keeping
D) stripping
Fig. 1-79
E) partial fixed braces
F) lingual crib
G) myofunctional trainer
Fig. 1-80
H) lip bumper
I) palatal bar
J) palatal expansion

1-78

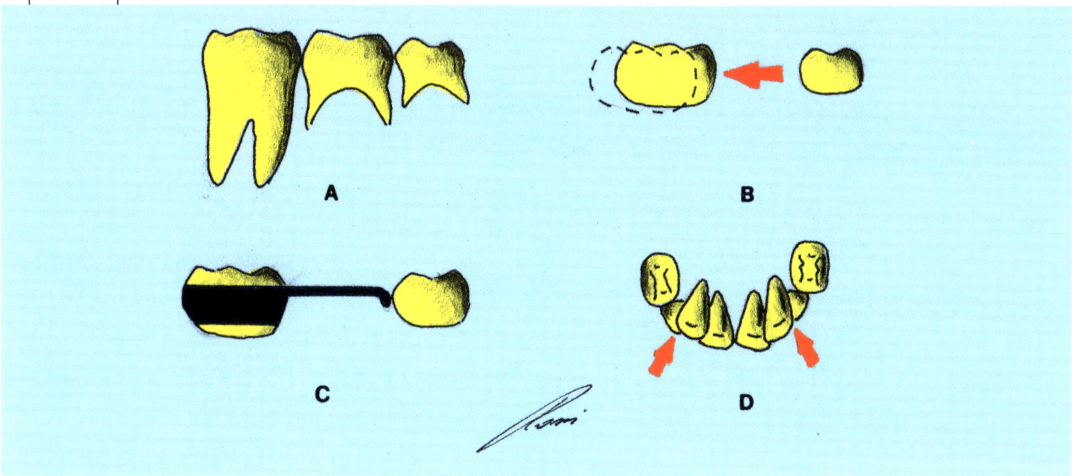

1-79

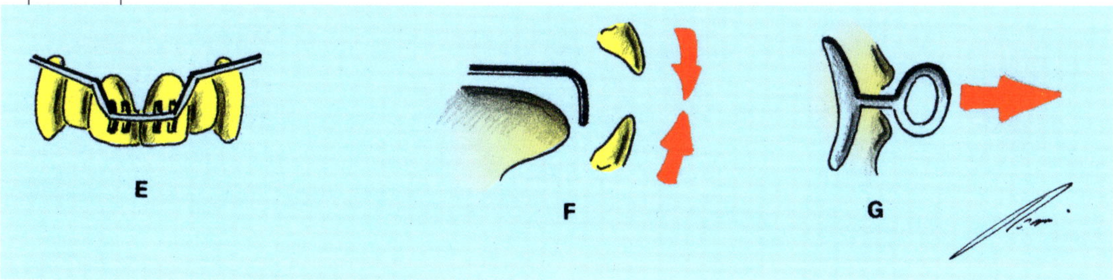

1-80

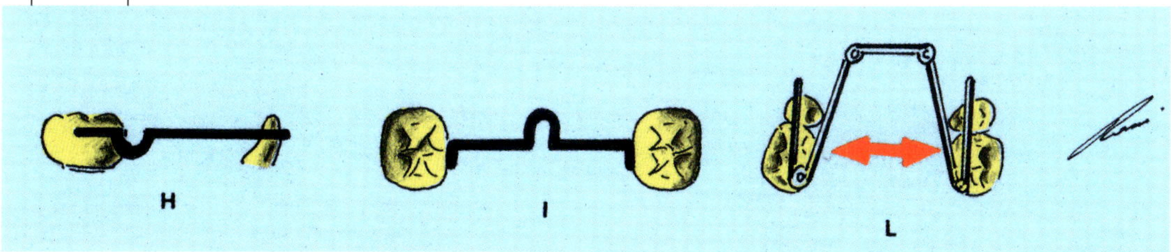

Don't forget the importance of simple procedures like those shown here below.

1-81

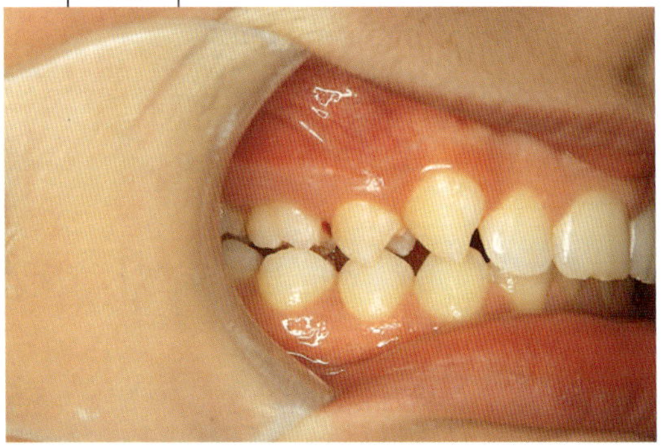

1-82

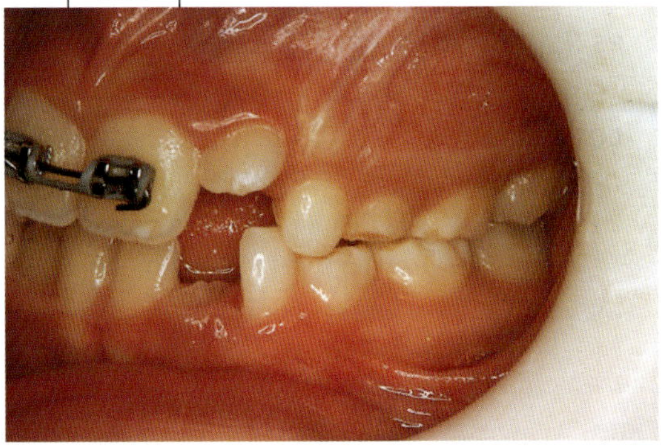

1-83

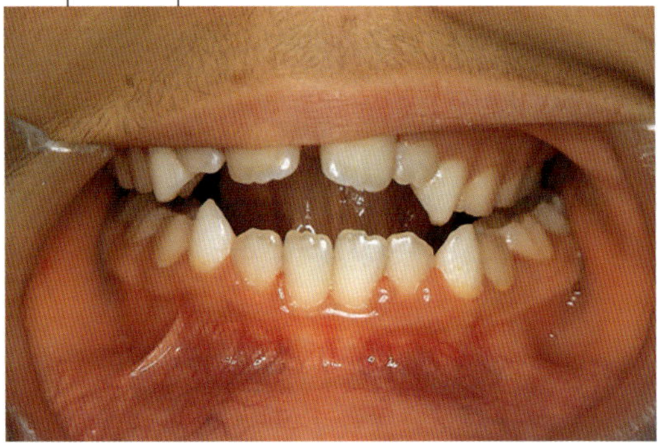

1-84

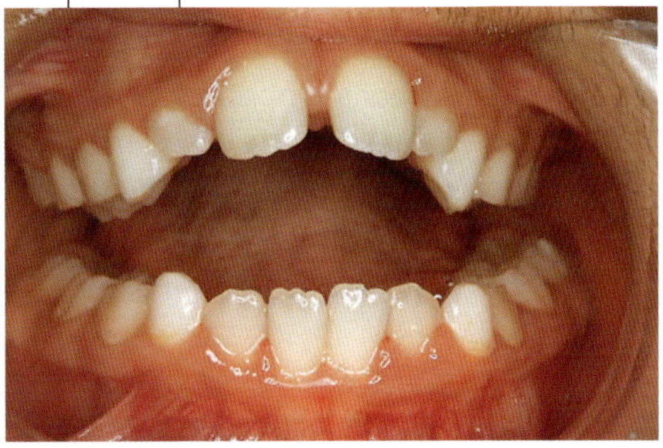

Fig. 1-81
The air rotor stripping of the mesial second deciduous molar surface allows the first permanent premolar to shift distally. This way the permanent canine can also move distally in a dental Class I relationship.

Fig. 1-82
A sectional elastic wire (NiTi) tied to two brackets on the upper central incisors is enough for their derotation. The mesial air rotor stripping of the deciduous canine allows the permanent lateral incisor alignment.

Fig. 1-83 & Fig. 1-84
A mandibular lateral displacement can usually be corrected with a maxillary expansion and deciduous teeth grinding can help the stability of the result. Note in this case the lower deciduous canines and (Fig. 1-84) their remodeling.

MYOFUNCTIONAL EXERCISES

In this book there are many cases that show the influence of the tongue and other muscles on some malocclusions. Theoretically, muscular activity education could lead to the improvement of those malocclusions.

Personally I do not deny that this can happen, but in my practice I obtain good results with braces, above all with removable ones (see for example Chapter V – Open Bites).

So, just in those cases with a high risk of relapse, I suggest the following exercises:

TONGUE

Put a small elastic band on the tip of the tongue and ask the patient to swallow, keeping the elastic in contact with the anterior part of the palatal surface. This exercise must be done swallowing 6-12 times, 3 times a day. Put another elastic band behind the previous one in order to educate the mid part of the tongue. With one more placed behind, it becomes the turn of the posterior part of the tongue.

The patient must pronounce the letters T, D, L, N slowly at the beginning, then increasing the speed, in order to educate the anterior part of the tongue. He must reproduce the gallop sound "clop, clop, clop" in order to educate the median part of the tongue. By pronouncing "ghi-gug-gag", instead, he can re-educate the posterior part of the tongue.

OROFACIAL MUSCULATURE EXERCISES

- A weight is tied to a button. Looking down to the floor, the patient must support the weight while keeping the button between the lips. The weight is gradually increased. Similar to this exercise is one done by two patients. Two buttons are tied together with a string. The patients, facing each other, hold the buttons with their lips and pull in a sort of tug of war. These exercises must be repeated 3 to

10 times in three different moments of the day.
This way, the labial musculature increases its strength.

- A series of labial and other areas' contractures are useful in increasing muscular tone.
- The market now offers a wide selection of "trainers" (silicone, polyurethane made) which can help with the correction of myofunctional habits.

REMOVABLE OR FIXED APPLIANCES?

Removable appliances are most known for their use in functional orthopaedic treatments (as will be shown later), but they can also be used as space keepers or retainers, in the classic acrylic plate form or as transparent polycarbonate splints (Fig. 1-98). With the addition of springs and screws, anterior arches can also be used for teeth displacement (orthodontic use) including transverse upper arch expansion (Figs. 1-99 to 1-103).
There is a prevalence of 2 Dimensional control, therefore orthodontic removable appliances are indicated for minor teeth movements. They are more hygienic, but when it comes to wearing them, the patient needs to be cooperative and efficient.
Fixed appliances displace teeth with optimal 3 Dimensional control. They work all day long so the teeth move faster. Careful hygiene is required. Treatments with brace combinations are possible. For example, in cases of deep anterior cross bite a lower removable splint, opening the bite, allows an easy upper arch alignment with fixed appliances. Otherwise, an initial phase is possible using a removable appliance, followed by a phase with a fixed one (Figs. 1-85 to 1-89).

RECOVERY OF A TRAUMATIZED UPPER CENTRAL INCISOR

According to many previous studies, dental traumas make up 8% of pediatric dental problems. A dental trauma can be followed by enamel and root fracture, tooth luxation or tooth loss. When a tooth is lost there are good chances of recovery if it can be re-implanted within two hours.
The following case shows the occlusion after a dental trauma that had happened five days before (Fig. 1-85). The upper right central incisor is extruded and it is in cross-bite with a weakly positive vitality test. X-rays do not offer additional insights. The patient and parents asserted that before the trauma it was not in cross–bite. Therefore, the traumatic injury is suspected to have caused its luxation.
A *first treatment phase* using a *removable* brace with an anterior sector screw offered the cross-bite solution (Figs. 1-86 and 1-87). During a *second phase* with a *fixed* appliance, the active intrusion and alignment of the right upper central incisor was achieved (Figs. 1-88 and 1-89).

1-85

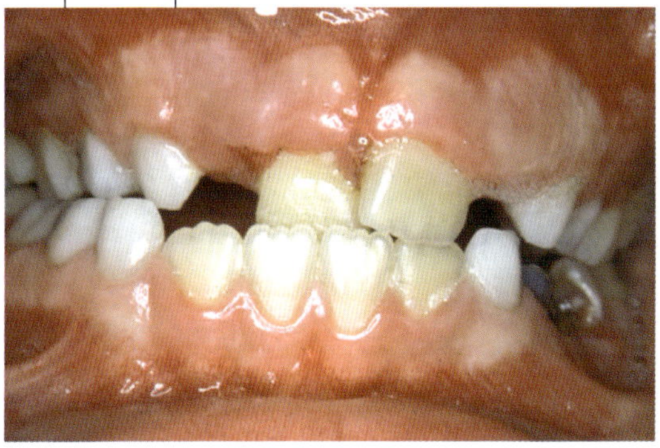

1-86

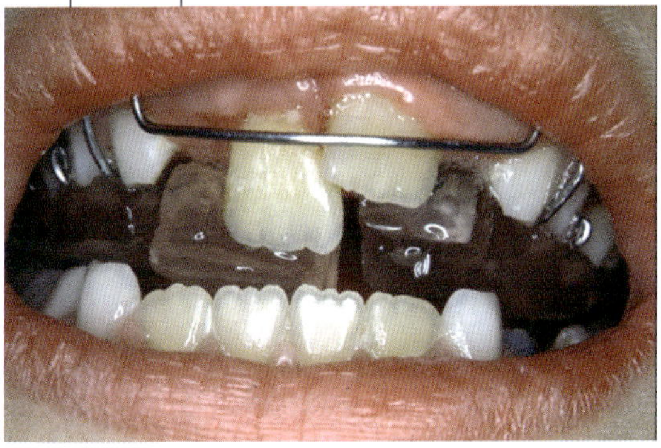

1-87

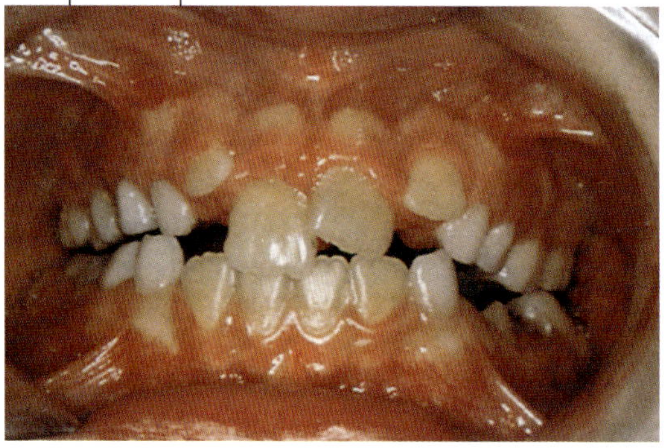

1-88

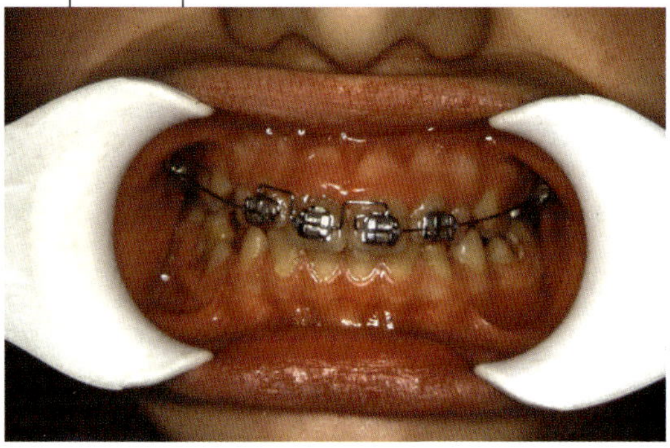

1-89

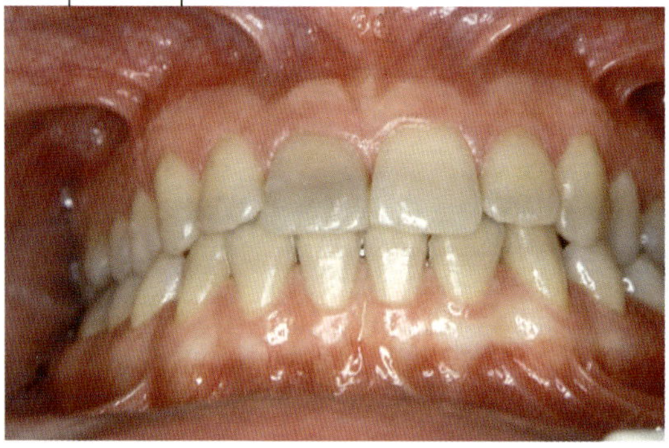

FIXED TECHNIQUES IN ORTHODONTICS

EDGEWISE

Edward Angle, frequently described as "the father of modern orthodontics", introduced his edgewise appliance in 1925. Teeth were moved by using arch wires tied to brackets welded to metallic bands. The bracket slots were all similar with rectangular sections, so that for a tridimensional control of the teeth into the space, the orthodontist needed to bend the arch wires (1st, 2nd, 3rd order bends). With the discovery of enamel bonding the use of bands is now very limited.

From a philosophical point of view, Angle refused to carry out treatment involving teeth extractions and this principle, for many years, was dogmatic. After a quarter of century different point of views merged.

TWEED[234]

Charles Tweed, in the 1940s presented his orthodontic philosophy and technique.

From the philosophical point of view:

- Tweed did not believe in the orthopedic treatment of malocclusions.
- Following his indications, treatments were based on the FMA-FMIA-IMPA angle analysis.
- The angles are those of the triangle formed by the Frankfurt plane, the mandibular plane, the lower incisor long axis. Until the early 1980s, according to this philosophy the lower incisor had to form a 90° angle with the mandibular plane.
- It was then evident that in many cases this limit was too rigid so Tweed's disciples increased the tolerance, admitting 94° in a brachifacial and 89° in a dolicofacial patient.
- Dental arch expansion is rarely admitted, especially when an expansion to gain space is performed.
- He strongly believed that in those cases the expansion altered a functional balance and it was the basis of a relapse.
- These basic elements explain why, according to this philosophy, there are a lot of extraction treatment plans (premolars and wisdom teeth).

From a technical point of view:

- Narrow single not pre-adjusted brackets are used. Therefore rotation control can be difficult to achieve and wire bending is necessary to obtain the correct dental crown: *in-out* (1st order bends), *up-down* (2nd order bends), *torque* (3rd order bends). The slots are usually 0.022" x 0.028".

- Classically the initial phase of alignment is obtained with a stainless steel round wire (0.016"). To increase the elasticity, wire bending to form loop springs is necessary.
- After the initial phase of alignment, rectangular arches are used.
- The final size of the rectangular arch is 0.215" x 0.275" stainless steel wire.
- The aim of the treatment is to achieve greater 3D teeth control, but usually that happens by developing forces heavier than in other techniques.
- Typical of this technique is, in Class 2, the application of inter–maxillary elastics. Thus, in order to increase the anchorage, the lower molars are distally tipped (like tent pegs). The occlusion obtained this way is called "Tweed occlusion".

Since contact among molars is lacking, mandibular advancement is favoured. At the end of the treatment, with a so called "guided relapse", the molars move to the new occlusion.

Among Tweed's disciples, Dr. L. Merrifield developed some modifications to the basic Tweed edgewise technique called the "directional force technique". One of the main aspects of that technique is the application of J-hooks to move canines distally in extraction spaces.

When it comes to that technique, I personally think that there are several no-compliance alternatives.

BEGG[20]

Dr. Begg conceived his technique while observing the Australian aboriginal occlusion presenting progressive teeth abrasion due to diet. There is a vertical reduction of crowns until the contact point is lost and is followed by mesial teeth movement. This movement determines a contact surface and an anterior edge to edge relationship which Begg considers physiological. There is no crowding and third molars are well aligned.

Begg's technique reflects these observations dividing the typical four extractions treatments in three phases:

PHASE 1

- Crowding correction.
- Rotations hypercorrection.
- Achievement of an edge to edge incisors relationship.

PHASE 2

- Space closure.
- Midline correction.

At the end of those two phases, the upper canines are distally tipped while the upper incisors are palatally tipped. Thus, uprighting and torque correction are necessary.

PHASE 3

- Cuspid and bicuspid uprighting.
- Upper incisors torque.

Begg's technique utilizes round wires only (0.016" during phase one and two, 0.020" during phase three).There are no ligatures, instead the brackets have lock pins to hold the wire in the slots. Class II elastics are widely used, thus their contraindication in Class II cases with increased verticality.

During phase 3 on a 0.020" arch, a 0.014" torquing spring for anterior teeth positive torque is applied. This spring is necessary to torque the upper incisors roots palatally, otherwise it would not be possible to achieve a root torque with a round wire.

Light forces are used in this technique. Begg is considered the father of light forces treatments.

ANDREWS – STRAIGHT WIRE[8]

In Edgewise standard and Tweed-Merrifield techniques the brackets have the same design and they are not pre-adjusted. Thus, in order to obtain a good alignment, the orthodontist must bend the archwire.

In the 1970s *Dr. Lawrence Andrews inverted the issue: no more archwire bending using straight archwires and pre-adjusted*

1-90

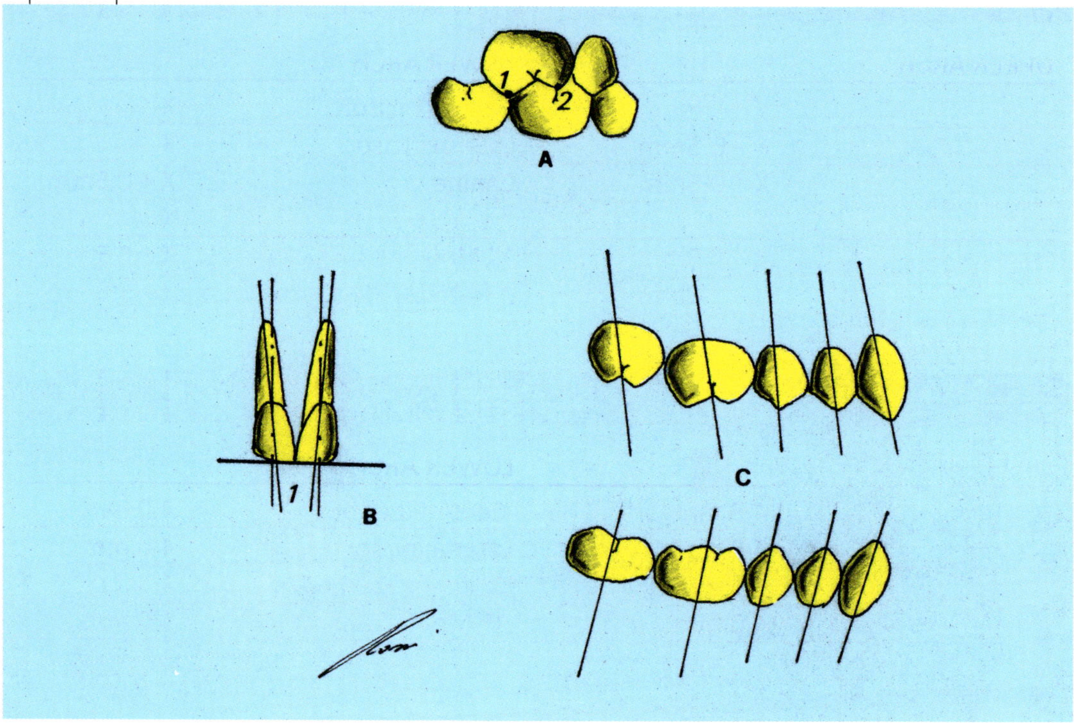

1-91

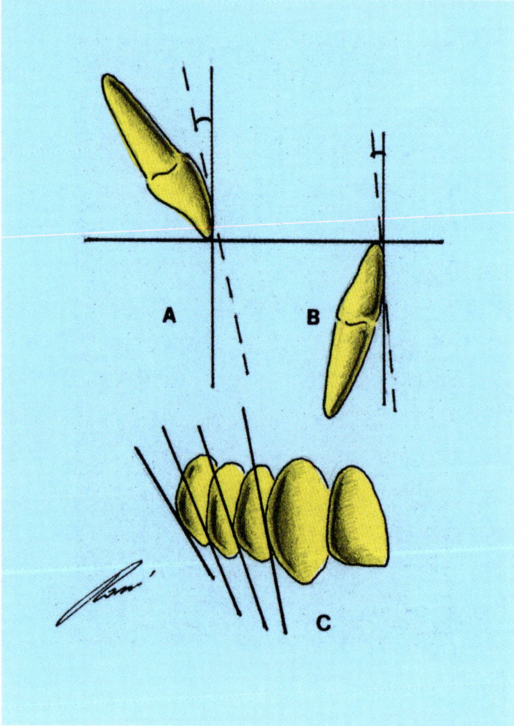

brackets. Nowadays, different brackets for different teeth make the job of an orthodontist easier and faster (see also Fig. 1-92).

To establish the brackets and slot adjustment values (in-out, angulations, torque), he analysed 120 very good bites of people who had not received orthodontic treatment. He defined six key elements for an optimal occlusion:

- molars and canines in a Class I relationship (Fig. 1-90: A)
- crowns mesially angulated (Fig. 1-90: B & C)
- torque (Fig. 1-91)
  - positive for upper incisors (Fig 1-91: A)
  - slightly negative for lower incisors (Fig 1-91: B)
  - negative for other teeth (Fig 1-91: C)
- absences of rotations
- absences of spaces
- Spee curve – flat or slightly concave

One of the main differences compared with the other techniques is bracket placement.

Andrews centred the slots on the FA point, which is the middle point of FAAC (facial axis clinical crown). In this way, at the end of treatment teeth would be positioned on Andrew's occlusal plane. Twin brackets are used with 0.018" and 0.022" slots. As with many other techniques there is an initial levelling and alignment phase, which is obtained using light force delivering wires, like nickel titanium ones.

In premolar extraction cases, the canine retraction with sliding mechanics follows.

BRACKET POSITIONING VALUES IN ROTH TECHNIQUE

UPPER ARCH		LOWER ARCH	
	X	Central incisor	X
	X – 0.5mm	Lateral incisor	X
	X + 0.5mm	Canine	X + 0.5mm
	X	Premolars	X
	X – 0.5mm	1st Molar	X – 0.5mm
	X – 1.0mm	2nd Molar	X – 0.5mm

X is the distance from the incisal edge and from the cusps.

BRACKET POSITIONING VALUES IN BIDIMENSIONAL TECHNIQUE

UPPER ARCH		LOWER ARCH	
	4.5 mm	Central incisor	4.0 mm
	4.0 mm	Lateral incisor	4.0 mm
	4.5 mm	Canine & Premolars	4.5 mm
	4.0 mm	1st Molar	4.0 mm
	4.0 mm	2nd Molar	3.5 mm

Distance in mm from the incisal edge and from the cusps.

Round stainless steel arch wires (0.016" – 0.018") with elastic tractions are used. Also, the anterior teeth retraction is achieved with sliding mechanics and elastic tractions. In this phase, rectangular arches are used (0.019" x 0.025" with 0.022"x 0.030" slots).

Many authors followed Andrews' original idea, modifying the pre-adjusted brackets values with their personal prescriptions, so we can probably speak of a "straight wire family".

Other differences in the "family" are represented by biomechanics. Bennet and McLaughlin,[21] for example, move the teeth on the arch with a tip-uprighting sliding mechanism. For anterior teeth retraction Roth[214] uses arches with closure loops.

Gianelly[103] in his "bidimensional technique' applies pre-adjusted brackets with two dimension slots 0.018" x 0.025" anteriorly, 0.022" x 0.030" posteriorly.

In this way there is good anterior teeth control with an easier lateral sliding movement.

There are no doubts that " the straight wire" is a milestone in orthodontic progress, but some criticism must be made. Many orthodontists think that a pre-adjusted appliance is a sort of automatic pilot that guides the treatment, but this is only partially true. Unfortunately, *no bending* does *not* mean *no thinking*.

The brackets must be well positioned otherwise there will certainly be problems. The inclination of the slots can cause a loss of anchorage and an anterior teeth extrusion.

If the positioning of the brackets is well performed then at the end of the treatment the teeth will be ideally positioned.

There are so many situations where, in the past, Andrews indicated 12 sets of brackets with alternative values for different cases. This complicates the orthodontics treatment management and causes criticisms. In my opinion other criticisms come when the technique is not well understood and sometimes is badly used without paying attention, for example, to those elements pointed out by Burstone. [36, 40, 41]

ALEXANDER[3]

In lower arch extraction cases, usually of first premolars, canine distalization is often necessary before the incisor alignment. R.G. "Wick" Alexander begins this treatment by applying a fixed brace on the upper jaw and suggests waiting before applying it on the lower jaw. Depending on the amount of crowding, after 2-6 months

X is the distance from the slot to the incisal edge and to the cusps..

BRACKET POSITIONING VALUES IN ALEXANDER TECHNIQUE			
UPPER ARCH		LOWER ARCH	
	X	Central incisor	X – 0.5mm
	X – 0.5mm	Lateral incisor	X – 0.5mm
	X + 0.5mm	Canine	X + 0.5 mm
	X	Premolars	X
	X – 0.5 mm	1st Molar	X – 0.5mm
	X – 1 mm	2nd Molar	X – 1 mm

there is a spontaneous distal movement towards the first premolar space, without the mesial advancement of the lower molars.

Alexander calls this movement "driftodontics", remembering that it is more active in younger patients with great crowding. Once it is happening, the lower brace can be applied. The brackets are pre-adjusted and mixed: twins on upper incisors, single Lang type on canines, single Lewis type on premolars and lower incisors. Those brackets, with 0.018" x 0.030" slots, are positioned along the long axis of the teeth. The distance from the slot to the incisal edge of the anterior teeth and the cusps of the posterior ones is shown in the above scheme:

In dental open bite cases, the distance from the anterior teeth is increased by 0.5 mm while that from the posterior ones is decreased by 0.5 mm. As with many other techniques, the initial phase of alignment is achieved by using elastic memory wires (NiTi).

In extraction cases, canines are moved distally with sliding mechanics (traction with an elastic chain on a 0.016" stainless steel arch). The upper incisors are retracted by using a 0.018" x 0.025" arch with closure spring loops. The lower mechanism is similar, but for the anterior teeth retraction a 0.016" x 0.022" arch size is used.

The treatment is finished with 0.017" x 0.025" arches on both upper and lower..

SEGMENTED ARCH[37]

With the segmented arch technique, Burstone [37]offers an alternative to those treatments where continuous arches are used.

As shown back in Fig. 1-70 and Fig. 1-71 a wire and two brackets can be a complex force-delivering system. Burstone believes that this complexity increases with a continuous arch wire and that the orthodontists easily lose control of a correct teeth movement. In order to avoid this he suggests segmenting the arch in three parts, an anterior one and two posterior ones.

Typical of the technique is the intrusion arch for the upper anterior unit. The use of springs delivering low forces is the base of the so called "forgiving therapy". This definition means that wrong spring activation producing very low forces does not have important negative effects. A palatal bar is present in most cases.

When two upper first premolars are extracted, unlike with the other techniques, the space is closed by moving distally the whole anterior unit (canine – canine) using "T" loop springs.

Burstone elaborated a sophisticated biomechanical analysis which can prevent many undesired effects that are typical of a continuous arch treatment. It is true that these effects can happen. However, it is also true that a skilled orthodontist, thanks to his experience, can avoid them.

BIOPROGRESSIVE[209]

In the 1950s, R.M. Ricketts gave this name to his technique and philosophy, indicating a progression of events in sequential order.

Unlike many other orthodontic "gurus", Ricketts understands the possibilities of an orthopaedic treatment and carefully controls the musculature function (tongue, lips and chin musculature). He also considers wider dental arches "normal", suggesting the lower third molars' germectomy at 9-10 years of age. Thus, in those cases characterized by crowding and treated with extractions by many orthodontists, Ricketts believes that there is enough space for a good alignment.

Technically, pre-adjusted twin brackets with 0.018" x 0.030" slots are used. The bite opening in deep bite cases or the levelling of a deep curve of Spee is one of the main features of this technique.

In order to achieve these goals, Ricketts, like Burstone, divides the arch into three sections and uses the "utility arch" to intrude the lower incisors. For the intrusion of these teeth, a light force of 60-80 g is ideal. The intrusion of upper incisors is obtained with an arch similar to the one used by Burstone, developing 80-100 g of force. In extraction cases, space closure is obtained with sliding mechanics or retraction wires with spring loops (a famous one is the "Las Vegas loop"). Those mechanisms develop light forces decreasing the anchorage need, but it is necessary to bend the wire (usually cobalt–chromium).

BRACKET POSITIONING VALUES IN BIOPREGRESSIVE TECHNIQUE

UPPER ARCH		LOWER ARCH	
	X	Central incisor	X
	X – 0.5 mm	Lateral incisor	X
	X + 0.5 / 1 mm	Canine	X+0.5/1mm
	X	Premolars and molars	X

X is the distance from the slot to the incisal edge and the cusps.

Does a bite opening with a continuous arch increase the lower facial more than Ricketts' bioprogressive technique? Does it have the same stability?

It is useful to consider Dake and Sinclair.[59] The purpose of their study was to compare the effectiveness and long term stability of arch levelling and overbite correction carried out by the Ricketts and Tweed modified techniques.

These techniques are an example of sectional wire alternatives to continuous arch levelling.

The sample comprised 60 Class II, deep bite, low angle adolescent nonextraction cases, 30 each from the office of Robert Ricketts and Fred Schudy, with cephalograms taken before and immediately after treatment and an average of more than 4 years post treatment.

Both techniques were successful in overbite correction, producing only minimal increases in mandibular plane angle and anterior facial height. Mandibular incisors in Ricketts' group demonstrated more flaring and anterior bodily movement during treatment, with a greater amount of post treatment uprighting and overbite relapse than the Schudy group. The Ricketts group demonstrated slightly more than 1 mm of true lower incisor intrusion; this change was very stable after treatment.

Both techniques produced a similar amount of mandibular molar extrusion during treatment.

These changes remained stable after treatment.

COMMON CONSIDERATIONS ABOUT BRACKETS

Most orthodontists (70% in the USA) use pre-adjusted brackets that have different in-out, slot inclination and torque, which avoid the bending of the wire that is necessary with Edgewise standard brackets. I want to remind you that with no pre-adjusted brackets, in order to obtain a correct teeth alignment, as many as 76 1st, 2nd and 3rd order *bends might be required* (Fig. 1-92).

Besides those differences, for all types of brackets we must remember the following.

ANTERIOR TEETH

- An incorrect vertical bracket position causes a bad vertical teeth alignment (Fig. 1-93: A correct, B incorrect).
- Brackets with incorrect mesio-distal position can cause undesired rotations (Fig. 1-93: C).
- Torque value changes when the bracket is more gingivally or occlusally positioned (Fig. 1-94: A).
- Torque value changes when the bracket is positioned at the same height on those teeth with a different crown curvature (Fig. 94: B)
- Brackets that are not well positioned on the long axis can lead to undesired mesio-distal movements (Fig. 1-95: A correct, B incorrect).

POSTERIOR TEETH

- An incorrect vertical position causes a bad vertical alignment and often an undesired bite opening.

1-92

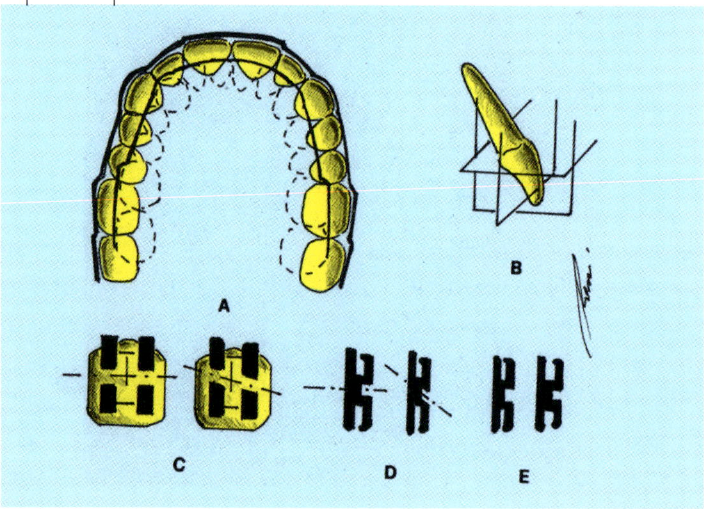

Fig. 1-92 Archwires need 3 order bends, (A) to determine an optimal occlusion in 3 space dimensions (B) when no pre-adjusted brackets are used (C-D-E left). With (right) pre-adjusted brackets C (tip), D (torque) and E (in/out) no bends are necessary.

1-92A

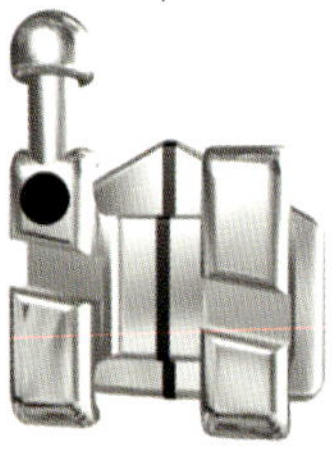

Fig. 1-92A Examples of brackets with preadjusted values by Leone Orthodontic Products

1-92B

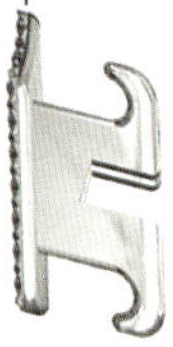

Fig. 1-92B Examples of brackets with preadjusted values by Leone Orthodontic Products

1-93

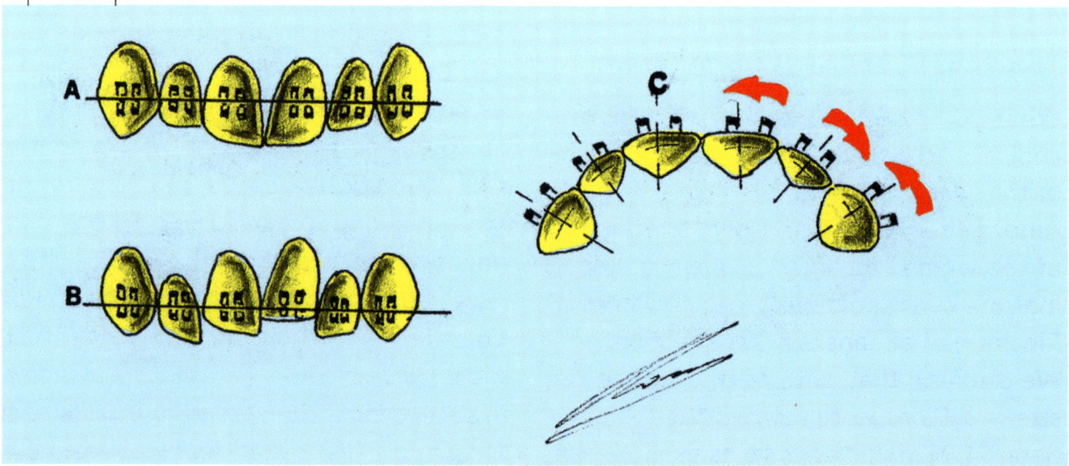

1-94

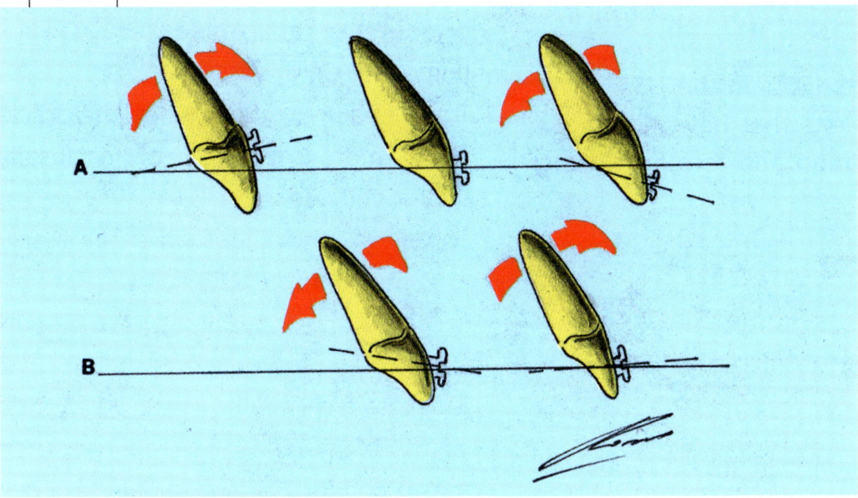

1-95

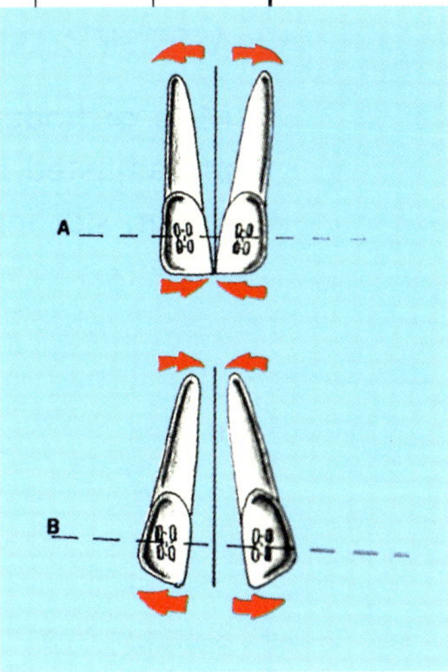

1-96

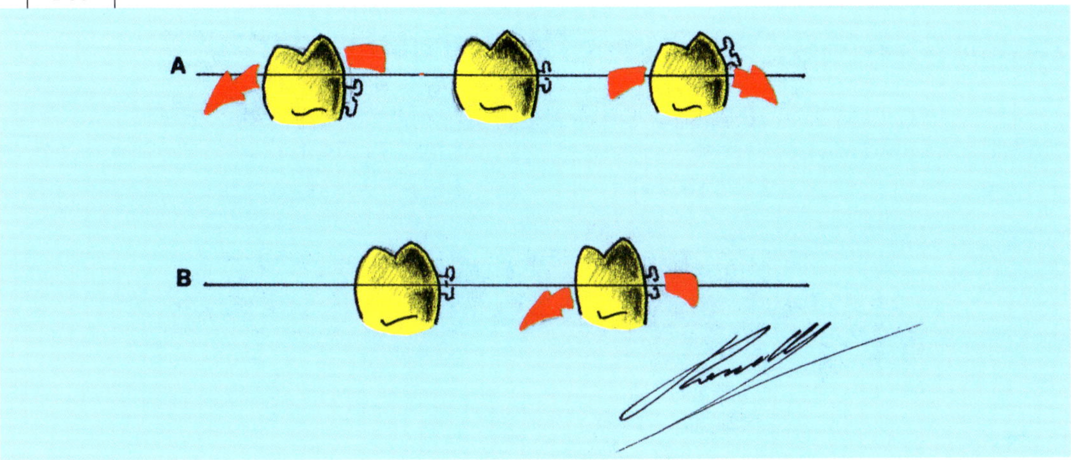

- Torque value changes when a bracket or tube is more occlusally or gingivally positioned (Fig. 1-96: A).
- Torque value changes with more or less crown curvature (Fig. 1-96: B).
- Brackets that are not well positioned on the long axis can lead to undesired mesio-distal movements (inclinations).
- Brackets with incorrect mesio-distal position can cause rotations.

THE "BEST" TECHNICAL SYSTEM

What pushes an orthodontist to make a choice of techniques? Is it the best analysis or the best advertising?

Among the positive and negative aspects of the various techniques, are we able to indicate what the best technical system is? Rinchuse et al.* answer this question.

We can read that, with respect to the slot size, a 2002 report provided the following data: 54.2% of orthodontists used 22-slot, 40.5% used 18-slot, 4.3% used bidimensional and other slot sizes. Another report revealed that 53% of clinicians based their decision about bracket specifications on what they believed to be correct for most of their patients. The remaining 43% simply chose a pre-adjusted brackets technique, most favouring a Roth prescription. When it comes to narrow versus wide brackets it appears that with wide ones there is greater teeth movement control. However, it is not clear what pushes the orthodontist to choose between them.

Furthermore, as far as filling the bracket slot, a significant number of orthodontists indicated that they did not fill the slots and finished with 0.019" x 0.025" stainless steel wire in a 0.022" x 0.028" slot. Considering that the bracket – wire interplay is one of the most important factors in determining the appropriate amount of torque in a bracket, it clearly appears that the orthodontists' choice of a fixed appliance is often based on some elements that do not rely on logic or scientific evidence.

Another factor which influences the torque, reducing its amount, is the use of rectangular wires with rounded or bevelled corners. The insertion of undersized wires related to adjacent teeth can result in various effective torque values: using a 0.019" x 0.025" stainless steel wire in a stainless steel 0.22" slot bracket, about 10° of effective torque is lost.
Considering that most orthodontists routinely use 0.018" x 0.025" rectangular wires, I personally agree with Proffitt and Field (Contemporary Orthodontics) when they suggest the use of 0.018" x 0.025" brackets slot. Thus the slot can be fully filled easily and the values of torque correspond to the prescription.
Torque prescriptions are quite variable, depending on the author's philosophy. In fact, I can understand the great difference between Ricketts' torque values (more non-extraction treatments) and other authors' (more extraction treatments). However, can a few degrees, more or less, in pre-adjusted appliances really determine different outcomes? I do not think so.

SELF LIGATING - LOW FRICTION

The magic words in orthodontics of the last few years seem to be "self ligating" and "low friction". That is the name of a family of brackets that do not need any ligature and permit, thanks to their design, a low friction dental movement (Damon, Speed, Time, Smart Clip, In-Ovation R etc.). Thus, with the use of wide arches developing light forces, there is a gain of space which leads to many non extraction cases.
One particular question is fundamental. *Where does the advertising end and where does the scientific evidence begin?*
Rinchuse and Miles** remind us that:

- *Self ligating brackets are not new to orthodontics. In the 1930s the Russel attachment was an attempt to enhance clinical efficiency by reducing ligation time.*
- *Harradine and Eberting in two different studies reported reduced treatment times using self ligating brackets. However, those results, compared to the times indicated by Fink, Smith, Skidmore using conventional brackets, are contradictory.*

Pandis et al.*** point out:
"There was no difference in the time required to correct mandibular crowding between self-ligating Damon-2 and conventional edgewise brackets...there was an overall increase in the proinclination of the mandibular incisors associated with crowding correction in both brackets group"
Scott et al.**** conclude:
"Damon-3 self-ligating brackets are no more efficient than conventional ligated pre- adjusted brackets during tooth alignment."
Sorry if I am not an enthusiastic supporter of self ligating/low friction phenomena but I cannot ignore what follows. In the August 2010 issue of the *American Journal of Orthodontics and Dentofacial Orthopedics*, ."Traditional braces vs Self – Ligating Braces" (Damon, Smart Clip, Speed, In-Ovation) an article was written about claims made by the manufacturers of various self ligating braces. The American Association of Orthodontics' Council on Scientific Affairs looked at this topic from the standpoint of the evidence available for these claims. They considered a number of questions such as:

1. ***Does lateral expansion of the dental arch by self ligating (SL) brackets "grow" buccal alveolar bone?***
   There is no peer reviewed material on this subject.
2. ***Is lateral expansion of the dental arch by SL brackets comparable with the lateral expansion gained by rapid maxillary expansion followed by conventional brackets?***
   There is no peer reviewed material on this subject.

3. ***Is lateral expansion of the dental arch gained by SL brackets stable in the long term?***
   There is no peer reviewed material on this subject.
4. ***Are SL brackets more efficient and more effective than conventional bracket systems?***
   Current evidence DOES NOT support this assertion.
5. ***Do SL brackets provide less friction between the archwire and the bracket?***
   Current evidence shows this under specific lab conditions, which does not represent real life conditions.
6. ***Do SL brackets produce lower clinical forces compared to traditional brackets?***
   No in-vivo studies have been shown to answer this question.
7. ***Do patients treated with SL brackets experience less pain during treatment?***
   There is not a lot of data to compare, yet there is a study reporting that patients with SL brackets experienced greater pain than those with traditional brackets.
8. ***Are conventional brackets less hygienic than SL brackets?***
   Evidence does not support this claim.

In conclusion, *most of the notable assertions made by SL bracket companies are* <u>*not*</u> *backed up by evidence in scientific studies.*

AESTHETIC TECHNIQUES

The number of orthodontic adult patients is growing and there is now a larger demand for aesthetic treatments. Consequently, there is a huge range of plastic and ceramic aesthetic brackets on the market. The plastic brackets were initially constructed from acrylics and later polycarbonate but they soon showed many negative aspects (lack of strength and stiffness resulting in bonding problems, tie wing fractures, permanent brackets slot deformation with loss of torque, staining and odours).

To solve those problems, high-grade medical polyurethane brackets and polycarbonate brackets reinforced with ceramic or fibreglass fillers and/or metal slots are now available.

The performance of these brackets is significantly better than in the past and they probably will challenge the ceramic brackets in the future.

Ceramic brackets offer higher strength, more resistance to wear and deformation, better colour stability and superior aesthetics. All currently available ceramic brackets are composed of polycrystalline or monocrystalline oxide. The monocrystalline ceramic bracket is much more translucent.

Many advantages are countered by disadvantages such as:

- Bonding/debonding: Ceramic brackets are applied thanks to a chemical retention which results in extremely strong bonds that cause the enamel/adhesive interface to be stressed during debonding, risking irreversible enamel damage in the form of crack and delamination that often require dental restorations.[131] Thus, the majority of new ceramic brackets have mechanical retention, which allow the use of common adhesives. Mechanically retained brackets have adequate bond strength and appear to cause less enamel damage at debond.
- Frictional resistance: Conventional ceramic brackets produce significantly greater friction forces. To reduce this friction, metal insertions in ceramic bracket slots have been introduced.
- Iatrogenic enamel wear: Ceramic is significantly harder than enamel. Severe enamel wear to the opposite dentition has been reported when ceramic brackets were placed on the lower arch. It is very important to avoid contact with the opposite teeth.
- Fractures: There are a greater number of fractures compared to metal brackets.

LINGUAL ORTHODONTICS

The best answer to orthodontic aesthetic demand is lingual orthodontics. However, it is not commonly used. That is because when compared to traditional techniques, it produces considerable difficulties, takes more work time and, of course, is more expensive. Indirect bonding is the standard in lingual orthodontics because a correct direct bonding is very difficult. Most of all, in complex cases when 3 dimensional teeth control is needed, it is highly recommended to evaluate the complexity of certain treatments, the patients and the case selection. All things considered, the results can be excellent.

There is greater use for minor teeth movements when 2 dimensional teeth control is enough for an acceptable result. That is the case when 2D brackets are used to align crowded lower incisors. The appliance can then be maintained as a retainer.

CLEAR ALIGNERS

The past ten years have seen clear aligners emerge. These braces made with clear polymer have their most known example in the Invisalign system. With this system, displaced teeth are moved in the wanted position using a series of aligners.

The progression of teeth movements in the aligners is determined by a computer program. The aligners must be worn 22 hours per day and changed after two weeks. They are removed to eat, drink and when the teeth need to be brushed.

Invisalign has initially been reserved for simple cases in adult patients. I have tried it under those circumstances and I can say that it works. More recently it has been proposed for the treatment of patients who are still growing and for more difficult cases.

Boyd***** concludes:

"In this report, patients were treated with Align Technology's new best practices protocol.

These three patients' treatment demonstrate that a variety of complex malocclusions are able to be successfully treated using this protocol..." Then the pictures of 3 cases follow.

I have no comments regarding the "protocol". I can simply observe that *if those are considered "complex malocclusions", in my practice I probably treat " crazy malocclusions" daily.* I don't share Boyd's total confidence in the product.

ELASTICS

After evaluations of many techniques, I think that the elastics deserve to be mentioned. They are inexpensive and they work so well! They are used as:

- *ligatures or elastic chains to close the spaces.*
- *traction in one jaw (Class I traction) (Fig. 1-97: A)*
- *traction between the jaws (Class II – Class III tractions) (Fig. 97: B-C).*

Remember to change:

- elastic ties, usually after one month.
- elastic chain, after 10-15 days.
- traction elastic, after 4-5 days (their strength in the mouth decreases by 10% after 1 hour and 20% after 3 days).

1-97

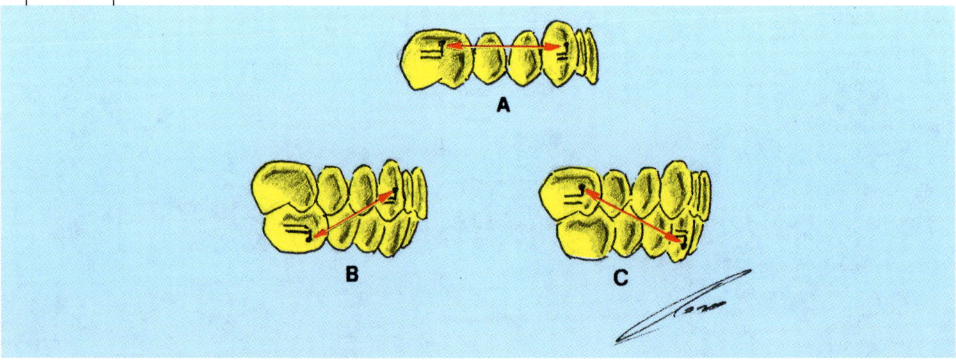

1-98

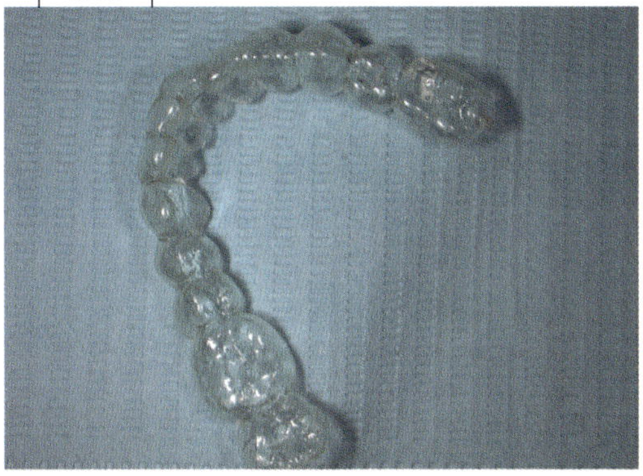

1-99

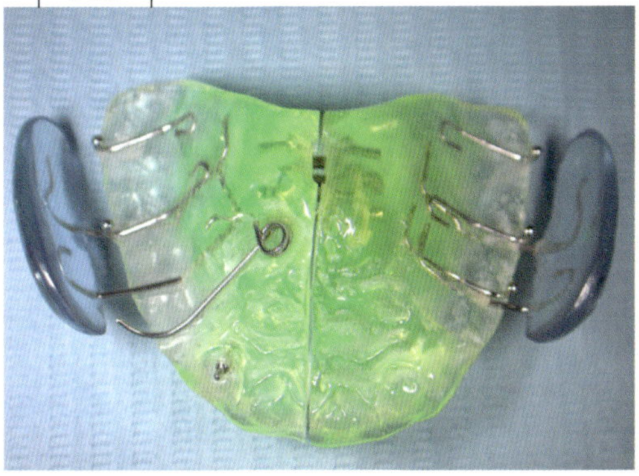

1-100

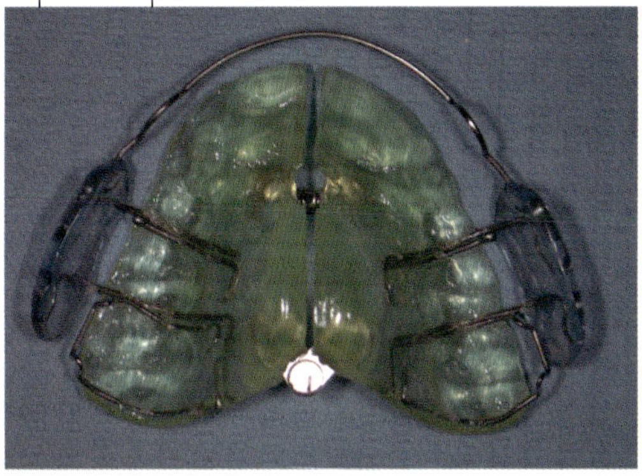

1-101

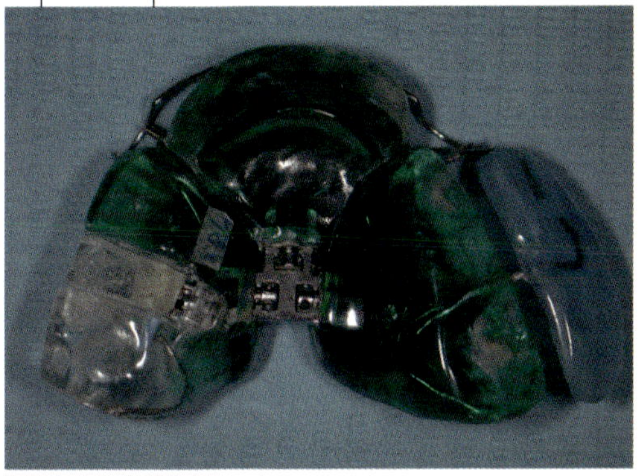

1-102

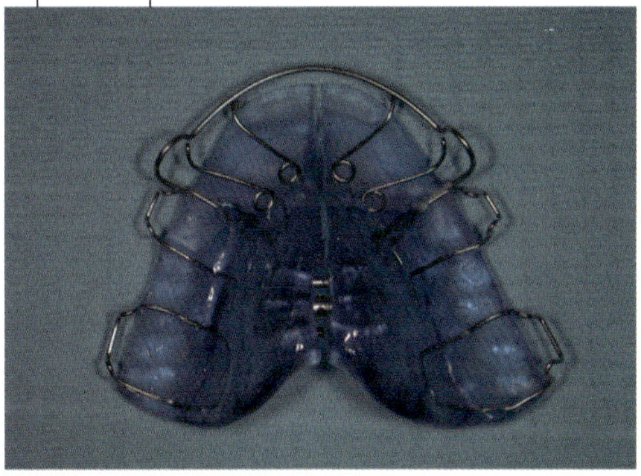

1-103

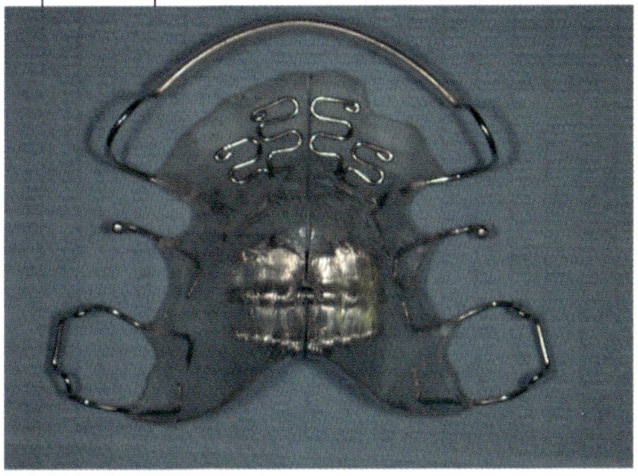

EXAMPLES OF REMOVABLE ORTHODONTIC APPLIANCES

Fig.1-98
Polycarbonate retainer and/or aligner.

Fig. 1-99
Maxillary acrylic plate with transverse expansion screw. Micro spring screw to move the upper right lateral incisor buccally Finger spring to move distally the first right upper premolar.

Fig.1-100
Maxillary acrylic plate with median "V" screw for antero-lateral expansion.

Fig.1-101
Maxillary acrylic plate with "3 ways screws" for transverse expansion, anterior dental advancement, posterior dental displacement.

Fig. 1-102
Maxillary acrylic plate with transverse expansion screw and finger springs to move the upper incisors mesially.

Fig. 1-103
Maxillary acrylic plate with transverse expansion and mattress spring to move the upper incisors buccally.

PARTS OF FIXED APPLIANCES

1-104

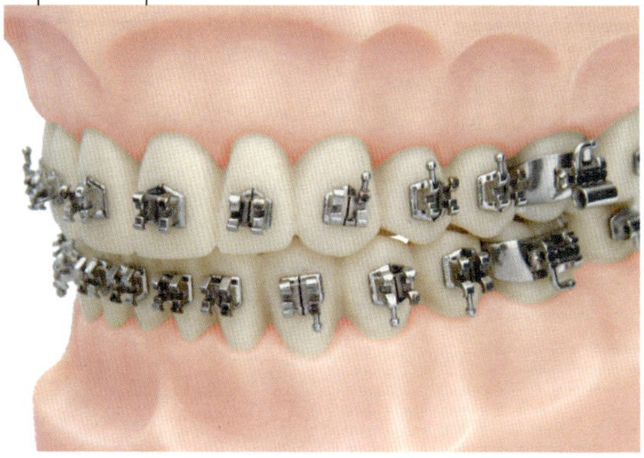

Fig.1-104
1 case with Logic STEP Line brackets

1-105

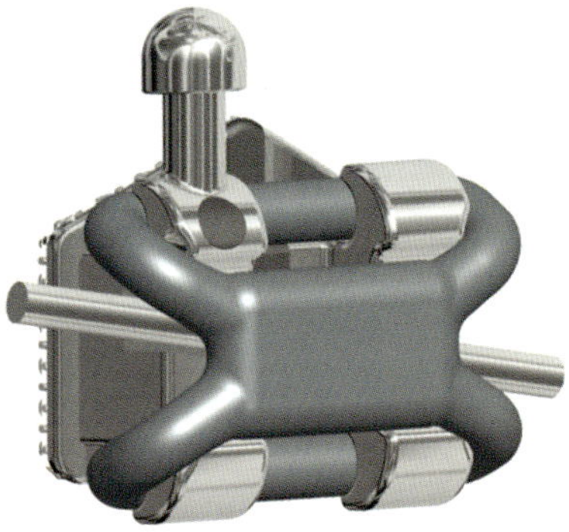

Fig. 1-105
Step Line with SLIDE ligature (Low friction)

1-106

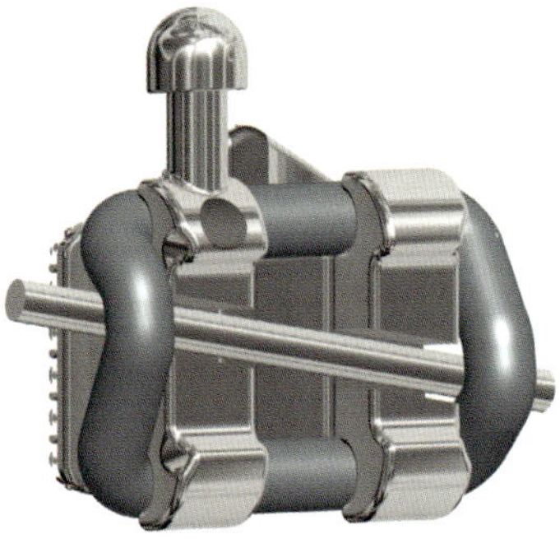

Fig.1-106
Logic STEP Line with standard ligature

1-107

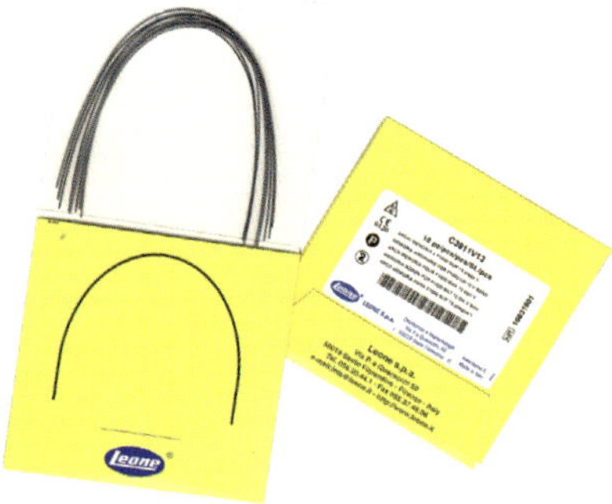

Fig.1-107
NiTi Arches

1-108

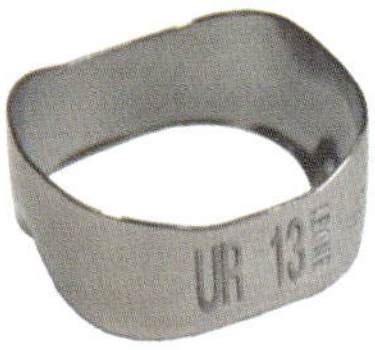

Fig. 1-108
Molar band

1-109

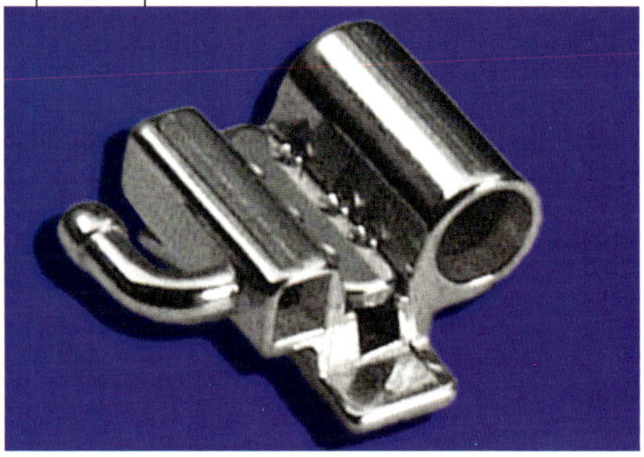

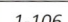

Fig. 1-109
Upper buccal tube

1-110

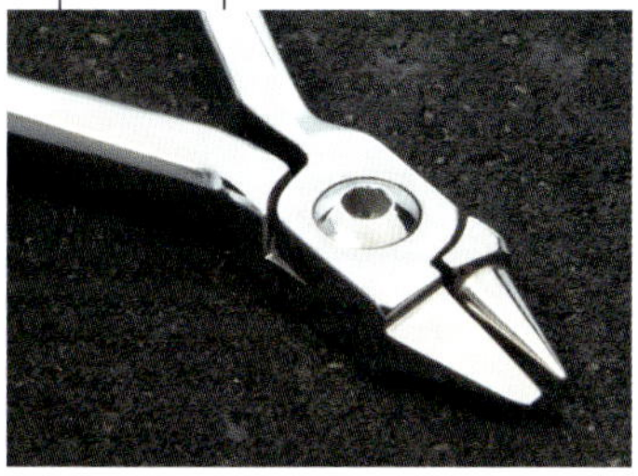

1-111

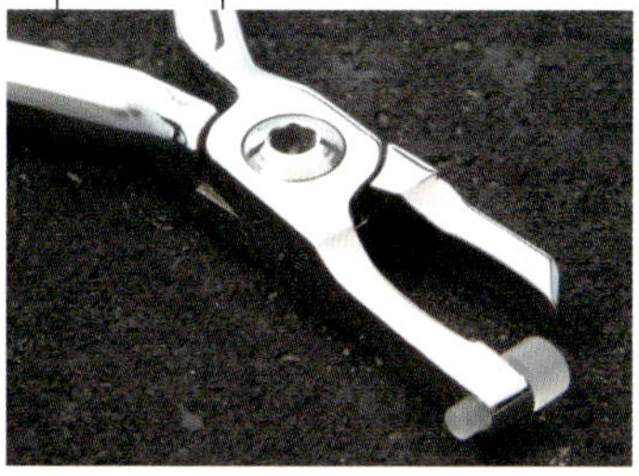

1-112

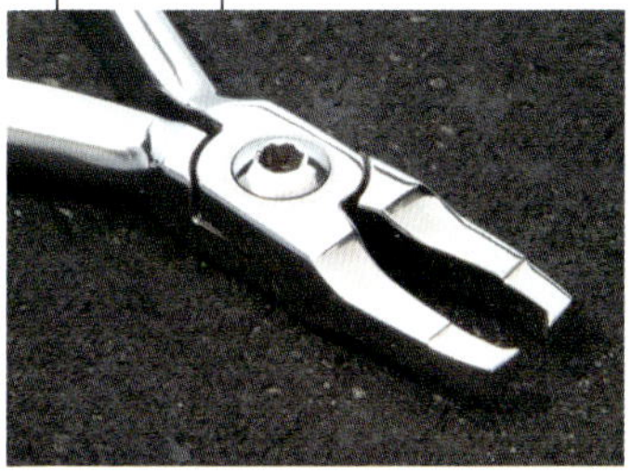

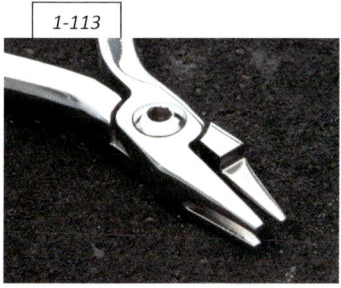

1-113

1-114

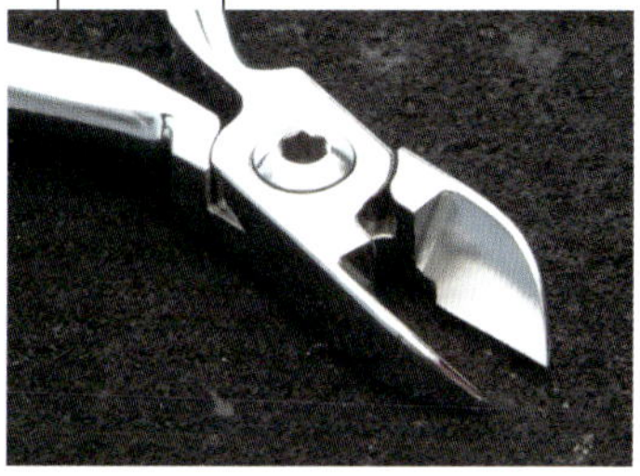

1-115

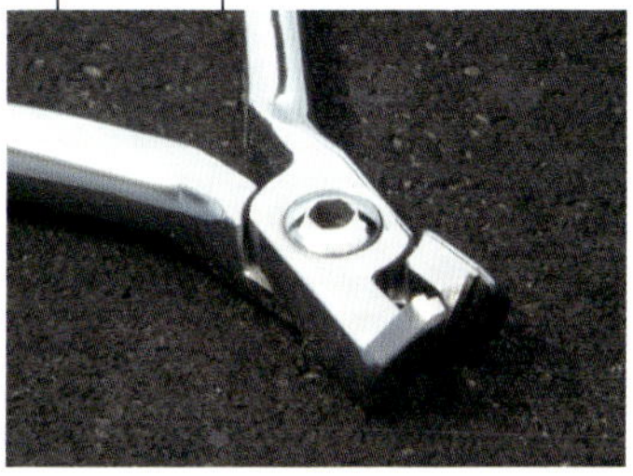

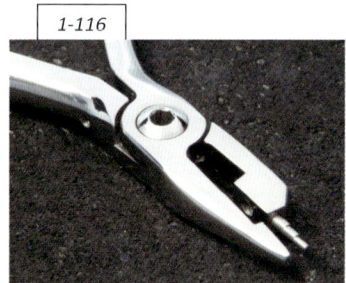

1-116

1-117

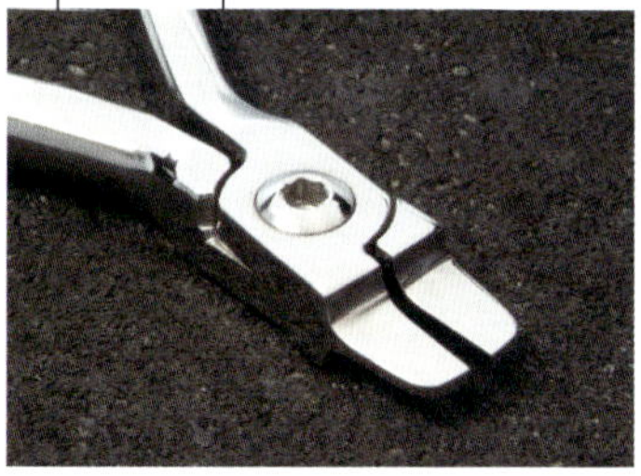

1-118

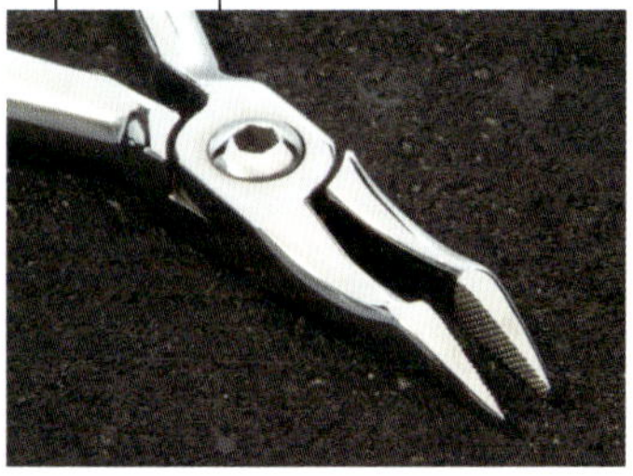

Orthodontics Pliers (Manufactured by Leone)

Fig.1-110
Bird Beak (Angle style)

Fig.1-111
Posterior band remover

Fig.1-112
Direct bond metal bracket remover

Fig.1-113
Three jaw

Fig.1-114
Ligature cutter

Fig.1-115
Distal end cutter

Fig.1-116

Loop forming (Tweed style)

Fig.1-117
Rectangular arch forming (Tweed style)

Fig.1-118
Weingart

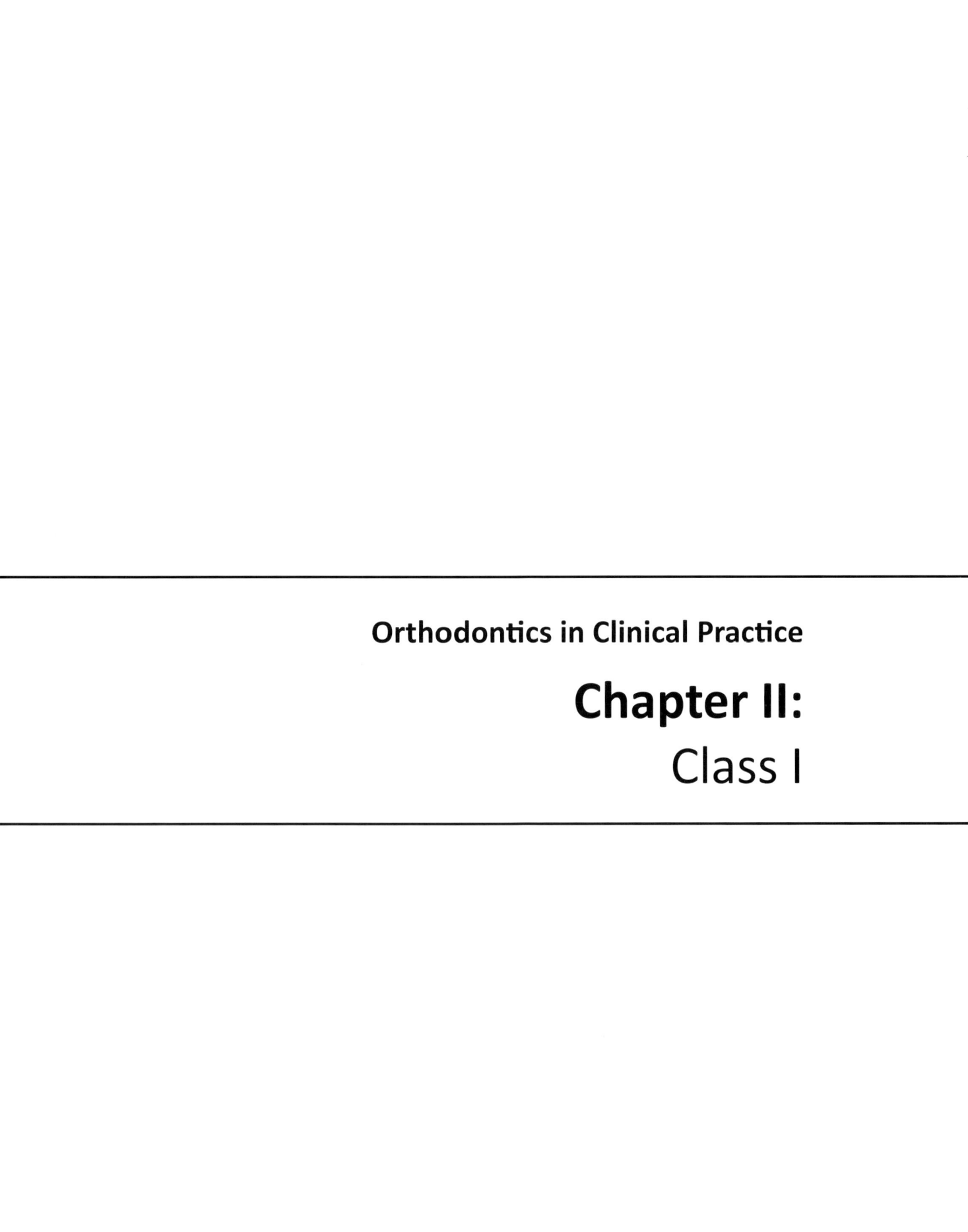

Orthodontics in Clinical Practice

Chapter II:

Class I

CLASS I

In a lateral view of skeletal Class 1 the relationship between the maxilla and mandible is good and the ANB angle is 2° ± 2.

There are no orthopedic problems but instead mainly orthodontic (dental) ones: dental crowding, cross bites, dental deep and open bites. These cases can be corrected both with or without the extraction of permanent teeth: expanding the dental arches, moving molars distally, and reducing the mesio-distal diameter of teeth (stripping).

2-1

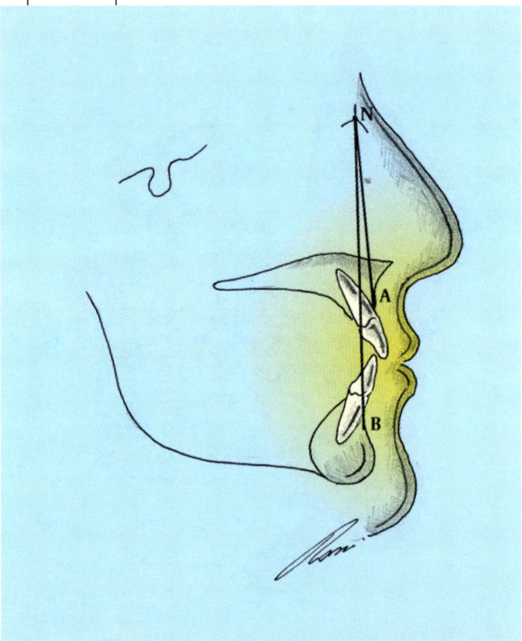

Fig. 2-1
Skeletal Class I
ANB = 2° ± 2

EXPANSION IN ORTHODONTICS

The topic of expansion in orthodontics has been under discussion for many years. For some people it is a never-ending story. Thinking logically, it is necessary to expand something that looks narrow. However, that is not always correct since there are situations where what one person considers narrow, others consider normal.

Usually the standard reference model is the lower dental arch. For many authors its expansion is considered unstable. In a normal situation, skeletal and dental parts show the posterior view, as in Fig. 2-2: the correct dental cusps–fossa relationship, coincidence of dental and jaws midline.

It is useful to remember the distinction between skeletal and dental aspects be-

2-2

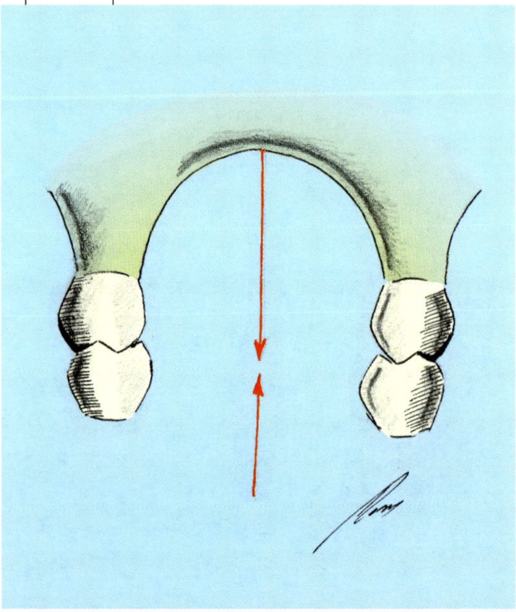

2-3

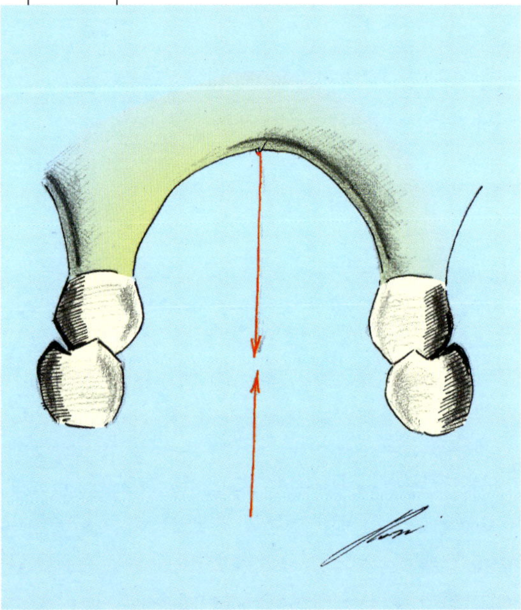

Fig. 2-2
Correct jaw relationship, posterior view.

Fig.2- 3
Bilateral cross bite. Midlines coincidence. Posterior view.

2-4

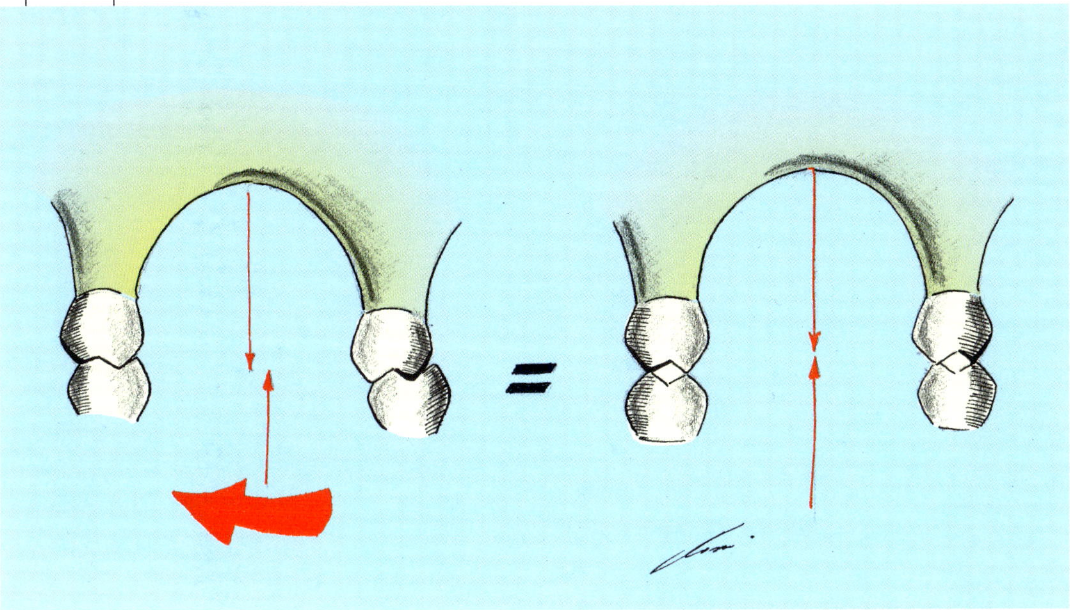

Fig. 2-4
Unilateral cross bite with lateral shift of the mandible. Midlines do not coincide (left). Posterior view.
If the mandible shifts as indicated by the arrow and there are no incorrect inclinations, midlines are coincident, with a dental cusp to cusp relationship. This occlusion is unstable and must be corrected by expanding the maxillary arch. Posterior view.

cause it is possible to expand a dental arch by modifying its skeletal base or changing the teeth's buccal/labial or lingual/palatal inclination (torque), or both.

MAXILLA

Transverse expansion

A narrow upper dental arch is the main cause of a posterior cross-bite, which can be unilateral or bilateral.

When it is bilateral and midlines are in alignment it is evident that the maxillary dental arch needs to be widened (Fig. 2-3). Usually there are no TMJ problems (such as clicks) indicating an internal derangement.

When the cross bite is unilateral, it is often because there is a maxillary transverse deficiency and when the mandible is correctly centred there are unstable teeth contacts which cause a lateral mandibular shift. There is not a midline coincidence and usually TMJ clicks are present (Fig 2-4). For many authors, the facial asymmetry following this situation must be corrected as soon as possible because from "positional" during the growth it can become "structural" at the end of growth.

I have personally successfully treated four year old patients (see Figs. 4-47 & 4- 48 Chapter IV). At the end of growth if the asymmetry becomes structural only surgery can change it.

Finally, there are dental cross bites without involvement of the jaws. In these cases only the teeth must be treated. A maxillary expansion which follows malpositioned lower teeth could be incorrect (Fig. 2-5, see also Figs. 2-6 to 2-11).

2-5

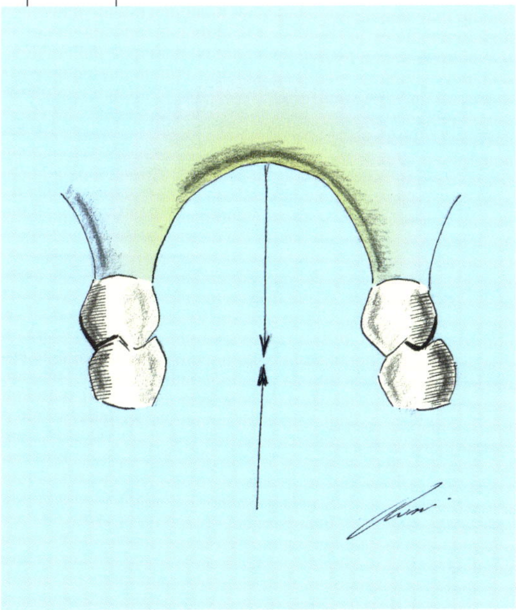

Fig. 2-5
Unilateral cross bite without facial asymmetry (dental). Posterior view.

The upper arch is crowded and narrow when looking at the second molar position. An alignment with extractions would be a big mistake as it could cause a Class III dental relationship. Following the second molar transverse width, the best approach is to align the upper dental arch without skeletal expansion.

What has been demonstrated until now refers to a skeletal Class I situation. In a skeletal Class III a minimal jaw cross bite can be corrected with maxillary protraction, while in a Class II, a treatment that is not followed by maxillary expansion causes a posterior cross bite.

2-6

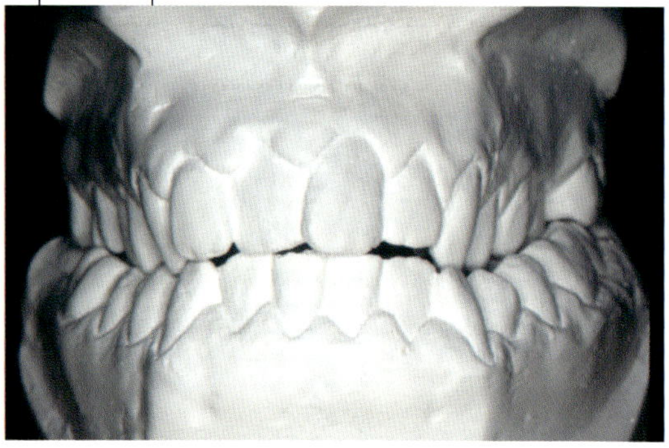

2-7

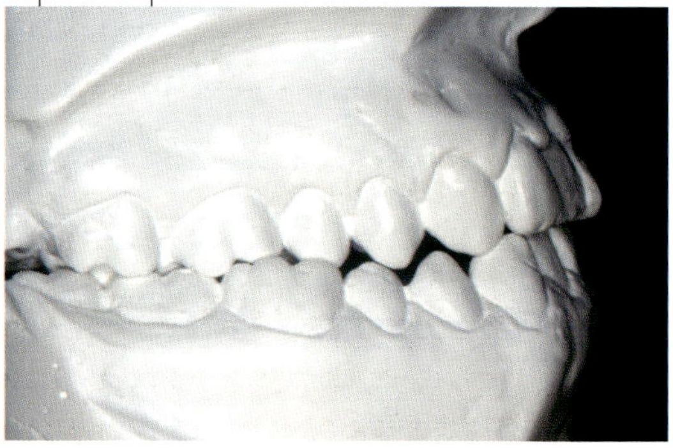

2-8

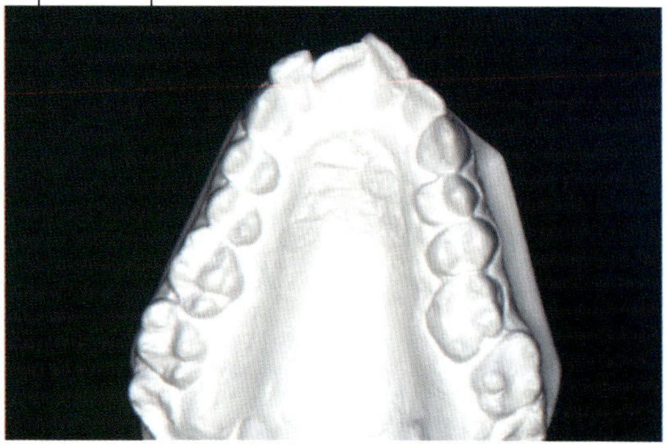

2-9

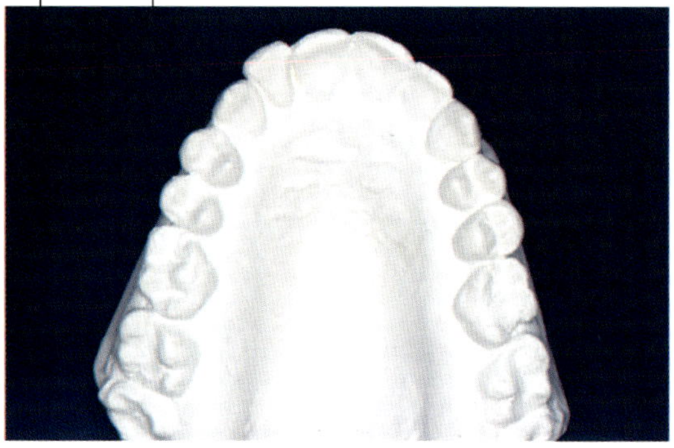

2-10

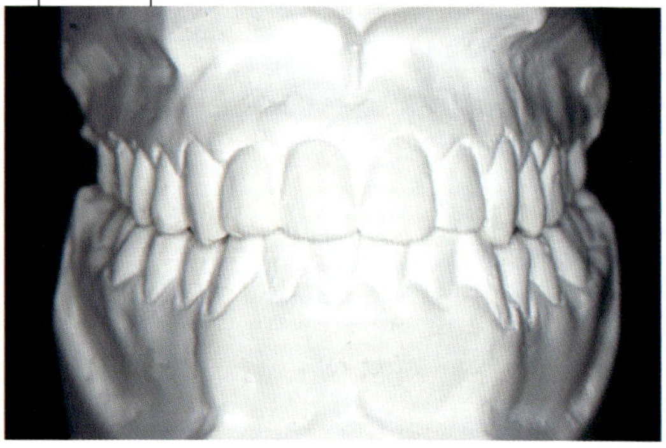

2-11

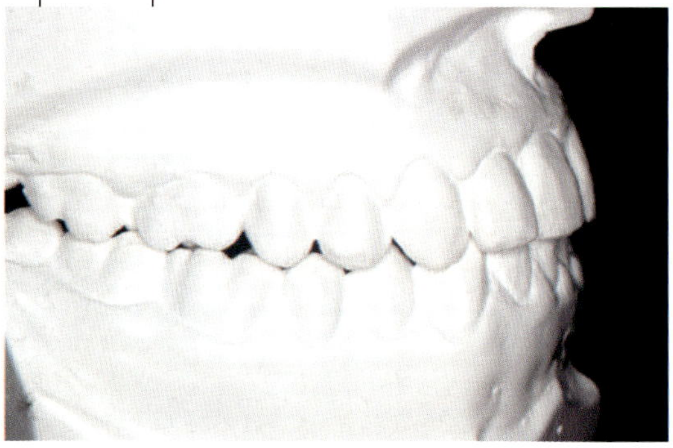

Fig. 2- 6 / 7 /8
Pre-treatment dental casts.

Fig. 2- 9 /10 /11
Post treatment dental casts.

TYPES OF EXPANSION

Which are the most common types of expansions? For many authors a palatal expansion can be rapid, slow or ultra-slow. The choice depends on many factors including the doctor's preference, different philosophies of treatment, different indications in different cases, the patient's compliance and time of treatment.

RAPID EXPANSION

Rapid palatal expansion is obtained using a device basically consisting of a screw fixed to four teeth: the upper first molars and the first premolars (or others available like in Figs. 2-12 & 2-13). There are also devices available which fix only to two teeth: the upper first molars.

Different authors indicate various means of activating them. I personally follow this one: turn 2/3 of the screw every day for no longer than 10–12 days. A complete turn of the screw gives about 1 mm of expansion, thus providing on average 5–7 mm in total.

When activated, the system develops heavy forces (from 1.5 kg to 5 kg) with hyalinization of the dentoalveolar bone without teeth movement. Thus the heavy force is transmitted to the midpalatal suture.

After about two weeks an osteoclastic activity of resorption of hyalinized tissue begins.

Therefore, it is necessary to use heavy forces for a short period of time (approximately two weeks maximum). After such period, the teeth risk moving out of the bone.

(Some people are critical of rapid palatal expansion because they believe that the heavy forces engaged will disturb the suture cellular activity, creating the possibility of a relapse. But this has not yet been demonstrated.)

2-12

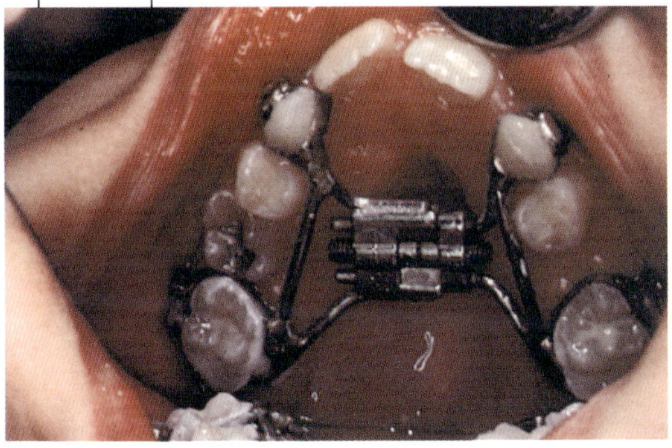

2-13

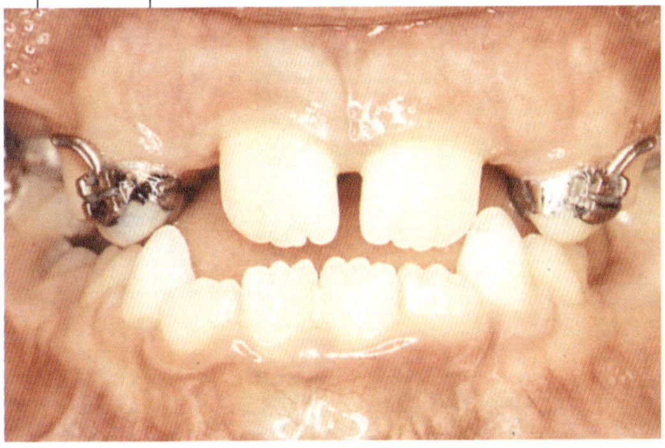

2-14

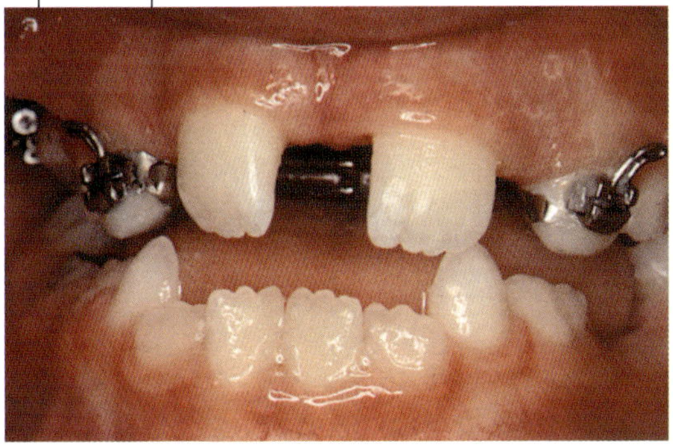

2-15

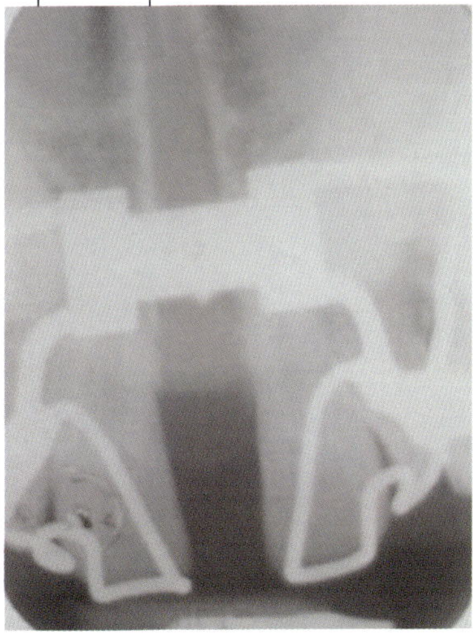

Fig. 2-12
Rapid palatal expander applied to the first upper molars and deciduous canines

Fig. 2-13
The activation begins

Fig. 2-14
After one week of activation. The large space between the central incisors is caused by the expansion of the maxillary suture. Usually after one month it returns to the starting width due to the elasticity of the transeptal fibres.

Fig. 2-15
X ray which shows the expansion of the maxillary suture.

After the active treatment is the containment phase, which usually lasts three months. During this period the device remains passive in the mouth. It is not possible to turn the screw because it is tied and fixed with acrylic or composite.

In my opinion the main indicators of rapid palatal expansion are those cases in which we do not expect good compliance, and those in which speed is an important factor. Even though some authors do not agree, Dr. Haas[113] and others believe that with rapid palatal expansion there is a downward dislocation of the maxillary and a consequent clockwise rotation of the mandible.

This is a positive effect in a Class III deep bite (hypodivergent), while it is negative in a Class II open bite (hyperdivergent). Therefore, caution is advised when choosing an appliance, so that the risks of undesired effects can be reduced (Figs. 2-16 to 2-19).

2-16

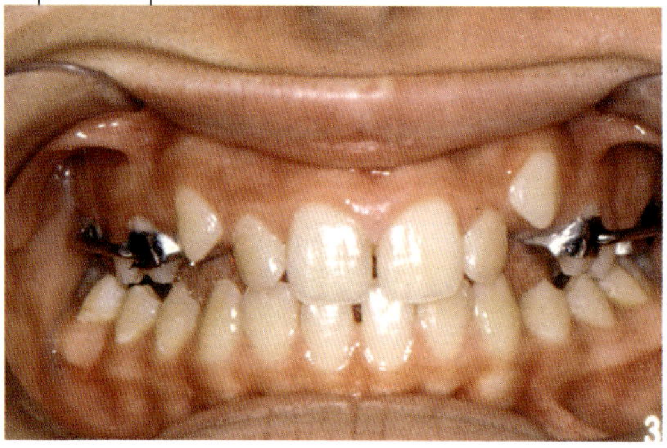

2-17

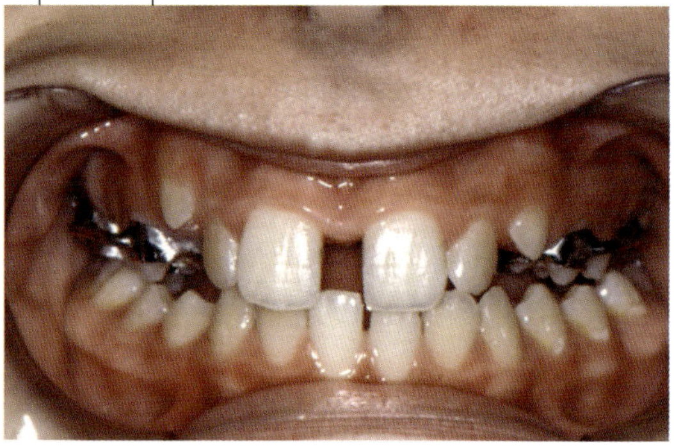

Figs. 2-16/17 Class II Hyperdivergent. Posterior crossbite partially corrected with rapid palatal expander.

2-18

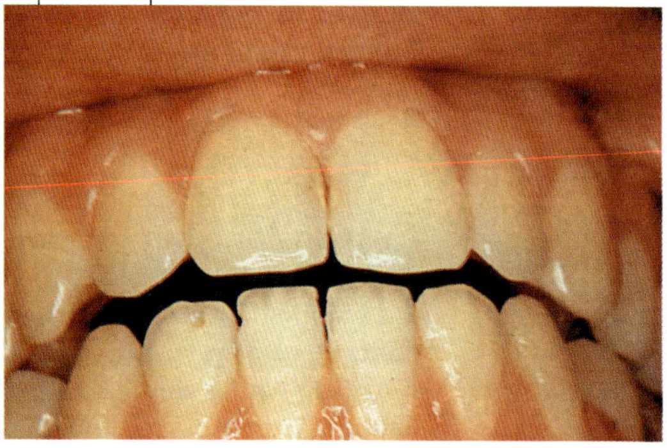

2-19

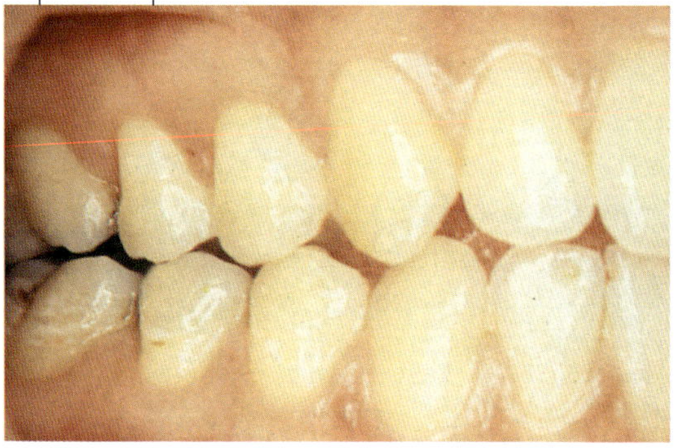

Figs. 2-18/19 The crossbite now is a cusp-bite and the Class II hyperdivergent worsened. A skeletal and dental open bite is present

SLOW EXPANSION

It is also possible to obtain palatal expansion in other ways and with other appliances.

For example, a Quad Helix[204-209] in 2-3 months can give results that are even more stable than those of a rapid expansion, according to those who use it..

Slow expansion also achieves good results using removable appliances with a median screw, as practised on the braces worn by millions of children.

When there is an acceptable patient compliance these are my favourite, especially in the cases of unilateral crossbite with mandibular shift, because they can work as a gnathologic splint and let the masticatory muscles relax, producing the correct jaws relationship. In other words, by eliminating the interferences of the occlusion they can immediately bring about a positional crossbite and indicate the correct way of expansion.

Dr. Chateau[49] states that with both rapid and slow expansion there is a widening of the nasal base, which improves nasal respiration. This is very good if we remember that many cases of palatal expansion deficiency are caused by a low posture of the tongue during swallowing.

2-20

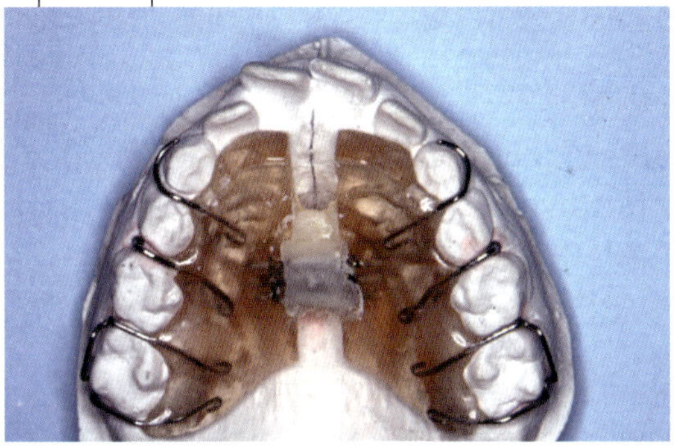

Fig. 2-20
Class I, mixed dentition with bilateral crossbite. Expansion with a simple acrylic plate. After the final turn of the screw more expansion is necessary.

2-21

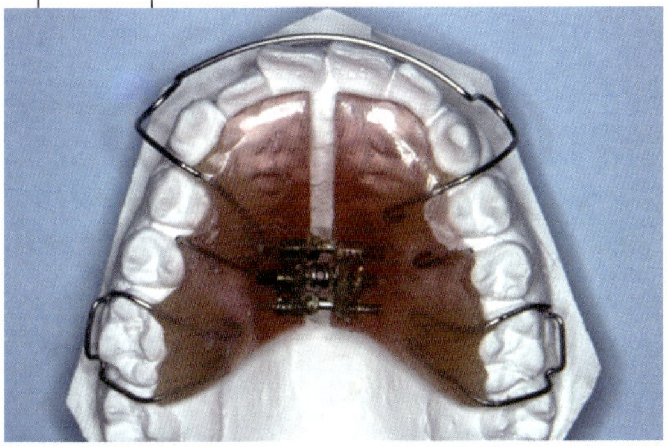

Fig. 2-21
The expansion obtained with the first appliance is increased with another appliance.

2-22

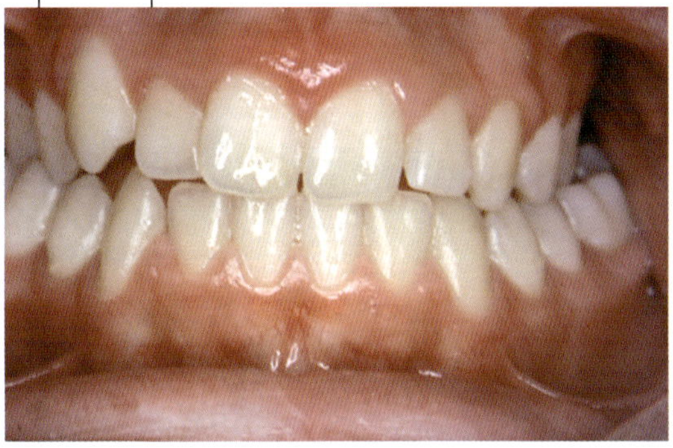

2-23

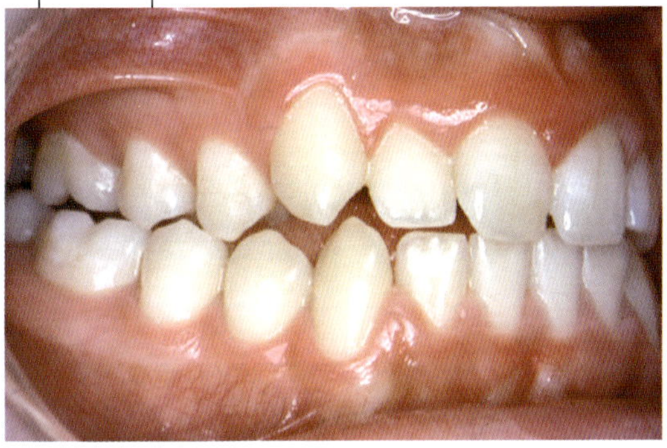

Fig. 2-22/23
Occlusion after the removal of appliances. More expansion is necessary, despite the previous treatment.

2-24

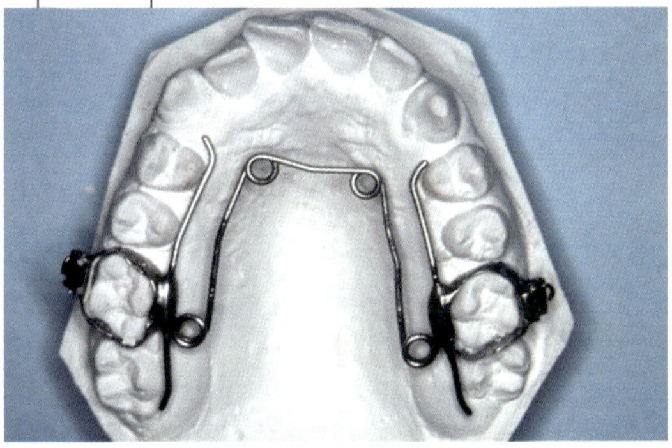

Fig. 2-24
Before placing an edgewise appliance it is better to use a Quad Helix.

2-25

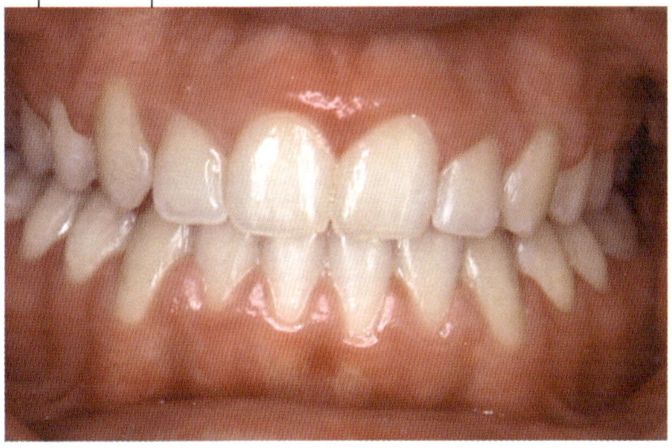

2-26

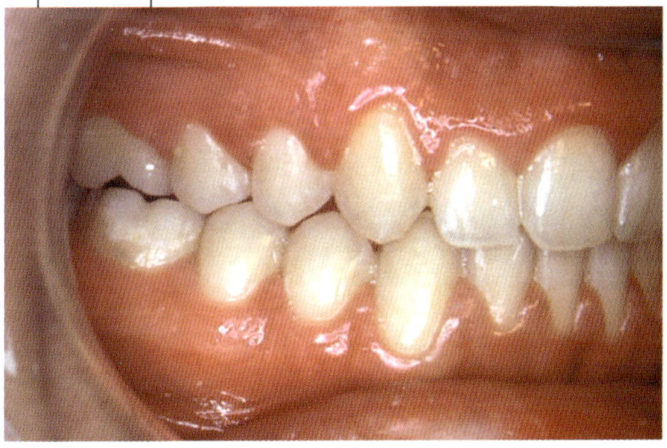

Fig. 2-25/26
Occlusion at the end of the treatment. Imagine the situation without the expansions.

ULTRA-SLOW EXPANSION

An ultra-slow expansion is a maxillary expansion caused naturally by the action of the tongue during swallowing while the cheeks oppose it. In this case, the suggested appliances are the following: Frankel, PCF, Bionator without clasps and with buccal shields. The tongue is activated to keep the appliance in place, meanwhile the buccal shields oppose the cheeks.

Under these circumstances, Owen[187] believes that the expansion is not only dental but also skeletal.

UNTIL WHAT AGE IS IT POSSIBLE TO PERFORM A MAXILLARY EXPANSION?

Once again it is important to remember the difference between skeletal parts and teeth. The majority of authors believe that until 14–16 years old the midpalatal suture is a fibrous synarthrosis. Then its calcification begins and around the age of 25 it is a synostosis. However, there are also some authors who are convinced that facial sutures remain open for many decades (Wright, Sicher).[228-258] Others like Scott[225] suggest that in old skulls they seem to be open but, in reality, they are so tight that they do not allow for widening. In that case prudence is essential.

In particular, when it comes to rapid palatal expansions, we can go ahead and perform them without any risks in very young patients before puberty. After puberty, it is important to ask for a detailed informed consent, since undesirable effects like fenestrations and dehiscences can occur.

No need for concern, but this curious case is listed in literature.....Lunder and Warunek[1**] reported the clinical appearance of a nasal-palatal duct in a 13 year old patient after a rapid palatal expansion. (Since 1881, 36 similar cases have been reported.)

My own personal suggestion is to activate the screw for 3–4 days and then take an X-ray.

If both the X-ray and the clinical exam show no signs of widening with the increase of the diastema of the central incisors, stop the activation and discuss with the patient or his relatives whether to continue or not evaluating, among other things, a surgically assisted expansion.

Until this point I have listed briefly the main maxillary expansion procedures in the presence of crossbites, which indicate a transverse discrepancy between jaws. When there is no crossbite, can maxillary expansion be useful?

Maxillary expansion can be in a Class II when mandibular advancement is wanted, otherwise there would be a crossbite. In other situations it is unclear, for example in cases with crowding where the expansion is performed to increase the available space.

Before providing more details, it is important to talk about the mandible. What we want in the end is the best relationship between upper and lower arch.

EXPANSION TO GAIN SPACE.

At this point it is very interesting to consider Gianelly:[2**]

"In the absence of a crossbite, is rapid palatal expansion necessary to gain arch width and avoid extraction treatment? If so, then is the maxillary arch perimeter the determinant in the extraction – non-extraction decision?"

He concludes that:

"the data indicate that a transverse expansion of the mandibular arch in selected areas is unstable. An alternate more conservative and less demanding strategy to resolve crowding is to simply maintain the arch length during the transition period."

Under these conditions 68% of patients with crowding will have adequate space for alignment, while another 19% will have adequate space with only marginal arch length increase (up to 1 mm per side).

He agrees with Grayson in saying that *"the use of rapid palatal expansion as a method of increasing lower arch length cannot be justified"*.

THE MANDIBLE

TRANSVERSE EXPANSION

A transverse expansion of the mandible is basically a dental expansion. There are no sutures so the skeletal part can be expanded only with surgery.

Many orthodontists in their treatment plan consider the lower intercanine distance modifiable, but only in a slow steady manner. As a matter of fact, the distance can be increased, but too many relapses occur.

2-27

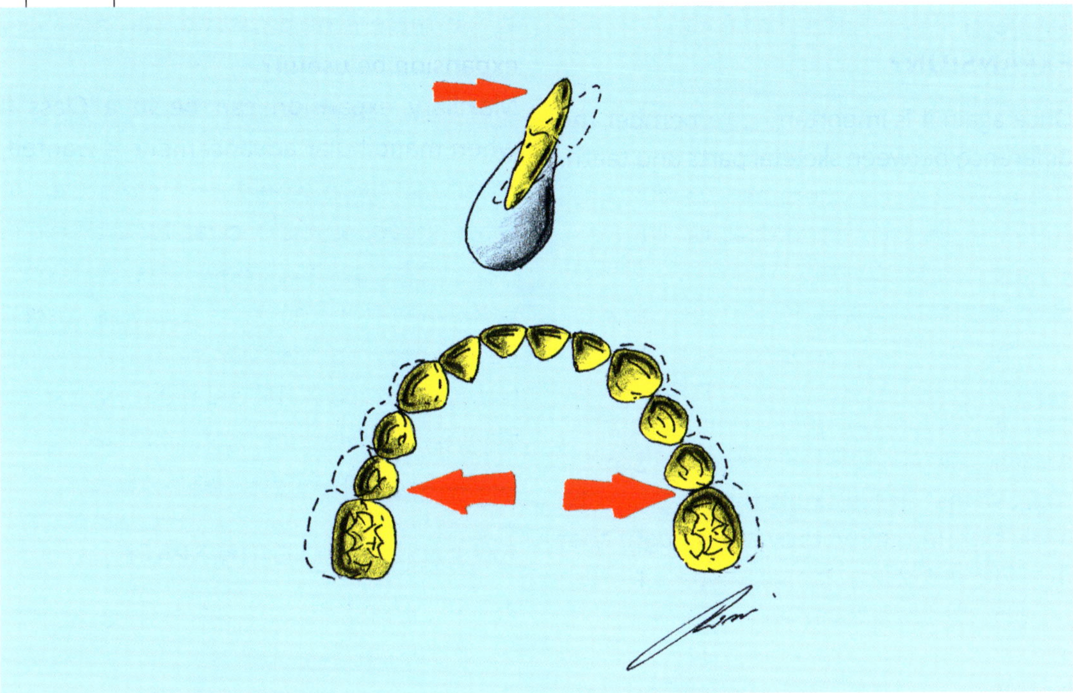

Fig. 2-27
Top
Every mm of lower incisors' proclination creates 2mm. of space on the arch.
Bottom
To gain 1 mm on the arch it is necessary to have an expansion of:
1 mm between canines
2 mm between the first premolars
3 mm between the second premolars
4 mm between the first molars

I follow this "classic" orthodontic vision even though there are more permissive authors like Cetlin and Ten Hoeve[49] who, by using a lip bumper in 50 cases, reported that the transverse distance between canines increased 2.5 mm, between the first premolars 4 mm, between the second premolars 4.5 mm and between the first molars 5.5 mm. But some critics are doubtful about the reliability and predictability of these results.

Whatever the method, these are the circumstances when seeking to gain space on the arch perimeter in order to avoid extractions if crowding is present.

TO EXTRACT OR NOT TO EXTRACT?

Just like "to be or not to be" for Hamlet, whether to perform an extraction or not is one of the major professional questions facing an orthodontist. I think that *there is great confusion on the subject* and it is therefore necessary to clarify a few things.

Whenever we speak of crowding we commonly imagine teeth that are not well aligned. However, that can be misleading if no analysis is made of the limits of the dental arch.

DENTAL ARCH LIMITS

Even after everything that has been said until now, I still agree with mandibular arch-based diagnosis and treatment planning.

A distal limit is indicated by the presence of the wisdom tooth. With its extraction it is possible to obtain a little bit of space. However, in order to obtain more space, it is necessary to expand laterally but mainly frontally with the incisor proclination.

The conflict between the philosophy and technique of two historic gurus of modern orthodontics, Tweed and Ricketts, is based on that theory. They represent the extremes of the question, while the other opinion leaders remain in the middle. For Tweed, the lower incisors must be more vertical on the mandibular plane than for Ricketts.

In cases of crowding this means that less space is available for a non-extraction treatment.

In a funny article, Dr. Jacobs emphasized the amount of anaesthetic that an orthodontist must buy. If he's a disciple of Tweed he will extract in 70% of cases, if he's a disciple of Ricketts only in 30%. Jacobs R.M.- " Treatment objectives and case retention: Cybernetic and myometric considerations". A.J.O Vol.58, n°6, December 1970 . 552-564

WHO IS RIGHT?

Remember that crowding is not necessarily represented by teeth that are not aligned. *When lower incisors are crowded, if they are proclined they look straight.* Therefore, when we look at apparently well aligned teeth we must wonder if they are actually hiding crowding, which is something to consider, particularly in borderline situations.

Those in favour of expanding the dental arch to gain space think that those who choose to extract in similar cases are doing something unnecessary which will flatten the facial profile and cause TMJ problems. On the contrary, the "extractors'" reply that carrying out expansion to gain space is unnatural and it can cause occlusal instability and relapse. As a matter of fact, the teeth erupt in a balanced neuromuscular system, which cannot be violated without consequences. Therefore, the expansion of the arch to gain space, not the extraction method, might lead to a relapse, periodontal disease, craniomandibular disorders...

I personally believe that the truth lies in the middle ground.

I remember when during a meeting in Venice in 1985 Dr. Ricketts showed a case treated with four extractions: the result was excellent. However, according to his analysis it could have been treated without extractions! When I asked him why he had chosen to extract the premolars, he answered that he had to do so because a dentist had already previously extracted one.

That was evidently a borderline case in which both solutions, extraction or non extraction, were acceptable.

On the other hand, Dr. Horn, a disciple of Tweed's philosophy, presented in Cernobbio in 1993 some cases where a degree of lower incisor proclination followed – Ricketts' indications!

When it comes to extraction versus non-extraction we must also remember that in many non-extraction treatments wisdom teeth are removed. Therefore, are they always considered non-extracting cases?

Later on we will see how an interproximal enamel reduction (stripping) can influence the decision whether to remove some teeth or not.

The following three clinical cases show how important it is to also evaluate the facial aesthetic and the periodontal situation. For all of them there was a detailed informed consent about treatment alternatives.

CLINICAL CASES
CASE NUMBER 1
PREVALENCE OF FACIAL AESTHETIC EVALUATION IN A BORDERLINE CASE

2-28

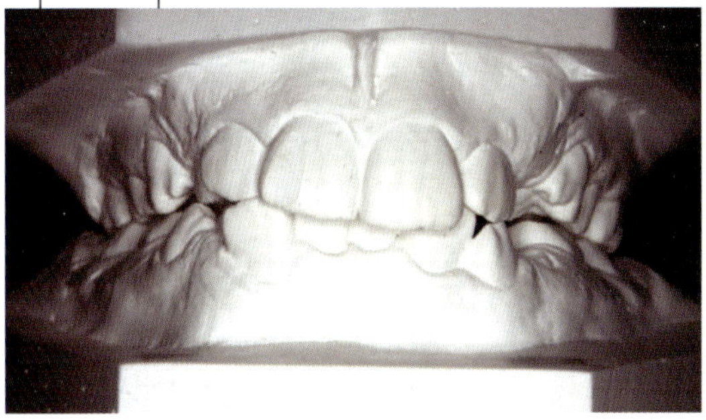

2-29

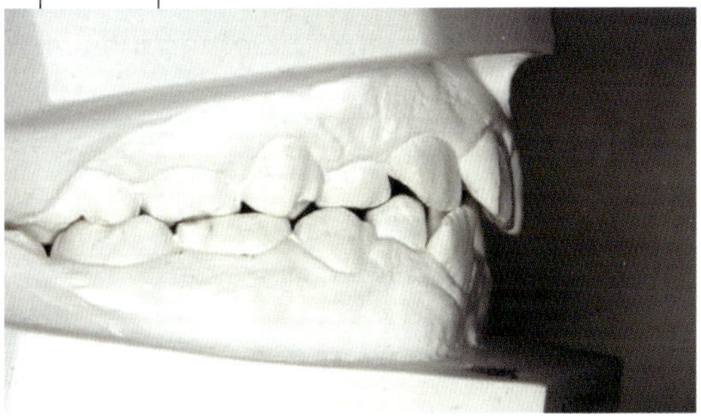

Figs. 2-28 & 2-29
Class I with crowding. Dental casts. Note the cross bite of the upper right lateral incisors.

2-30

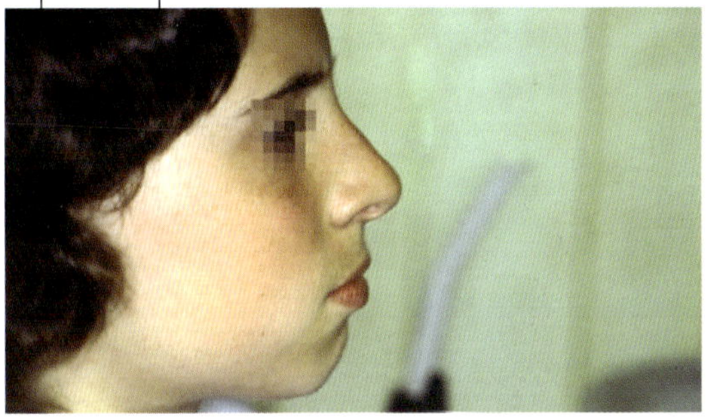

Fig. 2-30
Patient's profile. Labial seal is obtained only with excessive contraction of the chin musculature.

2-31

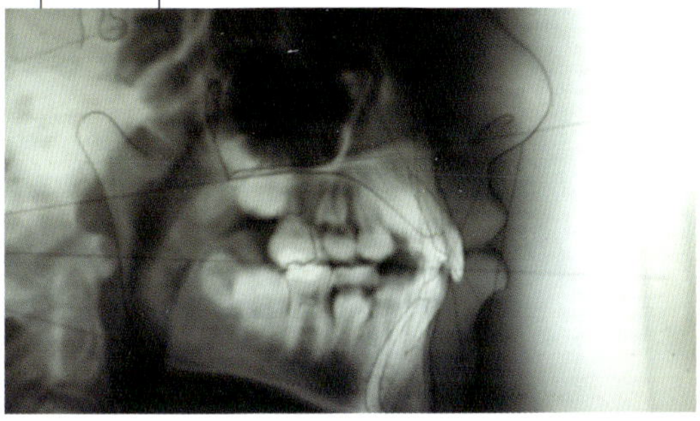

Fig. 2-31
Pre-treatment lateral cephalogram. When it comes to a tracing following Ricketts' philosophy it is possible to achieve a good alignment of the teeth without extractions. According to others, four extractions are necessary.

2-32

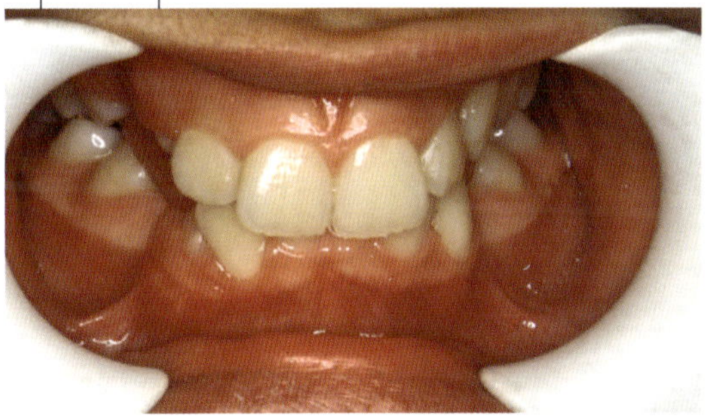

2-33

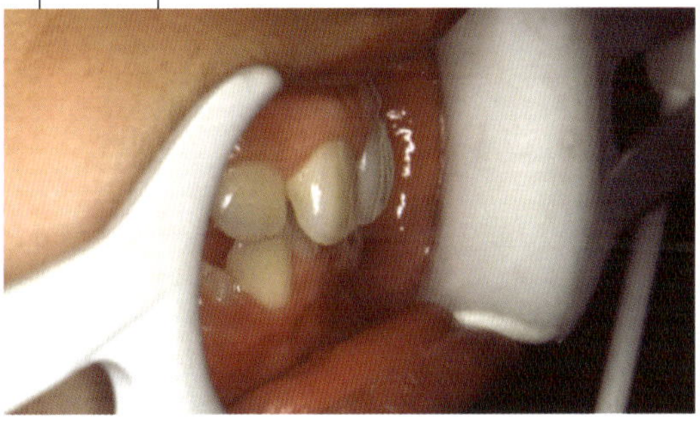

Fig. 2-32 / 33
If we do not extract, we will not expect any improvement of the facial profile. Therefore, the parents agree to the extraction of the upper first premolars and the lower second premolars. Right after the extractions there is a spontaneous correction of upper right lateral incisor crossbite.

2-34

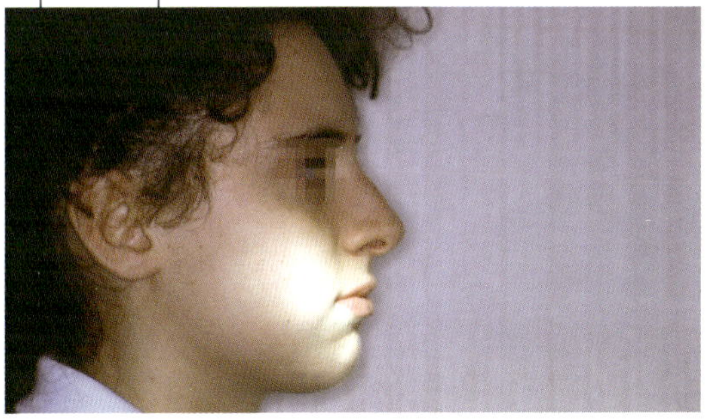

Fig. 2-34
Post treatment patient's profile. The musculature of the chin now is relaxed.

2-35

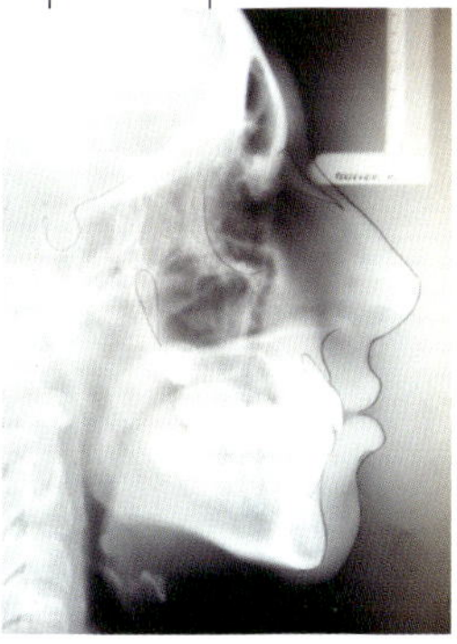

Fig. 2-35
Post treatment lateral cephalogram.

2-36

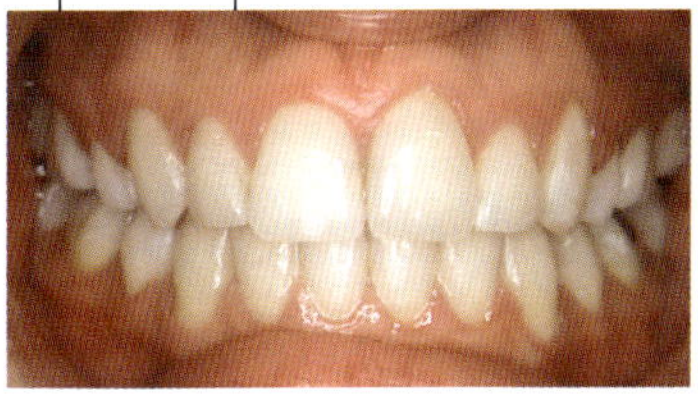

2-37

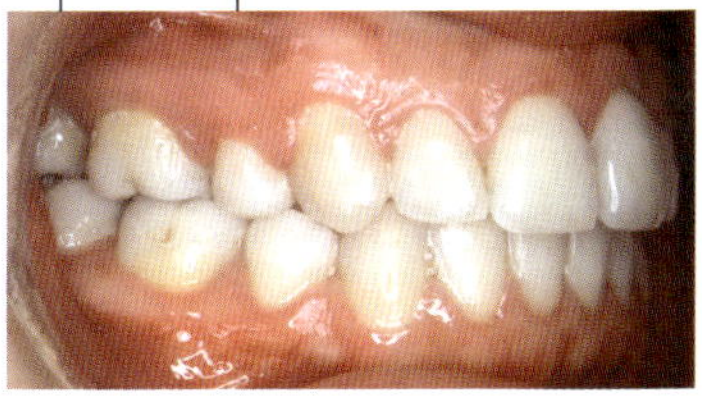

2-38

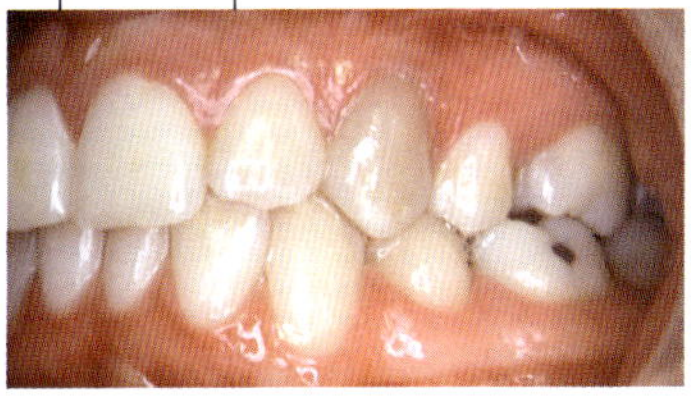

Figs. 2-36 to 2-38
Post treatment occlusion.

CASE NUMBER 2

FACIAL AESTHETIC AND CEPHALOMETRIC EVALUATION ALLOWING A NON-EXTRACTION TREATMENT

2-39

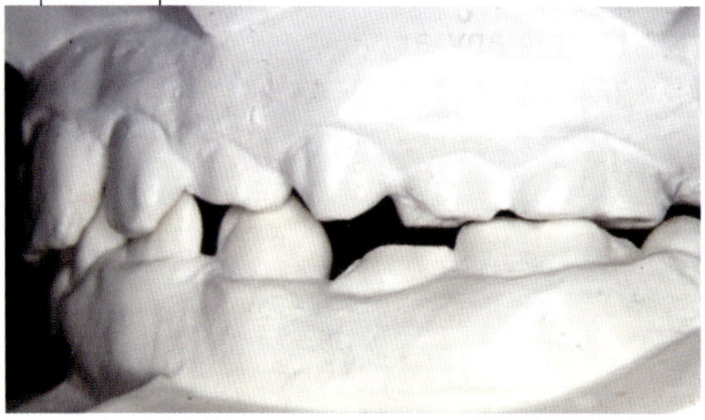

2-40

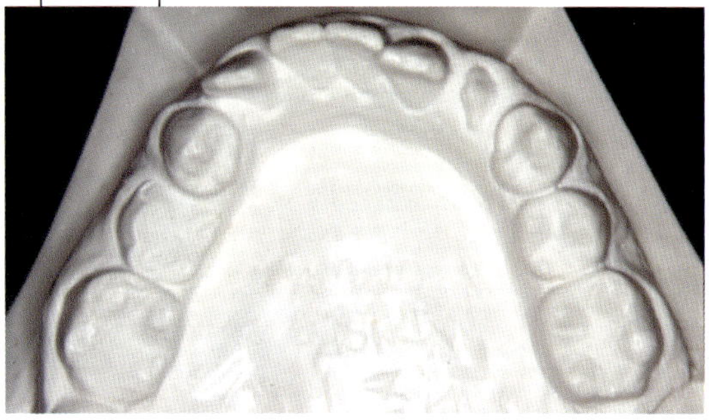

Figs. 2-39 & 2-40 Dental casts of a Class I with crowding. Note the lack of space for lower left canine (33) eruption.

2-41a

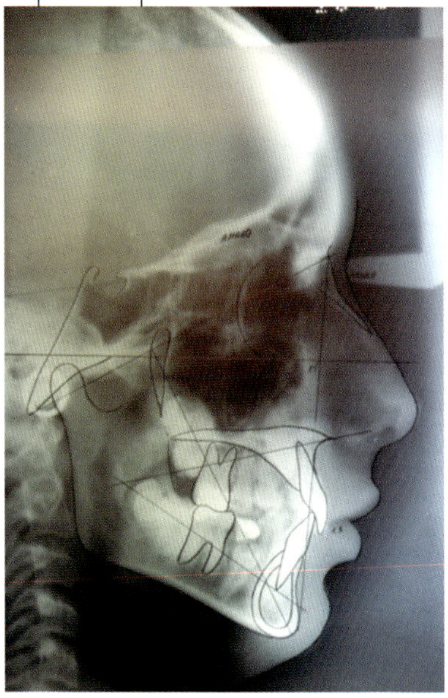

2-41b

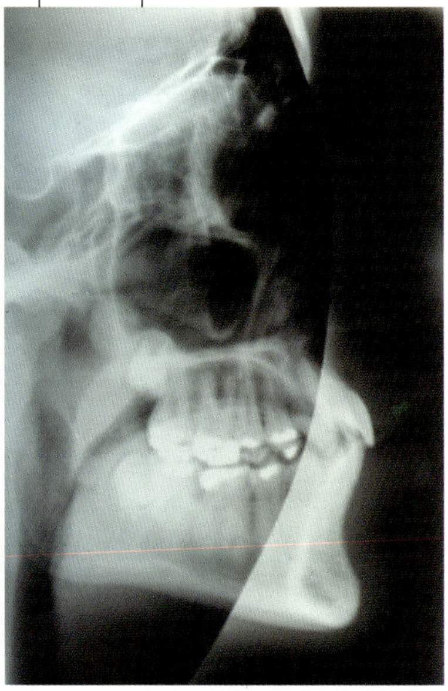

Fig. 2-41a Pre-treatment lateral cephalogram. For Ricketts' analysis it is possible to procline the lower incisors. This and the leeway space are the basis of a non-extraction treatment.

Fig. 2-41b Post treatment lateral cephalogram.

2-42

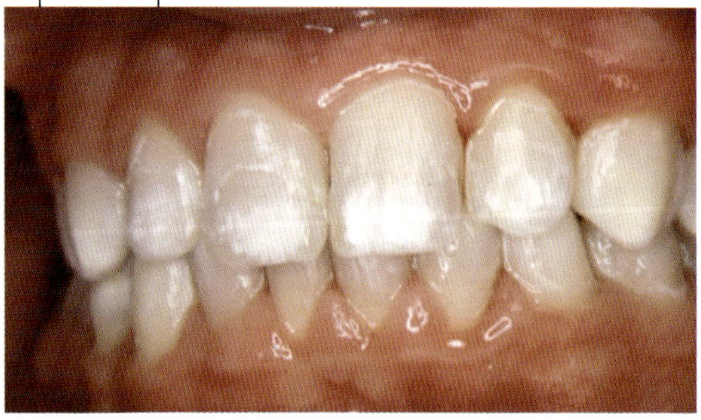

2-43

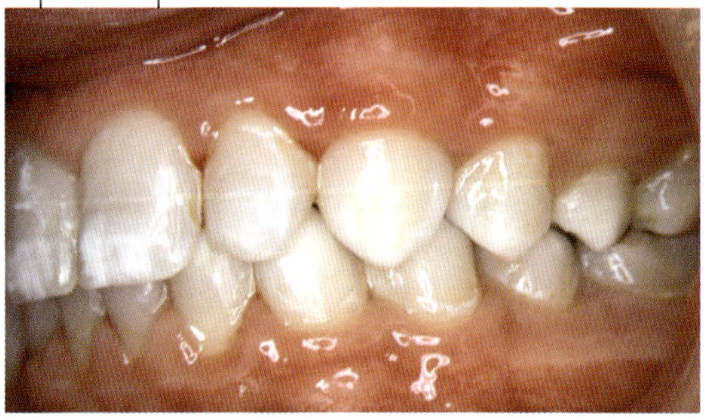

Figs. 2-42 & 2-43 Post treatment occlusion.

2-44

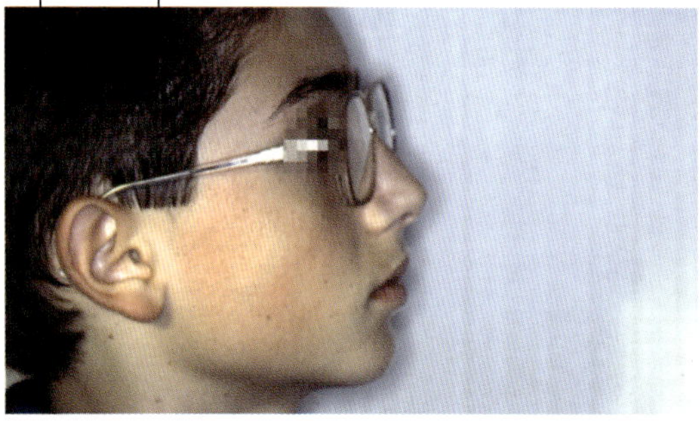

2-45

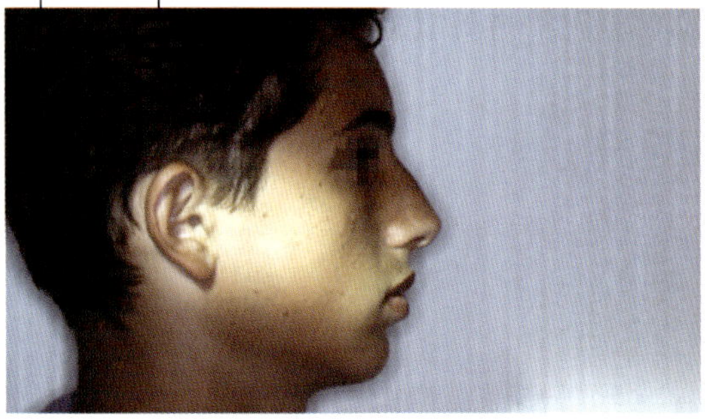

Fig. 2-44 Pre-treatment profile.

Fig. 2-45 Post treatment profile, 3 years later.

CASE NUMBER 3

PERIODONTAL CONDITIONS SUGGEST AN EXTRACTION TREATMENT.

The case, Class I dolico, is borderline. A thin periodontium covers the lower incisor roots that remind us of “organ pipes”. Notice the gingival recession which appears during the treatment where an appliance is *not placed on the lower incisors.*

Even though there are different and contradictory opinions on the relationship between orthodontics and periodontal status, I recommend caution, preferring not to put any appliance on those teeth because I would expect a worsening of the situation. Moreover, it would be difficult to deny that the outcome is not caused by the orthodontic treatment.

2-46

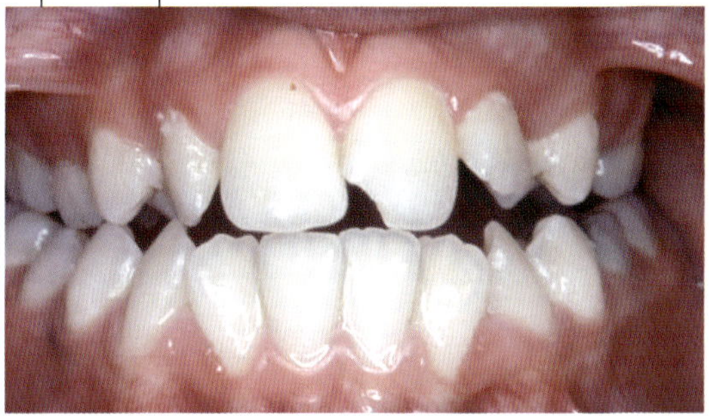

2-47

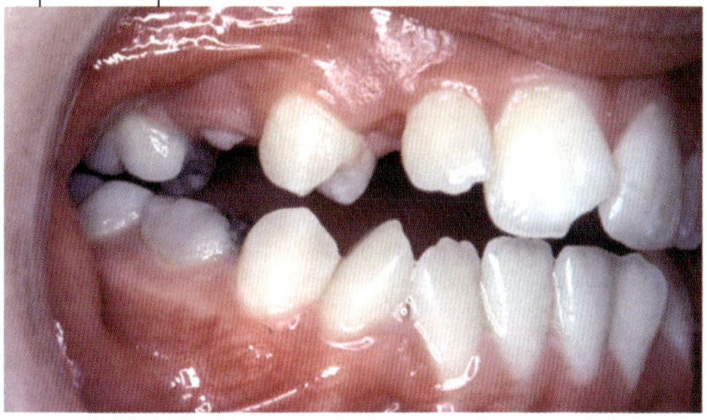

2-48

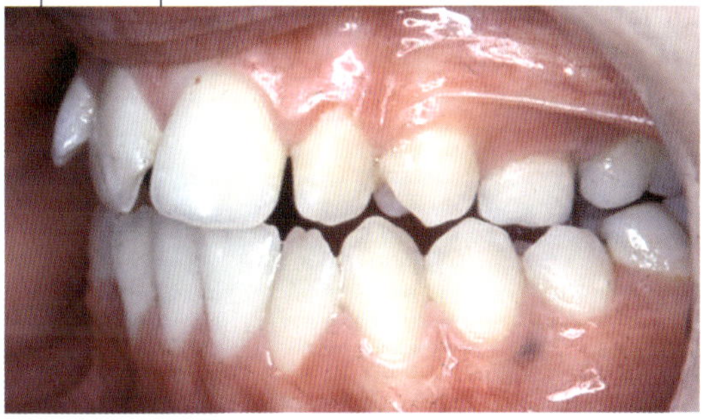

Figs. 2-46 to 2-48 Pre-treatment occlusion. Where are the spaces for upper canine eruption? The extractions of the upper first premolars and, later, of the second lower premolars will follow.

2-49

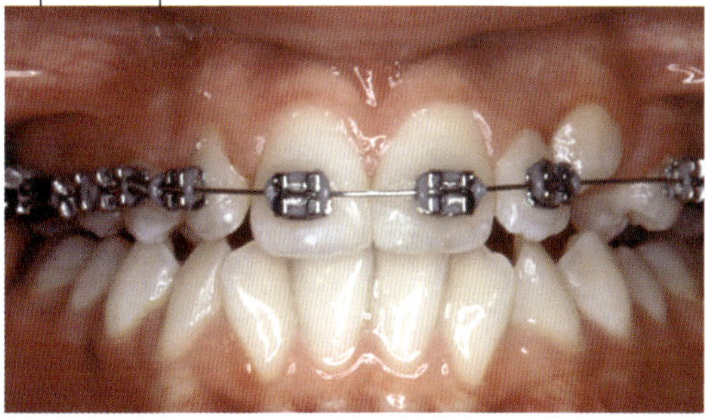

2-50

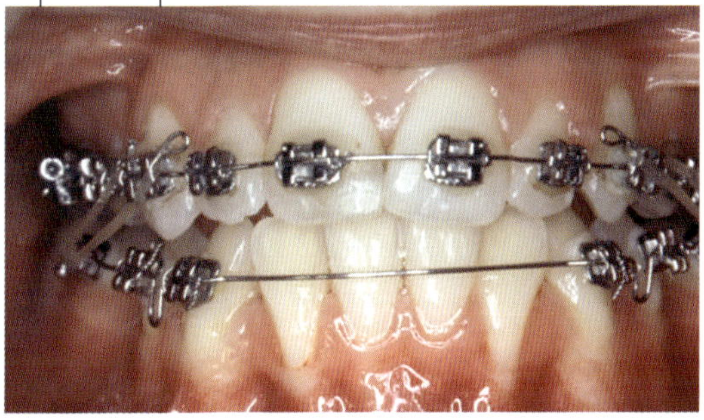

2-51

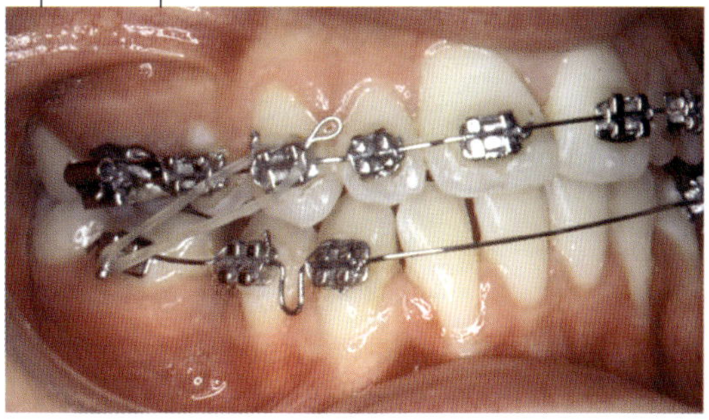

2-52

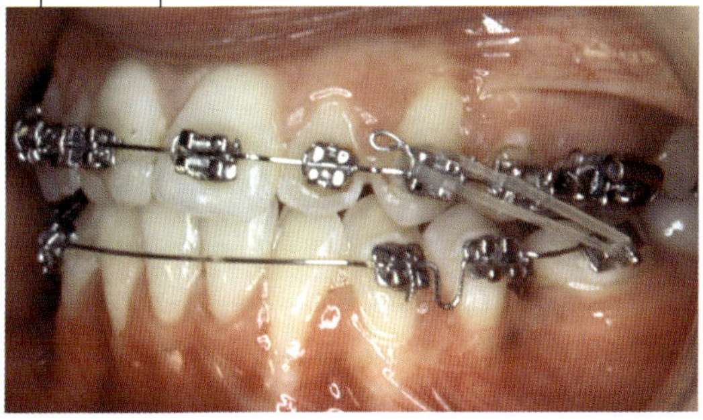

Figs. 2-49 to 2-52 Phases of treatment with edgewise appliance. Note the gingival recession of the lower lateral incisors.

2-53

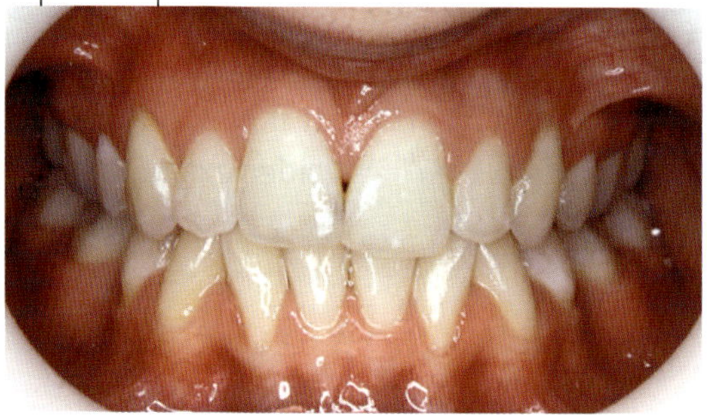

2-54

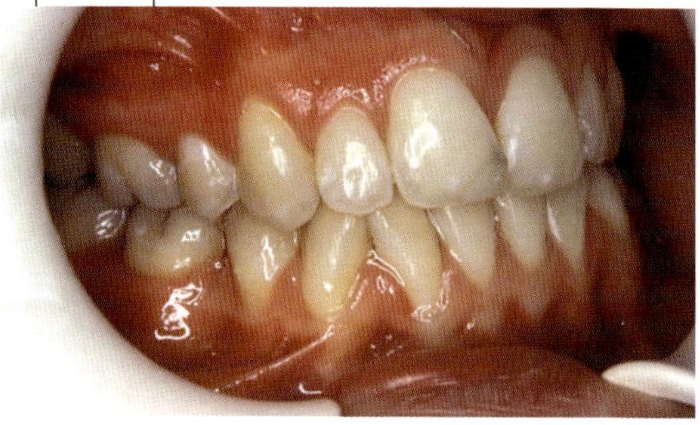

2-55

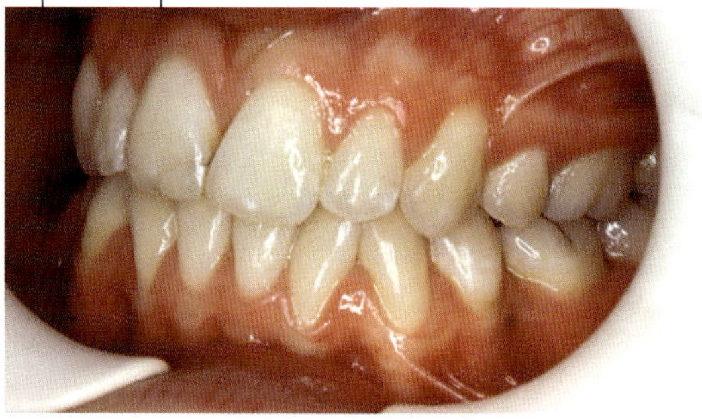

Figs. 2-53 to 2-55
Post treatment occlusion.

2-56

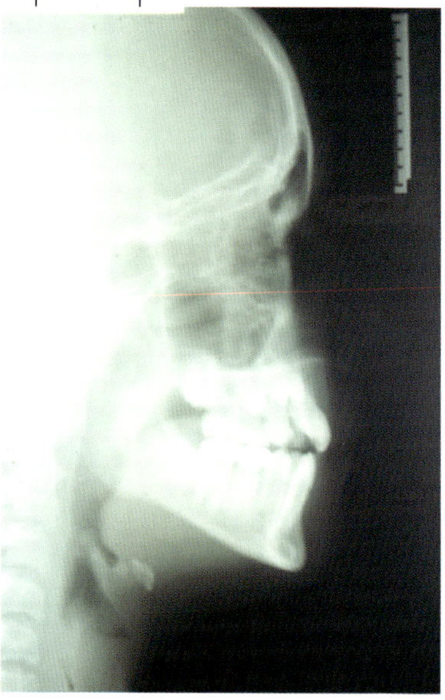

2-57

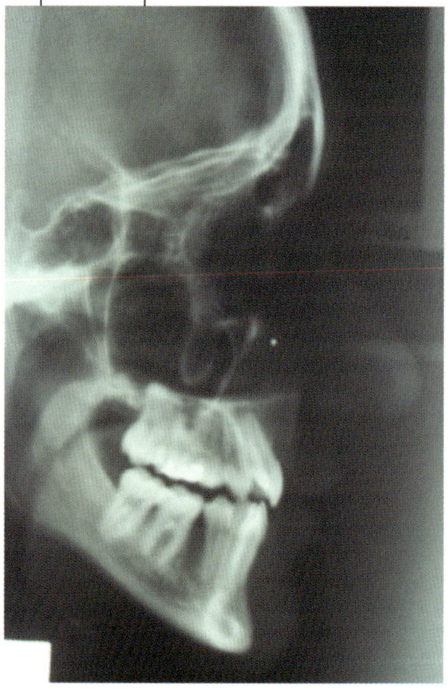

Fig. 2-56
Pre-treatment lateral cephalogram.

Fig. 2-57
Post treatment lateral cephalogram. The mouth is slightly open but that does not change the global evaluation.

NATURALLY BEYOND THE LIMITS: BIALVEOLAR PROTRUSIONS

On the subject of non-extraction treatments, when expanding the arch we must remember the importance of stability, periodontal conditions and TMJ health. However, in modern orthodontics I stress the importance of the facial aesthetic since there are people who naturally have a stable Class I occlusion without periodontal or TMJ problems, but they want to change their smile because it is too protrusive.

More protrusive incisors are very common in many Far East and African individuals. They represent a balance between the opposite pressure of the tongue and of the perioral soft tissues, muscles included. We could also consider them the natural correction of a crowding situation.

In western countries less protrusive incisors with a more relaxed musculature are preferred (Figs. 2-58 to 2-62). Keeping in mind that Ricketts is the most permissive when it comes to incisor advancement, we can label as "too protrusive" an occlusion where frontal teeth are more proclined than what its analysis indicates.

To correct a protrusive smile we must retract teeth and *to do so we need space distally.*

If there is no space available we must consider extractions.

CASE NUMBER 4

2-58

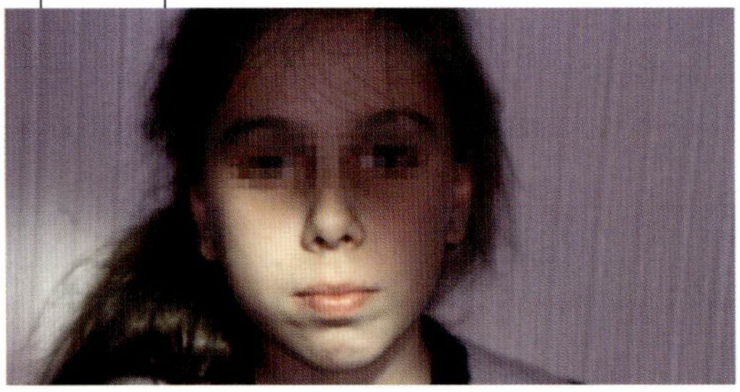

2-59

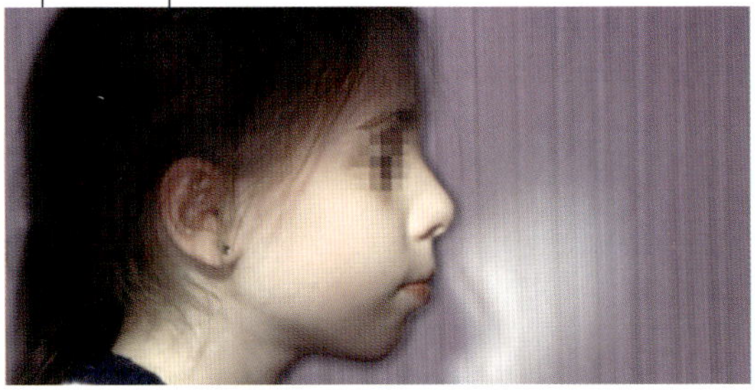

2-60

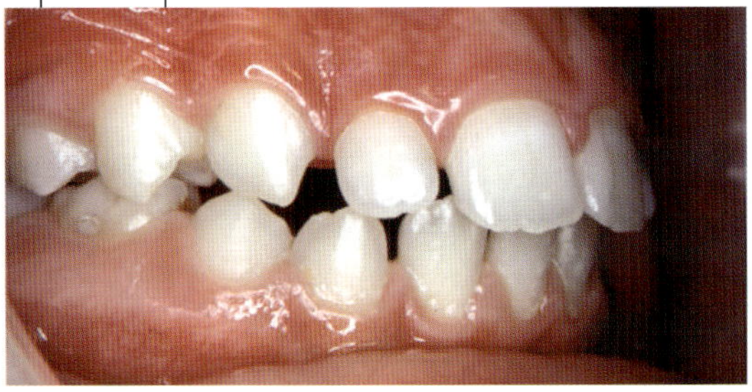

Figs. 2-58 to 2-60
Patient with bialveolar protrusion. Note the impact of the teeth on the patient's profile.

2-61

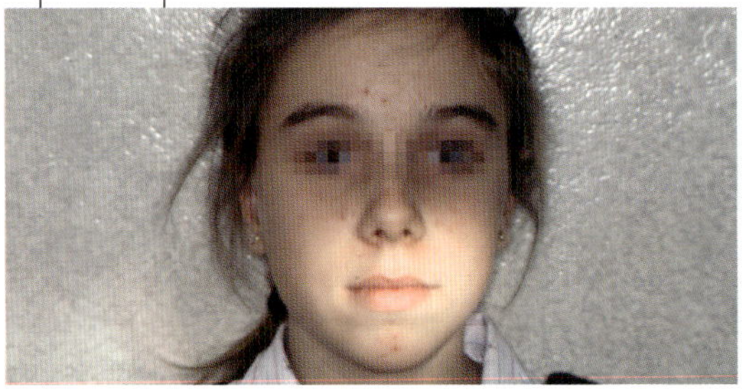

2-62

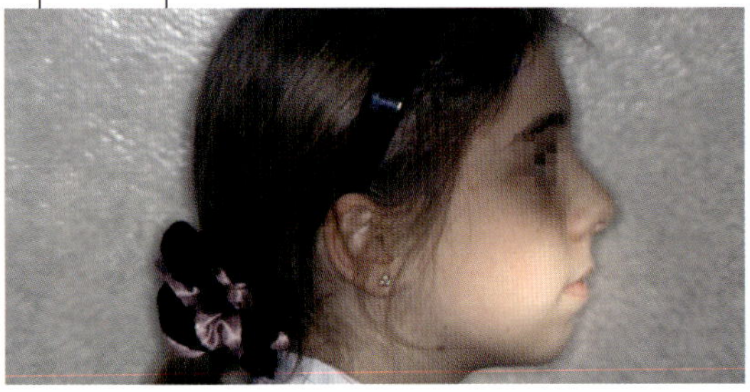

2-63

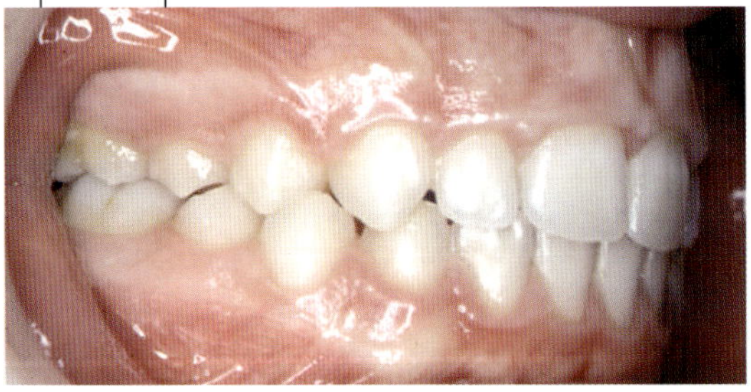

Figs. 2-61 to 2-63
The patient, one year after treatment. The change of occlusion and profile obtained with the retraction of frontal teeth and closure of interdental spaces is evident.

2-64

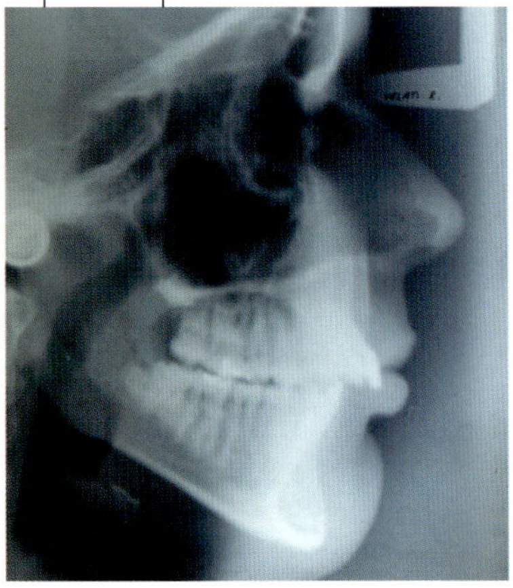

2-65

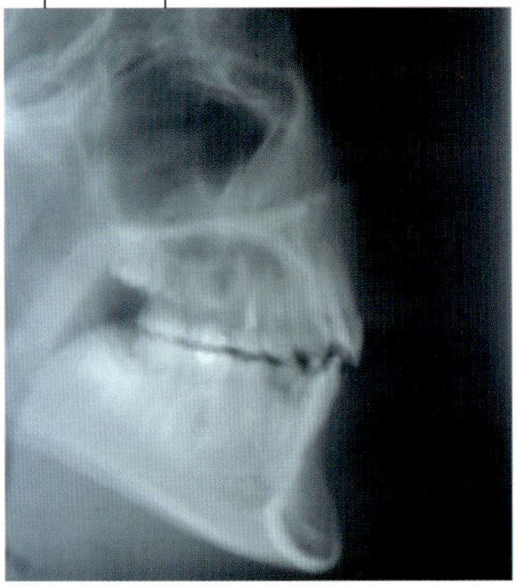

Fig. 2-64
Pre-treatment lateral cephalogram.

Fig. 2-65
Post treatment lateral cephalogram.

CASE NUMBER 5

2-66

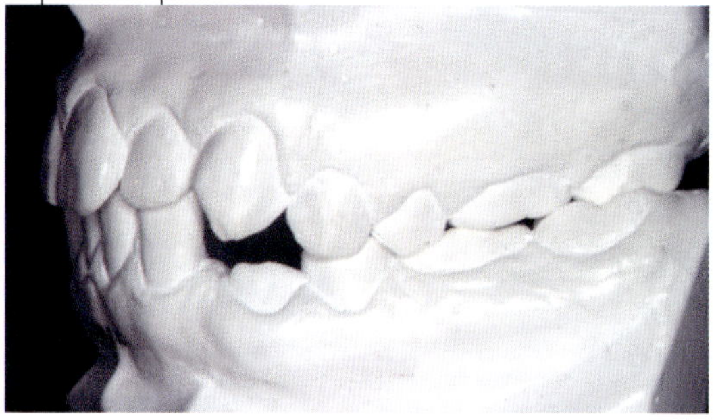

2-67

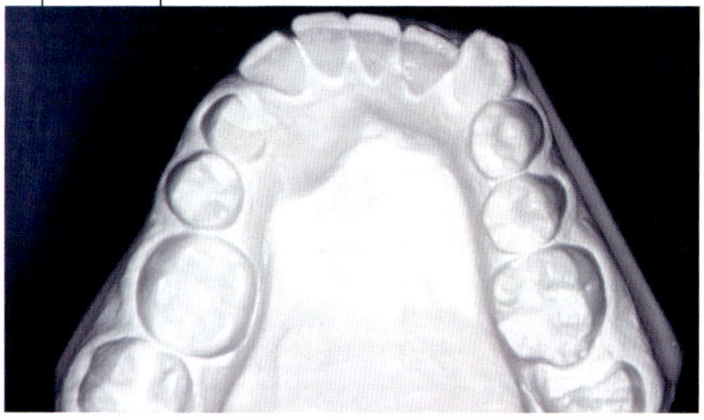

Figs. 2-66 &67
Dental casts of a bialveolar protrusion with crowding. Note the lack of space for lower left canine (33) eruption. Without doubt this is an extraction case.

2-68

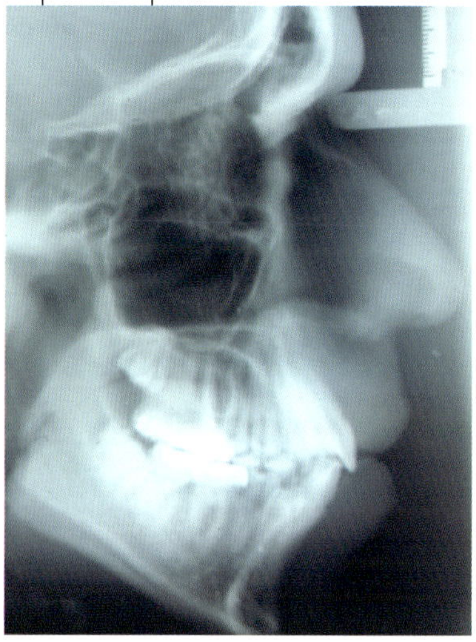

2-69

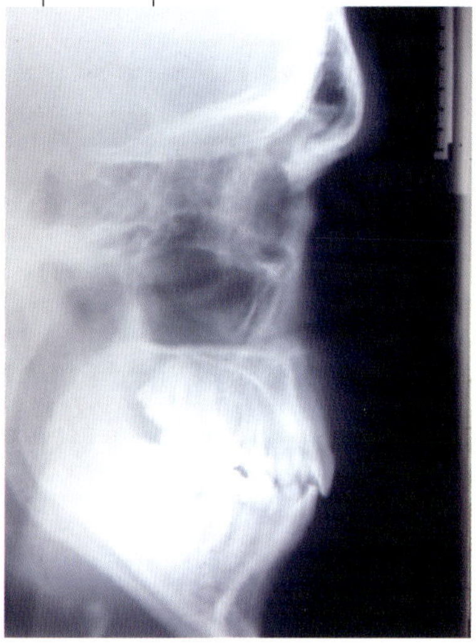

Fig. 2- 68
Pre-treatment lateral cephalogram.

Fig. 2-69
Post-treatment lateral cephalogram. The difference from the pre-treatment is evident.

2-70

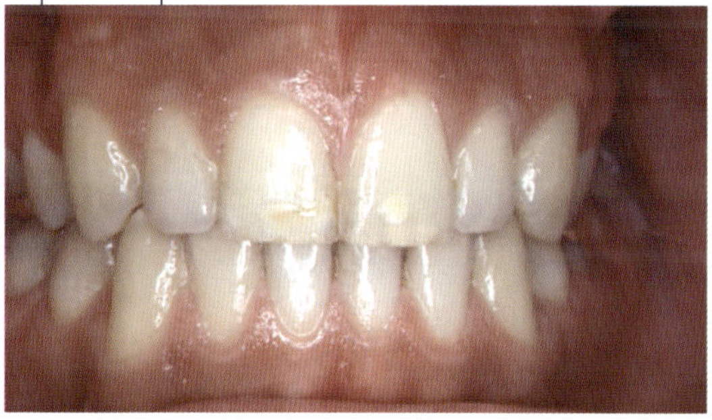

2-71

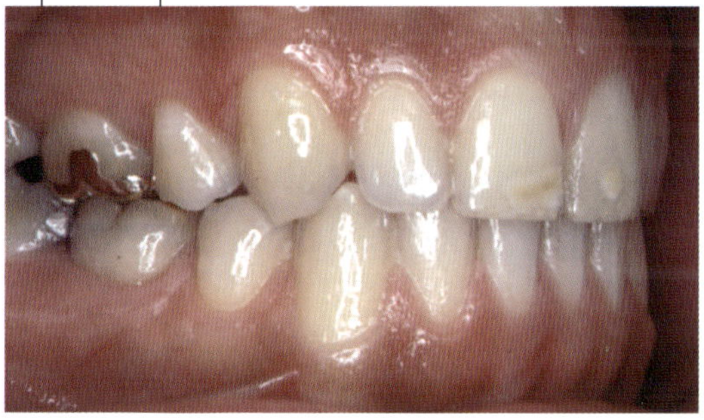

Figs. 2-70 & 2-71
Occlusion after a four extraction (first premolars) treatment.

- In the matter of extractions versus non-extractions there was a book by Duterloo with some famous orthodontists' opinions. For example:
- A. Gianelly: even though in many cases an early treatment can avoid extractions, there are some cases where they are necessary.
- D. Grobéty: even though he treats many cases with extractions, he admits that they can be avoided by using orthopaedic appliances in patients who are willing to cooperate.
- D. Grummons: proclination of the incisors, molar rotation, changing the curve of Wilson etc. can avoid extractions in 90% of the cases.
- N.M. Cetlin: it is also possible to carry out treatment without extractions on adult patients affected by crowding and a high value of vertical angles.
- R. Slavicek: whether to extract or not depends on an accurate diagnosis.
- T.E. Christie: it is actually possible to predict the growth, to move the teeth in all directions, to expand the dental arches, to change the oral environment. Therefore, the only reason for extractions is that, when the teeth have finished growing, there should be enough available space for a good alignment.
- W. Stockli: changing vertical, transverse, sagittal dimensions and functional appliances can be helpful to reduce the extractive treatments in borderline cases.

HOW TO GAIN SPACE DISTALLY (MOLAR DISTALIZATION)

Lower molars

The main indication to move lower molars distally is when they are mesially displaced. Otherwise, only Cetlin[48] with his technique suggests the use of a lip bumper to gain space by moving molars distally. Extraoral tractions are not used because, among other things, they can cause TMJ problems.

Upper molars

There are many ways to obtain a distal displacement of maxillary molars. When the patients are willing to cooperate, applying extraoral traction (Fig. 2-72) is a well-known method.

KLOEHN HEADGEAR (FIG. 2-72A)[136]

For a bodily distalization, extraoral arms are bent to obtain a vector of force passing through the centre of resistance.

Average application time: 12–14 hours a day.

Average force: 150 g per side.

For a more effective distal displacement of upper molars, Cetlin suggests the use of traction alternated to an acrylic plate with springs (Fig. 2-72b). This way the force is applied all day long.

To make the use of springs easier: three days before the first application of the plate he suggests widening the interdental space by putting separating elastics mesial to molars.

He also says that it is possible to obtain a bodily molar distalization of 5–6 mm in 4–8 months.

Other authors use different spring systems on edgewise appliances. However, keep in mind that every action is followed by a reaction. Therefore, when the goal is represented by the molar displacement it is important not to have an undesired movement of other teeth.

To avoid that, it is necessary to make sure to reinforce the anchorage units with, for example, a Nance button, intermaxillary elastics or micro implants (Fig. 2-73).

2-72

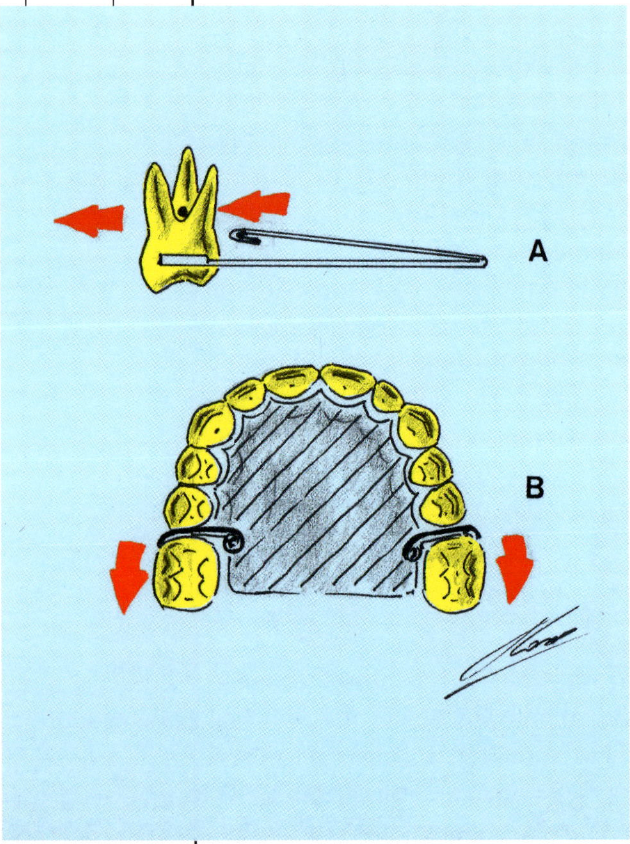

2-73

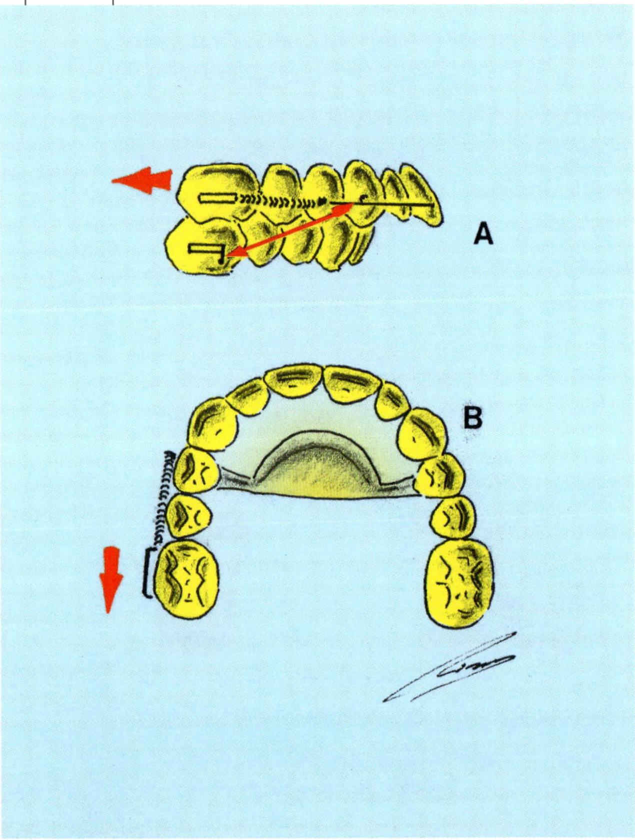

DISTALIZATION OF UPPER MOLARS WITH NON-COMPLIANCE APPLIANCES

The extraoral tractions alone or combined with other appliances can lead to good results. However, they also have a weak spot: the patient's cooperation. In order to bypass the problem of a lack of cooperation, a family of no-compliance appliances for upper molar distalization has been created: Distal Jet, First Class, Pendulum, etc..

These are basically fixed appliances with molar-premolar bands and palatal compressed coil springs which push molars distally. Wide spaces open partially because of molar distalization and partially because of upper incisor proclination (loss of anchorage).

To minimize the loss of anchorage usually there is some type of structure just like the Nance button. (Fig. 2-91). The button is also important for retaining the molars in the new position. This way it is possible to prevent a relapse by letting the frontal teeth move back.

These appliances are usually presented with the promise of great results and, of course, the end of extraction treatments. *But is it really that easy or are there still a lot of questions requiring an answer?* For example, *how much can we distalize the upper molars? Can that be done at any age and for all malocclusions?*

Gianelly[3**] reminds us that the first upper molars can be distally displaced by 1 mm a month easily before the second molar eruption. *After then it is more difficult.*

Ngantung et al.[4**] show the following data:

- **Force**: 240 g per side
- **Average age of treatment**: 12.8 ± 2.2 years
- **Total duration of treatment**: 25.7 ± 3.9 months
- **Class II molars relationship not more than** 3–4 mm
- **Average first molar distalization**: 2.1 ± 1.8 mm

The results of this study indicate that the Distal Jet is effective in distally displacing the first upper molars. Unfortunately, just like with other devices (Pendulum, Jones Jig), there is a lack of anterior anchorage. *Therefore, its reinforcement with intermaxillary elastics and extraoral traction is often necessary.*

Kizinger et al.[5**] conclude that the best period to begin a first maxillary molar distalization is before the second molar eruption. After which it is strongly recommended to carry out the germectomy of the third molar

Angelieri et al.[6**] reminded us that by 2006 there had been only seven clinical communications on the effects of the Pendulum appliance and the consequent loss of anchorage, and that there had only been one article about the Pendulum effects after an orthodontic treatment: an increase in the lower facial height with clockwise mandibular rotation was reported.

Together with molar distalization there is anterior teeth proclination. For its correction an anchorage reinforcement with a Nance button and extraoral traction is recommended. The clinician then faces the challenge of distally displacing the anterior teeth while maintaining the molars in 1st Class. In this case, it is often necessary to have a willing, compliant patient.

ARE WE ALWAYS TALKING ABOUT NON-COMPLIANCE APPLIANCES?

At the end of the treatment the molars have a Class I relationship. However, a lateral cephalogram will show that they moved forward probably because they followed a new mandibular position.

CONCLUSIONS

I am not against non-compliance appliances, I use them in selected cases (Figs. 2-88 to 2-102), but I think the trend is to exaggerate their results through advertising. *So, once again, I suggest caution.* I personally believe that only with implants is it possible to create real non-compliance devices.

CASE NUMBER 6

Skeletal Class I with dental Class II relationship and lack of space for upper right canine eruption. Non-extraction treatment. An edgewise appliance with the use of Class II elastics gives a good result.

2-74

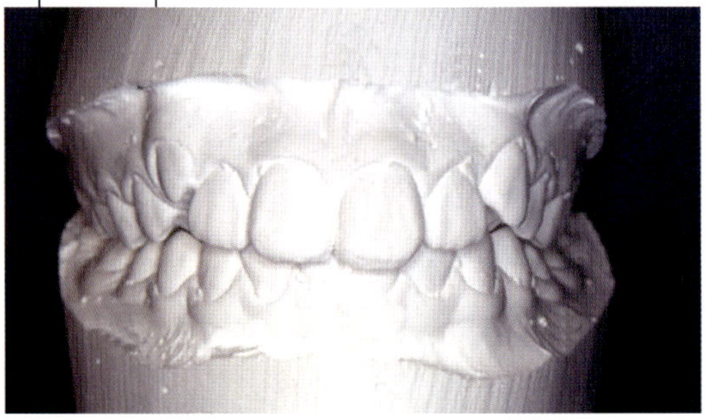

2-76

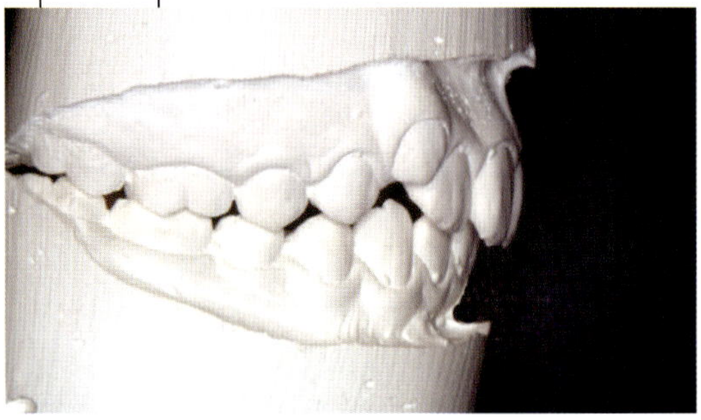

2-75

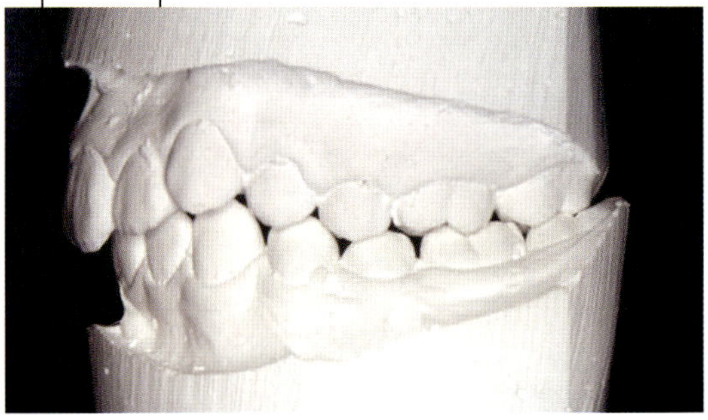

Figs. 2-74 to 2-76
Pre-treatment dental casts.

2-77

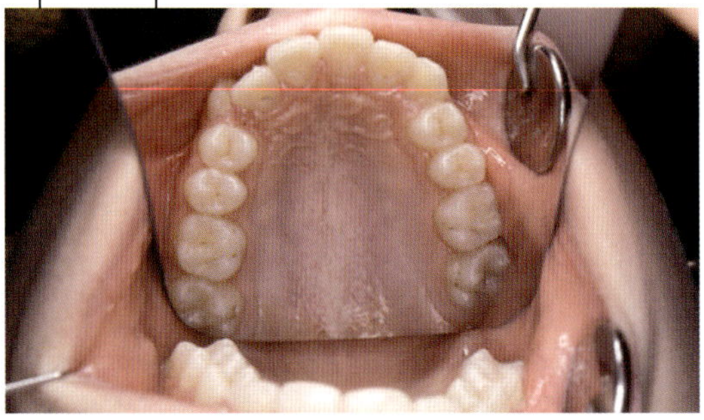

Fig. 2-77
Palatal view of upper dental arch.

2-78

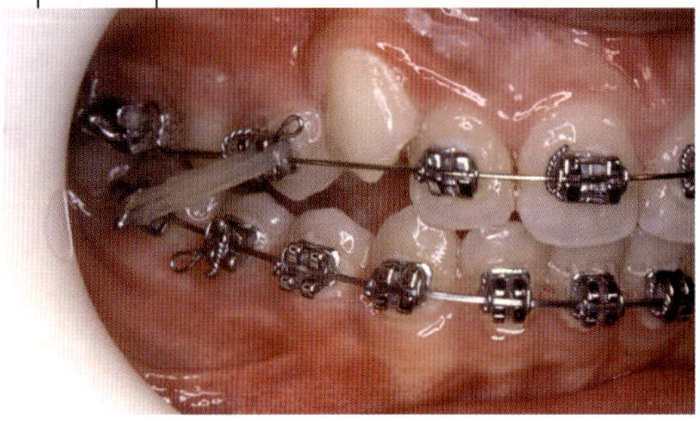

2-79

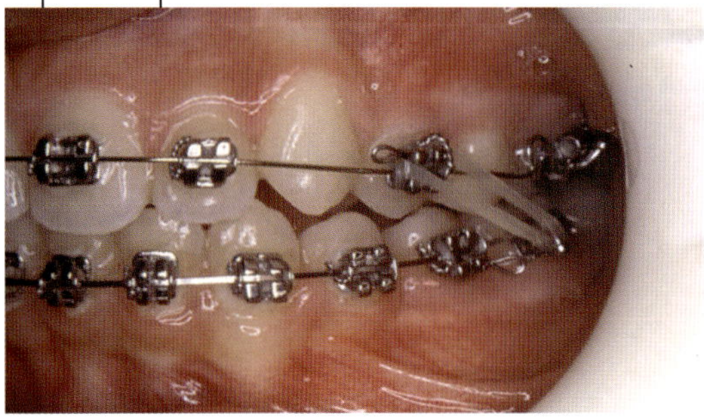

Figs. 2-78 & 2-79
A phase of the treatment.

2-80

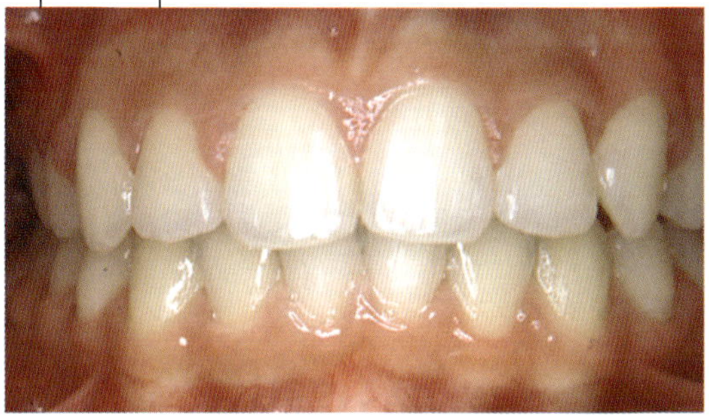

2-81

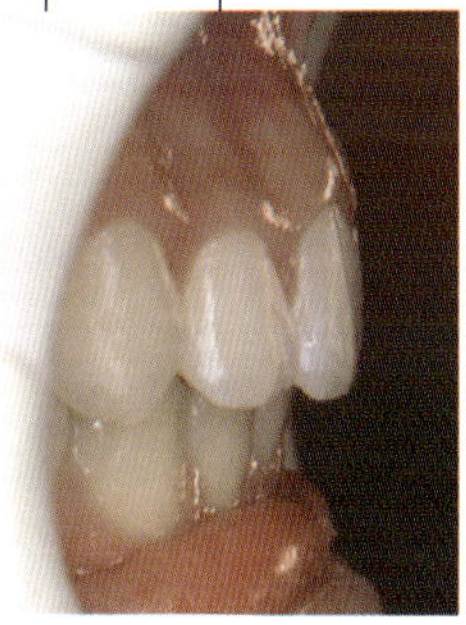

2-82

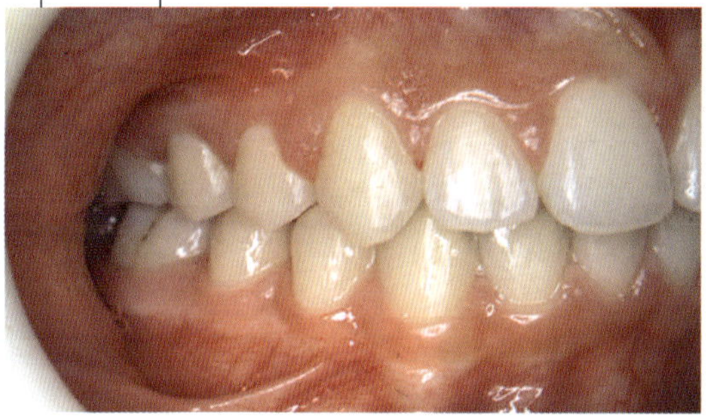

2-83

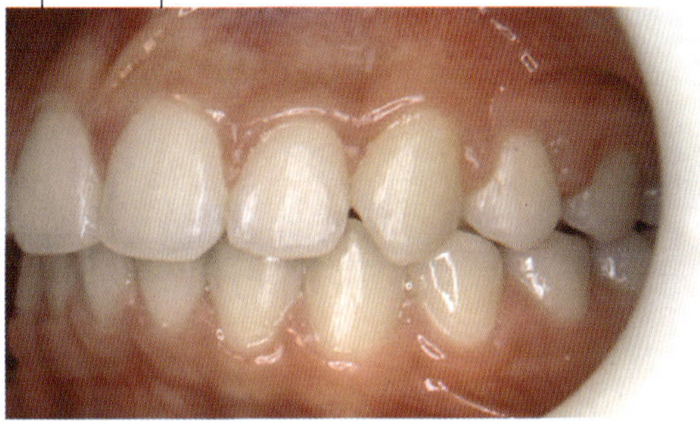

Figs. 2-80 to 2-83
Post treatment occlusion.

2-84

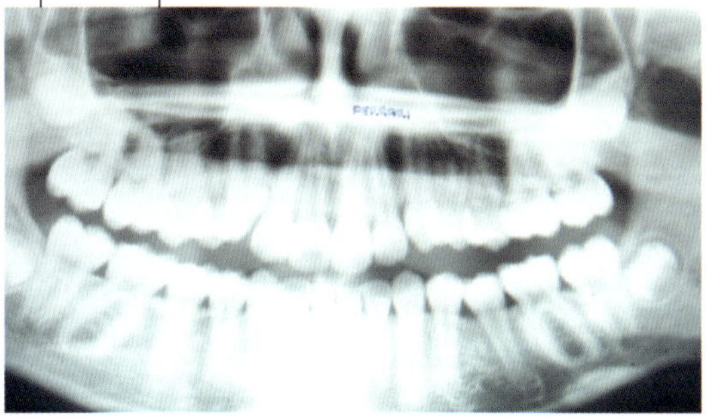

2-85

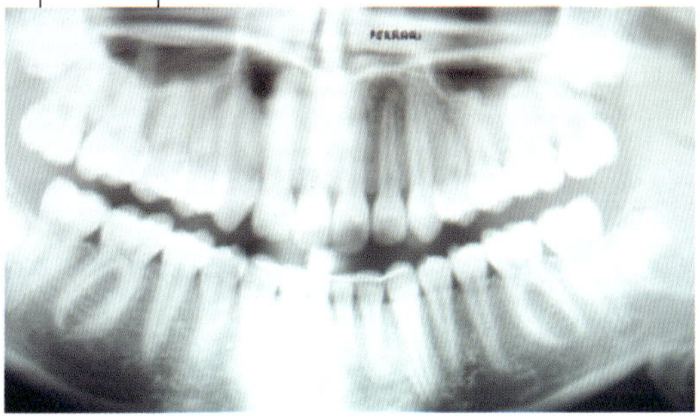

Fig. 2-84
Pre-treatment panoramic radiograph.

Fig. 2-85
Post-treatment panoramic radiograph.

2-86

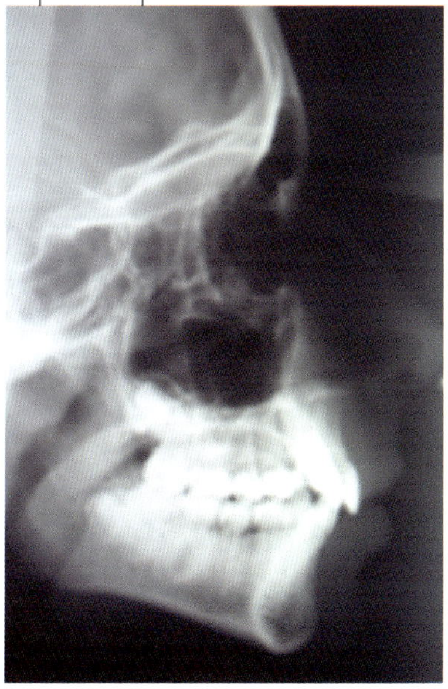

2-87

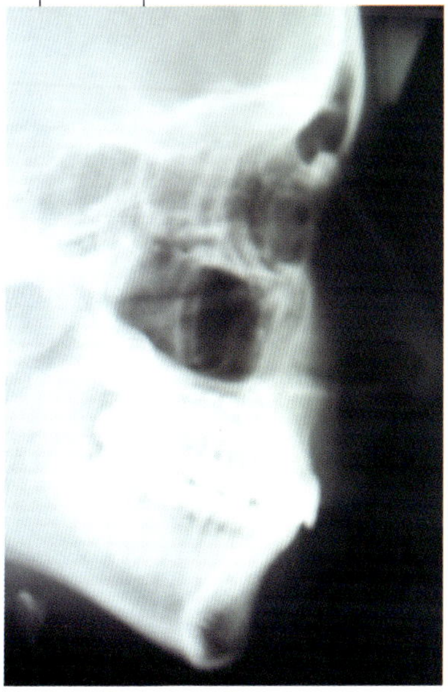

Fig. 2-86
Pre-treatment lateral cephalogram.

Fig. 2- 87
Post treatment lateral cephalogram.

CASE NUMBER 7

Class I borderline between normal and hyperdivergence; it is important not to increase the vertical values. It is also important to avoid an anterior loss of anchorage. The treatment begins with an edgewise appliance on the lower arch followed by the application of a RVD (Rossi–Vigotti distalizer) on the upper arch. Thus Class II elastics can be used to reinforce the anterior anchorage.

2-88

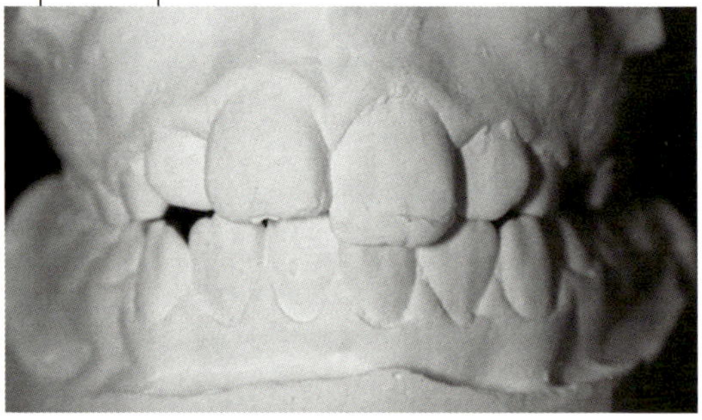

2-89

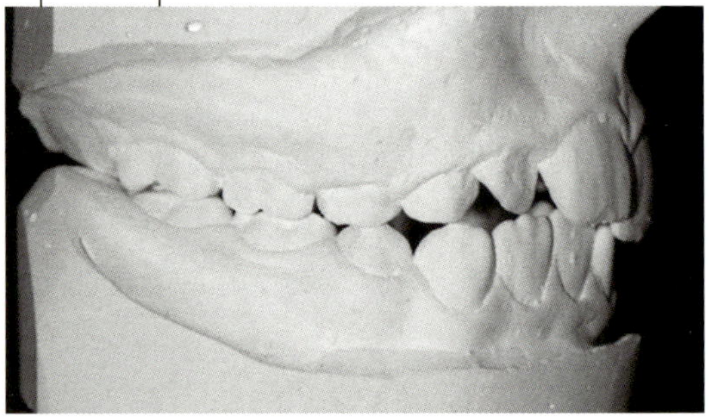

Figs. 2-88 & 2-89 Pre-treatment dental casts.

2-90

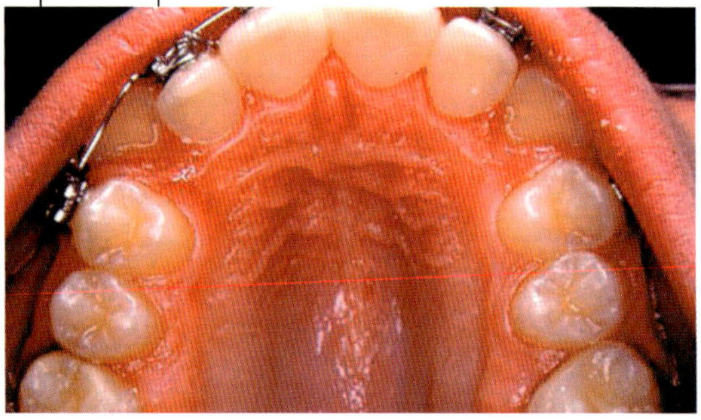

Fig. 2-90 Palatal view.

2-91

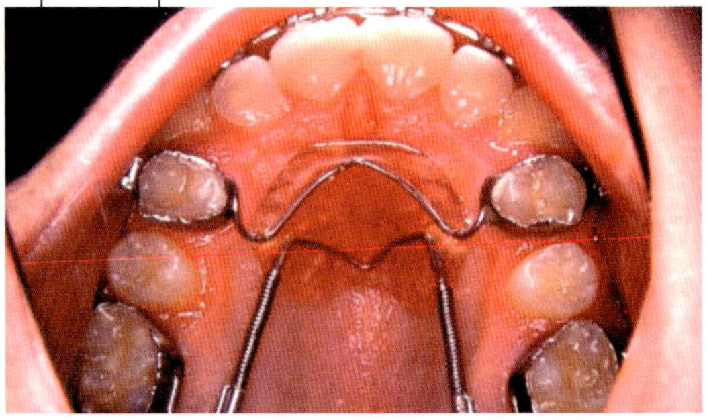

*Fig. 2-91. **RVD** appliance*

2-92

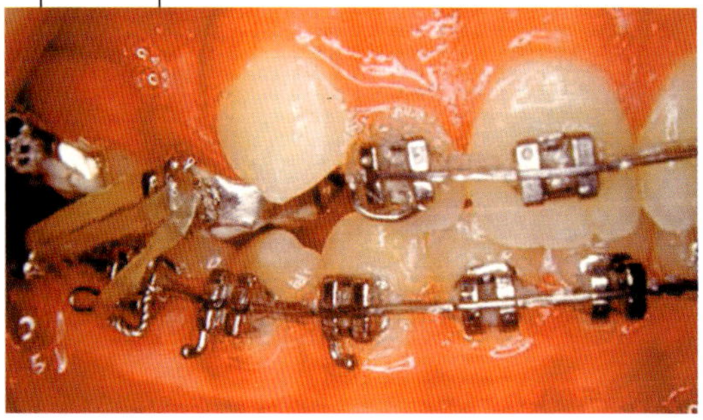

2-93

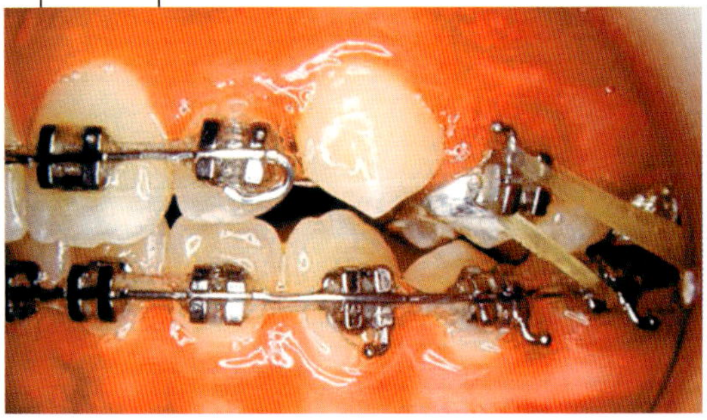

2-94

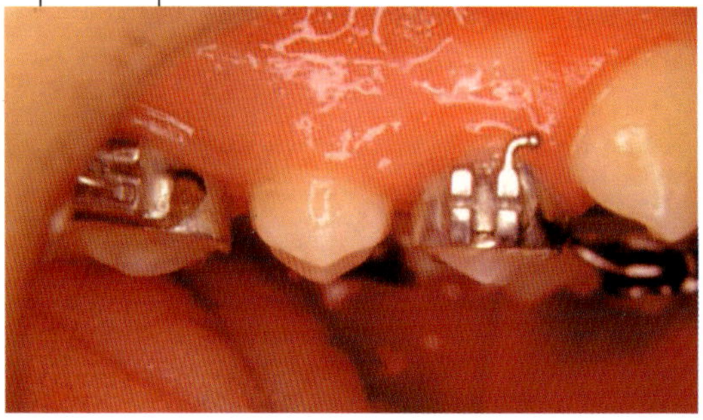

2-95

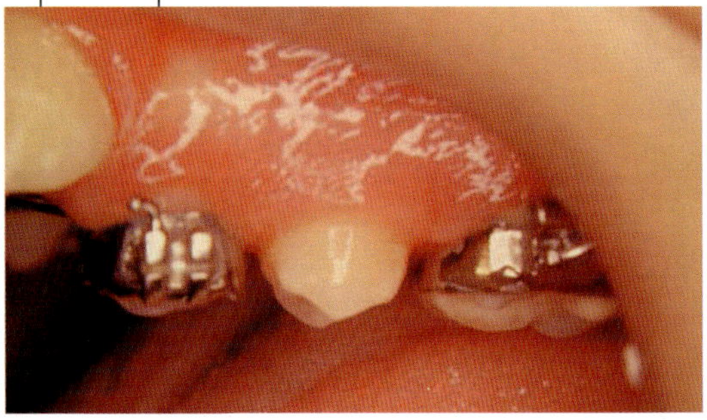

Figs. 2-92 to 2-95 Phases of treatment. Note the spaces opening without loss of anterior anchorage.

2-96

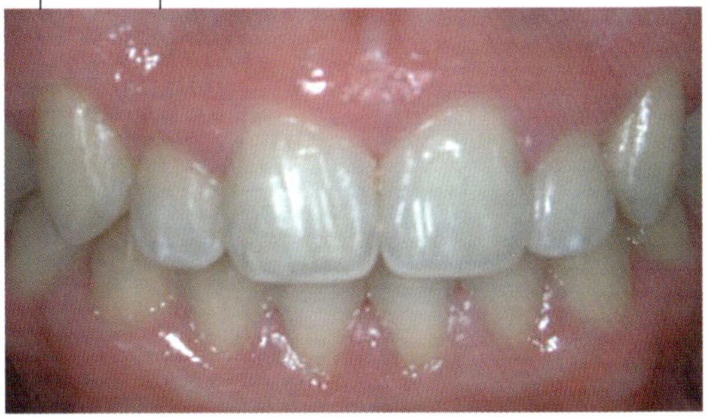

2-97

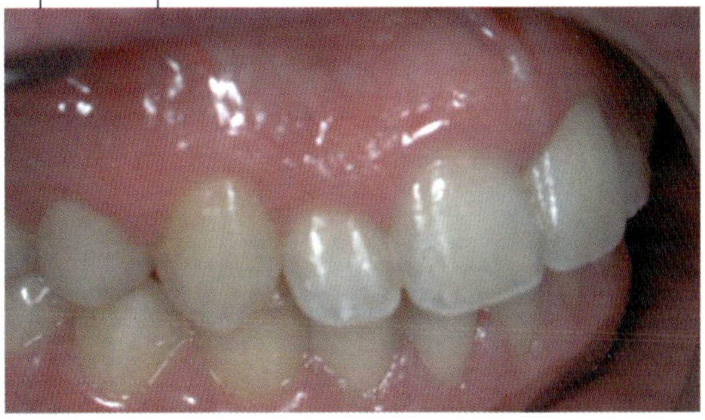

2-98

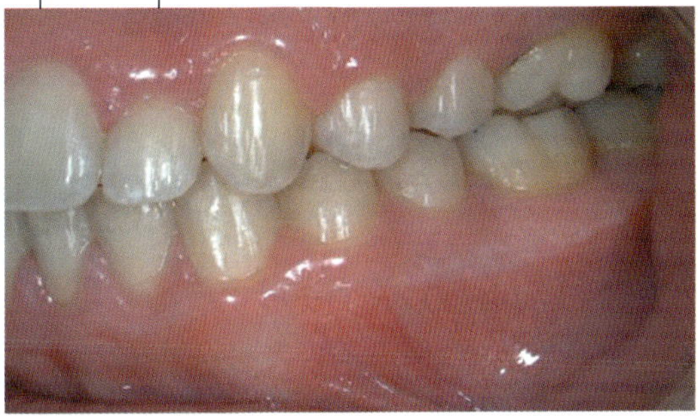

Fig. 2-96 to 2-98
Post treatment occlusion.

2-99

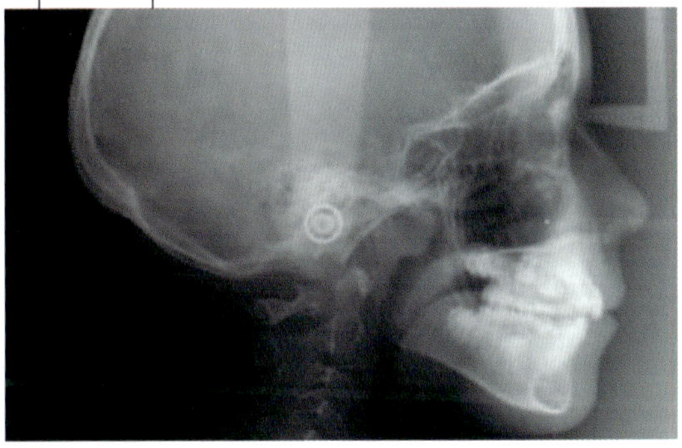

2-100

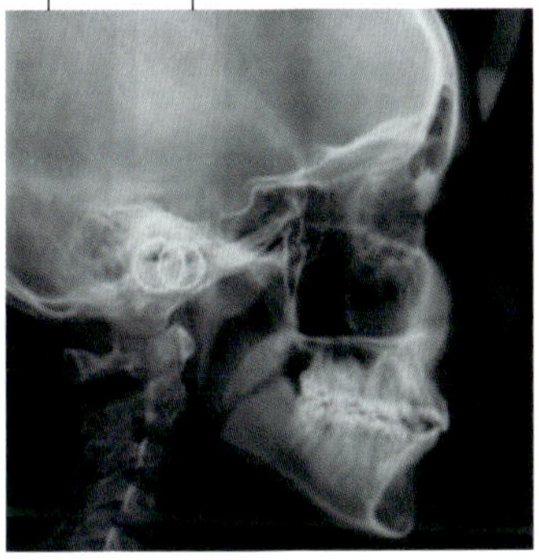

Fig. 2-99
Pre-treatment lateral cephalogram.

Fig. 2-100
Post treament lateral cephalogram. One can see a good relationship between the incisors with no excessive vestibular extension of the front group.

2-101

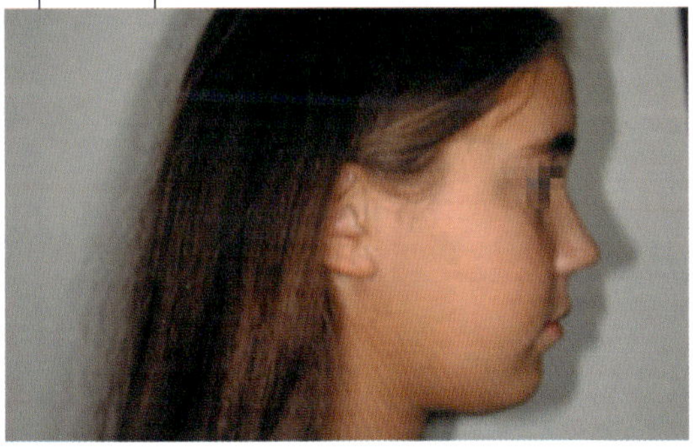

2-102

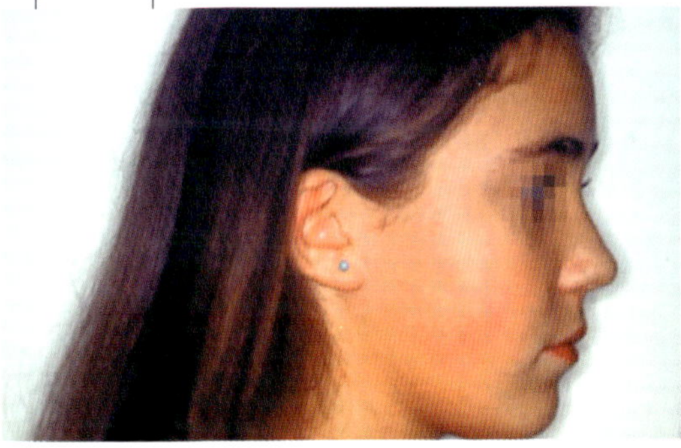

Fig. 2-101
Pre-treatment profile.

Fig. 2-102
Post treatment profile..

LIP BUMPER

Using this appliance, the force of labial musculature is transferred to lower molars to displace them distally. Its correct distance from the teeth is shown in Fig. 2-103: A.

Cetlin [48] indicates three vertical positions related to the lower incisors:-

Top: a distance of 1.5–2 mm from lower incisors. Lower lip goes under the arch and it will upright the molars while avoiding the proclination of lower incisors (Fig. 2-103: B & 2-104).

Middle: a distance of 2 mm from lower incisors. Distalization of lower molars with lower incisor proclination (Fig. 2-103: C & 2-105).

Bottom: a distance of 1.5 mm from lower incisors. Bodily distalization of lower molars without lower incisor proclination (Fig. 103: D & 2-106).

The best results are achieved when the lip bumper is worn 24 hours a day (excluding meals)

a) In early mixed dentition when there is crowding.
b) In late mixed dentition: the ideal time.
c) In permanent dentition as anchorage reinforcement during a treatment with edgewise appliances.

Cetlin states that it is possible to obtain:

a) Uprighting and derotation of lower molars.
b) Lower incisors alignment.
c) Correction of Spee curve.
d) Transverse increase:

from 3 to 3 – 2.7 mm
4 to 4 – 4.5 mm
5 to 5 – 5. mm
6 to 6 – 5.5 mm

However - **Beware of second and third molar impaction!**

2-103

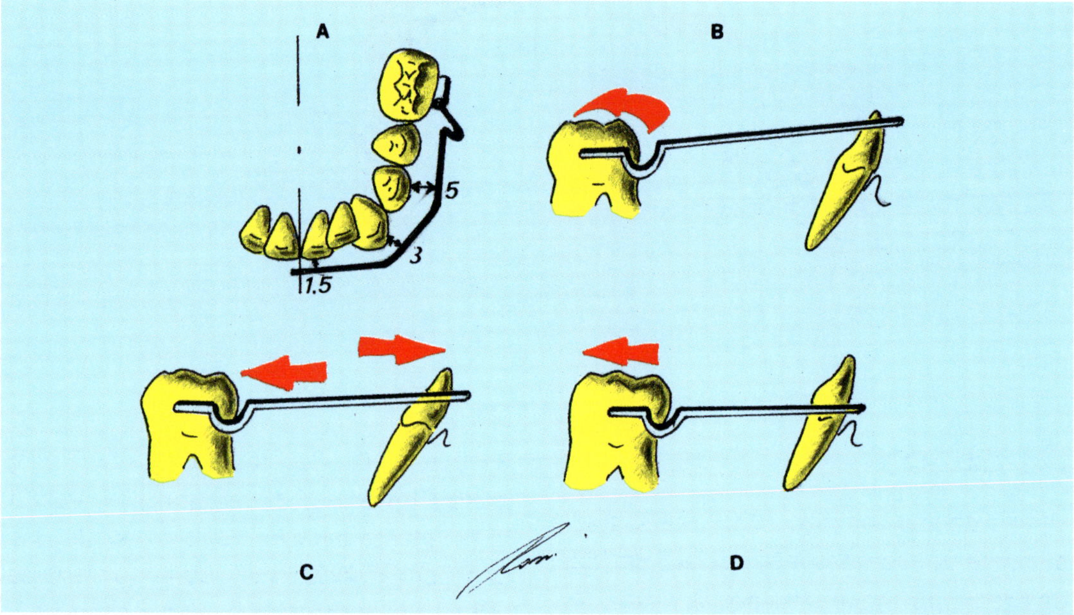

2-104

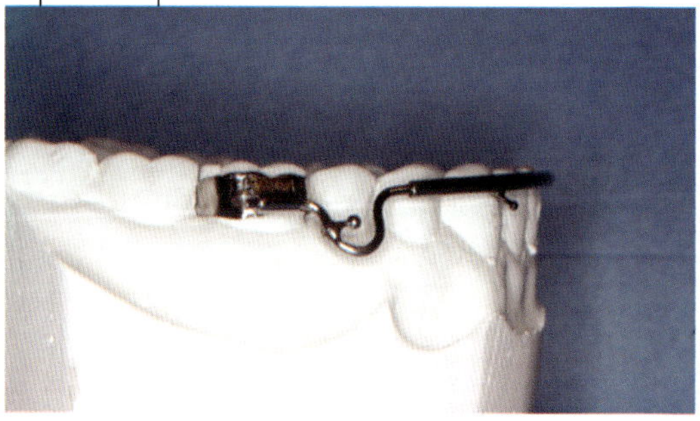

2-105

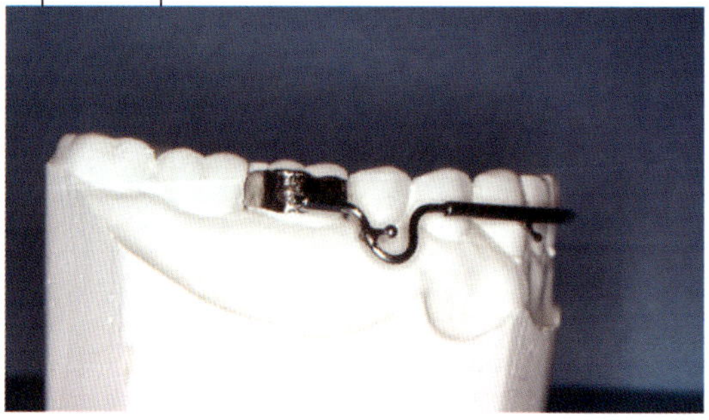

2-106

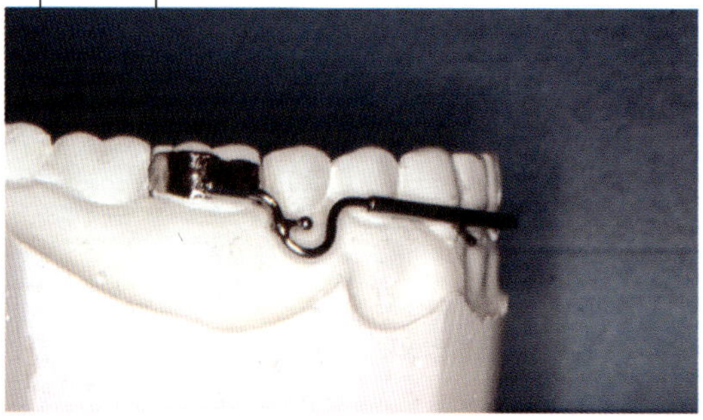

2-107

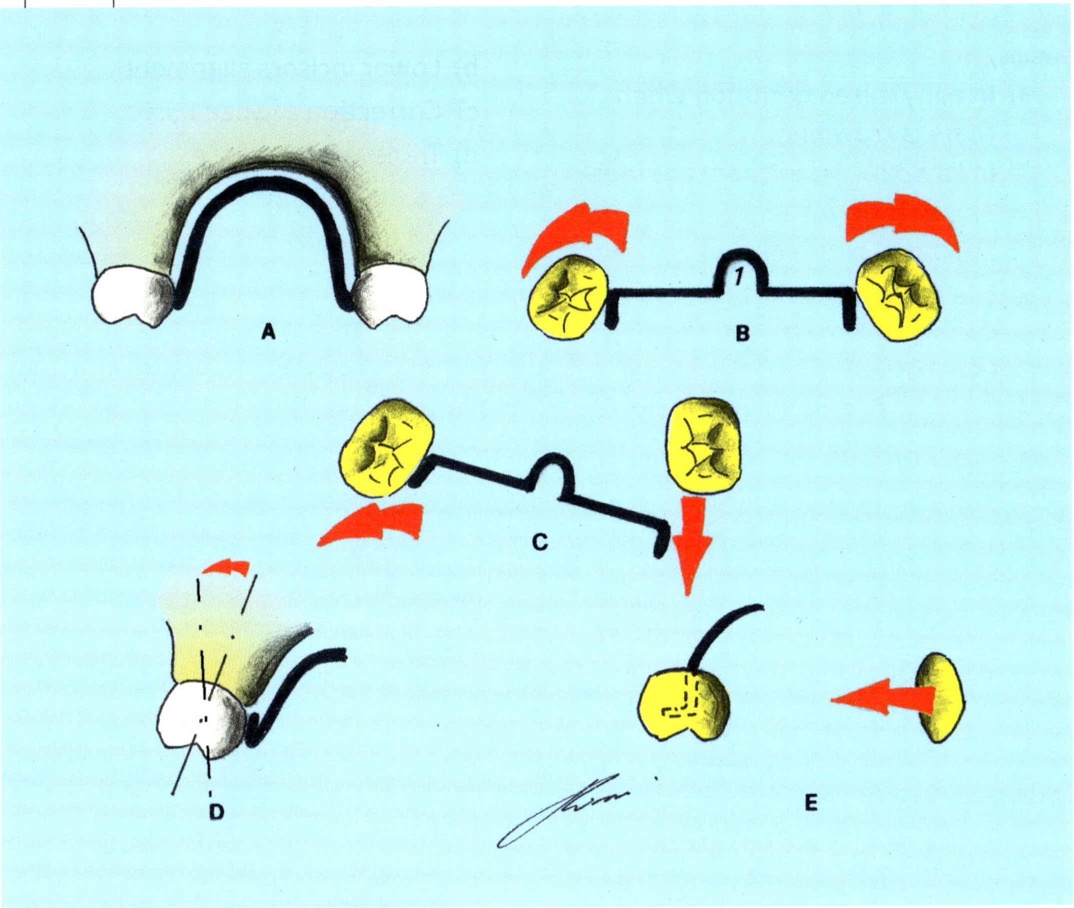

PALATAL BAR

With a palatal bar (Fig. 107: A) placed at a distance of 2 mm from the palatal surface, on the upper molars it is possible to:

a) expand or contract the intermolar distance
b) rotate the molars (Fig. 107: B)
c) displace distally one molar while the other moves mesially: there can also be a rotation of both (Fig. 107: C)
d) produce torque (Fig. 107: D)
e) increase the anchorage (Fig. 107: E).

STRIPPING

In the 1950s, Hudson described a procedure that would allow the gain of some millimetres of space by reducing the interproximal lower incisors dimension. Hudson AL. A study of the effects of mesio-distal reduction of mandibular anterior teeth. Am J Orthod 1956; 42 : 615-24

By the 1970s, Barrer and Paskow[191] suggested lower incisor stripping to prevent their relapse back to crowding, while Peck and Peck[194] fixed some rules for enamel reduction. In the 1980s, with the introduction of bonding and the end of the practice of using bands, Sheridan [226] introduced air rotor stripping on the entire arch, with a resulting gain of space of anything from 4 to 8 mm.

Nowadays stripping not only offers a simple way to control relapses but also gives an opportunity for non-extraction treatment. There are various methods including the use of stripping disks, diamond-coated metal strips, diamond or tungsten burs.

Critics of entire arch enamel reduction claim that it leads to more caries or periodontal problems, however there is no actual evidence for these claims. The general opinion among practitioners suggests an average reduction of 0.10 mm per side (lower incisors and canines), 0.20 mm (upper incisors and canines) and 0.40 mm (molars and premolars).

CONCLUSIONS

This chapter has described the analysis of space, ranging from skeletal and dental expansion to the distalization of teeth and stripping procedures. In particular, the vertical jaw relationship makes an important difference: extractions are more acceptable in a dolico than in a brachy patient. Bearing in mind all these factors, when speaking of extractions versus non-extractions, it is not possible to say (as was the case in the past) that we must remove teeth when, for example, more than 5 mm of space is necessary.

Our aim is to avoid extractions. But the decision does not depend only on numbers. There is also an aesthetic or periodontal evaluation which might suggest extractions when the "numbers" allow a non-extraction treatment. And vice versa.

Other factors influence the choice of a treatment. For example, a non-extractive one usually begins earlier, has a longer duration, needs a cooperative patient and it is often more expensive. Such are the criteria of detailed informed consent where the various possibilities of treatment need to be clearly explained.

Last but not least, I can't ignore that many orthodontists declare that in their practice they themselves abandoned extraction treatment but often their patient, before having braces fitted, would go to a dental surgeon to remove the wisdom teeth. (Especially the lower ones.) In such instances, can we therefore describe it as non-extraction treatment?

SUMMARY

After analysing the dental arch expansion, when it comes to the question "extractions versus non-extractions", please remember that:

a) for 1 mm of lower incisor proclination the space on the lower arch increases by 2 mm
b) to straighten a Spee curve of variable depth, 2–4 mm of space on the dental arch is necessary
c) rotated teeth can occupy both more or less space
d) in general, with a crowding of:
   less than 3 mm: non-extraction
   between 3 and 5 mm: borderline
   more than 5 mm: extraction

However, do not forget what you have read earlier: "numbers" depend on many factors. And if possible, avoid extractions in brachyfacial patients.

NON-EXTRACTION TREATMENT

Usual steps :

a) dental alignment with NiTi arches (Fig. 2-108: A & B)
b) correction of rotations (Fig. 2-108: C)
c) correction of midline with the use of intermaxillary elastics (Fig. 2-108: D)
d) correction of open bites with grids, intermaxillary elastics (Fig. 2-108: E).

EXTRACTION TREATMENT

More common situations:

a) Four extractions. Usually first premolars. Sometimes, for example for problems of verticality, it is better to extract the upper first premolars and the second lower premolars.

2-108

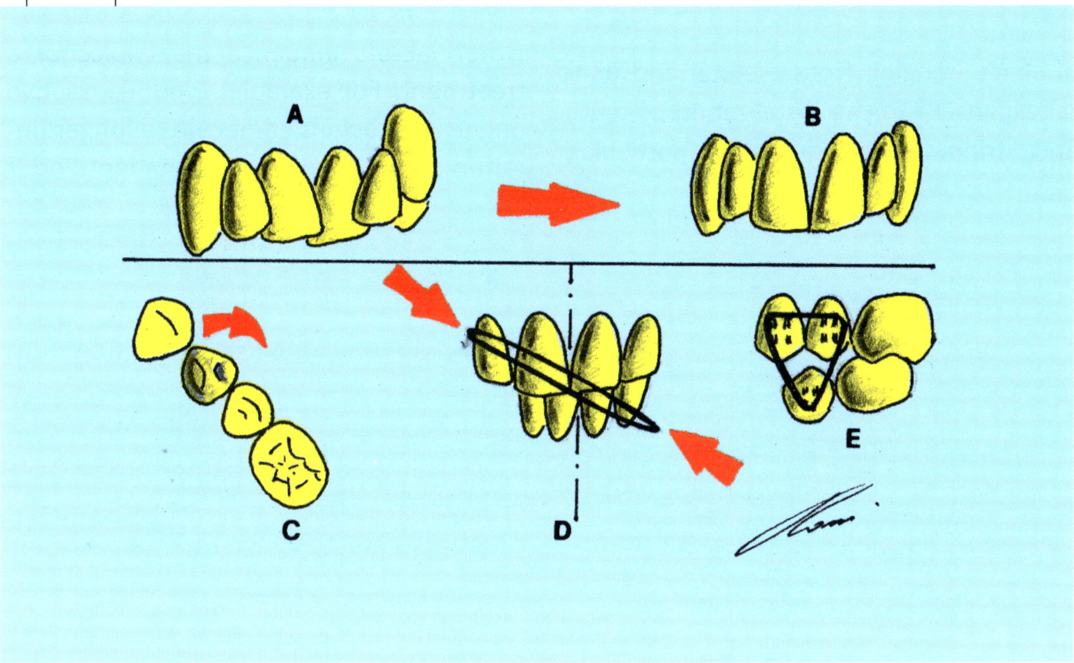

b) Two extractions. Usually upper first premolars in a Class II, lower first premolars in a Class III.

c) One extraction. The more commonly accepted is the extraction of one lower incisor. Otherwise, an asymmetric extraction is acceptable only in exceptional circumstances..

Suggestions regarding the practical application of a fixed appliance:

a) etch the enamel tooth surface, usually 1 minute for permanent teeth, 2 minutes for milk teeth.
b) use 0.18 x 0.25 brackets
c) optimum distance from the occlusal margin (according to Alexander) should be:

Maxillary	Mandible
Central incisors x (3.5 mm)	Central incisors x - 0.5 mm (3)
Lateral incisors x - 0.5 mm (3)	Lateral incisors x - 0.5 mm (3)
Canines x + 0.5 mm (4)	Canines x + 0.5 mm (4)
Premolars x (3.5mm)	Premolars x (3.5 mm)
First molars x - 0.5 mm (3)	First molars x - 0.5 mm (3)
Second molars x - 1.0 mm (2.5)	Second molars x - 0.5 mm (3)

a) the alignment starts with a 0.14 NiTi wire. When there are very crowded arches use a 0.12 NiTi wire
b) begin from distally positioned teeth because the crown of the second upper premolar is often shorter than that of the first premolar. This can influence the correct positioning of the brackets.
c) sometimes it's better to start the treatment on only one arch. The other will follow.
d) In some cases it is convenient not to put the brackets on all the teeth to begin with.
e) beware of undesired movements
f) pay attention to hygiene control and bacterial plaque
g) after the alignment with a:
 0.16 NiTi wire, it is time for stainless steel arches
 0.16 – 0.18 round for sliding mechanics
 0.16 x 0.22 – 0.18 x 0.25 rectangular when torque is needed
h) to open a bite "Spee curve" arches can be useful
i) stabilize after the final treatment for approximately three months.

EXTRACTIONS: WHICH TEETH TO EXTRACT?

When an extraction treatment is planned it is important to remember what Little et al. observed in 1988.[158] A twenty year follow-up of cases treated with four first premolar extraction found varied amounts of lower incisors crowding.
In 1994 Little[159] concluded:

a) When it comes to an extraction treatment, premolars are the most common teeth extracted.
   Even though the results are good with a cephalometric analysis, in only 30% of cases is there long term stability. Therefore, *in order to preserve the premolars, lifelong retention might be necessary.*
b) Serial extractions have long term results similar to those of conventional extractions for premolar treatments.
c) In cases of crowding, the extraction of one or two lower incisors can give more stable results than those treated with premolar extractions.
d) Lateral and anterior expansions of dental arches relapse in many cases. Only 10% maintain long term results that are clinically acceptable.

THIRD MOLARS

Many dentists believe that third molars cause anterior dental crowding, however, there is no evidence for this. Other factors such as growth, muscle forces or the anatomy of the patient probably affect anterior dental crowding as well.
If third molar extraction does not prevent possible anterior crowding, it can offer a few millimetres of space for a second molar distalization. In those cases where there is no space for a third molar eruption Ricketts [207] suggests its germectomy.
During the analysis of 160 orthodontically treated cases, Richardson[212] found more than 50% unerupted third molars. There were fewer in those cases treated with premolar extraction. All third molars erupted after first and second molar extractions.

FIRST MOLARS

There are not many cases where the first molars, considered the keystones of occlusion, are extracted. For many authors such as Giannì[106] first molar extraction is a procedure which is very useful to correct a skeletal open bite - by removing distal contacts there is a counterclockwise rotation of the mandible with a lowering of the facial height.
In cases where the first molars are decayed and the other molars have not yet erupted, their extraction could be an interesting choice considering that the second and third molars have many chances to erupt and close the extraction space with a bodily movement. And if an extraction is performed at a later time, the second and third molars will more easily undergo mesial tipping.

SECOND MOLARS

The removal of second molars to facilitate the eruption of third molars has been recommended by several authors..[126,129, 154, 156] Certainly the problems faced are not the same as with first molar extraction. But one has to be careful nonetheless – the third molar can behave unpredictably. There are recorded cases of "crazy" growth where the wisdom tooth changes its direction of eruption, for example by moving distally. It is not clear why this happens but the consequence can be the loss of two teeth.
According to Cryer,[58] when the third molar develops with an inclination of 30° or less against the second molar long axis, and the crown is calcified, then the likelihood of a good eruption is very high.

CASE NUMBER 8

Class I with crowding in an 11 year old patient is shown in Fig 2-109. An extraction treatment is planned. Usually four premolars would be extracted but the first molars are decayed and the third molars are evident on the X-ray.

By extracting the first molars there is an excellent result - together with the mesial bodily movement of the second molars enough space for third molar eruption can be created.

2-109

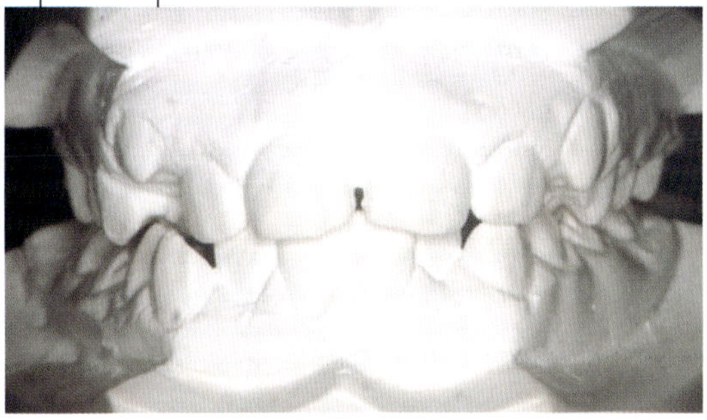

2-110

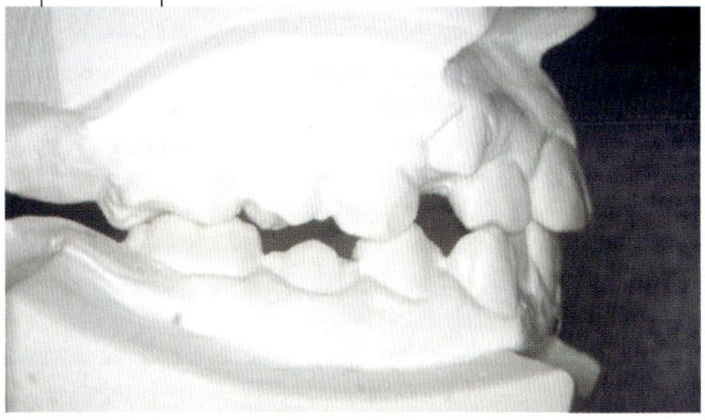

2-111

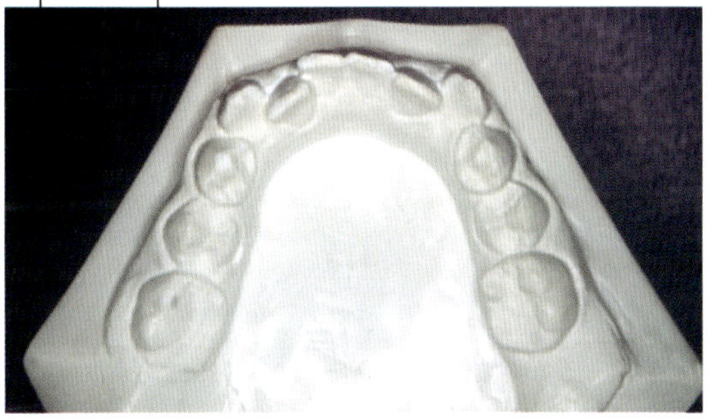

2-112

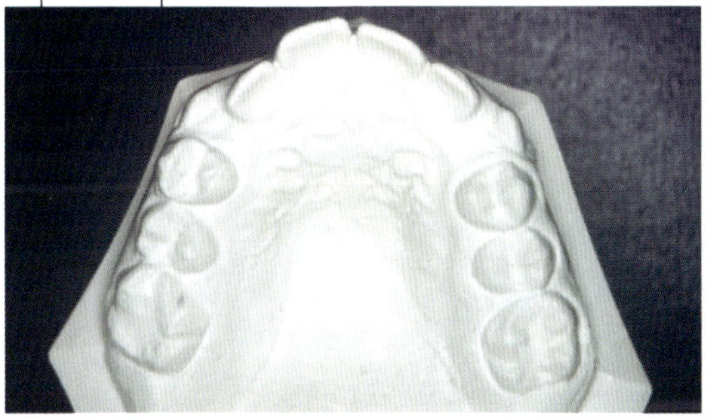

Figs. 2-109 to 2-112 Pre treatment dental casts.

2-113

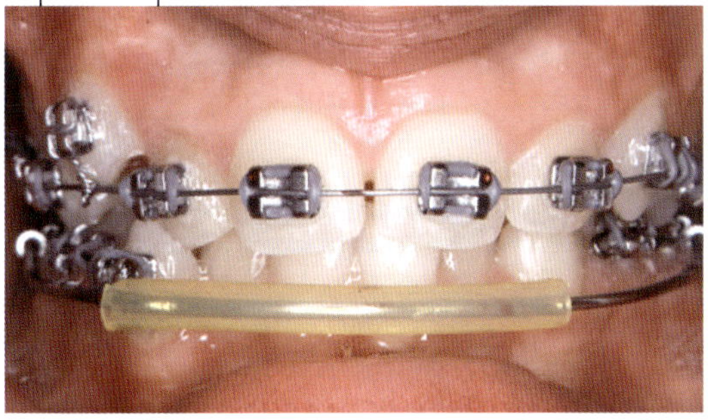

2-114

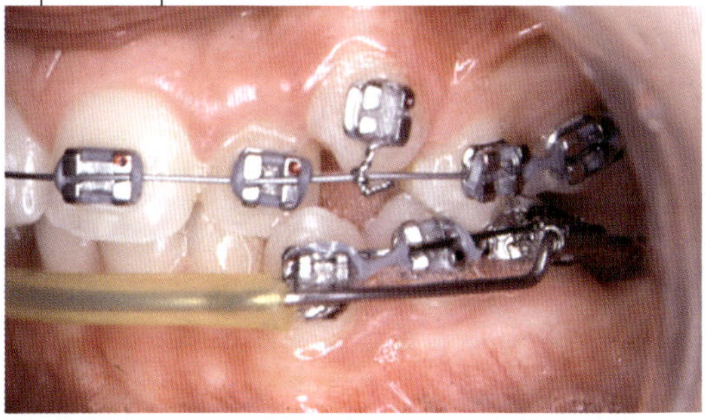

Figs. 2-113 & 2-114 Clinical phase. After the molars' extraction, a lip bumper is used to distalize lower premolars.

2-115

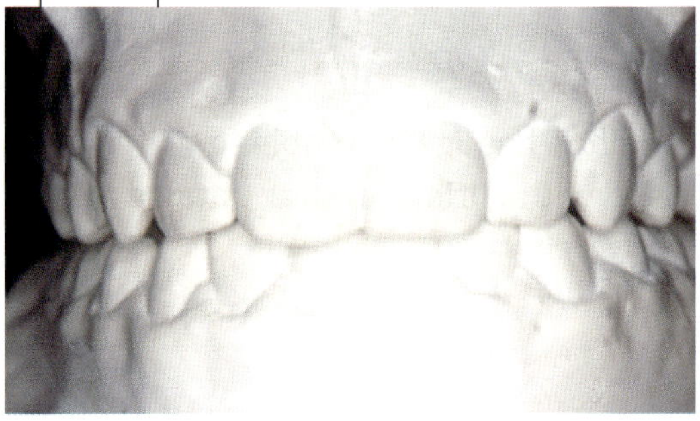

2-116

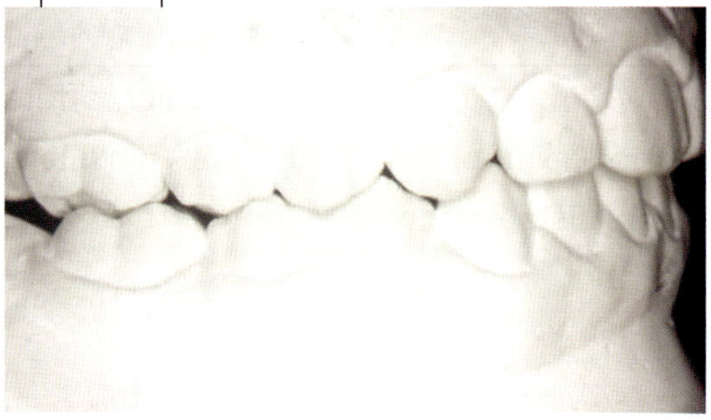

2-117

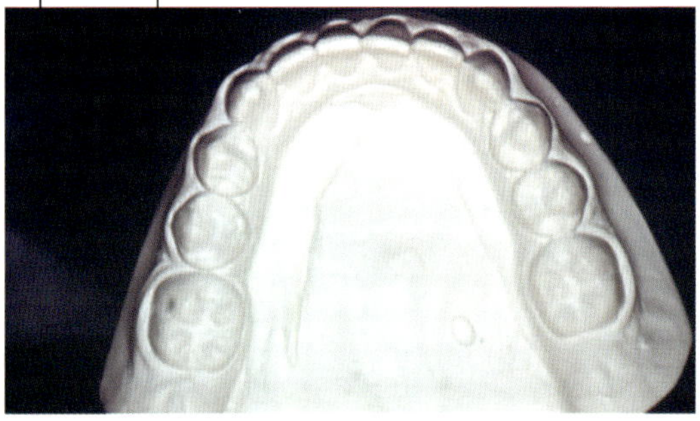

2-118

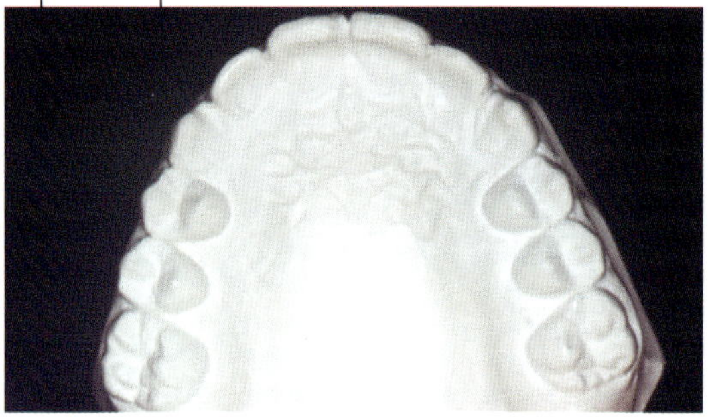

Figs. 2-115 to 2-118
Post treatment dental casts.

2-119

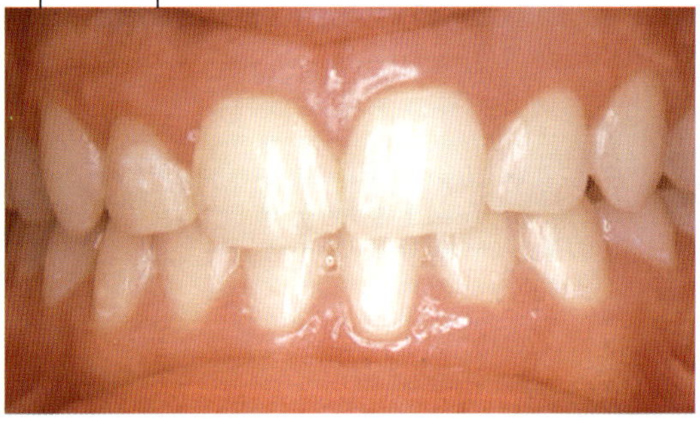

2-120

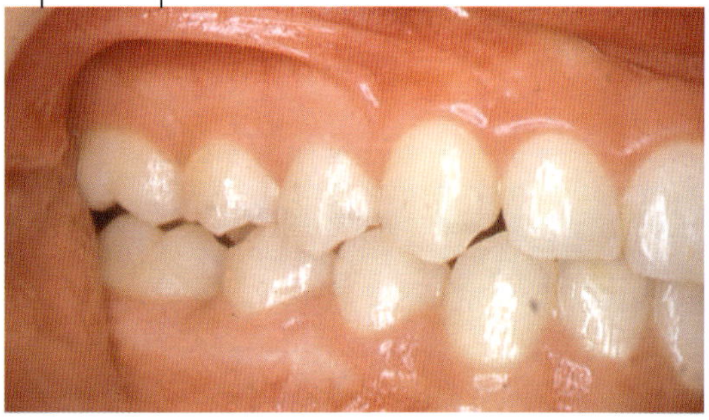

Figs. 2-119 & 2-120
Post treatment occlusion.

2-121

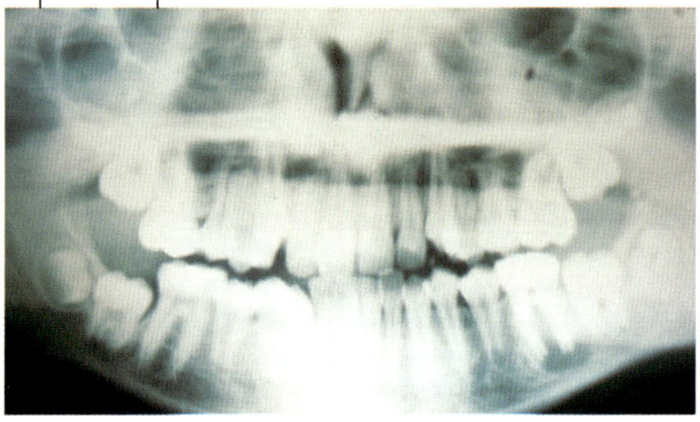

2-122

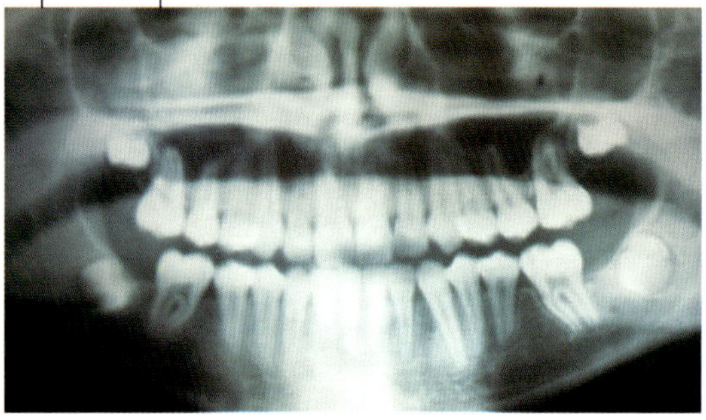

Fig. 2-121
Pre-treatment panoramic X ray.

Fig. 2-122
Post-treatment panoramic X ray. Notice the bodily eruption of second molars and the space available for third molars.

2-123

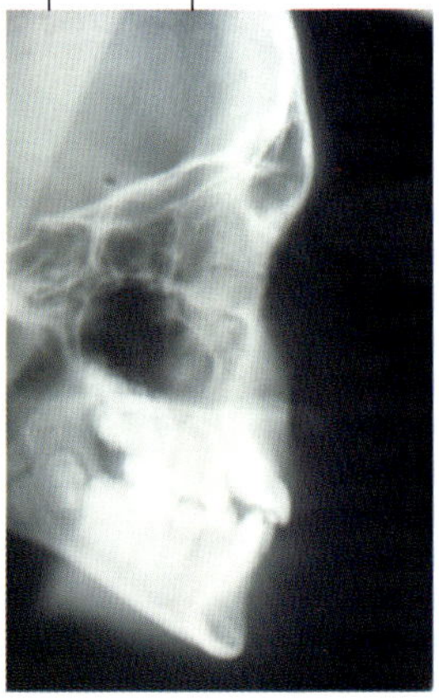

2-124

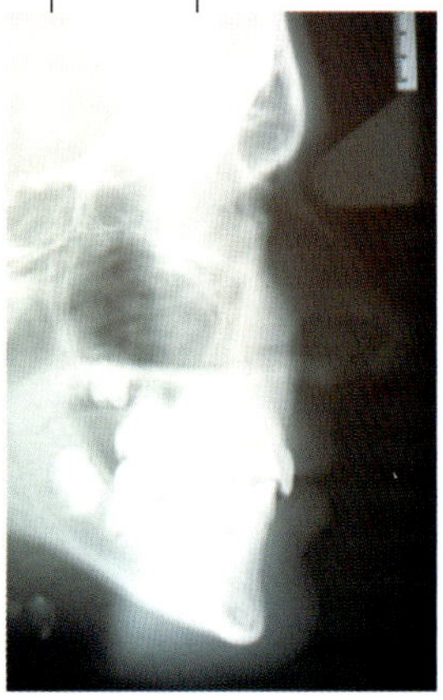

Fig. 2-123
Pre-treatment lateral cephalogram.

Fig. 2-124
Post-treatment lateral cephalogram.

CASE NUMBER 9

Case number 9 is a Class II division 2 shown in a Class I context , which offers a good example of "en masse" maxillary teeth distalization after upper third molars' extraction.

In this case the 22 year old patient refuses the simpler solution of two upper first premolars extraction and wants to try the much more difficult treatment described.

A Klohen headgear combined with palatal plate with spring (Cetlin) obtained 3mm of distalization per side. The application time was of 18-20 hours a day for 18 months.

Treatments like this can be successful only with an extremely cooperative patient.

2-125

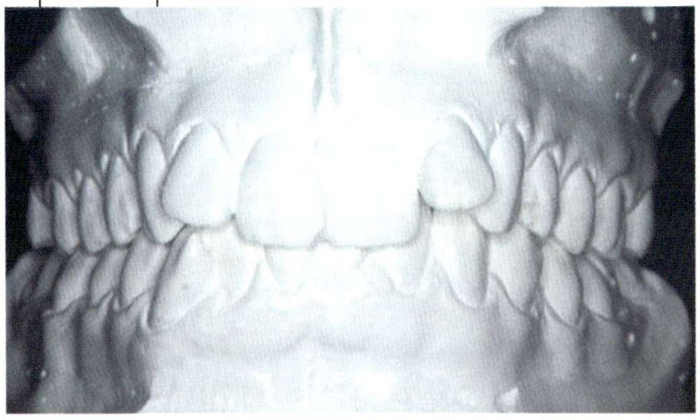

2-126

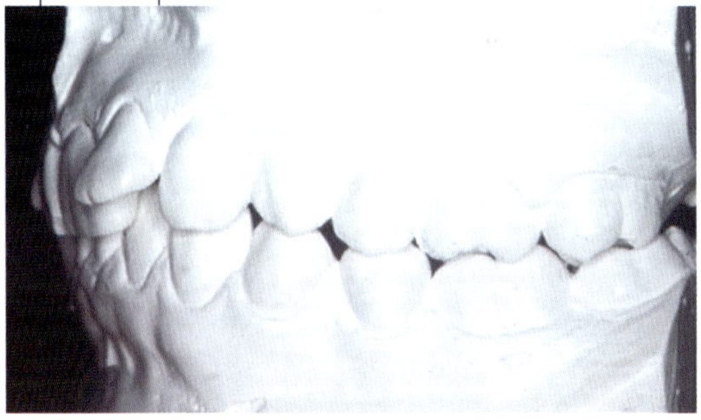

Figs. 2-125 & 2-126
Pre-treatment casts.

2-127

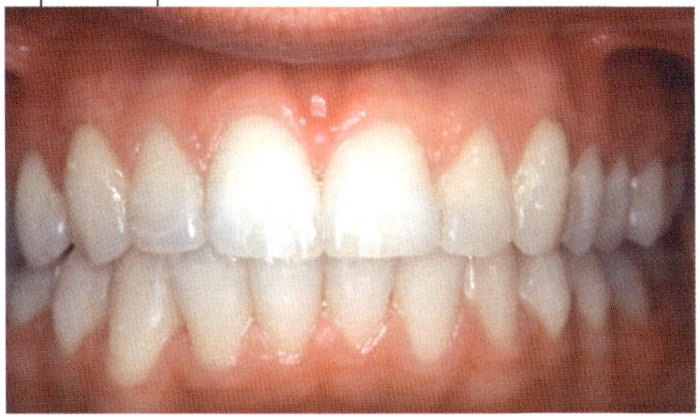

2-128

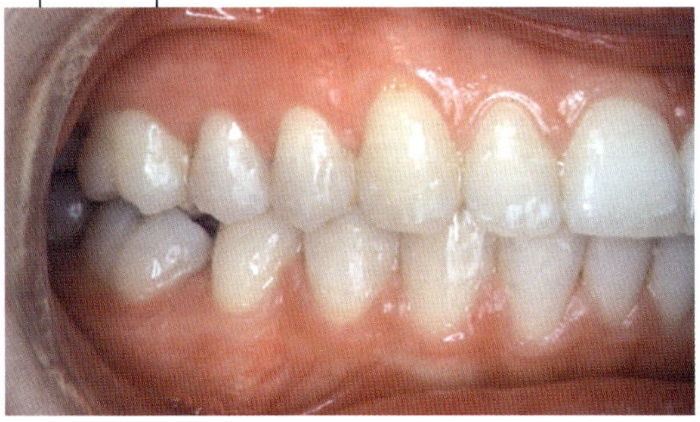

2-129

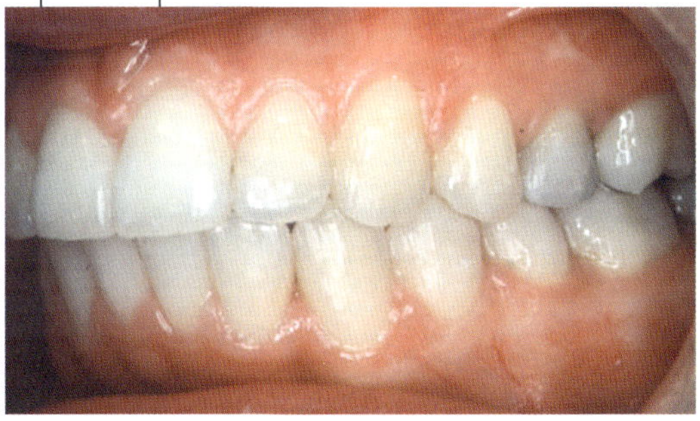

Figs. 2-127 to 2-129
Post-treatment occlusion.

2-130

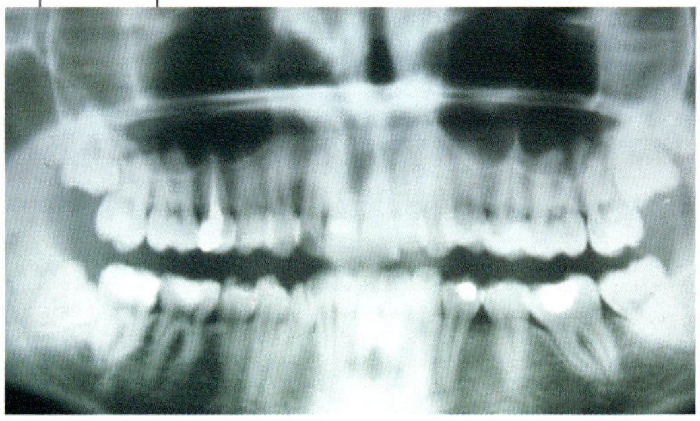

2-131

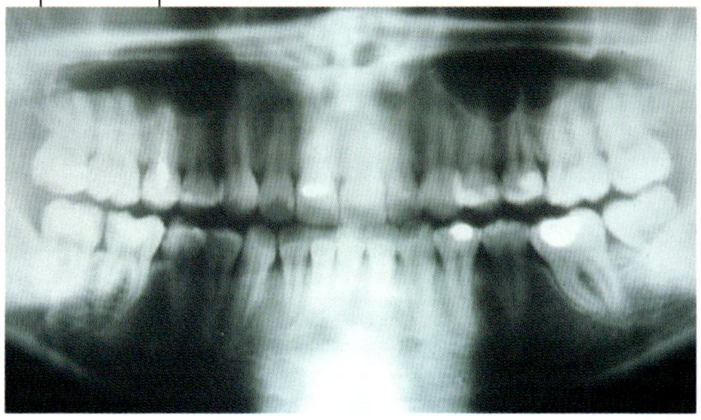

Fig. 2-130
Pre-treatment panoramic X ray.

Fig. 2-131
Post-treatment panoramic X ray.

2-132

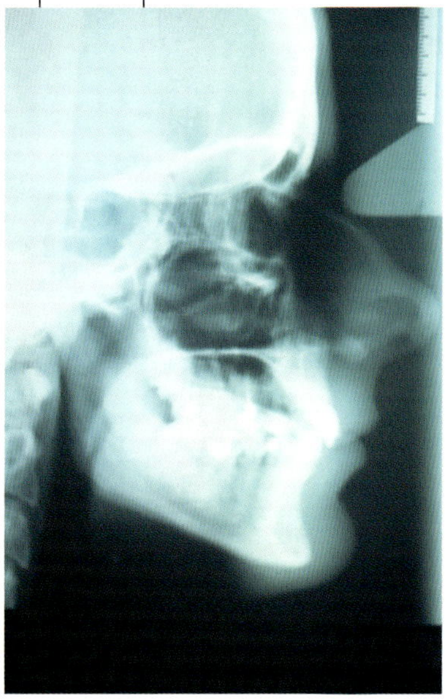

2-133

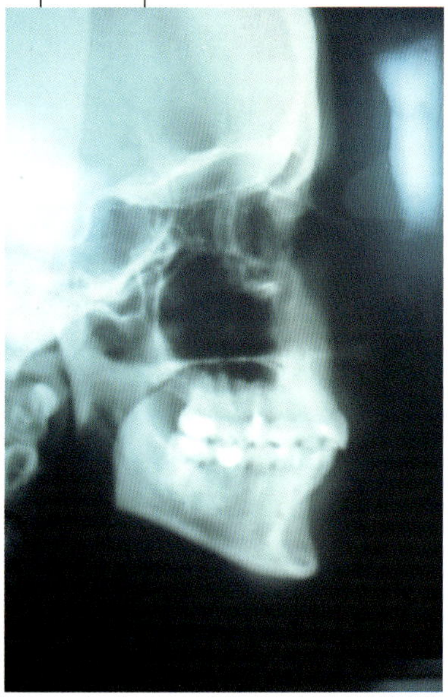

Fig. 2-132
Pre-treatment lateral cephalogram

Fig. 2-133
Post-treatment lateral cephalogram

CASE NUMBER 10

Class I with upper canine displacement. There is a lack of space for their alignment. After discussing the situation with the relatives of the 11 year old patient, the upper second molars are extracted in order to gain space distally.

With a fixed appliance on both arches, a compressed coil spring between the maxillary lateral incisors and first premolars and Class II elastics, there is a 3 mm distalization of the upper first molars and premolars. The treatment time was 20 months.

2-134

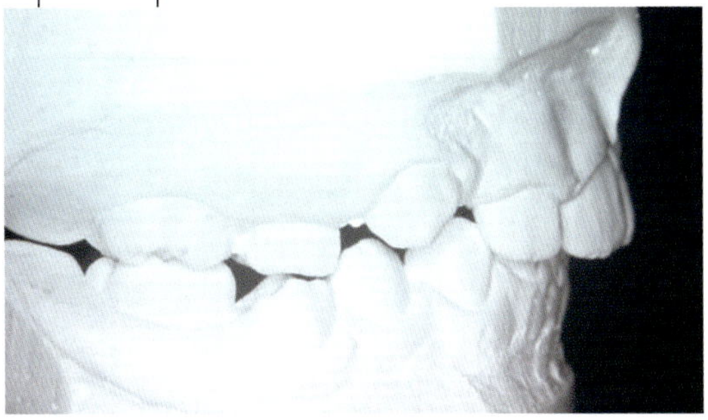

2-135

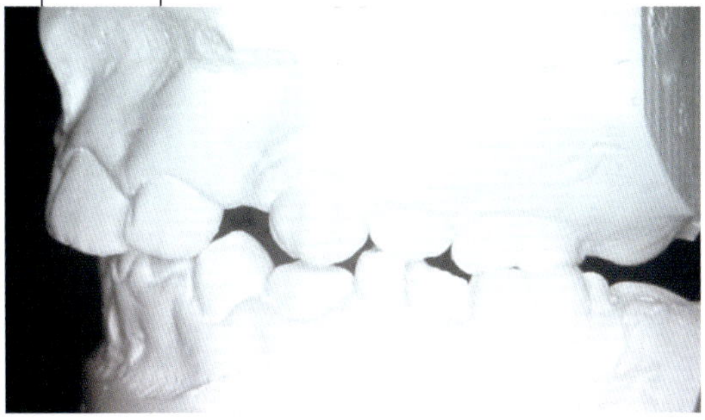

2-136

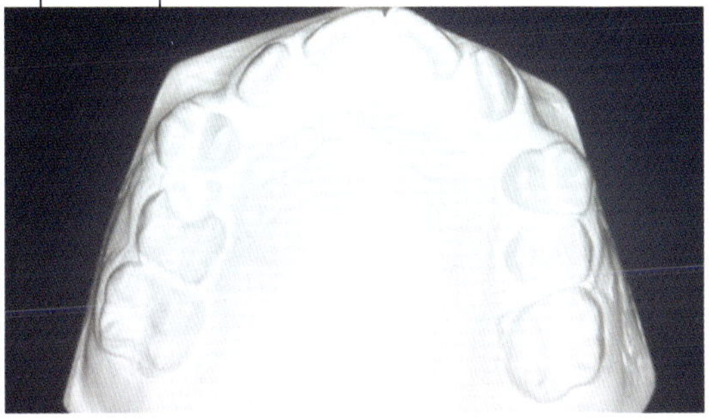

2-137

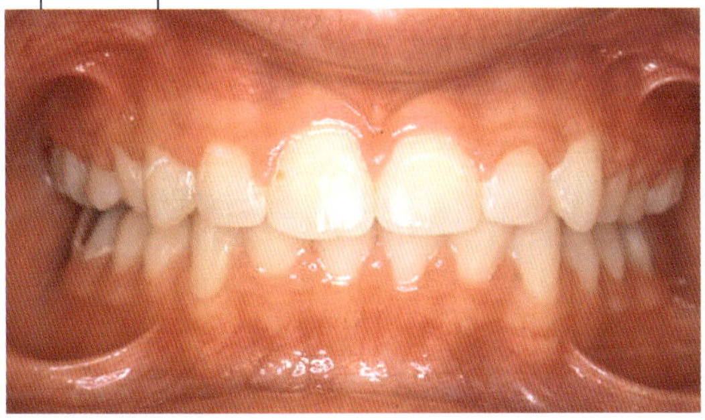

2-138

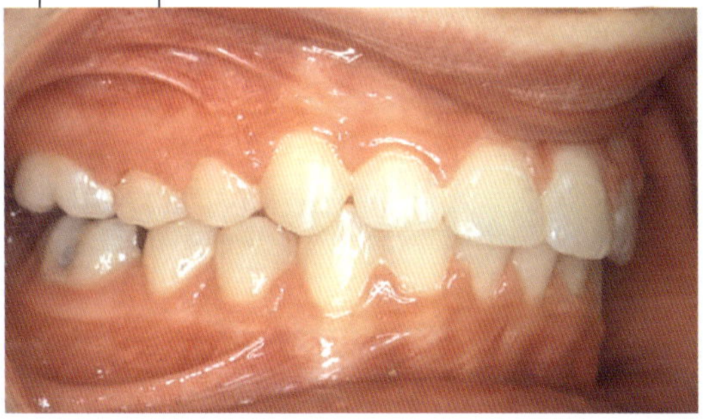

2-139

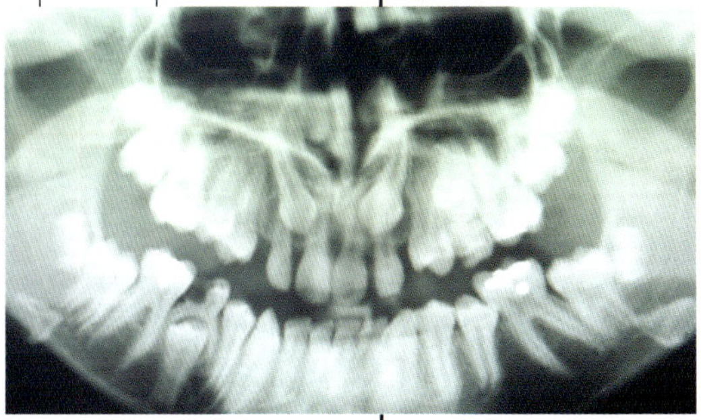

2-141

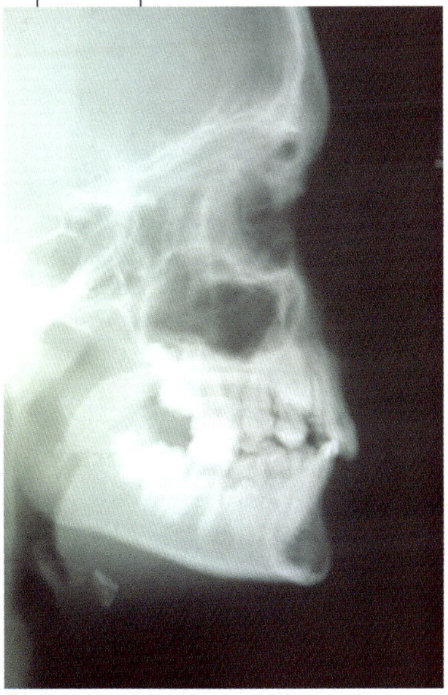

2-142

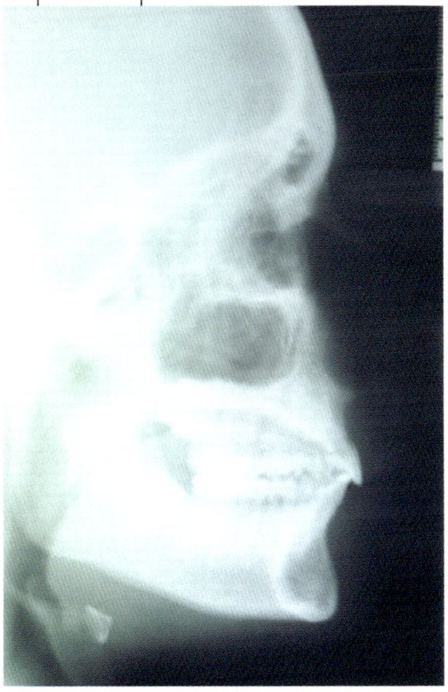

2-140

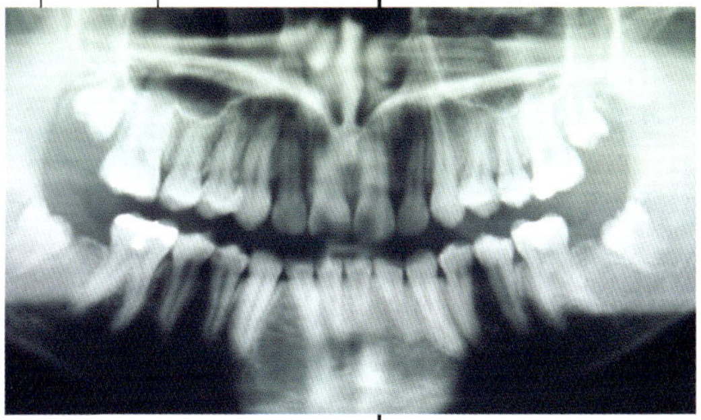

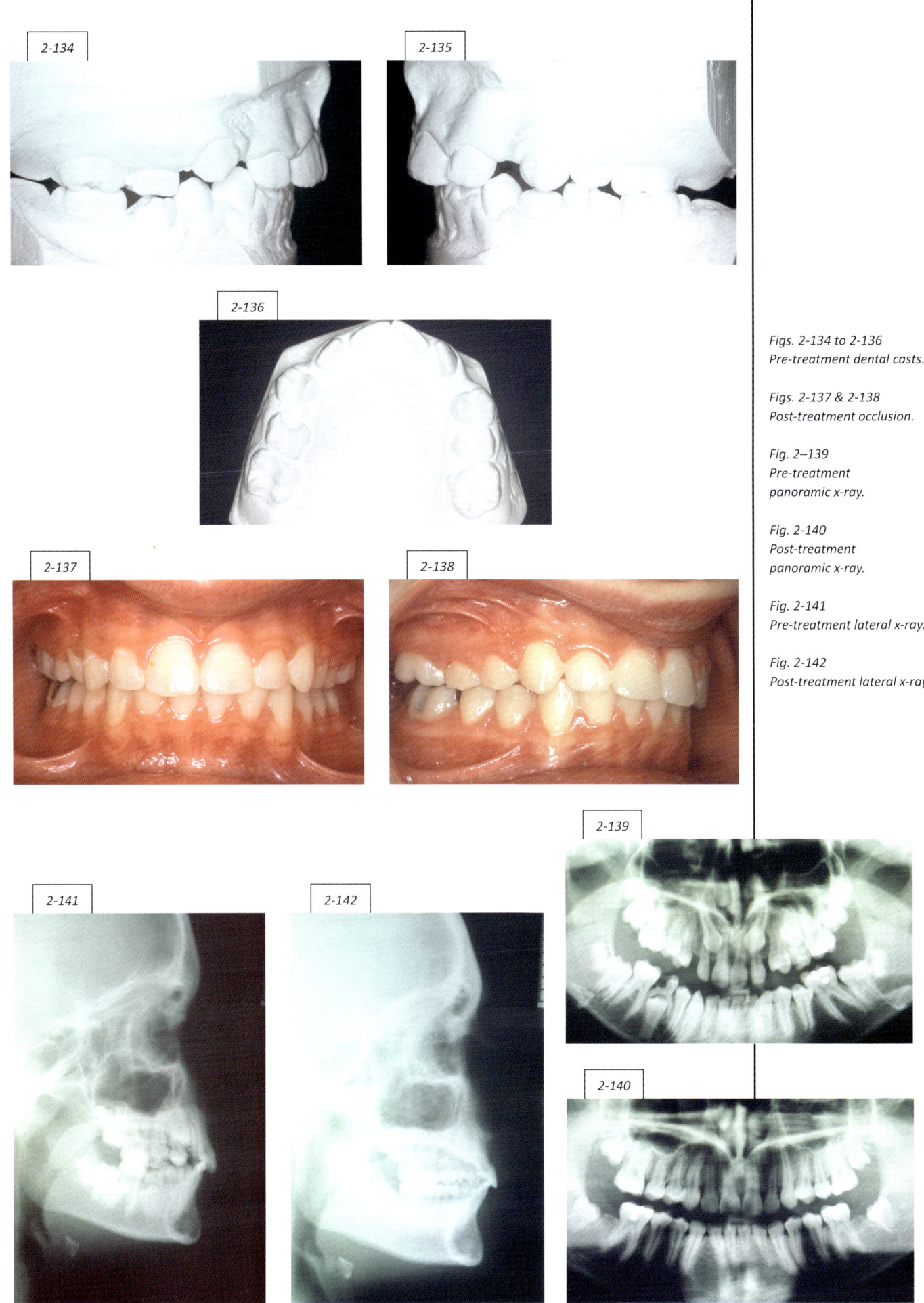

Figs. 2-134 to 2-136
Pre-treatment dental casts.

Figs. 2-137 & 2-138
Post-treatment occlusion.

Fig. 2–139
Pre-treatment panoramic x-ray.

Fig. 2-140
Post-treatment panoramic x-ray.

Fig. 2-141
Pre-treatment lateral x-ray.

Fig. 2-142
Post-treatment lateral x-ray.

CASE NUMBER 11

This is a Class I with a lack of space for upper canine alignment. It would be easier to extract the upper first premolars, however, the retrusive facial profile contraindicates it. Some space can be gained with anterior teeth proclination but it is not enough. Molars and premolars must be distalized a few millimetres after the second molar extraction, thus giving a good occlusion.

2-143

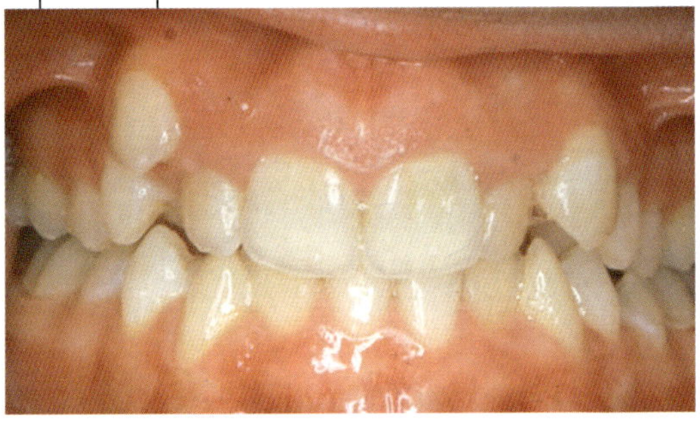

2-144

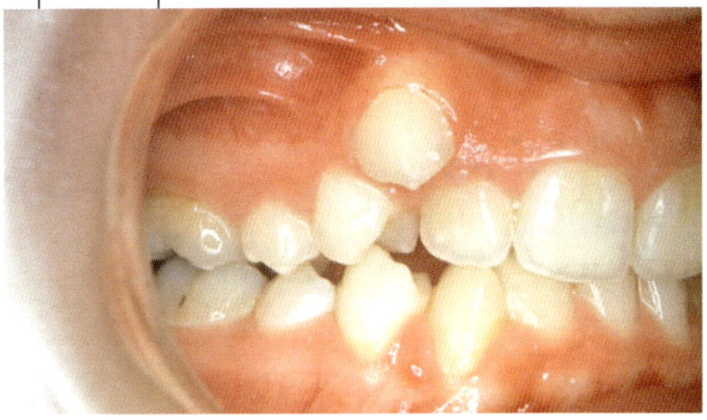

Figs. 2-143 & 2-144
Pre-treatment occlusion.

2-145

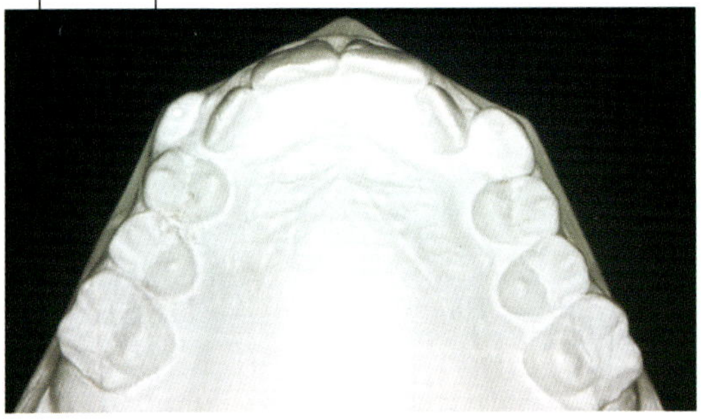

Fig. 2-145
Dental cast of maxillary arch.

2-146

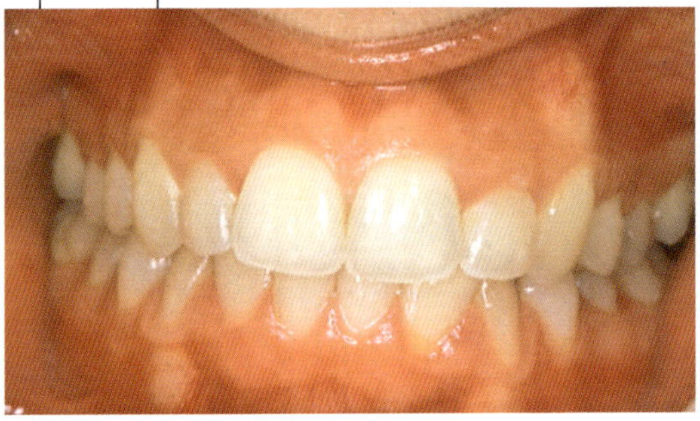

2-147

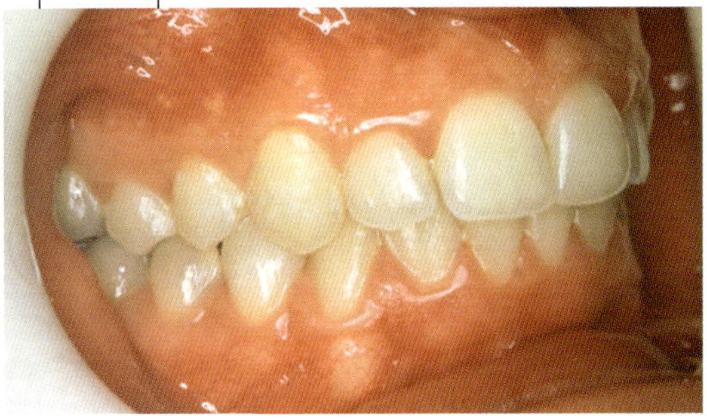

Figs. 2-146 & 2-147
Post-treatment occlusion.

2-148

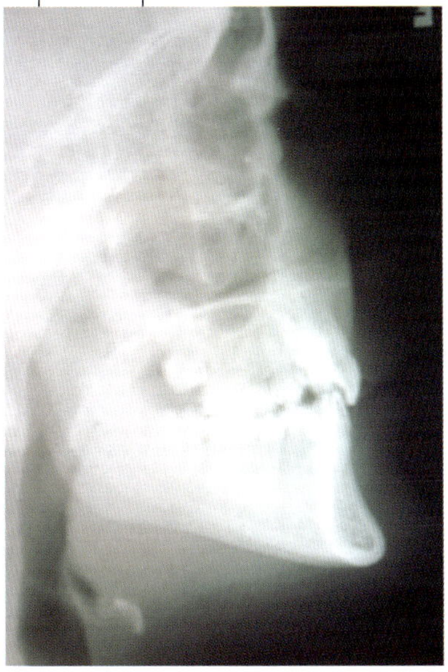

2-149

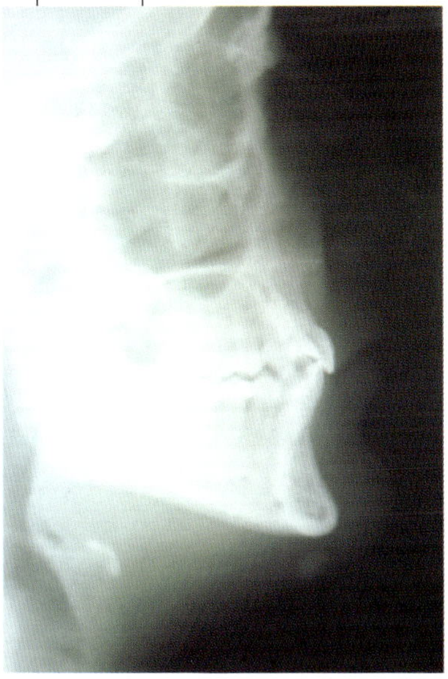

Fig. 2-148
Pre-treatment lateral cephalogram.

Fig. 2-149
Post-treatment lateral cephalogram.

2-150

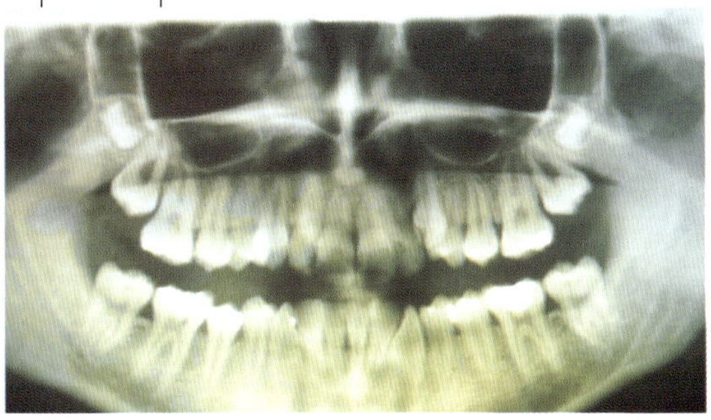

Fig. 2-150
Pre-treatment panoramic X ray.

2-151

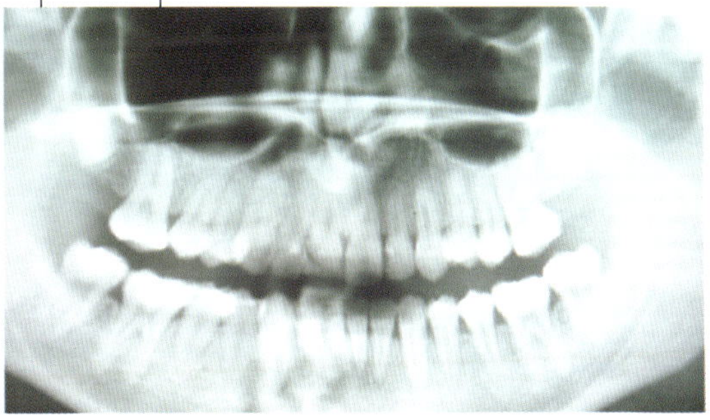

Fig. 2-151
Post-treatment panoramic X ray.

CONCLUSIONS

The decision on whether to extract or not to extract is an important choice based on many factors, including a correct informed consent. Teeth alignment, together with a good facial aesthetic , are the goals of modern orthodontics. On the subject of the facial aesthetic , I will now present two cases where the aesthetic evaluation leads to opposite treatment plans.

CASE NUMBER 12

Lower crowding is evident (Fig.2-156) but the patient's profile contraindicates extractions.

Well informed about the treatment choices, the parent agrees to a longer more satisfactory non-extractive treatment. With the use of a lip bumper on the very cooperative

2-152

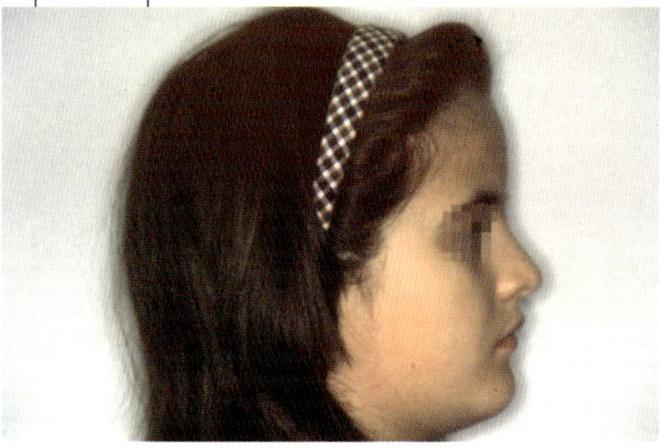

2-153

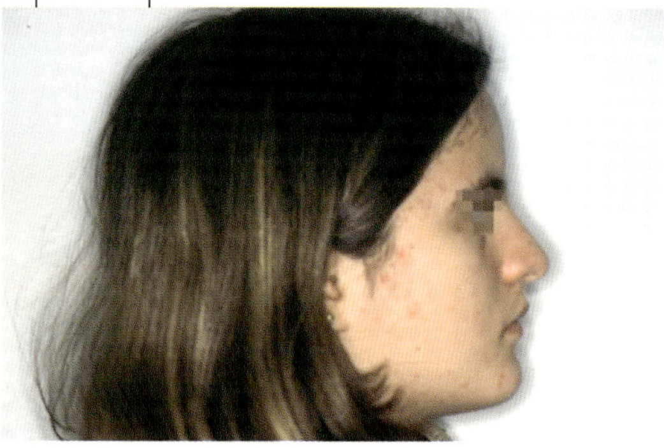

Fig. 2-152
Pre-treatment profile.

Fig. 2-153
Post-treatment profile.

2-154

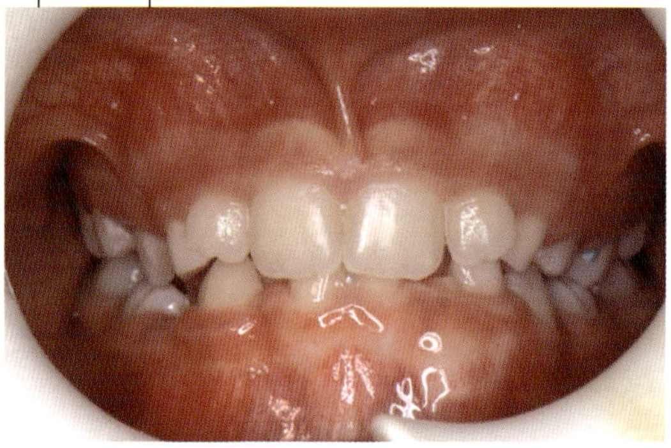

2-155

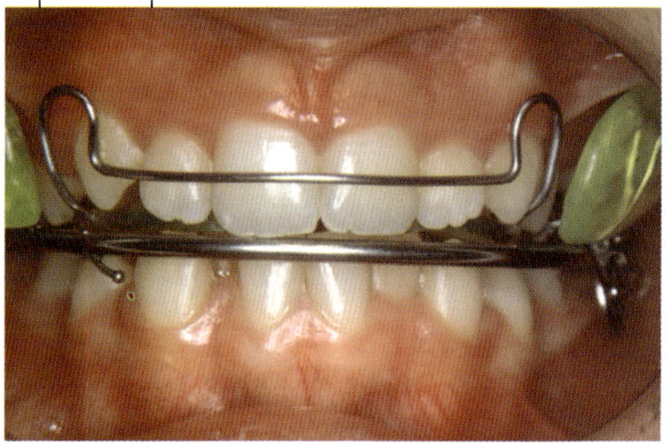

2-156

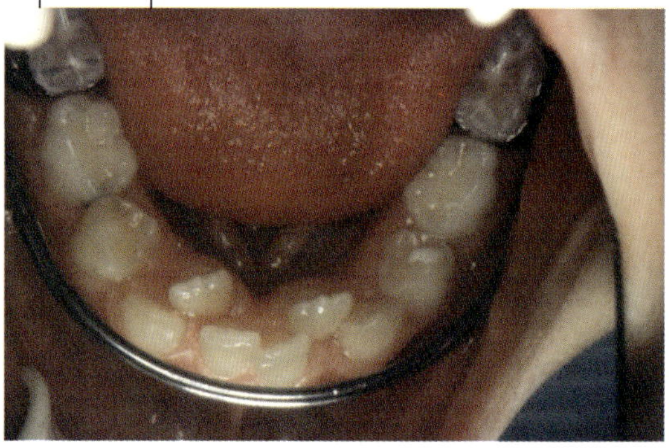

2-157

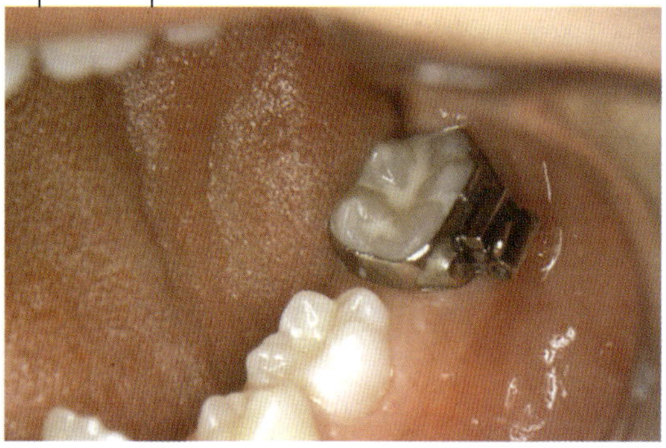

2-158

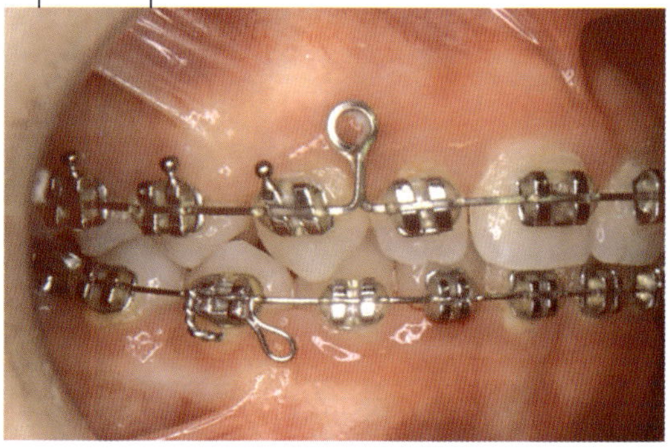

Figs. 2-154 to 2-158
Clinical aspects, before and during treatment. A palatal plate to control upper spaces and a lip bumper to distalize the first molars are used, before fitting the edgewise appliance. Notice the lack of space for lower lateral incisor alignment and the space gained with the lip bumper.

patient, the lower molars are distalized 2 mm per side without impaction against the second molars. After 20 months of treatment an edgewise appliance follows leading to an excellent result.

2-159

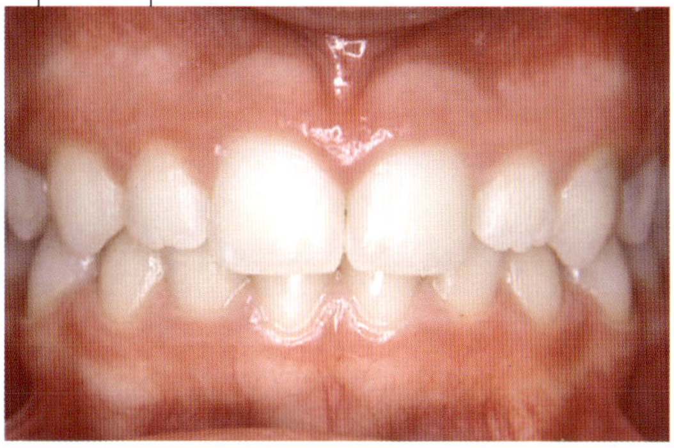

2-160

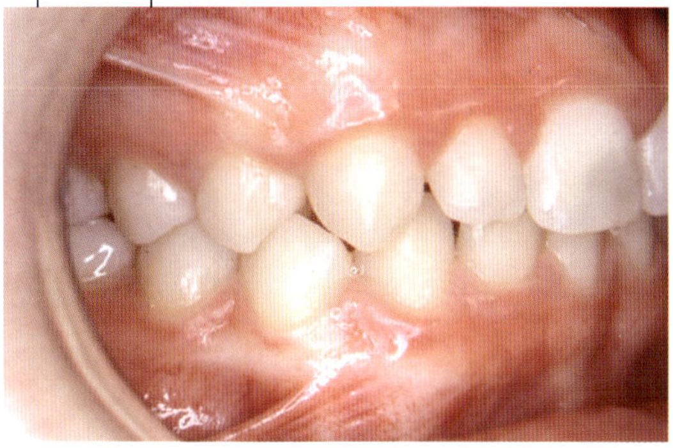

2-161

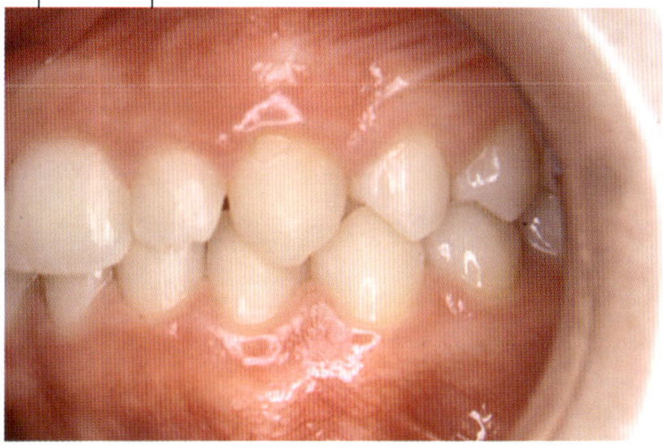

2-162

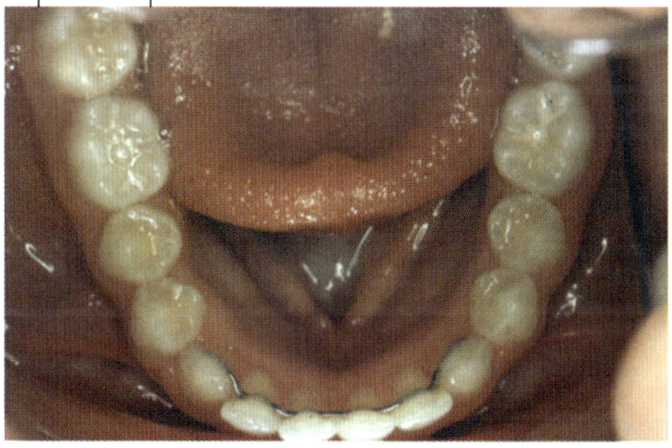

Figs. 2-159 to 2-162
Post-treatment occlusion.

2-163

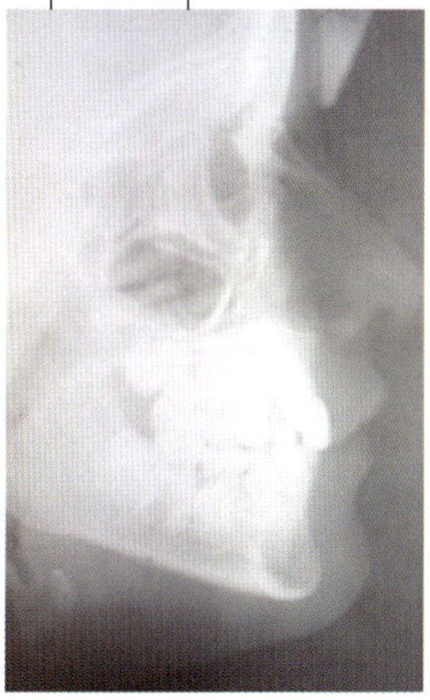

2-164

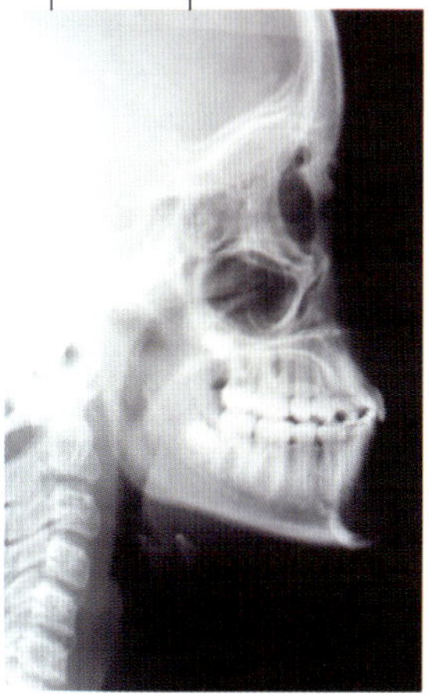

Fig. 2-163
Pre-treatment cephalogram.

Fig. 2-164
Post-treatment cephalogram.

CASE NUMBER 13

2-165

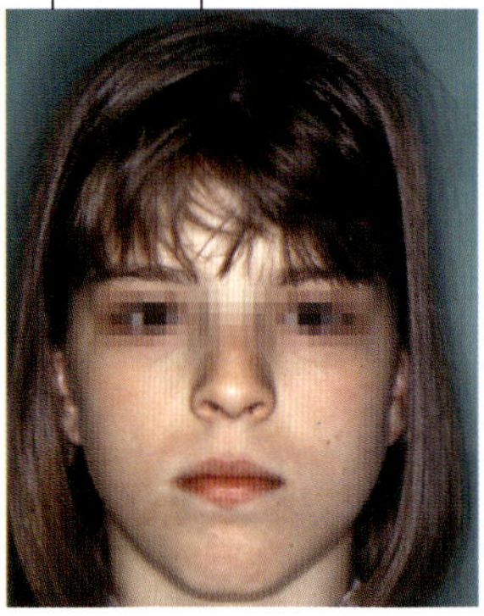

2-166

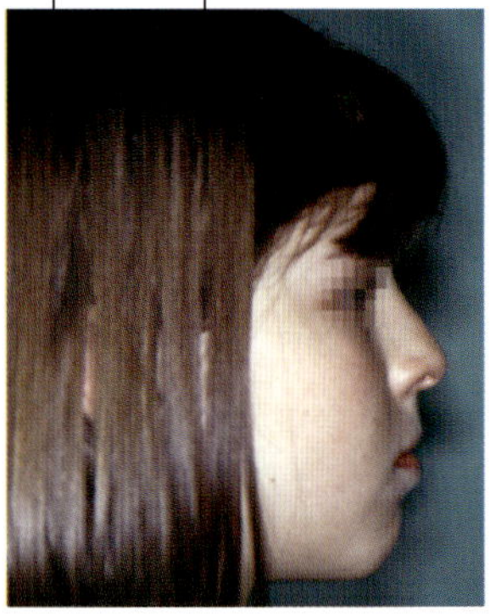

2-167

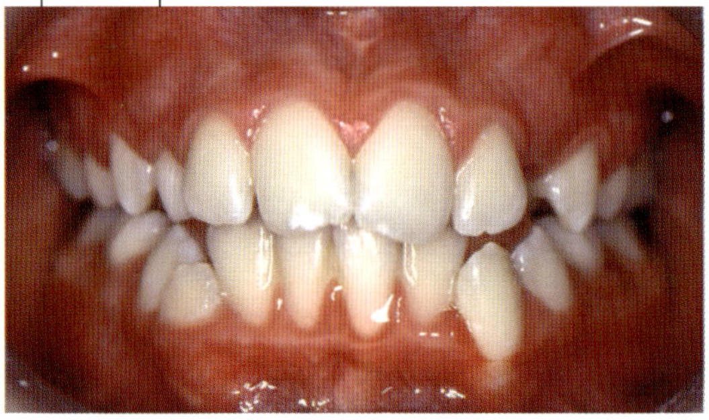

2-168

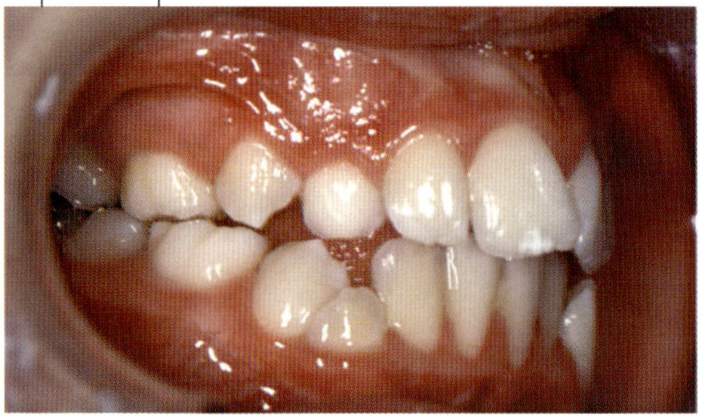

2-169

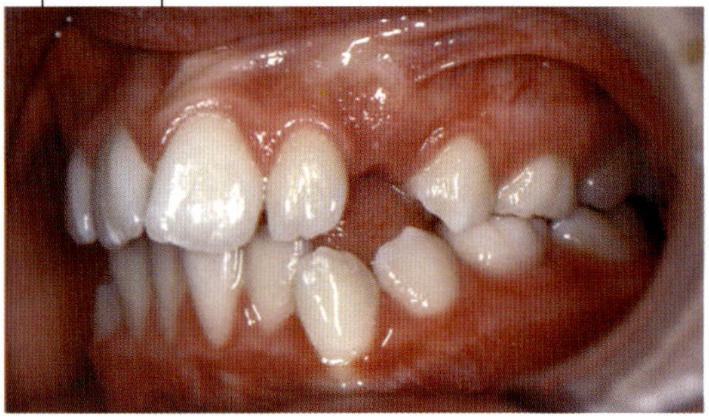

2-170

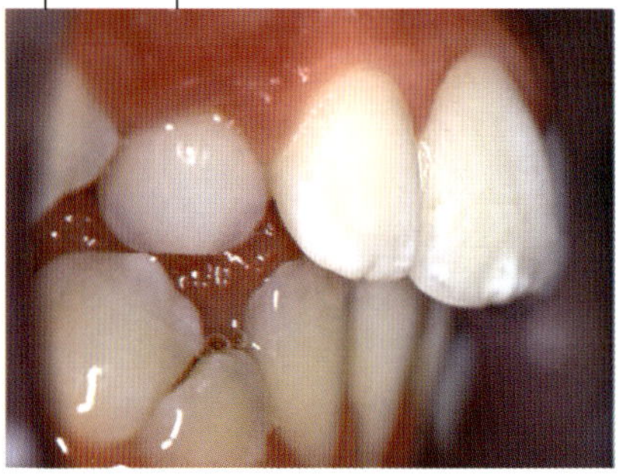

2-171

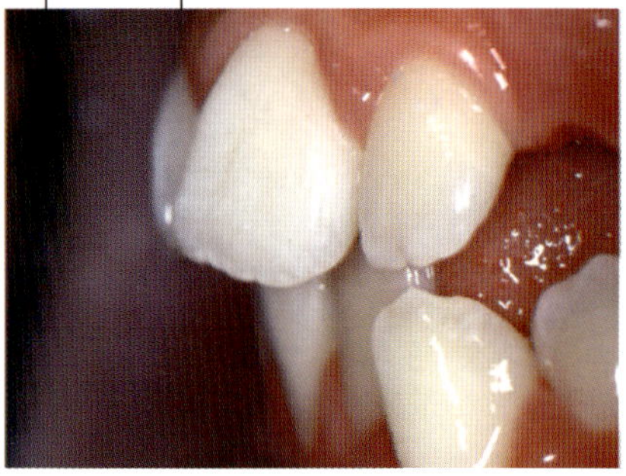

2-172

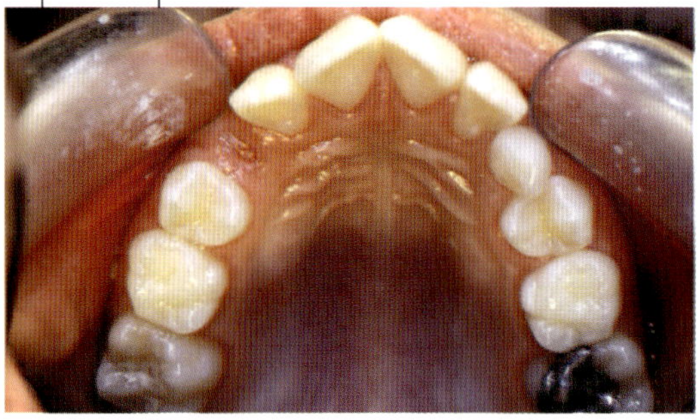

2-173

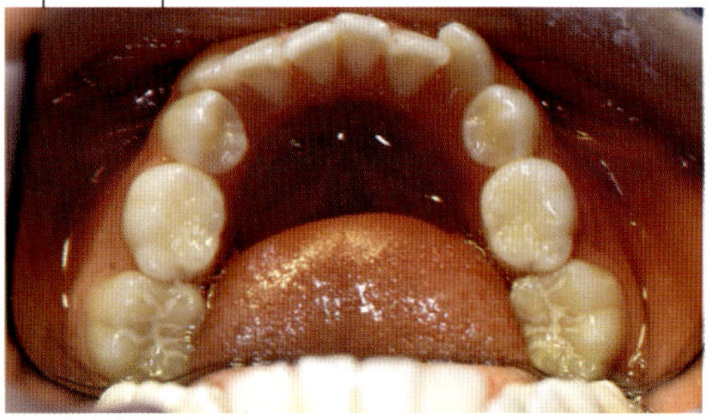

Figs. 2-165 to 2-173
First period of treatment.

2-174

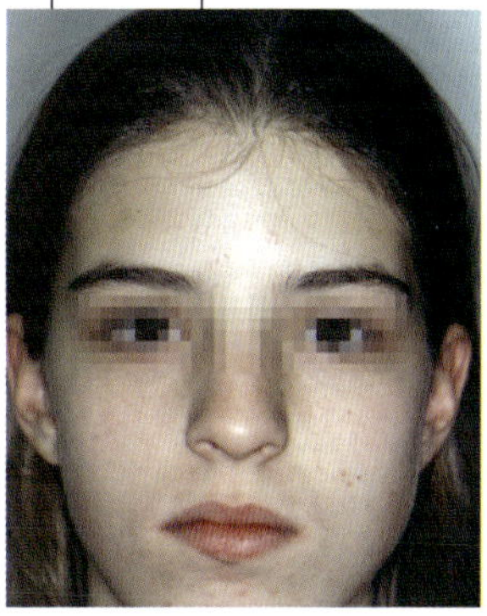

2-175

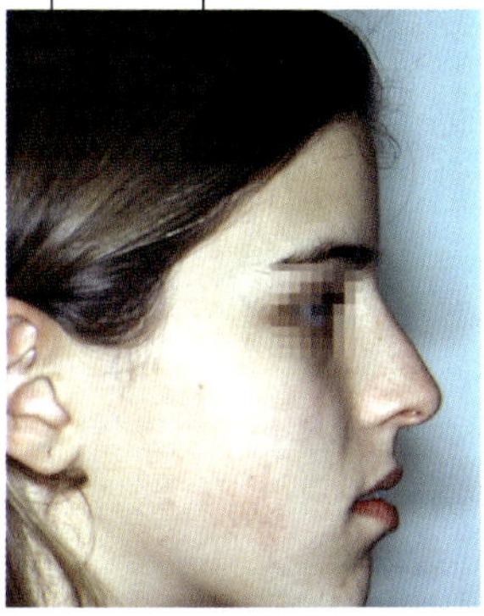

2-176

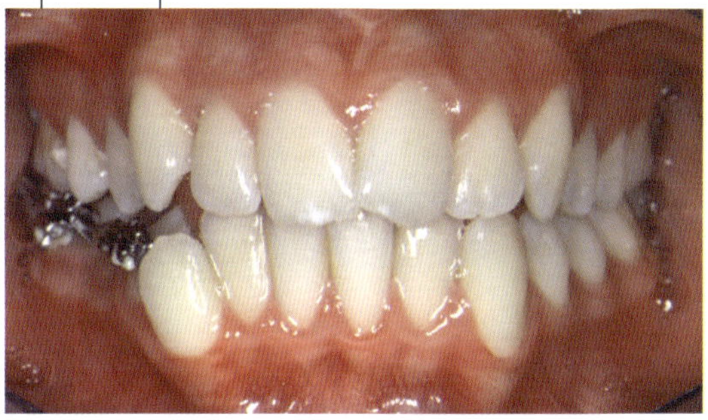

2-177

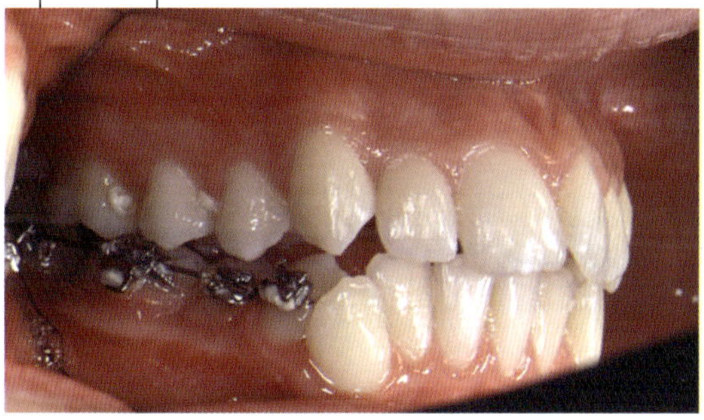

2-178

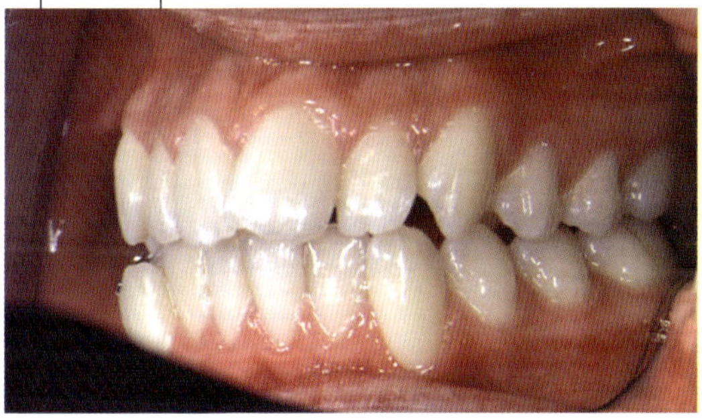

Fig. 2-174 & 2-178 Second period.

This is a typical example of the confusion that is still present among many orthodontists about the extraction versus non-extraction dilemma.

We can distinguish three periods of treatment. In the first period a very experienced orthodontist took wonderful pictures (Figs. 2-165 to 2-173) but *did not accomplish any results*. In the second period, after 18 months the lower third molars were extracted to correct the second lower right molar impaction with a sectional appliance (Figs. 2-174 to 2-178). *No results were achieved then either.*

The parents came to my office because they realized that the previous orthodontist did not know what to do. In this third period, I gave my opinion and they agreed with a four first premolar extraction treatment plan, the most suitable for the profile of the dolicofacial patient. You can see the result after 18 months of treatment with an edgewise appliance (Figs. 2-179 to 2-184). *Notice the change in the patient's profile.*

Since the problem was already evident in the first period and the treatment at that time was probably easier, the question is, what happened? The answer probably lies in the fact that the above mentioned "very experienced" orthodontist of 40 years had been a disciple of Cetlin, then a disciple of Tweed and currently is a disciple of Damon. Evidently his overall treatment plan was not clear.

2-179

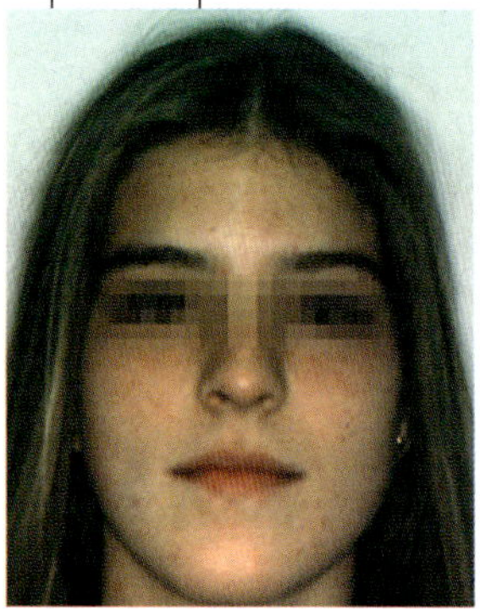

2-180

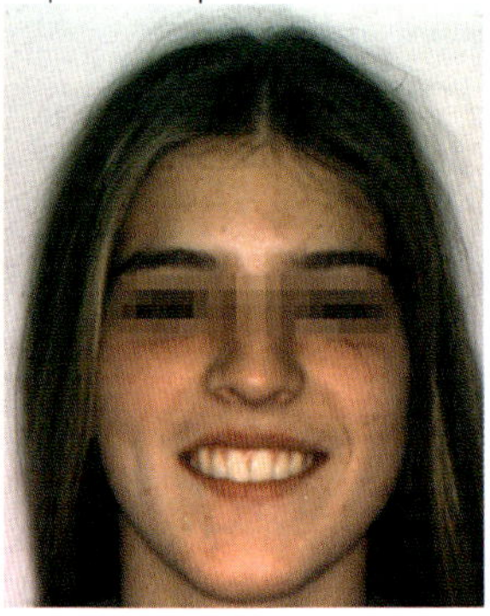

2-181

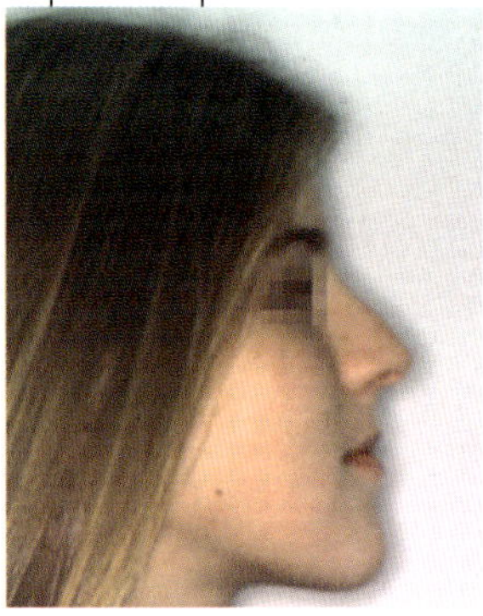

2-182

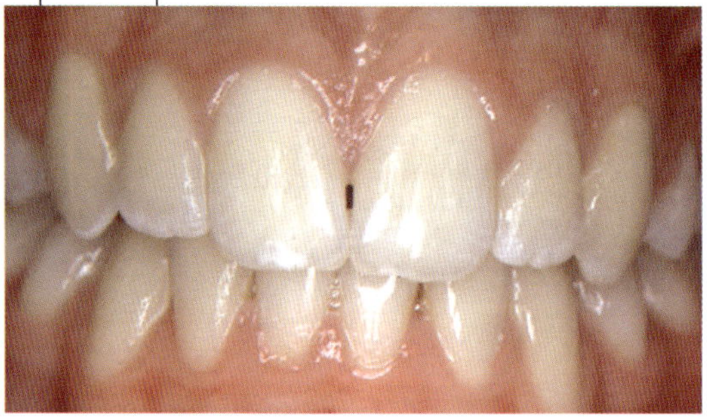

2-183

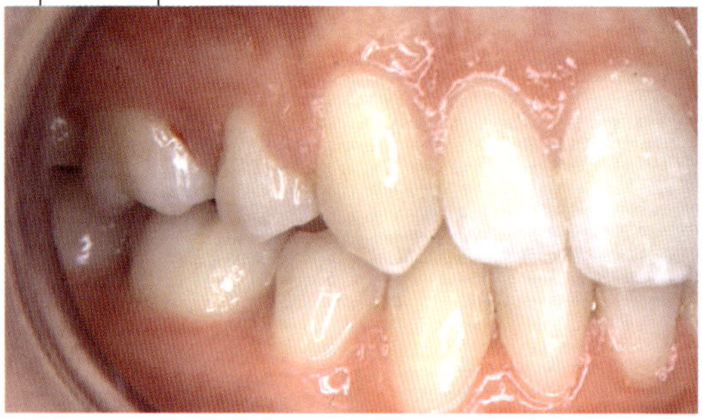

2-184

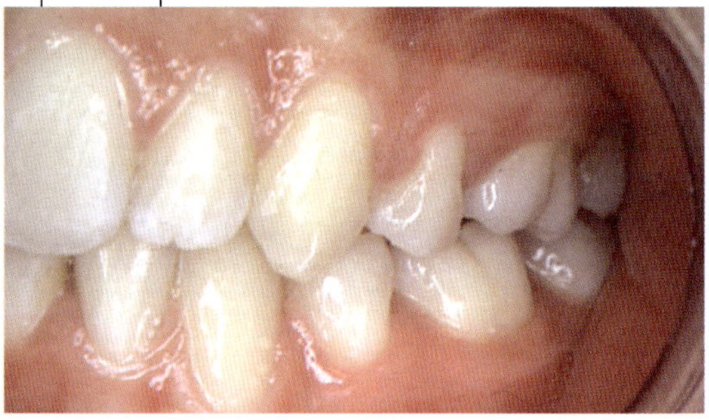

Fig. 2-179 to 2-184 Third period.

2-185

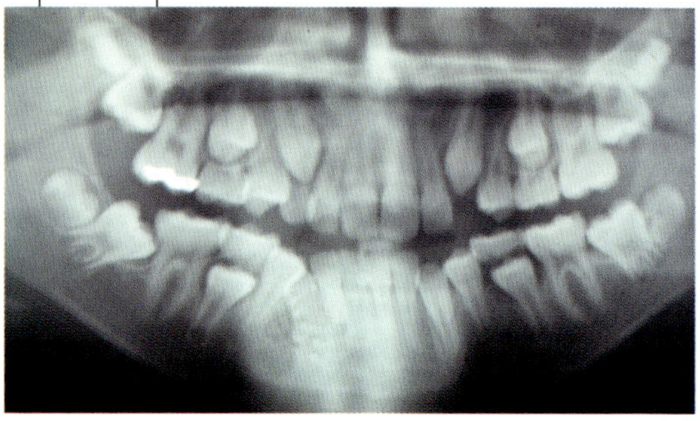

Fig. 2-185 First period panoramic X ray.

2-186

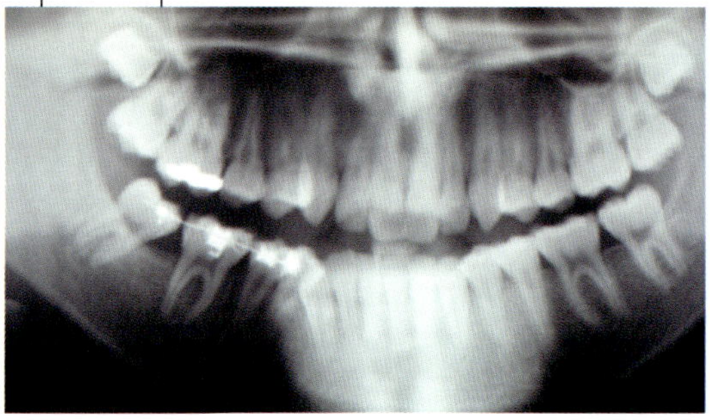

Fig. 2-186 Second period panoramic X ray.

2-187

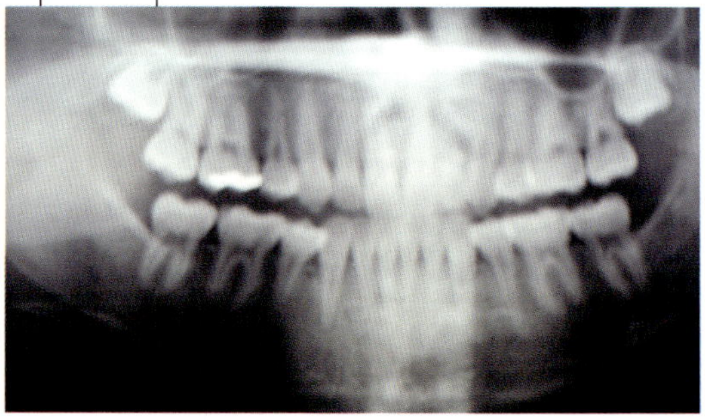

Fig. 2-187 Third period panoramic X ray.

2-188

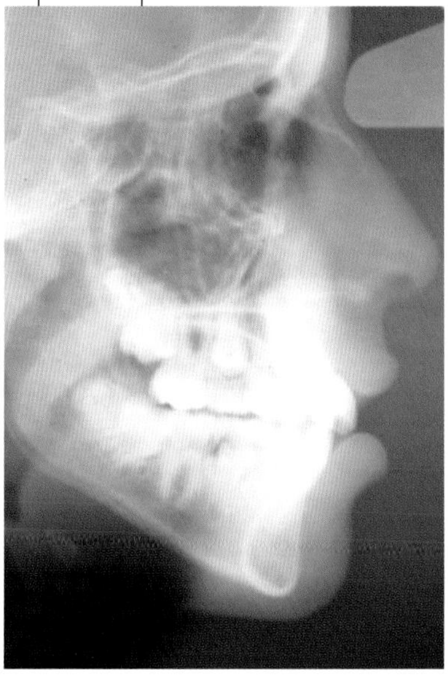

2-189

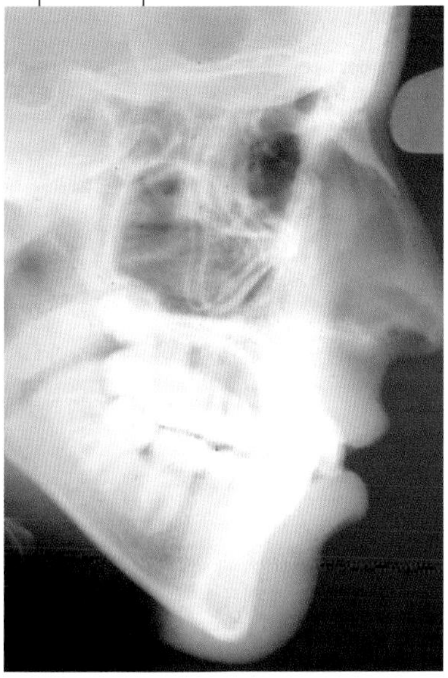

2-190

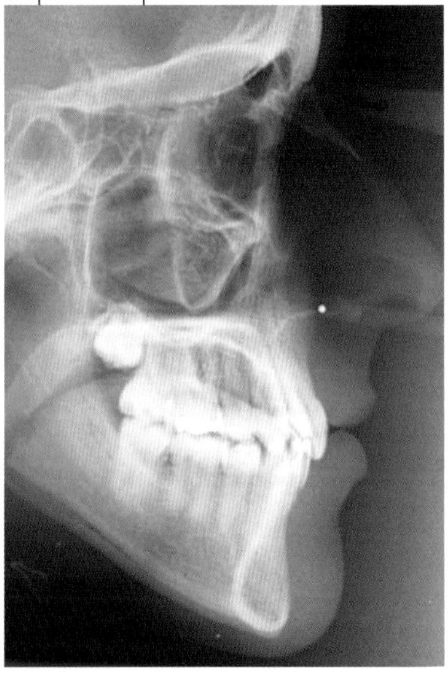

Fig. 2-188 First period lateral cephalogram.

Fig. 2-189 Second period lateral cephalogram.

Fig. 2-190 Third period lateral cephalogram.

SECTIONAL TREATMENTS

Often people refuse orthodontic treatment because they think the appliances are too invasive.

However, there are cases where sectional appliances can give good results. Of course such cases are very well received by the patients.

CASE NUMBER 14

A simple anterior cross bite in an adult patient treated with two sectionals, the upper one is lingual. The treatment took six months.

2-191

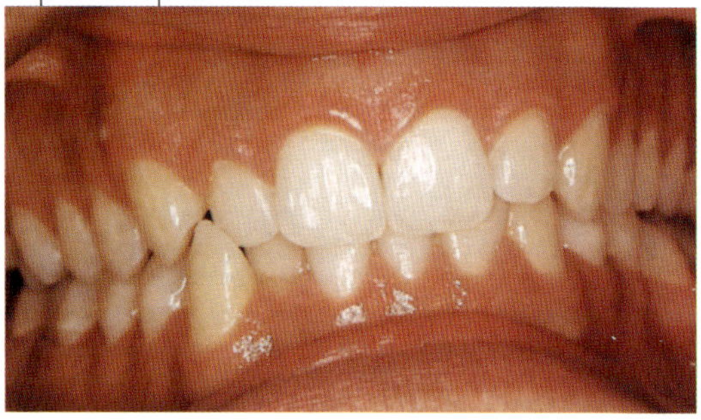

Fig. 2-191
Pre-treatment clinical view.

2-192

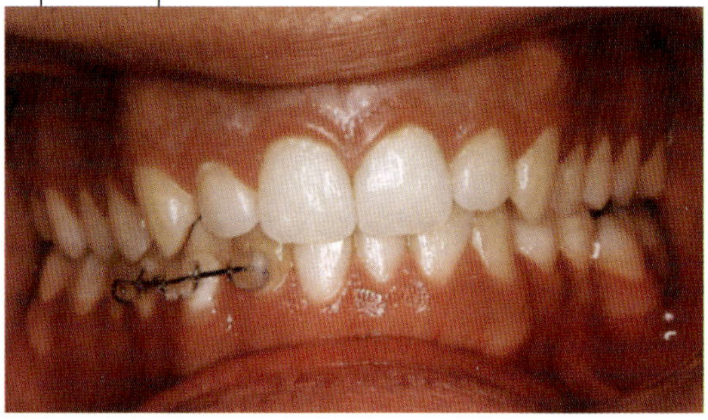

Fig. 2-192
During the treatment.

2-193

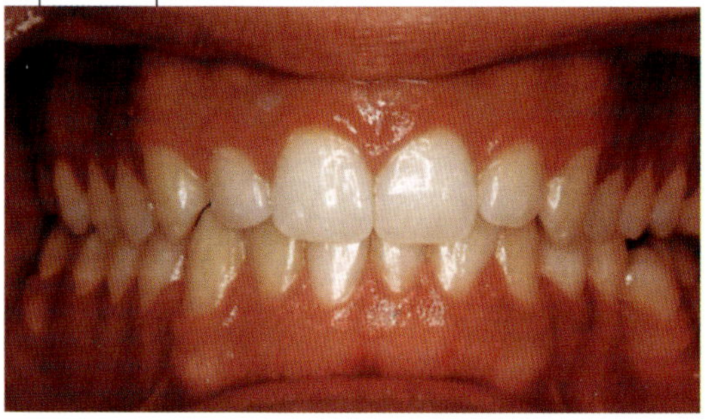

Fig. 2-193
Post-treatment clinical view.

CASE NUMBER 15

The patient is a fellow dentist who, after the extraction of the first left lower molar, wants to close the space with the alignment of the lower first premolar. He refuses a brace on the whole arch, preferring to be fitted with only a sectional appliance. After 18 months of treatment the first premolar is aligned, the space made by the extraction is closed, and the third molar has erupted well.

Notice (fig. 2 -196) that the left central incisor remains in the same position. Thus we can say that the biomechanic system of force has been applied to only the teeth actually requiring movement.

In my opinion it is an excellent result, impossible to achieve if a prosthetic dental replacement had been used. It is also an effective riposte to those who, in cases like this , do not consider the orthodontic option as a valid alternative to other treatments like bridges or implants.

2-194

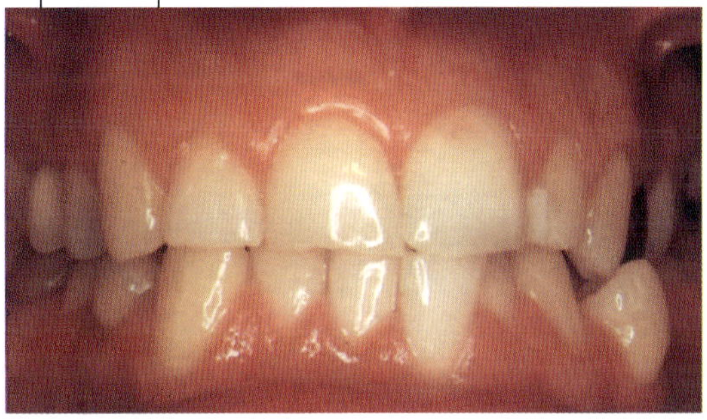

2-195

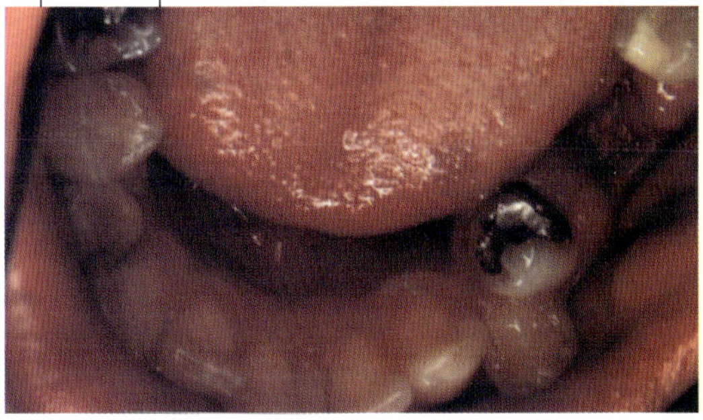

Figs. 2-194 & 2-195
Pre-treatment clinical view.

2-196

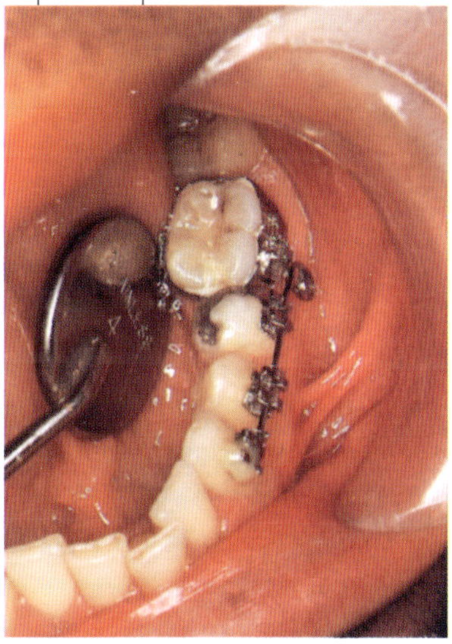

2-197

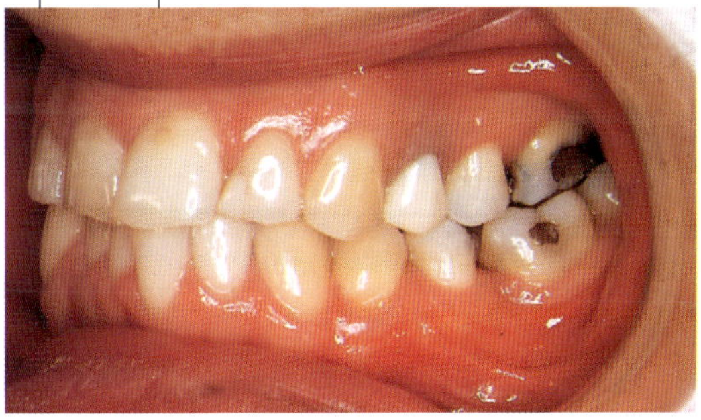

Fig.2-196
An advanced treatment phase.

Fig. 2-197
Post-treatment occlusion.

2-198

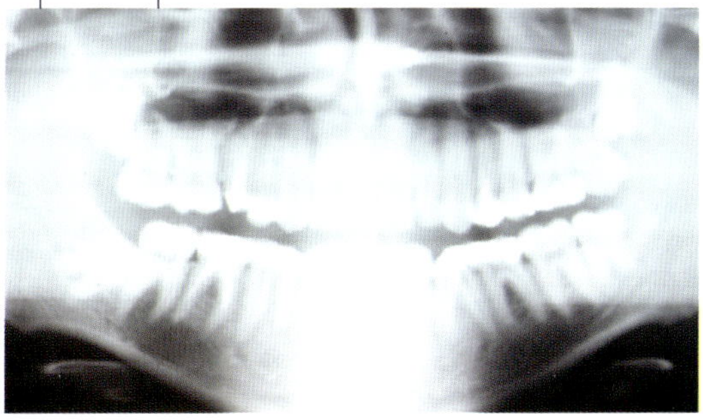

2-199

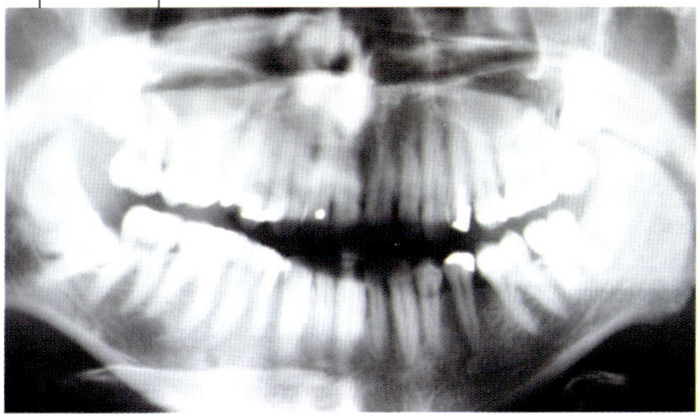

Fig. 2-198
Pre-treatment panoramic cephalogram.

Fig. 2-199
Post-treatment panoramic cephalogram.

Chapter III:

Class II

CLASS II

In a skeletal Class II, the maxillary is too advanced compared with the mandible. Just like other malocclusions, Class II cases are determined by genetics and by functional aspects.

Cases can be:

- **Maxillary Class II:** where the maxilla is too advanced compared to a normally positioned mandible.
- **Mandibular Class II:** where the maxilla is normally positioned, the mandible is too retrusive.
- **Mixed Class II:** where the maxilla is too advanced, the mandible is too retrusive.

The first indication of analysis is given by the ANB angle (in a Class II is more than 4°).

R.Slavicek - Clinical and instrumental functional analysis for diagnosis and treatment planning -J.Clin. Orthod .Ang. vol. 22 n.8 - 1988 says that the mandibular Class II cases are the most common, then maxillary cases, with mixed cases the least common. In the first group, be careful not to confuse a true skeletal Class II with a skeletal Class I with a protruded upper dental arch.

In the second group it is important to distinguish a retruded lower dental arch in a well dimensioned mandible from that with a short mandibular horizontal length, and also from a normal mandibular length which is distally positioned in the articular glenoid fossa.

We must also remember the importance of vertical growth, particularly of the condyle and the ramus, in order to balance the vertical growth of dentoalveolar processes. (The latter are necessary to maintain a good relationship between the maxillary and the mandible).

If that does not happen (for example due to a problematic genetic growth pattern, oral respiration or muscle dystrophy) the growing mandible can distally rotate, increasing the vertical height and the ANB angle. Should this happen the Class II would worsen and the facial profile would become more convex.

Many orthodontists think that a distal rotation of the mandible (clockwise growth) can also be provoked by an incorrect use of appliances (rapid palatal expanders, headgear, etc.).

When it comes to dentistry, a Class II Division 1 occurs when the upper arch is frontally protruding. A Class II Division 2 is when the frontal upper teeth are vertical or palatally inclined, either with or without crowding.

3-1

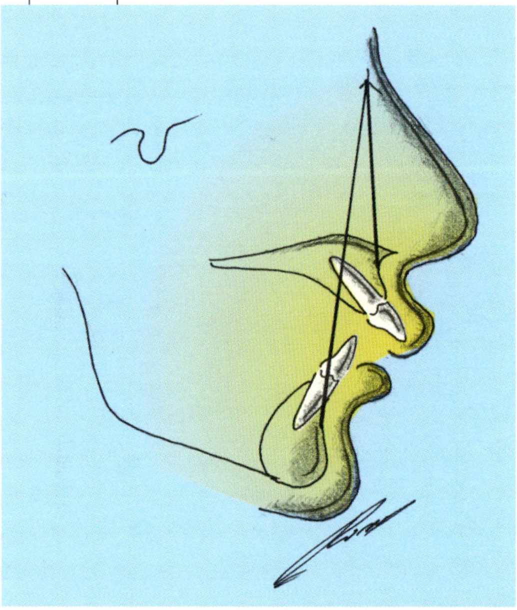

Fig. 3-1
ANB > 4°.

TREATMENT

In order to achieve an optimal result when attempting to correct a skeletal Class II malocclusion, it is necessary to use a treatment that achieves the best osteal relationship.

That is also the premise for good dental alignment and non-extraction treatment (Fig. 3-2).

The answer to the question "Is it possible to correct a Class II without extractions?" is "YES, after good orthopedic treatment and, of course, if there is not excessive crowding". However, not everybody agrees with this statement.

3-2

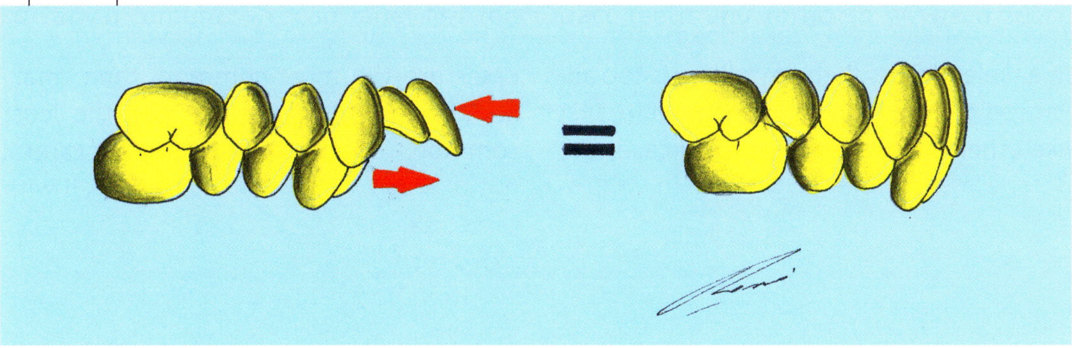

Fig. 3-2 schematic representation of non-extraction treatment.

Historically, European schools support orthopedic treatment. The American schools, on the other hand, move the teeth with fixed appliances believing that the osteal relationship can only be modified through surgery.

Over the years things have changed. Among the opinion leaders, the American Ricketts recognized the importance of orthopedics, unlike Tweed who followed his own philosophy.

As often happens, such discussions are problematic to the clinicians who strive to give the best to their patients.

Discussing a potential orthopedic growth control of about 1 mm or less is not very useful. However, it is hard to ignore an article written in 1953 by Dr. Beulah Nelson[184], mentioned by Ricketts, where it was described how a maxillary point A moved 5 mm backwards thanks to the application of extraoral traction.

So, what should a good orthodontist do?

I personally agree with Dr. Jarabak who, at the annual meeting of the American Orthodontics Association in 1980, stated "There are two ways of practising orthodontics: an orthopedic one, using basically removable appliances, and a mechanic one with fixed appliances. The first approach is mainly European, the second is American. Up to 30% of cases can be wonderfully treated with removable appliances, around 25% must be treated with either type of appliance. The rest have to be treated with fixed ones."

We could argue about the suggested percentages, but the principle is not in doubt - when there is no orthopedic treatment or where it fails, it is possible to effect some movement of the teeth according to the amount of the osteal discrepancy or to perform a surgical correction at the end of their period of growth.

FUNCTIONAL APPLIANCES

Premise

In a muscle we can have a contraction with shortening and movement (isotonic), or a contraction without shortening and movement (isometric).

The variation in muscular length is registered by the central nervous system and is regulated by neuromuscular fuses. If a muscle is stretched, the neuromuscular fuses activate and provoke a contraction which opposes the stretching - known as the myotactic reflex.

When the stretching is excessive, tendon receptors (Golgi receptors) are activated to put a stop to the contraction that thus acts as a safeguard for the integrity of the muscle (knife reflex). These reflexes can be triggered by removable appliances in different ways according to their various designs and elements of construction. They can also instigate muscular contractions which have sufficient force to effect skeletal and dental modification. Removable "functional" appliances have an essential role in the treatment of Class II.

They are not a new approach. In 1878, W. Kingsley presented in the USA a palatal plate tied to the upper molars with an anterior inclined surface that made the mandible move forward when it was closing. The treatment with this appliance was called "jumping the bite".

Since Kingsley's time, the principle of functional jumping has always been present in the various orthopedic-functional appliances, all of which try to modify functionally the soft tissues, the bones, the condyle and the occlusion. *By modifying the function we can modify the form.*

The correction of a skeletal Class II is similar in many procedures: stimulation of mandible growth, palatal inclination of upper incisors, labial inclination of lower incisors, mesial advancement of lower molars while the upper molars are stopped or moved distally, palatal expansion to compensate a mandibular advancement.

This does not mean that all the appliances are the same even if the choice appears at many times irrational. For example, in a case with proclined lower incisors it is better to use an appliance that does not come into contact (Fränkel) with them rather than one that does (Andresen). This is very important in order to achieve a good result. In fact, increasing the inclination of the lower incisors worsens the situation because it inhibits the skeletal mandibular advancement.

In a Class II division 2, only the appliances which allow the proclination of upper incisors (with springs, screws etc.) are effective. Otherwise it is not possible to advance the mandible.

Removable appliances are usually considered "easy" to manage. Many people believe it is enough to put them in the mouth as they will work automatically without particular attention being paid by the orthodontist. They think that it is enough to simply turn a screw from time to time.

Yet in order to obtain good results with these appliances, experience is required. It provides the knowhow for the strategic adjustment of the various components while the treatment proceeds and it helps to assure and motivate the patient.

ANDRESEN[7] ACTIVATOR (FIG. 3-3 & 3-4)

In the attempt to correct the syndrome named after him, the Frenchman Dr. Pierre Robin was the first to create a rubber-made appliance, which prompted Dr. Andresen to design the removable appliance known as the "Andresen activator" in Norway. The appliance is made with acrylics and a few parts of stainless steel.

Those who use the Andresen activator believe that by modifying the closure path of the mandible it is possible to obtain a neuromuscular adaptation which will eventually lead to an oral-facial muscular re-education. When the activator is placed in the mouth the mandible at closure is advanced while the muscles involved produce contrary forces that try to pull it back. These forces are transmitted to the upper and lower teeth by their contact through the acrylics, and to the upper incisors by their contact with the frontal steel arch. Theoretically these forces reach through the teeth to the bone to induce an inhibition of maxillary sagittal growth and a stimulation of mandibular growth, thus producing a new dental occlusion.

The original design of this appliance has no retention clasps so it is mobile in the mouth, requiring the patient to hold it in

3-3

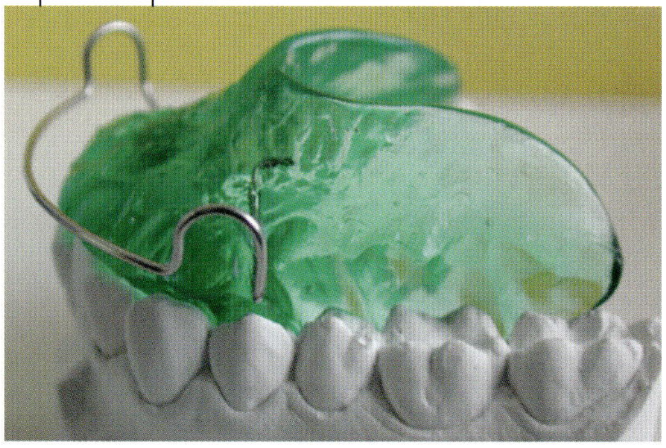

3-4

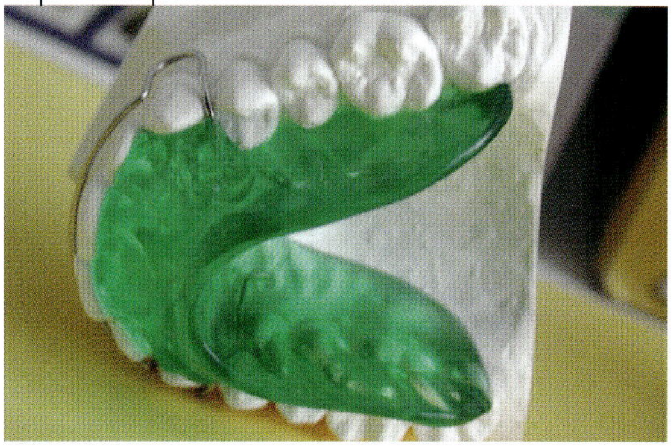

Fig. 3-3 and 3.4
For the removal appliances in this chapter, a special thanks to Wisil Laboratories Milan

place, which introduces the muscles and tongue into a new jaw relationship.
Over the years its design has been modified particularly with regard to its effect on the construction bite. This latter, in the opinion of Herren,[120] Harvold [117] and Woodside[257] is very important in order to be able to modify the skeletal front facial parts. The direction and opening of the construction bite influences the amount of reactive muscular forces which determine the structural changes. Construction bites with a minimum-to-moderate opening produce an active muscular tension, while construction bites with an extreme opening produce a passive muscular tension. We can say that a minimum-to-moderate opening (2-4 mm) is indicated when we want to increase sagittal forces, which should be c.315-395 g for good mandibular advancement, according to Witt[254].
When is mandibular advancement deemed to be good?
Many believe that mandibular advancement is good when the upper and lower incisors are edge to edge. It is excessive in cases with large overjet; so, in my opinion, it is better not to exceed 6-7 mm.
An alternative treatment could be progressive advancement. When there is an excessive vertical growth, which worsens the sagittal Class II relationship, a construction bite with small mandibular advancement (2-3 mm) and a greater opening (6 mm and more) is required. The Andresen activator is indicated in Class II where the lower incisors are not proclined because the contact with the appliance would increase their proclination. In such cases it is better to use an appliance with an anterior soft tissue contact (Fränkel, RV).
The best time for applying the treatment is during the passage of transitional dentition, with optimal application time of at least 14 hours a day (night included). A younger patient should build up to this amount of time slowly, beginning with 2-3 hours a day.

CASE NUMBER 1 (ANDRESEN)

	Before	After		Before	After
SNA	79°	79°	Angle of lower incisors		
SNB	74°	76°	on the mandibular plane	92°	94°
ANB	5°	3°			

Fig. 3-5
Dental casts of a male patient 12 years old. Two years after unsuccessful treatment the patient wants to try again. Since he is still growing, before opting for a camouflage treatment with two upper first premolar extractions, he accepts treatment with an Andresen activator.

Fig. 3-6
Lateral cephalogram before the new treatment, two years after the dental casts. Looking at the teeth and occlusion, the failure of previous treatment is evident.

Fig. 3-7
Lateral cephalogram at the end of treatment with the Andresen activator.

3-6

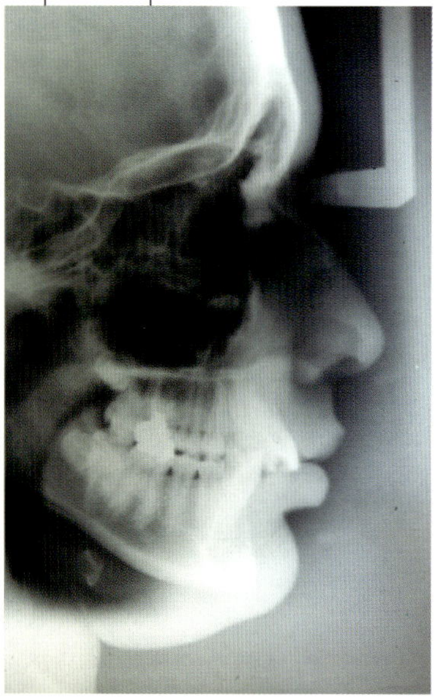

3-7

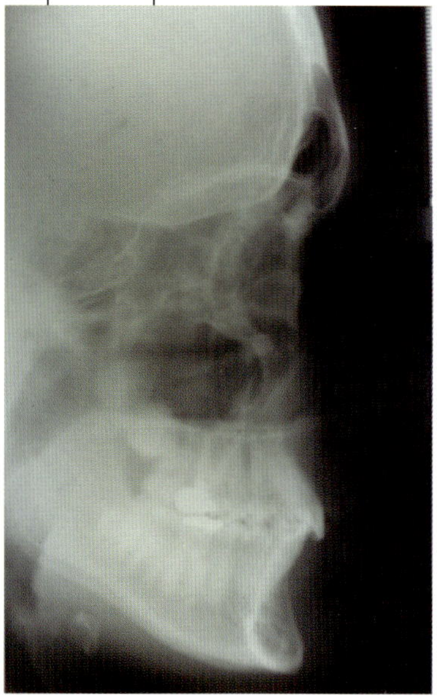

3-5

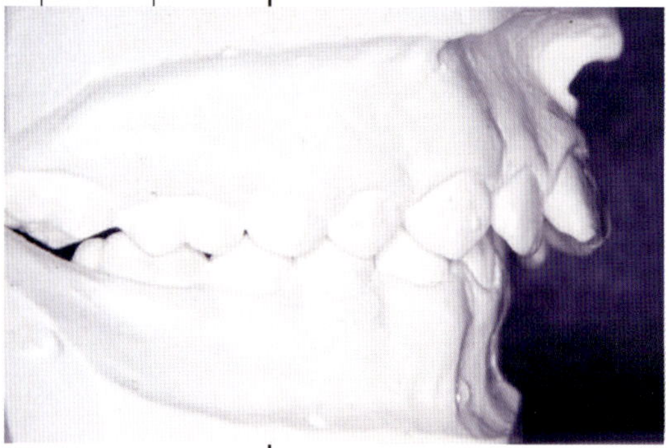

3-8

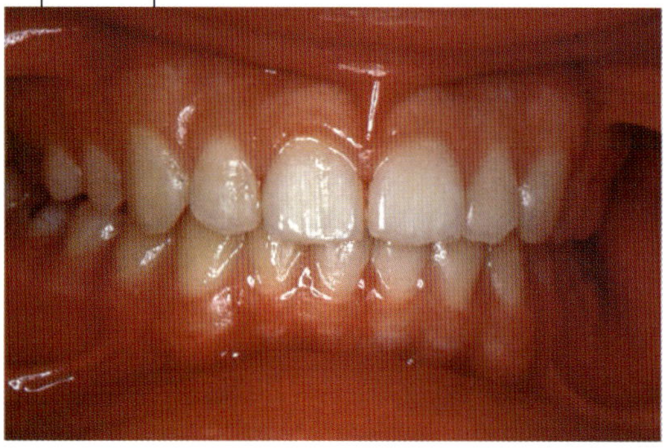

3-9

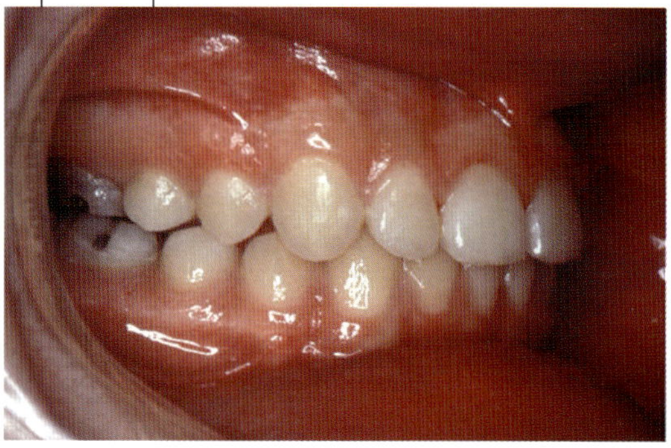

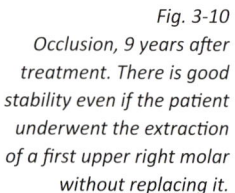

Figs. 3-8 & 3-9
Intraoral photographs at the end of treatment. The occlusion has been improved thanks to an elastic positioner.

3-10

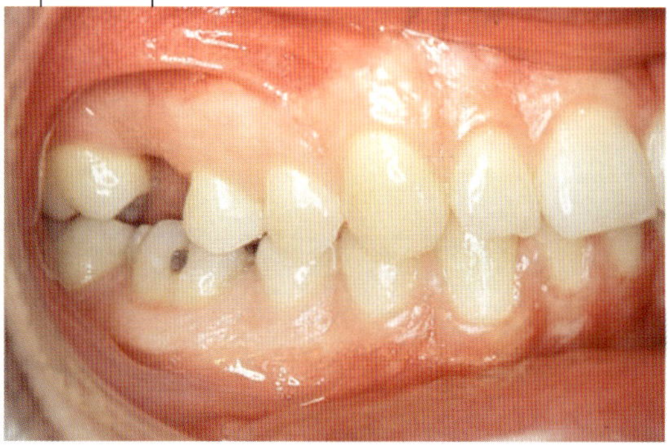

Fig. 3-10
Occlusion, 9 years after treatment. There is good stability even if the patient underwent the extraction of a first upper right molar without replacing it.

FRÄNKEL[96]

Fränkel designed his appliance following the principles of orthopedics that consider exercise and muscular activity very important in the development of bones and bone tissue. Fränkel believed that the growth of the jaws is based on genetic information transmitted indirectly by functional environment. If we modify the function we modify the form. In his opinion, Class II cases are mainly caused by wrong orofacial muscular activity and can be corrected with good muscle exercises.

Consequently, the Fränkel appliance has wide contact with soft tissues. It helps active muscular action and stimulates the muscles to advance the mandible gradually. It consists of acrylic lingual plates which are in contact with the alveolar mucosa and do not touch the lower incisors. When the mandible recedes, pressure on the soft tissue is painful. As an automatic reaction to the pain the muscles push the mandible forward again. Large acrylic lateral shields are inserted to counterbalance the cheek pressure, which inhibits maxillary lateral expansion.

The construction bite provides mandibular advancement of up to 2-3 mm and is increased during the treatment, according to Fränkel's recommendations. (There are also orthodontists like Graber Orthodontics Principles and practice. 2° edi, 1966 and McNamara [164] who declare good results with a wider advancement.) In any case, with a modest vertical increase, the mandibular advancement should not be greater than 6 mm.

The Fränkel appliance must be used night and day after its introduction - at the beginning for 2-3 hours, after two weeks for 4-6 hours, after four weeks for 10 hours, etc..

3-11

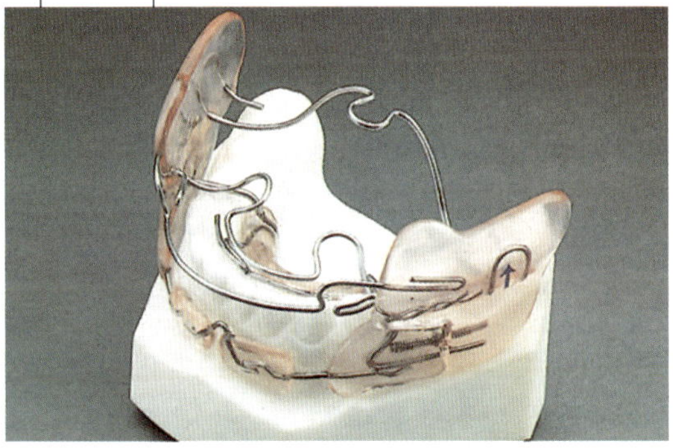

3-12

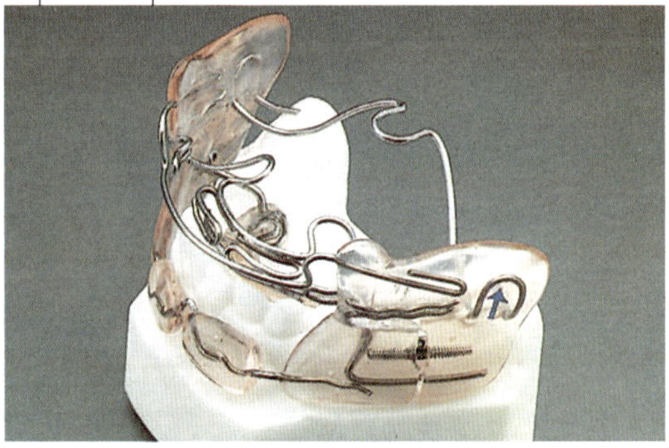

CASE NUMBER 2 (FRÄNKEL)

	Before	After		Before	After
SNA	*84°*	*84°*	*lower incisors inclication*		
SNB	*77°*	*81°*	*on the mandibular plane*	*110°*	*103°*
ANB	*7°*	*3°*			

Note the positional change of the mandible. The inclination of the lower incisors on a mandibular plane changed from 110° to 103°: they are now upright. This demonstrates the right choice of an appliance that was able to advance the mandible through soft tissue contact. Using another appliance in contact with the lower incisors would have increased their proclination, reducing the correct bone advancement.

3-13

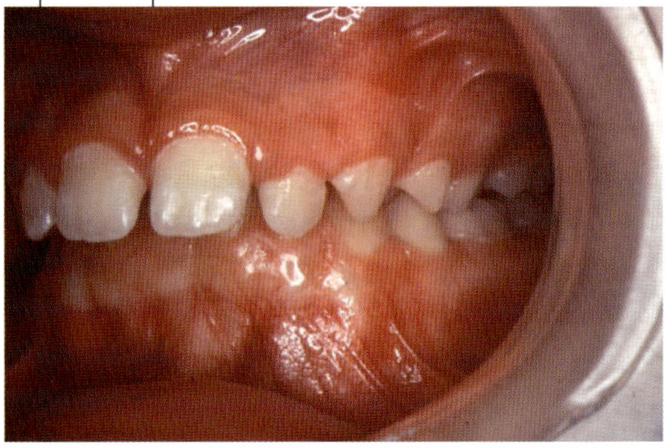

3-14

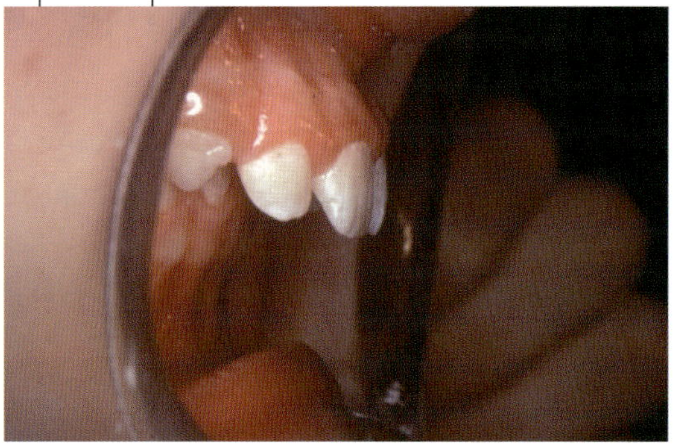

Figs. 3-13 & 3-14 Overbite and overjet. In a brachyfacial female, 8 years and 4 months old.

3-15

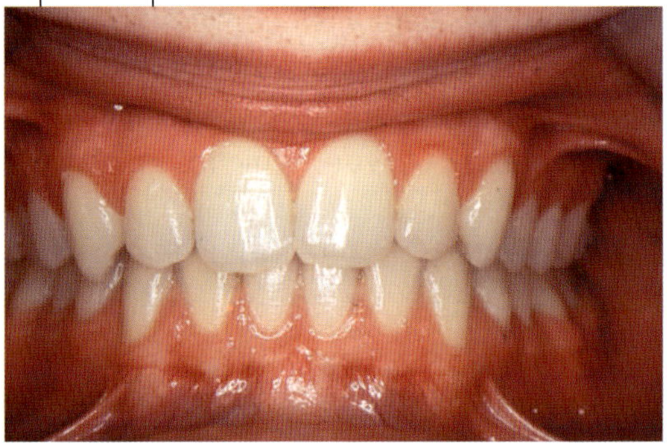

3-16

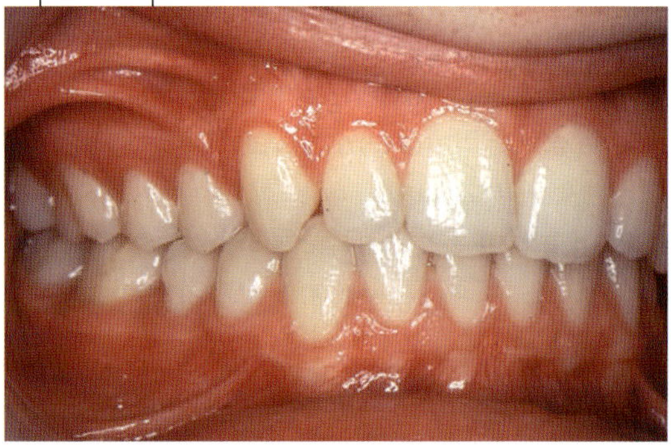

Figs. 3-15 & 3-16 Occlusion after 3 years and 3 months of treatment. The result is so beautiful that knowing whether or not the appliance had a real orthopaedic effect for a clinician is secondary. I just know that a Class 2 like this doesn't self correct.

3-17

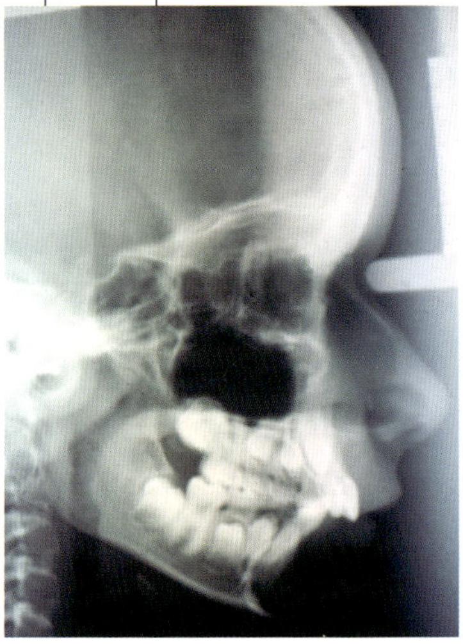

3-18

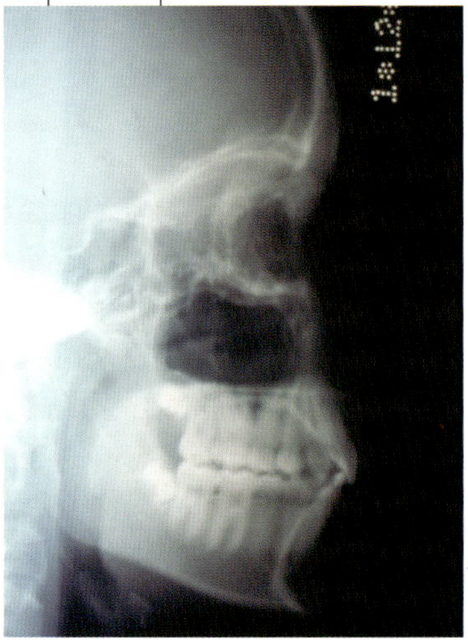

Fig. 3-17 Lateral cephalogram before treatment.

Fig. 3-18 Lateral cephalogram after treatment.

FUNCTIONAL PLATE OF CERVERA (PCF)[198] (FIG.3-19)

3-19

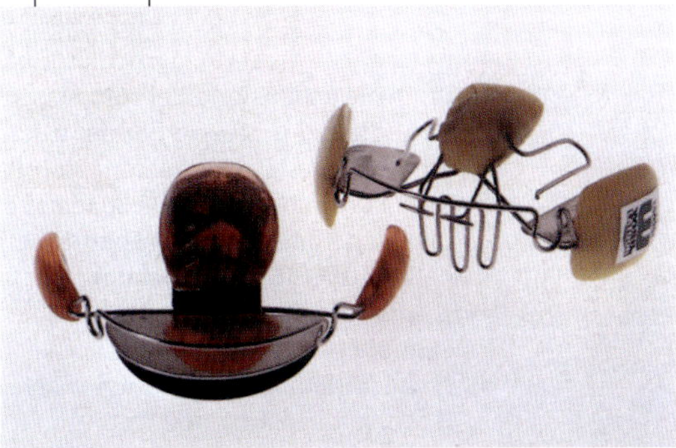

In Madrid, Dr. Cervera elaborated on the ideas of Dr. Planas who was the first to promote the use of a metallic plate between the anterior teeth. The PCF is free to move in the mouth. There are no clasps, so the PCF is kept in position by continuous activity of the tongue and other muscles, while there is an anterior contact with the lower incisors that prevents their extrusion and lets the mandible advance.

BIMLER

At the end of the 1940s, Bimler[24] described an appliance different from those used previously for the correction of a Class II division 1. His appliance was built using more elastic wire than usual, which helped to gain greater elasticity based on the supposition that reactive forces are more capable of changing the structural parts. In common with the other appliance inventors there is an attempt to determine structural changes through the modification of muscular forces.

The Bimler produces a construction bite with the teeth in a Class I relationship. The muscular activity of the internal pterygoid muscle activates the lateral part of the appliance by inducing a transverse expansion of the dental arch, and the vertical elements are activated when swallowing.

As well as the model described, other Bimler appliances are available for Class II division 2, and in Class III for crowded (extra 4) or double protruded (Bipro 6)occlusions, of both maxilla and mandible.

BIONATOR (FIG. 3-20)

This appliance[101] was designed by Balters in 1950 and even though it is based on the same principles as Robin and Andresen, some differences can be observed. While many opinion leaders admit the importance of the tongue for the occlusion, for Balters that was *the* most important factor. According to the concepts expressed by Van der Klaauw [246] about form and function, followed by Moss [178] with the functional matrix theory, the functional space of the tongue is necessary for the correct development of the orofacial system., Winders in his work, seemed to confirm the importance of the tongue, which can develop forces four times heavier than those of the oral and facial muscles. Am J Orthod V.42 n.9, p 645 - 57 Sept. 1956

Balters believed that without good tongue coordination, deformities and limitation of growth could occur. As happens, for example, in a Class II with a distal posture of the tongue. The appliance has a transverse palatal bar which stimulates the tongue activity vertically, while two lateral shields increase the transverse expansion, thereby avoiding the contact of soft tissues with teeth.

Those who believe in the Bionator think that this appliance is better than the others because it is smaller and therefore easier for young patients to use night and day, thus achieving better results.

There are three types of Bionator, for the Class II (standard), the Class III and for the open bite. The standard Bionator is indicated in a Class II with a slight sagittal discrepancy and a retruded mandible. It is not indicated in a Class II with maxillary protrusion, increased vertical growth and lower incisor proclination.

3-20

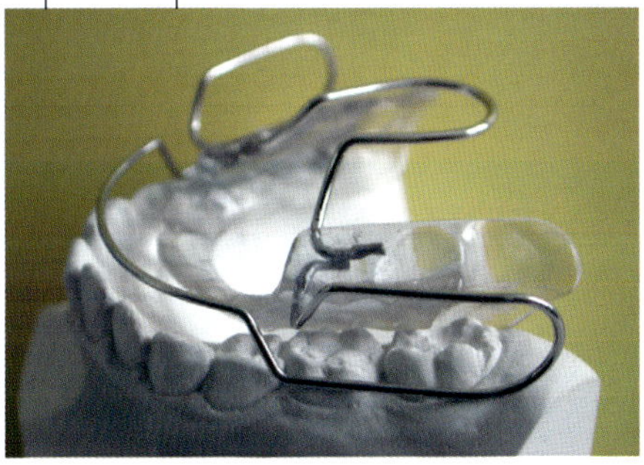

CASE NUMBER 3 (BIONATOR)

This case represents a classic "two phase" treatment of a Class II division 1.

The dental cast (Fig. 3-21) shows a Class II division 1 with mixed dentition at the beginning of a treatment with a Bionator ("first phase").

After 18 months the result is good (Fig. 3-22) but the occlusion is not ideal and it is improved by a fixed appliance for 8 months ("second phase") (Figs. 3-23 & 3-24).

3-21

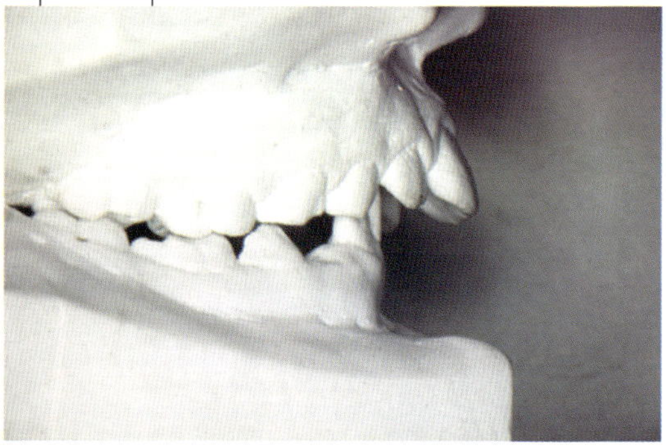

3-22

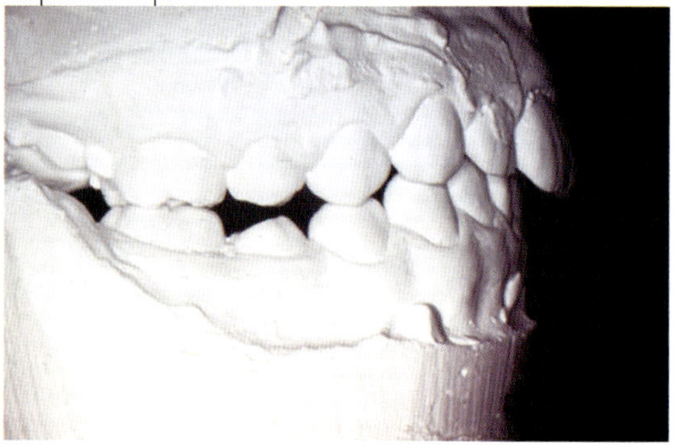

Fig. 3-21
Pre-treatment dental casts.

Fig. 3-22
Post-treatment dental casts.

3-23

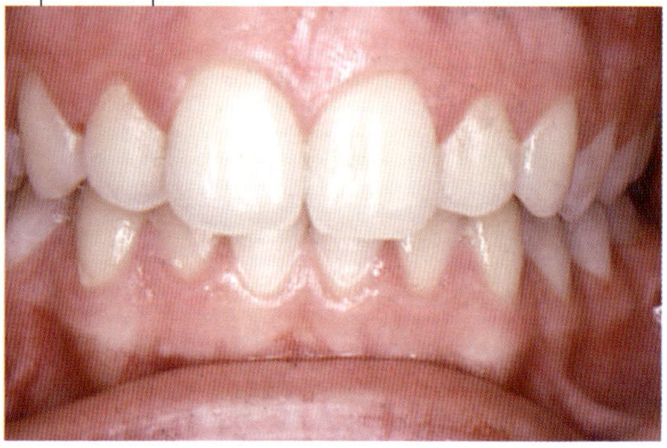

3-24

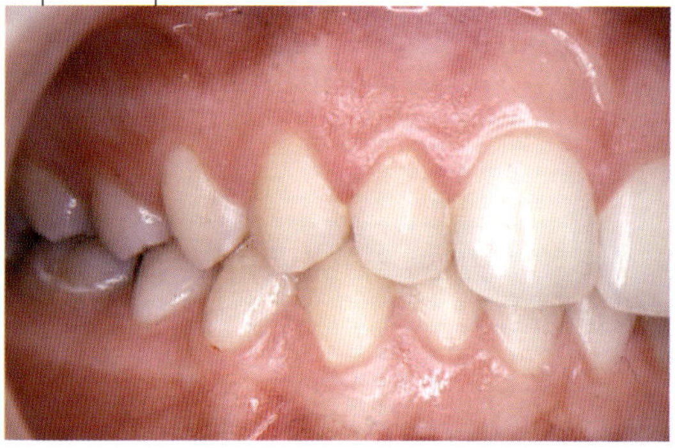

Figs. 3-23 & 3-24
Final occlusion.

3-25

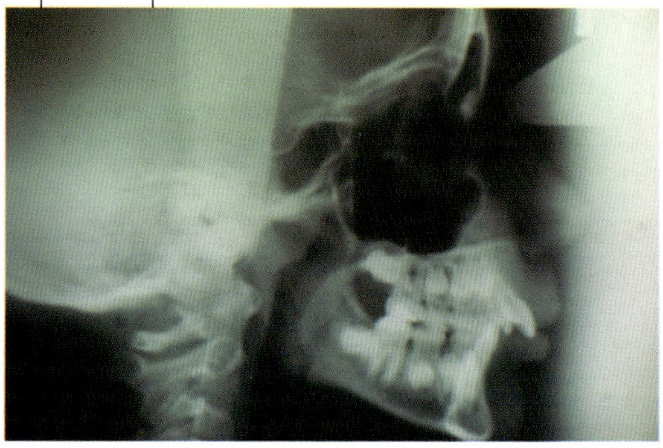

3-26

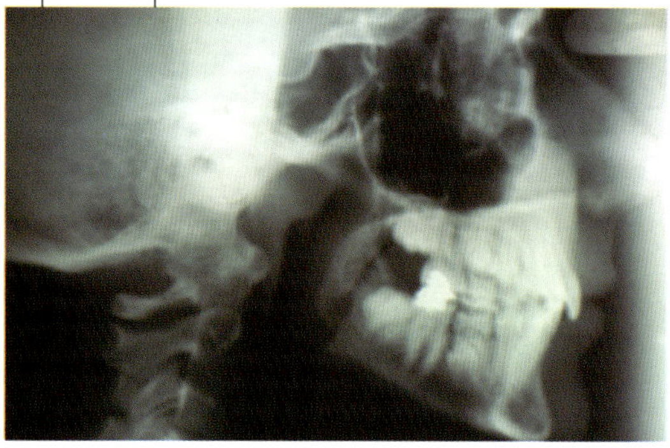

Fig. 3-25
Pre-treatment lateral cephalogram.

Fig. 3-26
Post-treatment lateral cephalogram. ANB from 6.5° to 4°.

KINETOR[236] (FIG. 3-27)

3-27

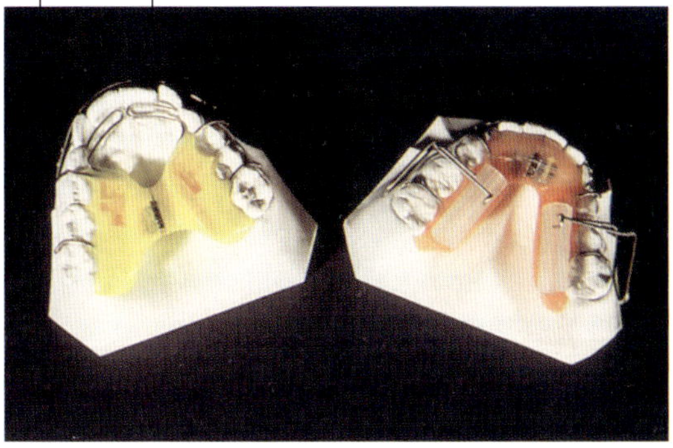

Dr. Stockfish's Kinetor [236] has many parts in common with other appliances (e.g. Andresen, Bionator, Fränkel). It has two dental plates with screws, coil springs, elastic tubes etc. which transmit the forces determined by functional activities.

It is mainly indicated in cases with excessive vertical growth.

SANDER'S APPLIANCES

a) Bite jumping appliance (Fig. 3-28)

3-28

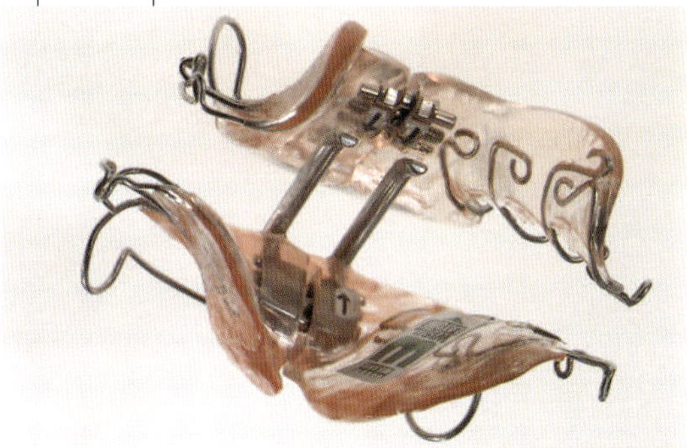

With this appliance, Prof. F G Sander (see Fortscher Kieferorthop. 1990 Jun ; 51 (3): 155-64 and Prakt. Kieferoethop. 1991 Mar; 5 (1) : 17 -28) modified a project of Dr. A.M. Schwartz, the advancement double plate[224]. There are two plates, a mandibular one and a maxillary one. When closing the mouth, the lower plate advances the mandible, sliding on two metallic guides fixed to the upper one. Its main usage is a Class II with a retruded mandible. All the teeth are in contact with the appliance and there is a labial retainer which counters the often undesired incisor proclination.

Those who opt for this appliance believe that it is more effective in late treatments and when a different action on the jaws is needed. Also it is possible to add micro screws to the appliance so that it can allow dental movement, tubes to extraoral headgear, and acrylics to avoid the development of bad habits, such as chewing the bottom lip.

This appliance tends to offer a construction bite with an edge to edge incisor relationship. In any case, it should not lead to more than 7 mm of mandibular advancement otherwise the appliance will not be effective.

b) Spring activator

In those cases where excessive vertical growth is present, Sander[218] suggests using the Spring activator. In this device there are, distally, two open coil springs which, developing 500 g of force when compressed, control the vertical dimension with intrusive vectors.

The construction bite does not exceed 5 mm of mandibular advancement, inducing an isometric contraction of muscles, which allows a condylar distraction.

This is the basis on which to contrast an undesirable, clockwise, mandibular growth.

If more control is needed it is possible to add two tubes from the upper plate to extraoral high pull headgear.

CASE NUMBER 4 (SANDER)

The statistics refer again to a typical Class II division 1, in this case a mesiofacial case study.

	Before	After		Before	After
SNA	*82°*	*81°*	*lower incisors on*		
SNB	*76°*	*78°*	*mandibular plane*	*88°*	*90°*
ANB	*6°*	*3°*			

This overjet and overbite has been caused, not only by skeletal characteristics, but also by the interposition of the lower lip between the lower and upper incisors, a typical bad habit.

3-29

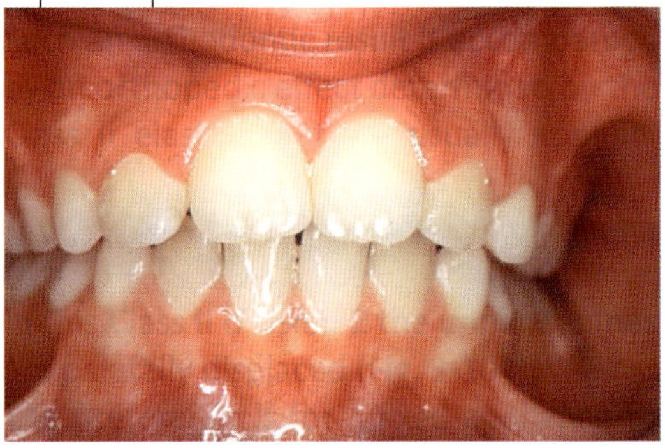

3-30

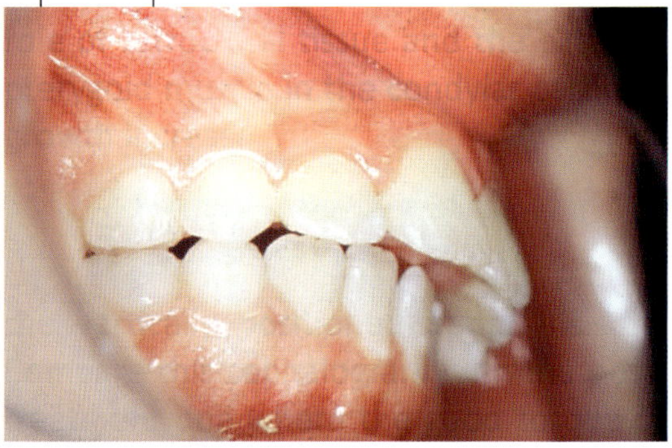

Figs. 3-29 & 3-30
Occlusion before treatment.

3-31

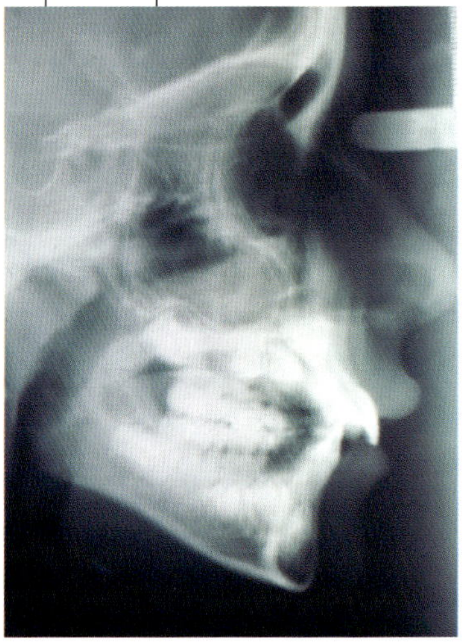

3-32

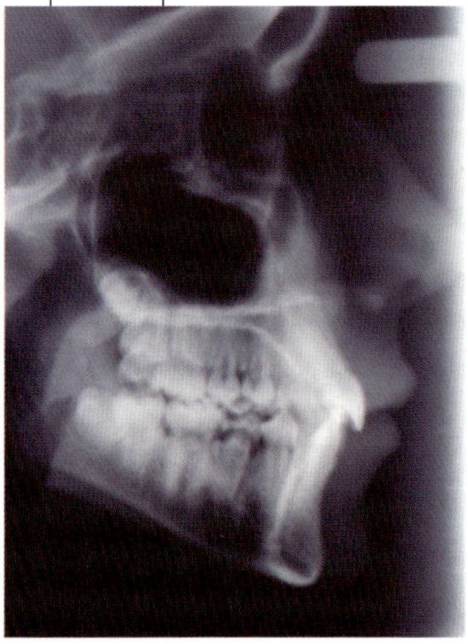

Fig. 3-31
Pre-treatment lateral cephalogram.

Fig. 3-32
Post-treatment lateral cephalogram.

3-33

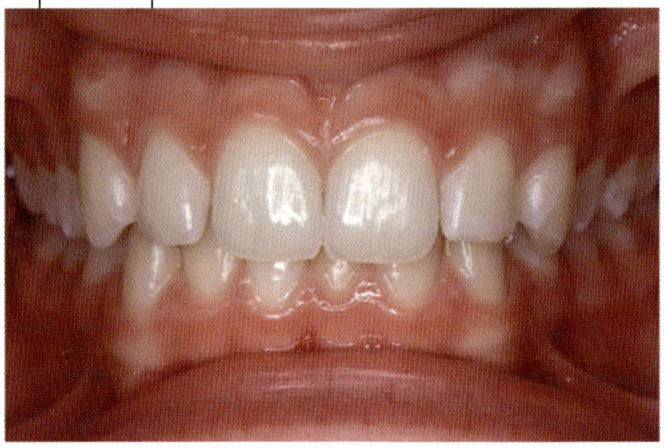

3-34

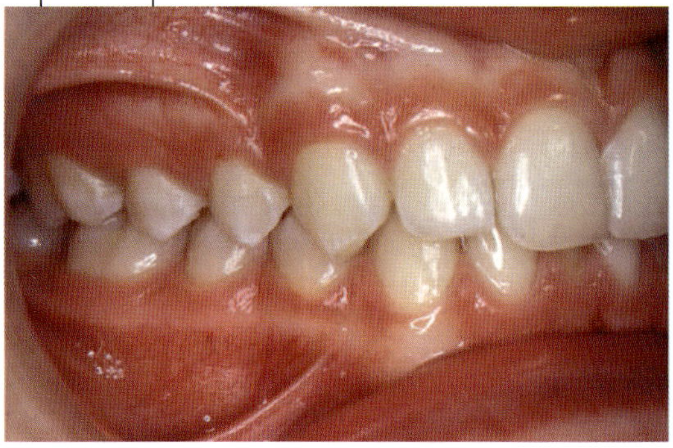

Figs. 3-33 & 3-34
18 months after treatment. The edge of the upper incisors has been softly ground (Ricketts called it dental manicure). It is an excellent result using only the removable appliance.

TWIN BLOCK (FIG. 3-35)

The Twin Block was also inspired by the Schwartz appliance. Just like in Sander's there are two plates, upper and lower. Each has an inclined plane. When the patient closes his mouth, the lower plate slides forward, guided by the inclined planes. Thus the mandibular advancement is instigated.

3-35

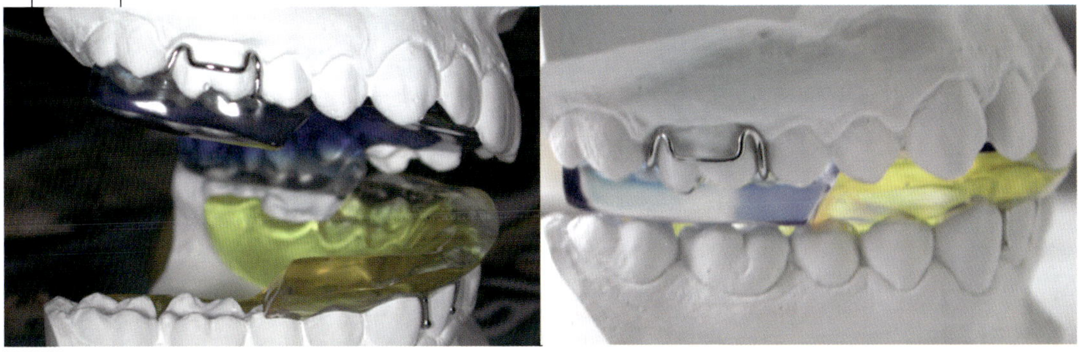

RV1 – RV 2 (FIG. 3-36 A & B)

The RV1 activator (Rossi - Vigotti) has in common with others, a mandibular advancement obtained by soft tissue contact using vertical "olives" or spurs (Fig. 3-36B).
In a treatment with RV1 I suggest a construction bite which brings the canines into dental Class I.
Mandibular advancement can be increased during treatment by adding extra acrylic material to the "olives". Transverse expansion is given by a palatal screw and buccal shields. There are clasps for intra-oral stabilization.
I prefer to use an appliance with palatal screw and clasps because they allow better management of the patient's cooperation. If some weeks after a well-fitting appliance has been applied the patient returns to the surgery and the appliance is unstable, it means that it has not been correctly used.
The main difference between the RV1 and the RV2 is the palatal three-way screw in Class II division 2. By pushing forward the upper incisors it allows anterior growth of the lower jaw.
In Class II with excessive vertical growth it is possible to add tubes for a high pull headgear.
I suggest the use of an RV for 14–16 hours a day, mostly during the night, when studying and watching TV.

3-36/A

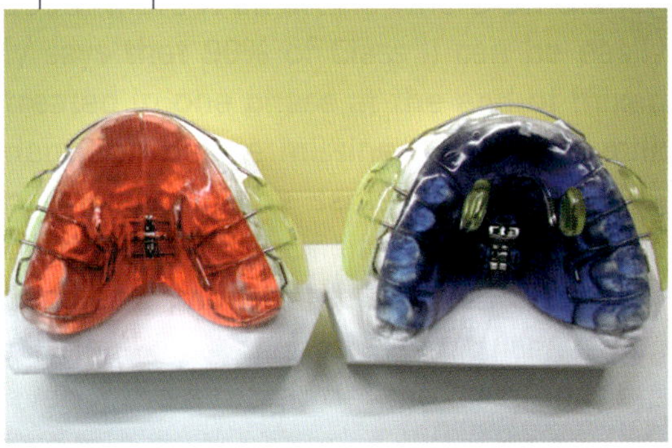

3-36B

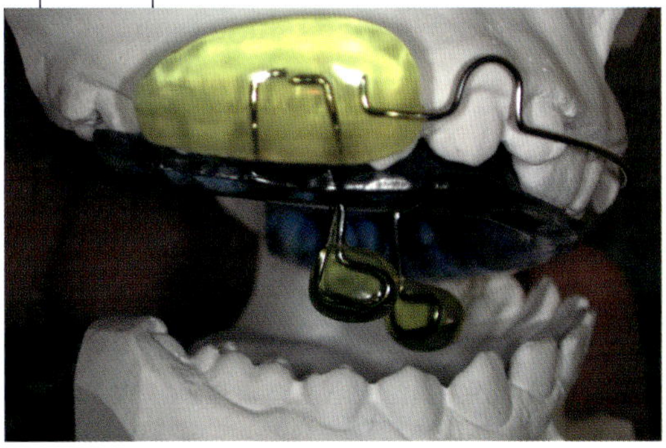

CASE NUMBER 5

This case is a Class II division 1 (ANB 11°) where the RV1 shows its effectiveness.
Notice the correction of the large overjet with a de-rotation of 11 – 21.

After one year, the good response stimulates the patient's compliance and allows a final result without an excessive proclination of the lower incisors.

	Before	After		Before	After
SNA	*80°*	*76°*	*lower incisors inclination*		
SNB	*69°*	*73°*	*on mandibular plane*	*92°*	*92°*
ANB	*11°*	*3°*			

3-37

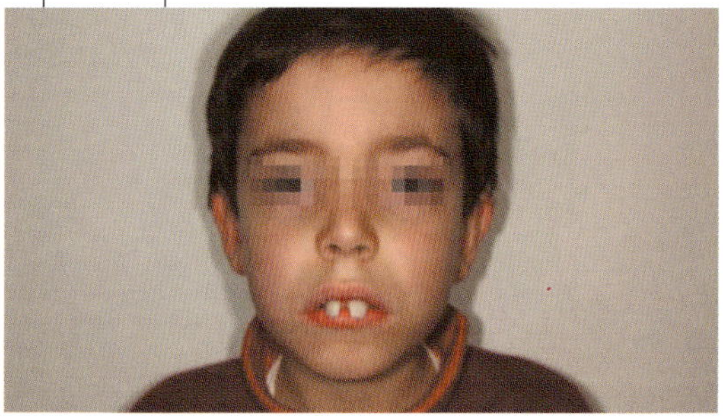

3-38

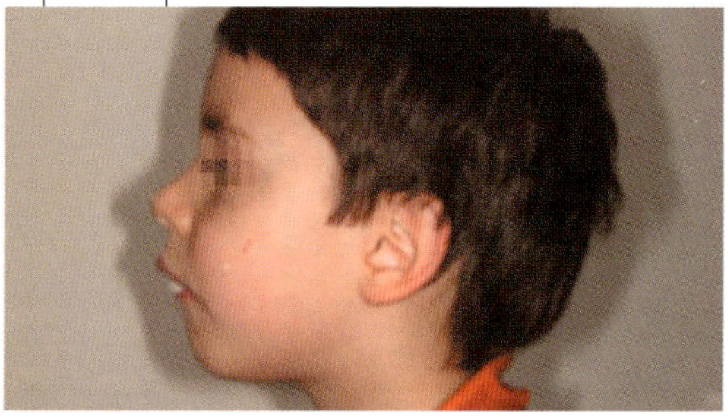

3-39

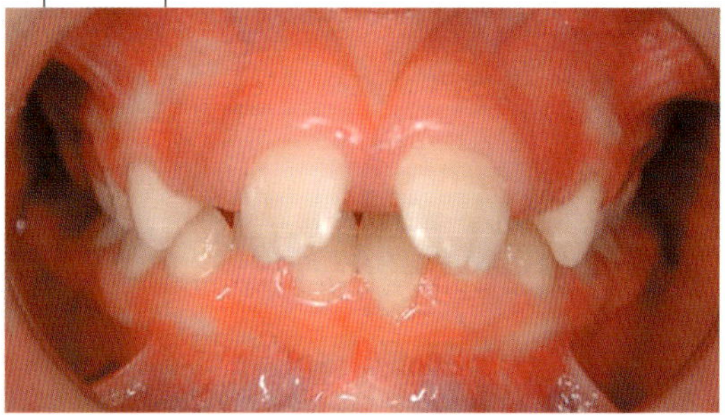

3-40

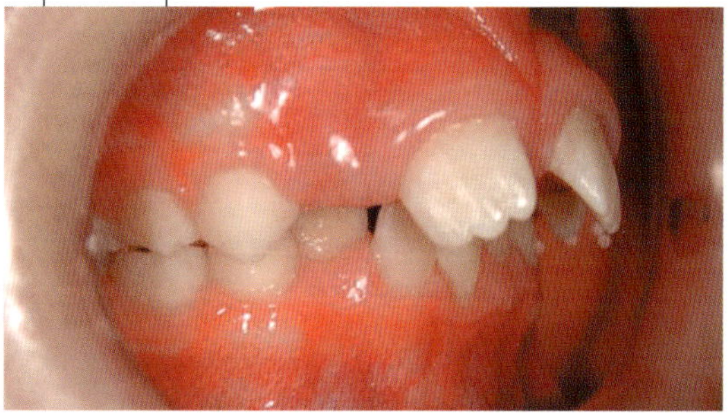

Figs. 3-37 to 3-41 Face and occlusion before treatment.

3-41

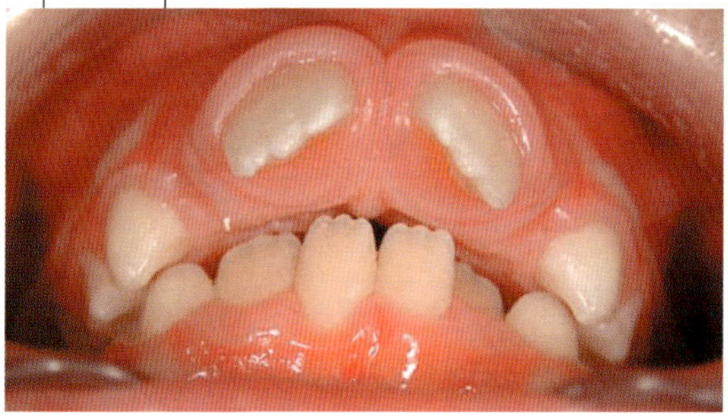

3-42

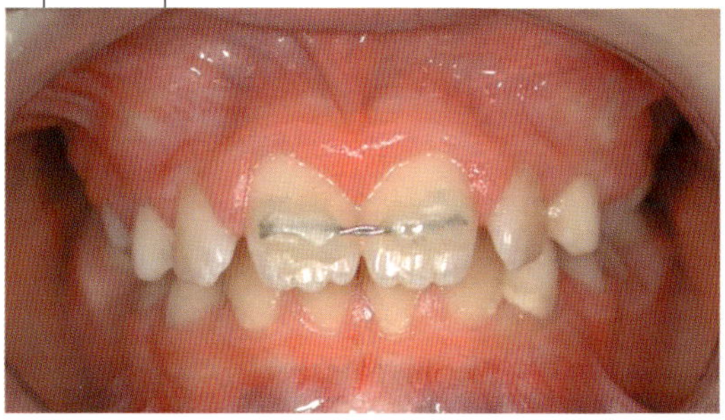

3-43

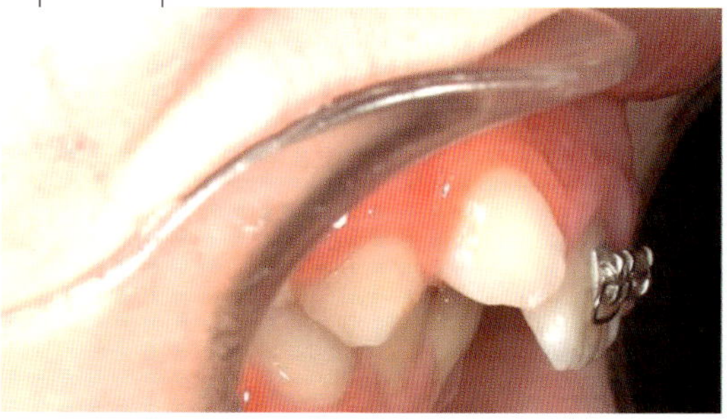

Figs. 3-41 to 3-43 Central incisors de-rotated with a sectional in NiTi.

3-44

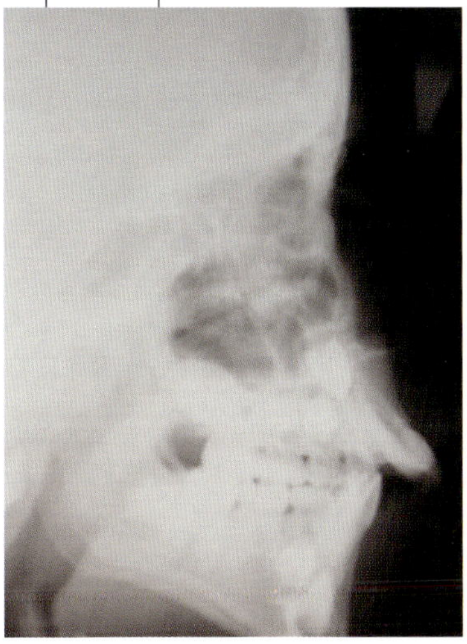

3-45

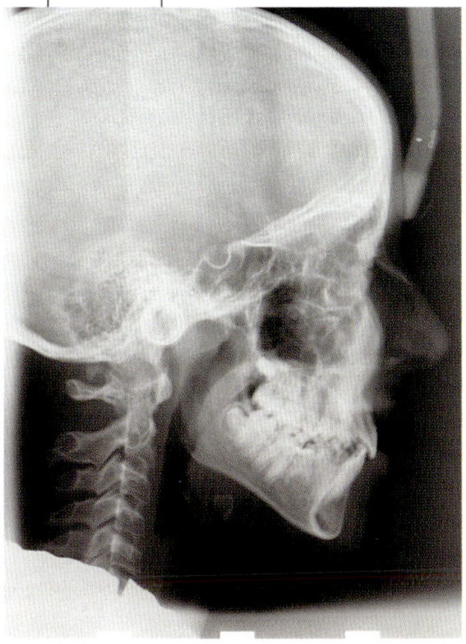

Fig. 3-44
Pre-treatment lateral cephalogram.

Fig. 3-45
Post-treatment lateral cephalogram.

3-46A

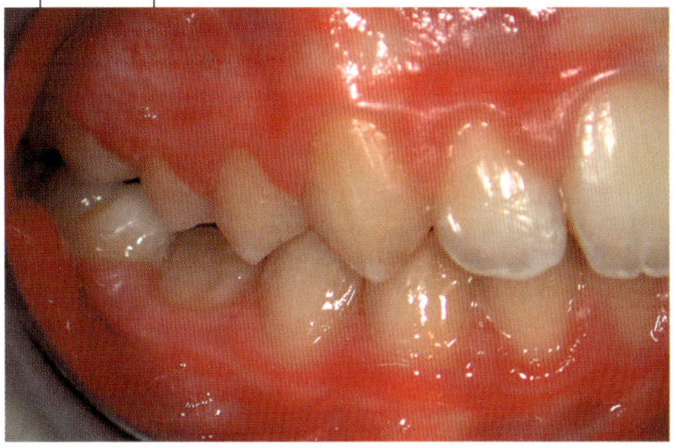

3-46B

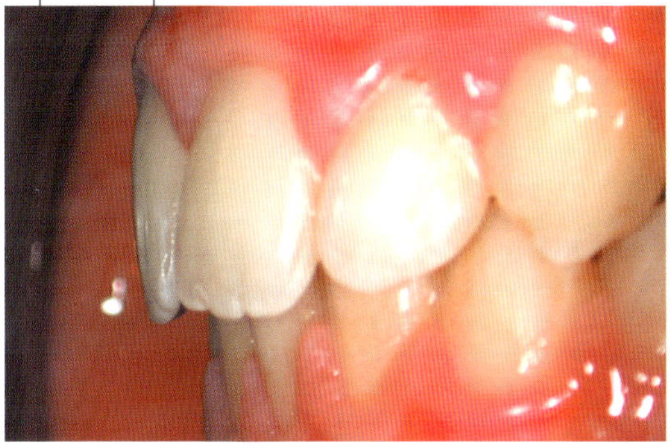

3-46C

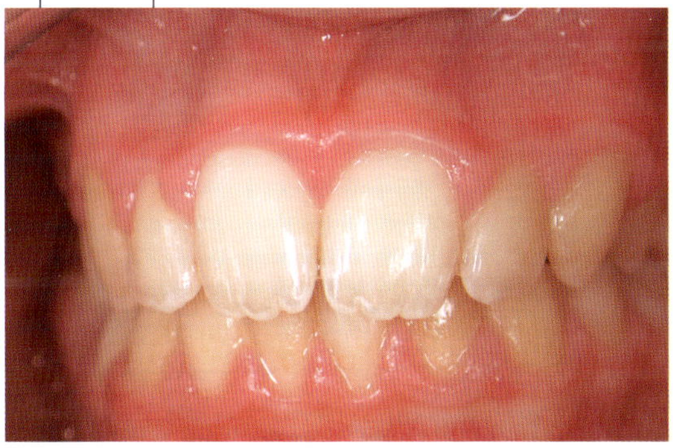

3-46D

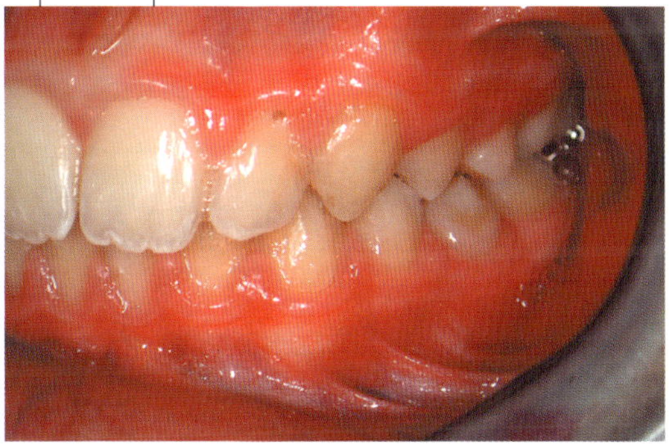

Fig. 3-46: A-B-C-D
Final occlusion.

HERBST APPLIANCE

The main criticism of functional appliances is that they are removable and therefore are effective only when in position, and if the patient is not compliant then good results do not show. With the Herbst appliance this does not happen because it is fixed in place securely and therefore patient compliance is not needed. Moreover, it is applied for only 6–18 months while a standard treatment with activators lasts 2–3 years.

Those who think that it is a new appliance are wrong. Dr. Emil Herbst presented it for the first time at the International Dental Congress in Berlin in 1905, but after a series of articles published in *Zahnärztliche Rundschau*[119] in 1934 the interest in this treatment decreased.

It was "discovered" in the USA at the end of the 1970s and the original design was modified - it has telescopic pistons fixed to molar and premolar bands, which push the mandible forward with steady permanent force to a Class I relationship. If the

appliance is inserted perfectly correctly, vertical and also lateral movements are possible. To avoid the posterior cross bite which follows a mandibular protrusion, a fixed palatal expander is useful.
When Dr. Pancherz compared 22 Class II division 1 cases treated with Herbst's appliance with 20 cases with the same malocclusion he found an increased mandibular growth (the Condylion – Gnathion length) during 6 months of treatment.[188]
These results show that the Herbst appliance can be used to advance a lower jaw with anticlockwise growth.
Such outcomes can be excellent, though some critics believe that treatments in mixed dentition need to be revised later. As a matter of fact, when the treatment is not followed by an active retainer (activator), a relapse can easily occur because the condyle-fossa relationship reached in 6-18 months of treatment is not stable.
Like Woodside's[256] research on animals, Pancherz observed during a study of lateral cephalograms not only a condyle remodelling but also a bone apposition on the posterior side of the fossa with a forward movement of the glenoid cavity and a thickening of the articular disc.
A process of remodelling needs time and this could explain the relapses in many "fast" treatments. Therefore I recommend the use of active retention until the final permanent occlusion is reached. Note that this latter is the primary element of stability.

CASE NUMBER 6

After 18 months of treatment of a Class II (Fig. 3-47), a young patient refuses to use the removable appliance even though it has improved the malocclusion.
More work is needed to reach a good Class I (Figs. 3-48 & 3-49), therefore the Herbst appliance has been utilized.

3-47

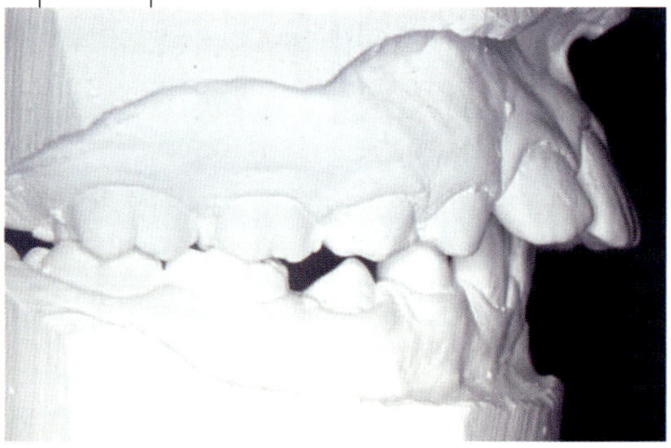

Fig. 3-47 Dental casts before treatment.

3-48

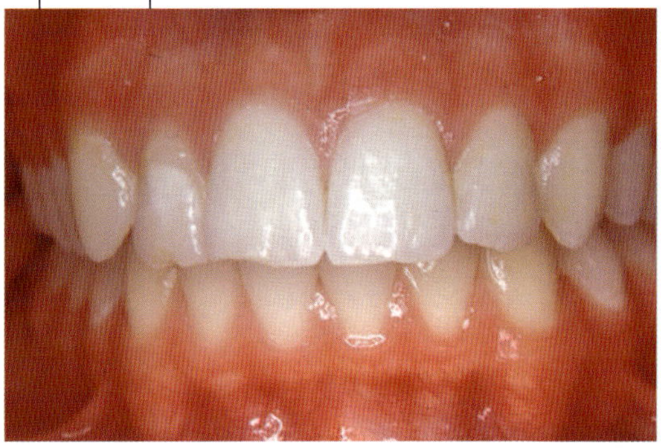

3-49

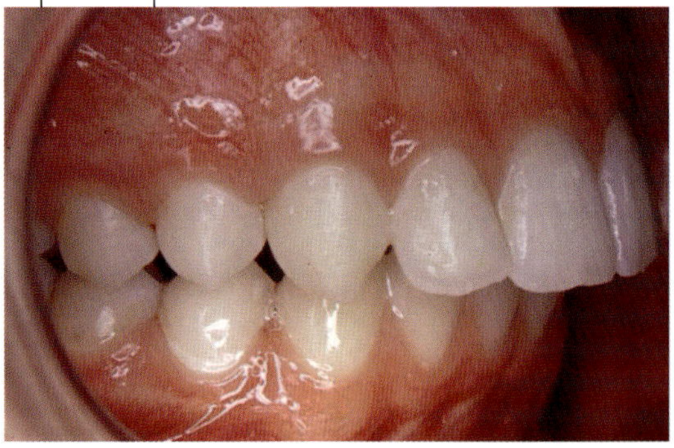

Figs. 3-48 & 3-49 Occlusion after the treatment with removable appliance.

3-50

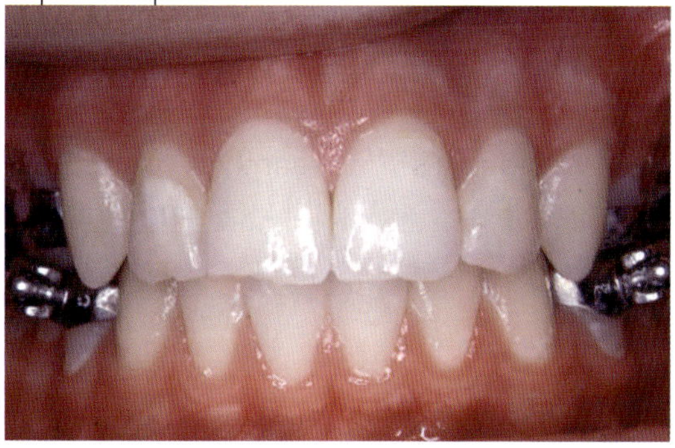

3-51

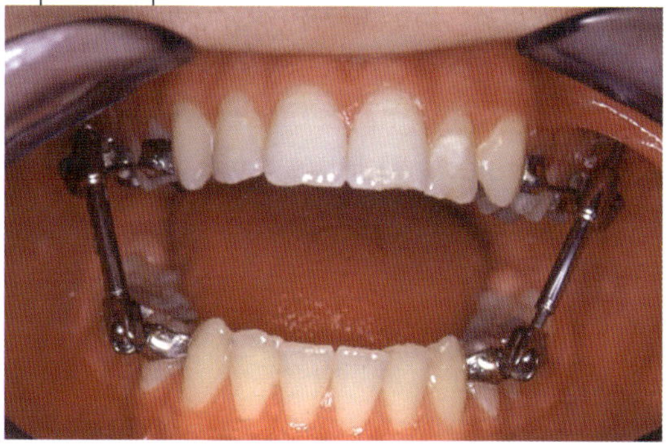

3-52

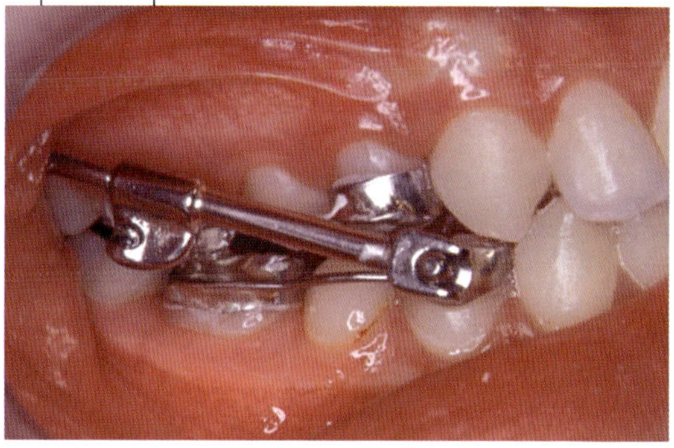

Figs. 3-50 to 3-52
Herbst appliance – clinical view.

3-53

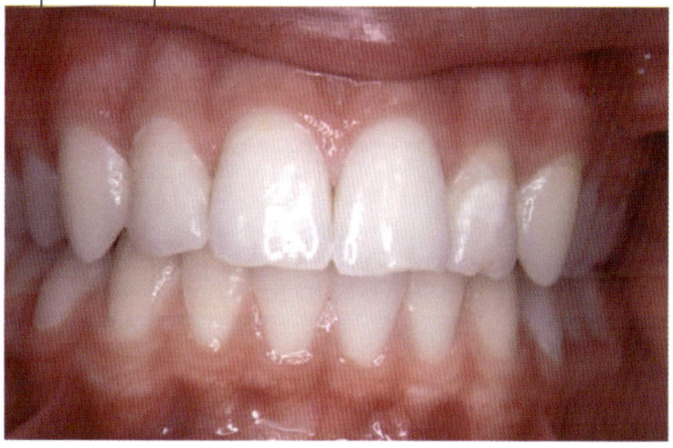

3-54

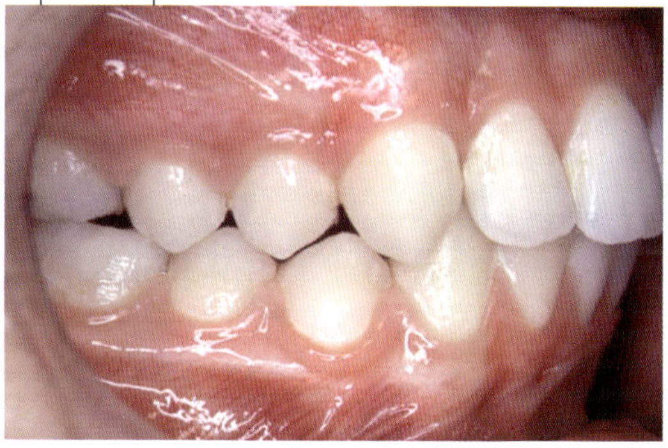

Figs. 3-53 & 3-54
Final occlusion after 9 months of treatment with Herbst appliance.

3-55

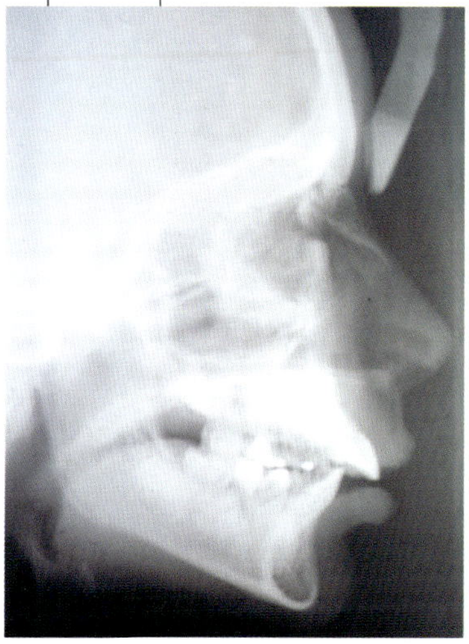

3-56

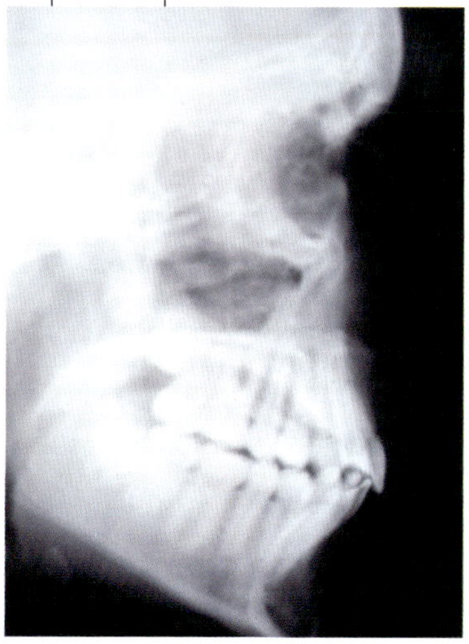

Fig. 3-55
Pre-treatment lateral cephalogram.

Fig. 3-56
Post-treatment lateral cephalogram.

THE HEADGEARS

Extra-oral tractions commonly known as headgears have been talked about for more than 100 years. Kinsley (in 1866) and Farrar (in 1870) used an intra-oral appliance combined with an extra-oral traction to retract proclined upper incisors. In 1888 Angle designed a headgear applied to two bands on the central upper incisors. In the same year, Goddard showed a device which is a combination of an extra-oral headgear connected to an intra-oral rubber made part. The rubber is in contact with the upper front teeth, which are retracted by the extra oral force.

In 1921, Case described the use of a headgear to distalize upper molars. In the 30s and 40s, Oppenheim, Nelson, Downs and others introduced the use of head cap tractions. In 1950 Fisher applied an extra-oral traction to the upper premolars. Soon afterwards, Kloehn[136] presented a cervical headgear which worked predominately on the upper molars, but also had positive effects on the lower arch.

A headgear can be used in an orthodontic or orthopedic way: **it is the forces of traction that make the difference**. When applied to the upper molars, remember that there is a bodily movement if the vector of force passes through the centre of resistance. The latter, with a good periodontal situation, is located at the root bifurcation. If forces are directed elsewhere than the centre of resistance then they become rotational forces. The centre of that rotation is determined by the direction of the force.

These forces are in turn effected by the length and angulation of the external facial bows.

For a precise application of headgear, Greenspan[110] suggests its adjustment on a lateral cephalogram while Kubein, Jäger and Bormann[146] use a compass that, when inserted in the buccal tube of the molar, marks externally on the cheeks the position of the centre of resistance (compasses of Gottingen).

BIOMECHANICAL EFFECTS OF THE HEADGEARS

My schematic representation is based on the model of Kubein, Jäger and Bormann.

CERVICAL PULL HEADGEAR

3-57

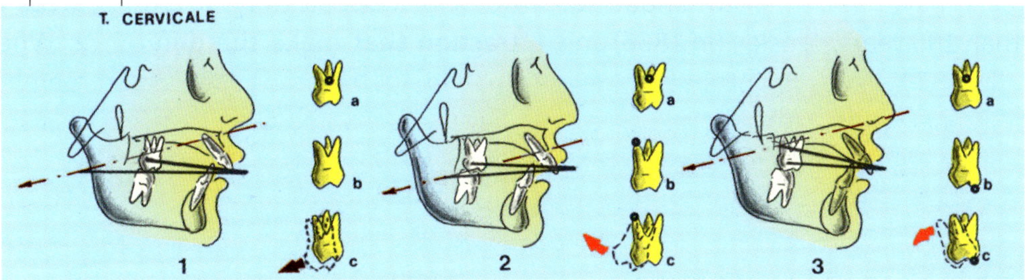

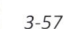

- Vector of force through the centre of resistance = bodily movement (distalisation and extrusion) with no rotation (centre of rotation at infinity).
- Vector of force below the centre of resistance = rotation with extrusion and crown distalisation. Centre of rotation at the roots apex.
- Vector of force above the centre of resistance = rotation with extrusion and roots distalisation. Centre of rotation at crown level.

3-58

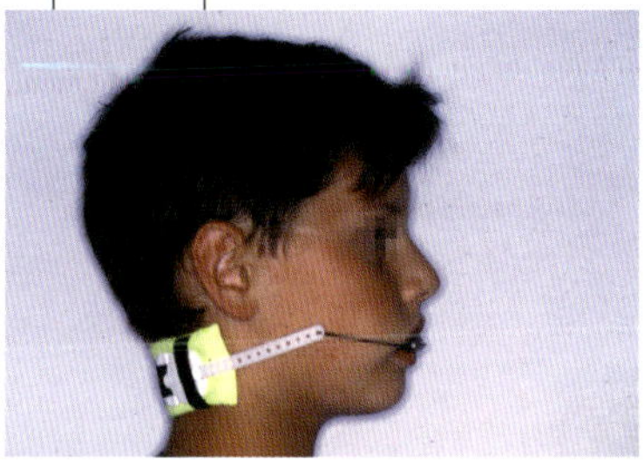

HORIZONTAL PULL HEADGEAR

3-59

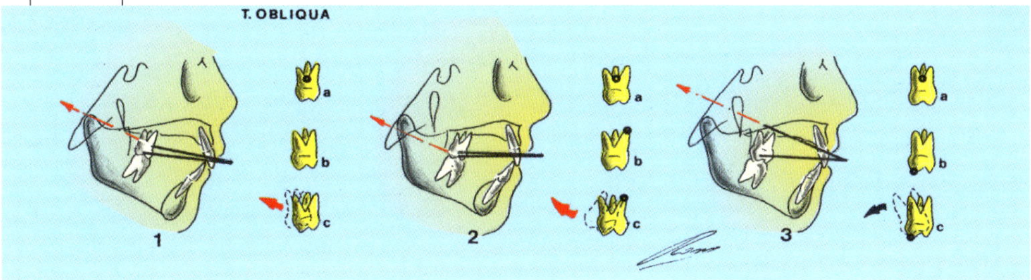

It is not easy to have a horizontal vector. Therefore many orthodontists obtain it with the resultant force of a combi (combination of cervical and high pull traction).

The force of the high pull traction is usually double the cervical one.

The same movement can be obtained as the cervical traction without extrusion of molars.

3-60

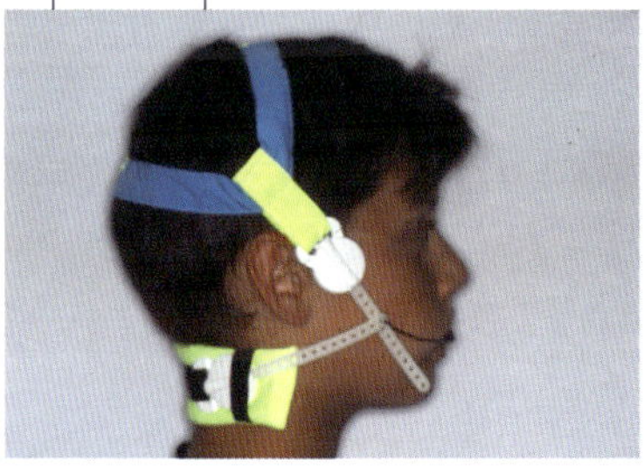

HIGH PULL HEADGEAR

3-61

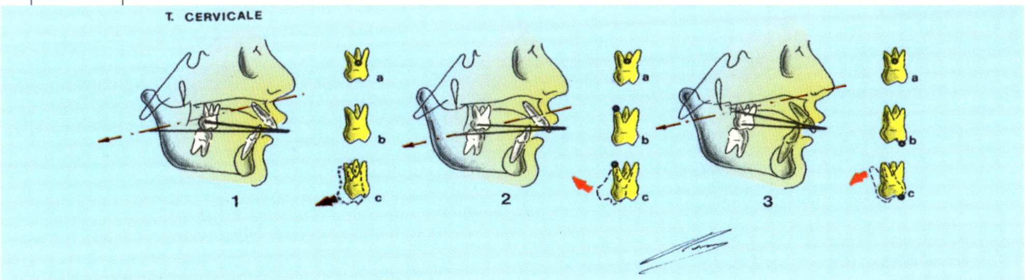

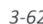

As above – distalisation takes place with molar intrusion.

3-62

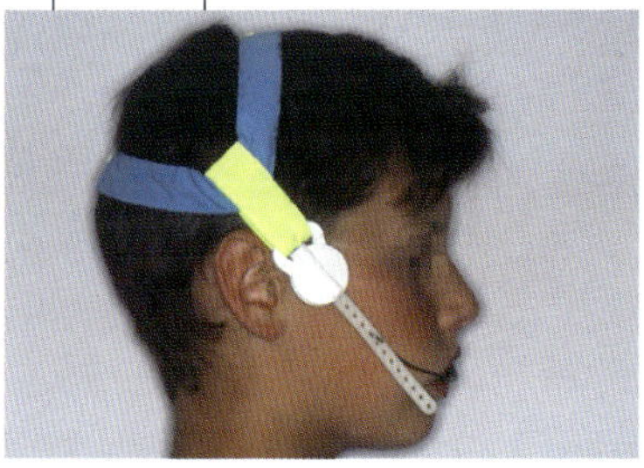

ORTHODONTIC USE

Headgears can be used orthodontically with forces less than 300 g. In these cases they are used as anchorage or to distalise upper molars in Class I with maxillary crowding and in Class II. At the same time, where there is a proclination of the frontal teeth, a traction with metallic bite as designed first by Gros[111] and later made popular by Cervera[47] as Equi. C can be used (Case Number 7, Figs. 3-63 to 3-69).

The retraction of the upper incisors is obtained by stretching an elastic from two hooks positioned on the appliance distally to the canines. Similar effects where an extrusion of the molars is not needed are obtainable with the traction included in thermoplastic splints (OPA, C modeller, etc.) and a high or combined pull.

CASE NUMBER 7 (EQUI-C)

3-63

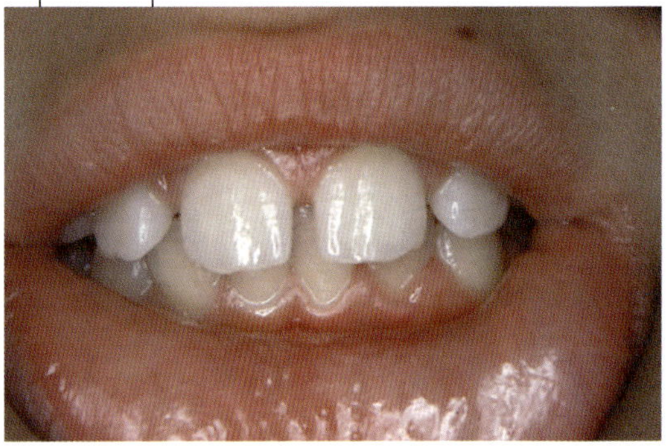

3-64

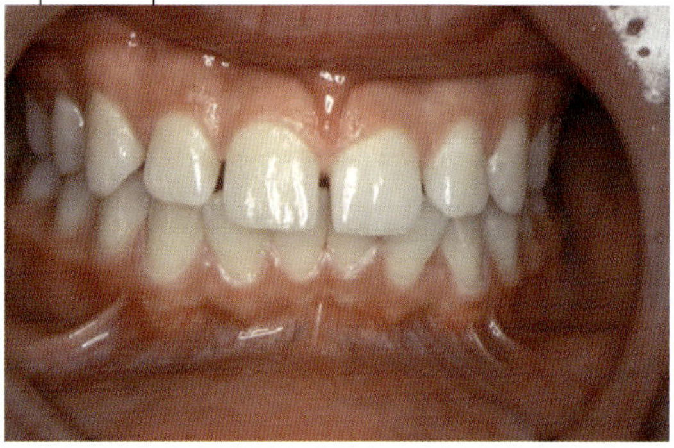

Figs. 3-63 & 3-64 Occlusion before treatment. It is a skeletal deep bite (brachi) Class II division 1 with evident upper teeth proclination.

3-65

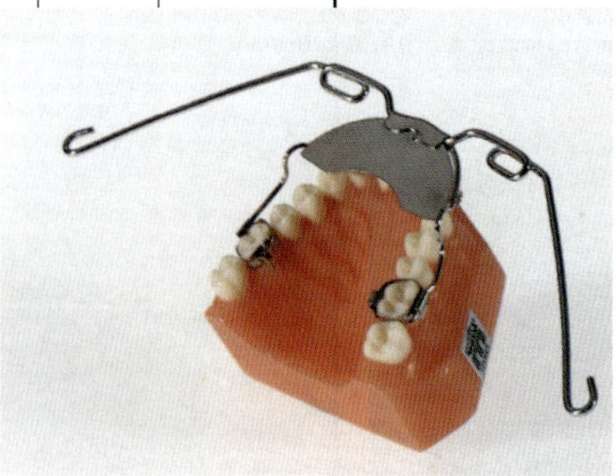

3-66

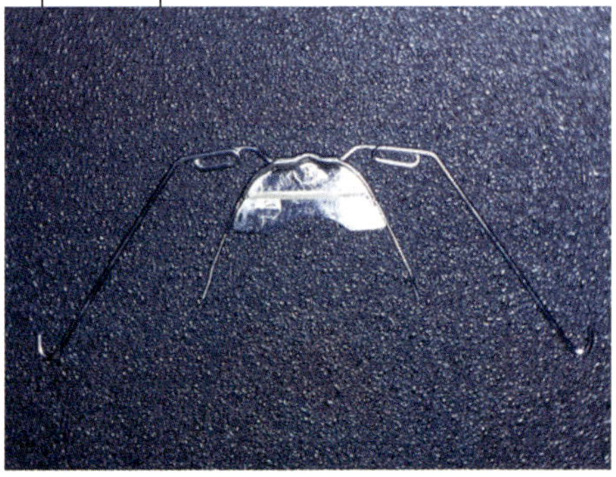

3-67

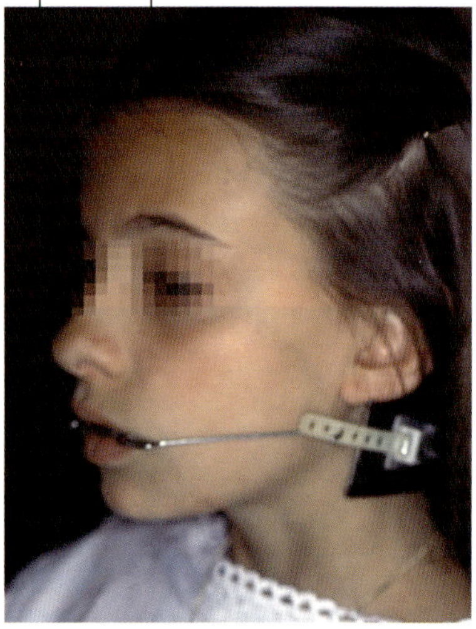

Figs. 3-65 to 3-67 A retraction of incisors with extrusion of molars correct the malocclusion. This is obtained with an Equi-C.

3-68

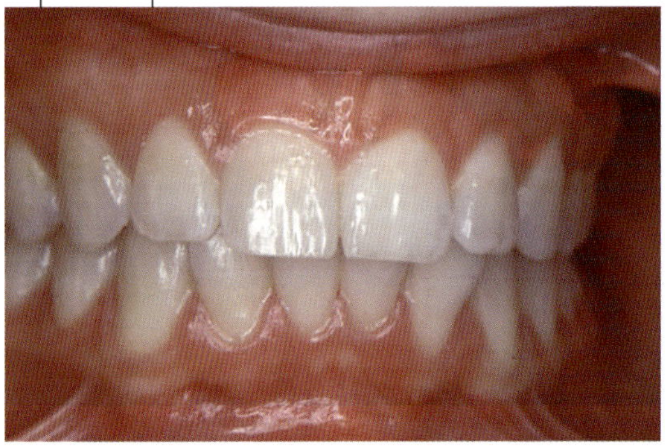

3-69

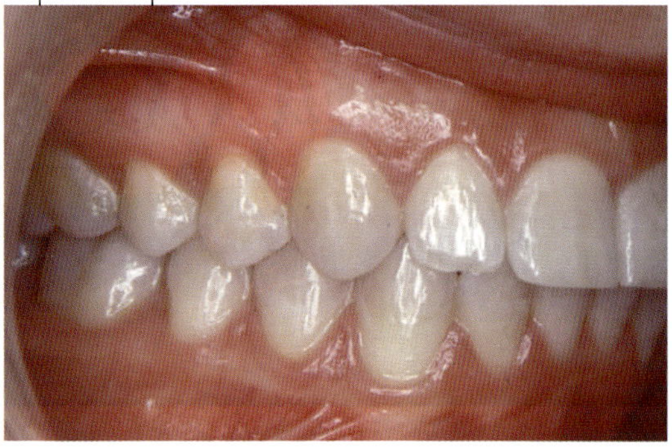

Figs. 3-68 & 3-69 Occlusion after 22 months of treatment.

Some orthodontists use a headgear for less than 12 hours in order to maintain an anchorage. To distalise the molars, a force is needed for 14-16 hours a day.

Since it is difficult to wear a headgear for many hours, in order to apply forces for a longer period of time they are often combined with other removable appliances (for example a Cetlin plate) or with Class II elastics. The force applied is the same on both sides. If more force is needed on one side, the external arm must be longer and straightened forward (Fig. 3-70).

Schudy suggested anterior J hooks to intrude on upper incisors. In my opinion, these braces are not commonly utilized (Fig. 3-71). Other orthodontists like Sassouni [219] and Merrifield[171] applied headgears on both jaws simultaneously. That type of technique is rarely used.

3-70

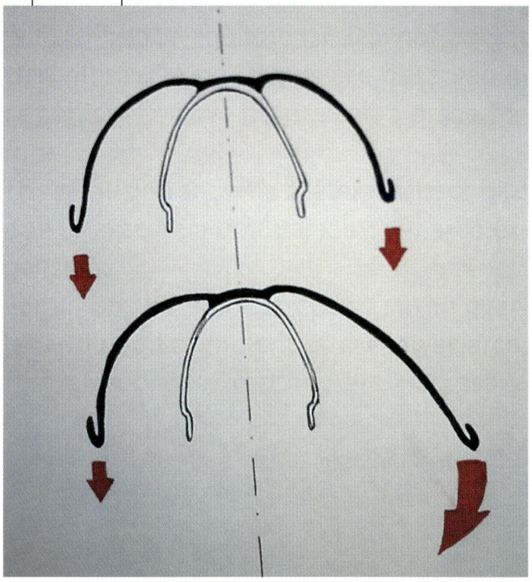

3-71

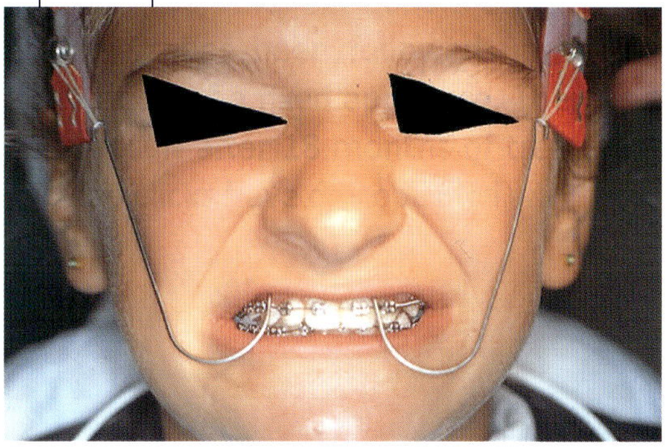

ORTHOPEDIC USE (WITH FORCES GREATER THAN 300 G)

Epstein,[85] Klohen,[136] Ricketts,[206] King,[134] Wieslander,[252] Sadowsky[215] and many others believe that by using a cervical headgear it is possible to stop maxillary advancement during growth, yet, as pointed out by Funk[99], the mandible not only goes on with its growth but also increases in length and improves its shape. In Ricketts' opinion, by applying a headgear to the maxilla, it is also possible to increase the ramus of the mandible.

Schudy[222] demonstrated that 73% of the growth of the lower third of the face is linked to the development of the maxillary and to the development of dental alveolar processes. Therefore, the vertical control of these aspects with a high pull headgear is orthopedic.

In a Class II dolicofacial the vertical control is very important because with a reduction of verticality, the mandible tends to have a counterclockwise rotation with a reduction of the ANB angle.

In other words, there is an improvement of the Class II.

HEADGEARS COMBINED WITH ACTIVATORS

When we want to influence the sagittal and vertical growth of the jaws, should we only use headgear? Why not use it with an activator and obtain more results?

Dr. Teuscher's activator (Zurich),[239] Dr. Joho's, Grobety's, Pfeiffer's Geneva activator (Geneva),[132] Dr. Bass' appliance (London),[11] Sander's appliance and the RV appliances are all based on this premise...

In common they have an intra-oral part (activator) with a tube on each side to apply the headgear. The latter has to be worn usually while sleeping, studying and watching TV.

The application time varies from 14 to 16 hours a day.

The differences are:

- in Teuscher's and Sander's the mandibular advancement occurs with tooth contact
- the Geneva, Bass and RV appliances have a soft tissue contact to avoid lower incisor proclination
- in the Geneva, Sander and RV appliances a buccal steel arch is in contact with the upper incisors
- in the Bass appliance there are two springs of torque on the central incisors while there are four in Teuscher's
- the tubes for the headgear are at first upper premolar level in Bass' appliance, at first premolar or first molar level depending on the maxillary rotation required in Sander's appliance and between the first and second upper premolars in Teuscher's and Geneva's.

The force applied on each side is usually 800 g. In order to avoid undesired maxillary and dento-alveolar rotations, the vector must pass through the maxillary and dental centre of resistance (Fig. 3-72). In this way it is possible to control the maxillary vertical growth inducing a positive rotation of the mandible with a reduction of the ANB angle.

Vertical control (headgear) and mandibular displacement (activator) give the best chances of correction of a Class II in dolicofacial patients.

CENTRES OF RESISTANCE

Teuscher believes that not only the teeth but also the maxilla (connected to surrounding structures by a sutural system) have a centre of resistance. Therefore, the middle part of the facial structures has two centres of resistance: a dental one between the upper premolar roots (A) and a bone one at the maxillary – zygomatic suture (B).

Again, in order to avoid undesirable rotations, the vector of force from the headgear must pass through the centres (Fig. 3-72).

3-72

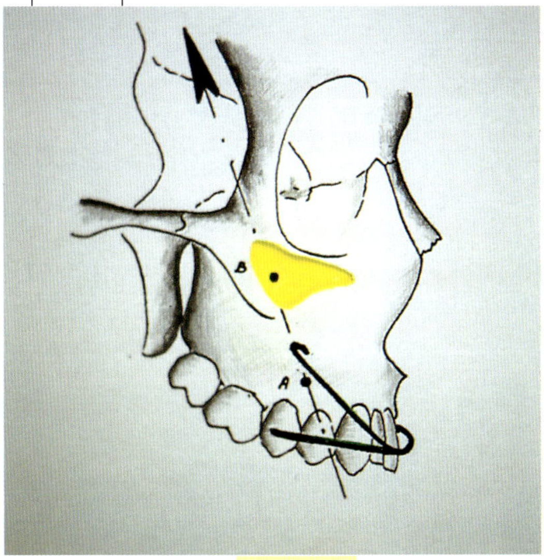

3-73

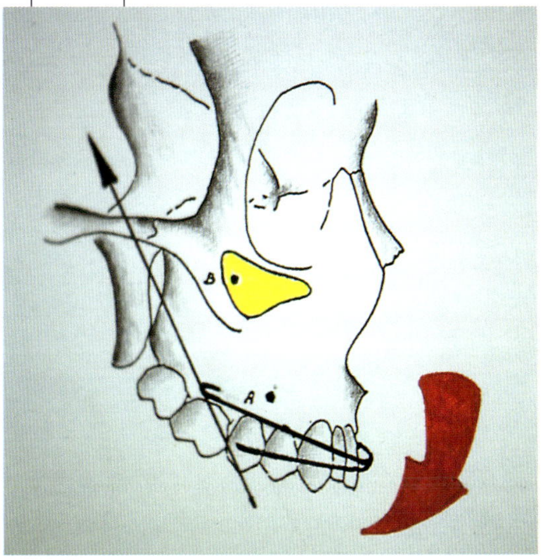

Fig. 3-73
When the vector of force passes behind the centres of resistance there is a tendency of the upper jaw to rotate clockwise. Positive in Class II open bites (dolico).

3-74

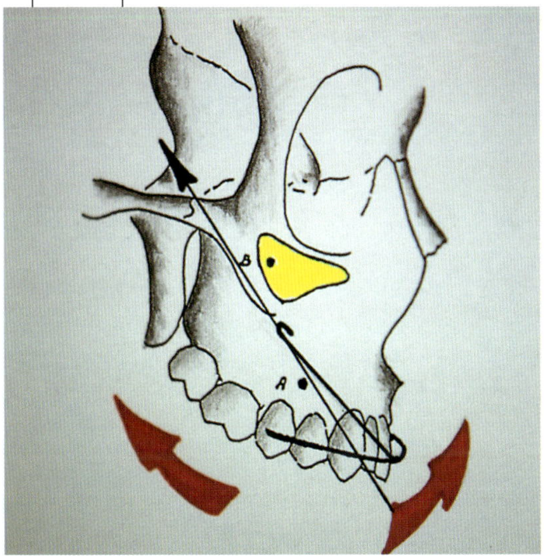

Fig. 3-74
When the vector of force passes between the two centres there is clockwise rotation of the palatal plane, counterclockwise for the occlusal plane. Positive in a Class II deepbite (brachi).

3-75

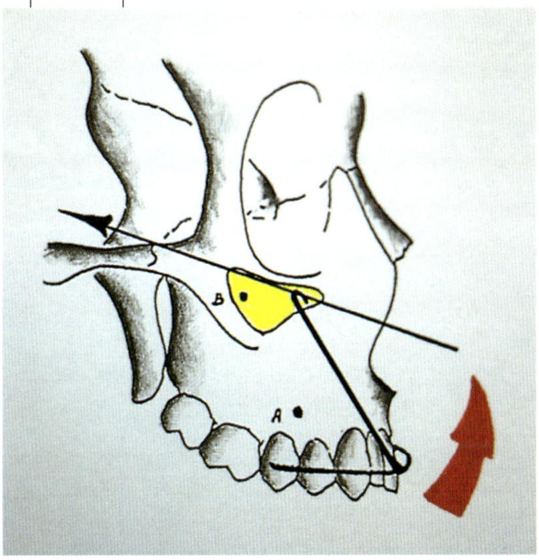

Fig. 3-75
When the vector of force passes above the centres of resistance there is anticlockwise rotation of the palatal and occlusal planes. If this anticlockwise rotation improves a deep dental bite it can inhibit an anterior displacement of the mandible. Such an outcome could be negative in a Class II open (dolico).

CASE NUMBER 8 (BASS)

	Before	After		Before	After
SNA	*86.5°*	*85°*	*lower incisors inclination*		
SNB	*79°*	*82°*	*on mandibular plane*	*91°*	*91°*
ANB	*7.5°*	*3°*			

With the correction of overjet and overbite, please note that the inclination of the lower incisors on the mandibular plane does not change.

Looking at the patient's profile (prominent nose, retrusion of the lower third) **the importance of a mandibular advancement is obvious.** Imagine the worsening of that profile if a case of conservative treatment (activator – headgear) failed, and thus necessitated a treatment characterized by two upper premolar extractions.

3-76

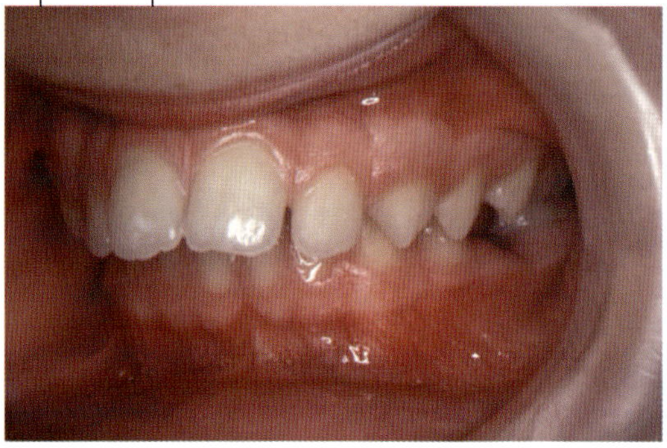

3-77

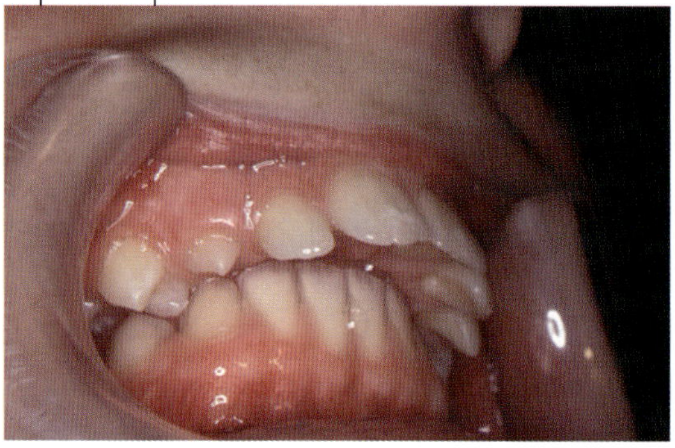

Figs. 3-76 & 3-77
Occlusion of a mixed Class II division 1 in a dolicofacial patient. We need an appliance that inhibits the anterior growth of the maxilla and gives a vertical control inducing a mandibular advancement.

3-78

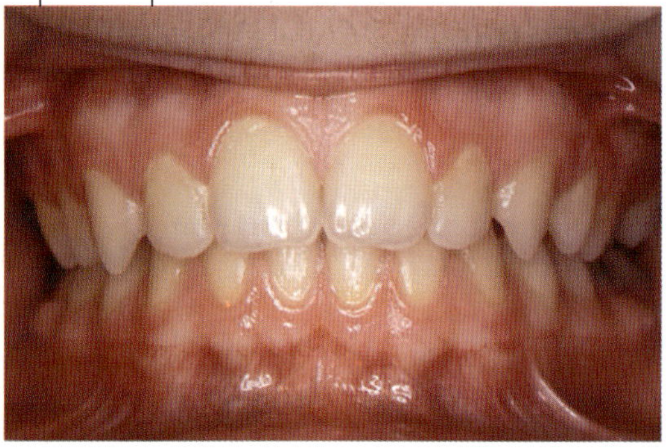

3-79

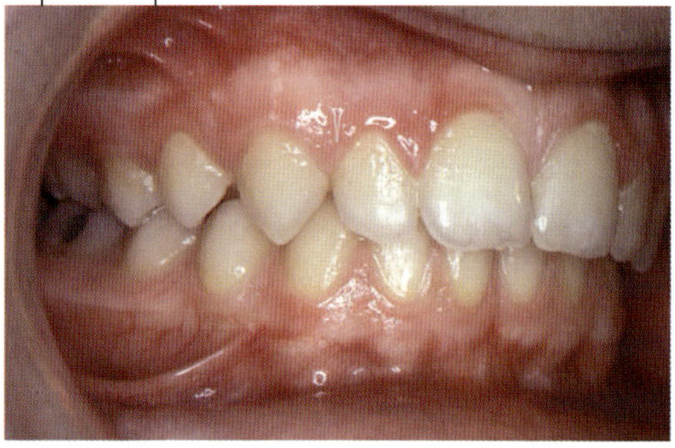

Fig. 3-78 & 3-79
Occlusion after 18 months of treatment with a Bass appliance worn 14 – 16 hours a day. The result is good.

3-80

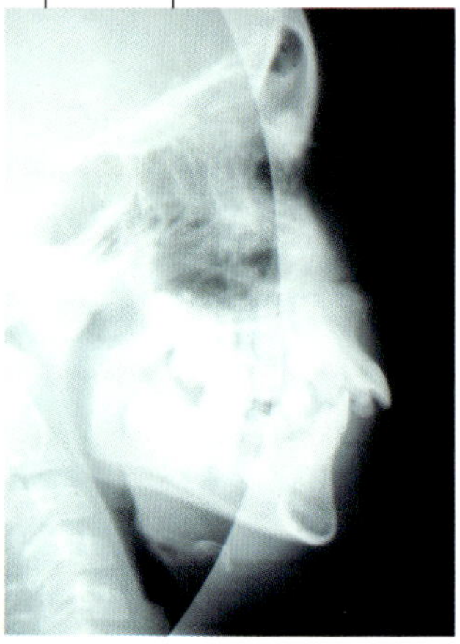

3-81

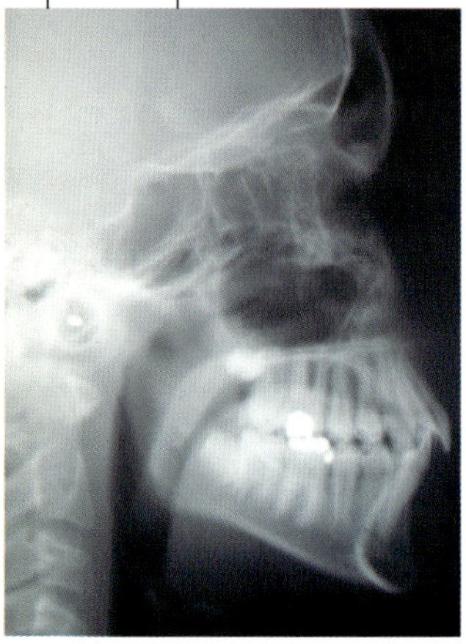

Fig. 3-80
Pre-treatment lateral cephalogram.

Fig. 3-81
Post-treatment lateral cephalogram.

3-82

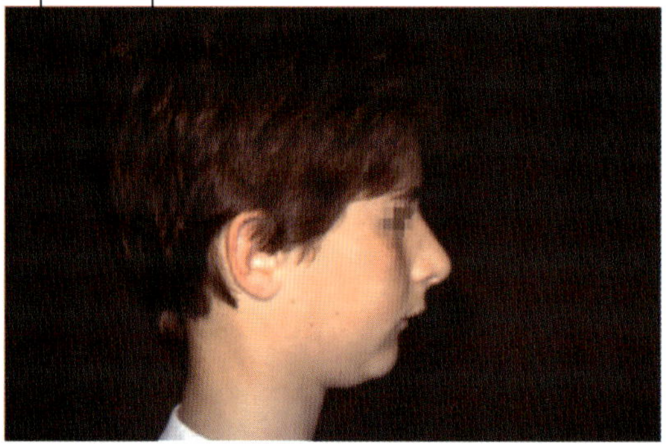

3-83

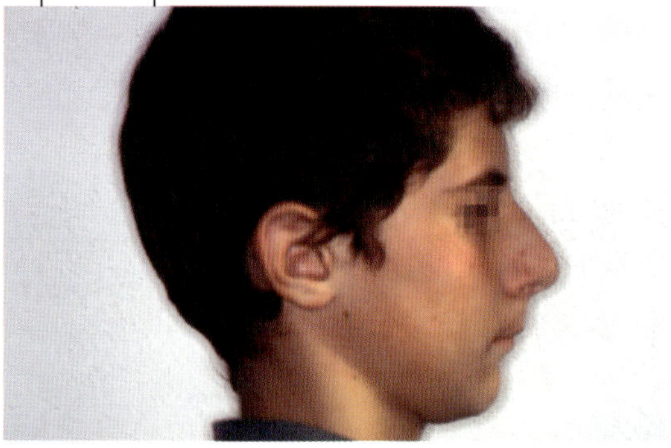

Fig. 3-82
Pre-treatment patient's profile.

Fig. 3-83
Post-treatment patient's profile.

CASE NUMBER 9 (TEUSCHER)

This case features a Class II division 1 dolico in an 8 year old female patient.

It is important to avoid clockwise growth of the jaws, which worsens the Class II and the facial profile. The use of a Teuscher activator was necessary for 30 months. This period of time is followed by treatment with a fixed appliance for 12 months. Please note the white spots caused by an initial dental plaque erosion.

3-84

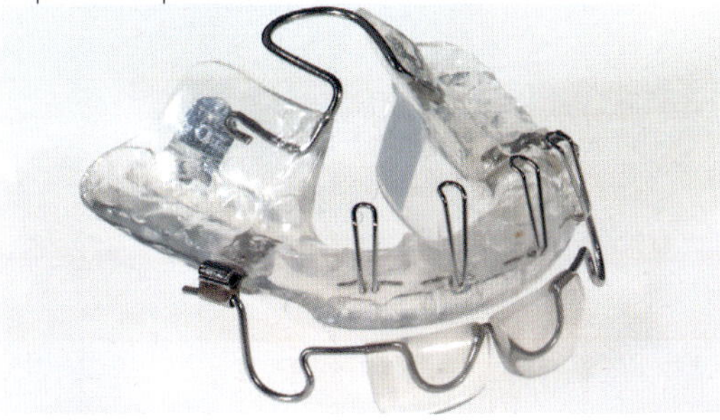

Fig. 3-84
Teuscher appliance with four upper incisor torque springs.

3-85

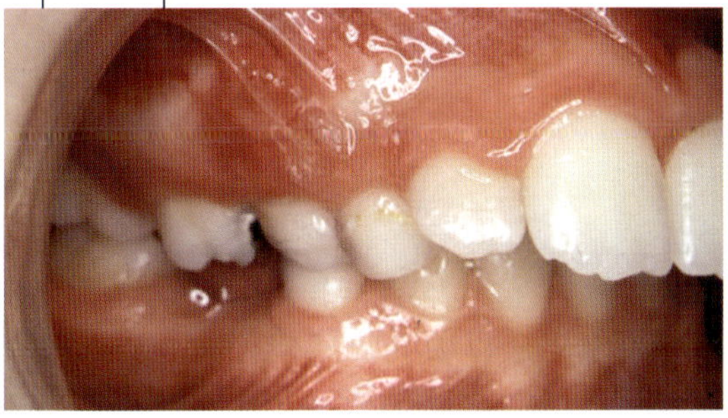

3-86

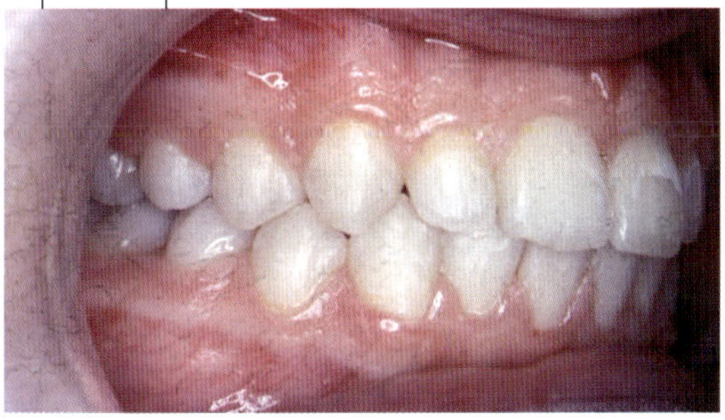

Fig. 3-85
Pre-treatment occlusion.

3-87

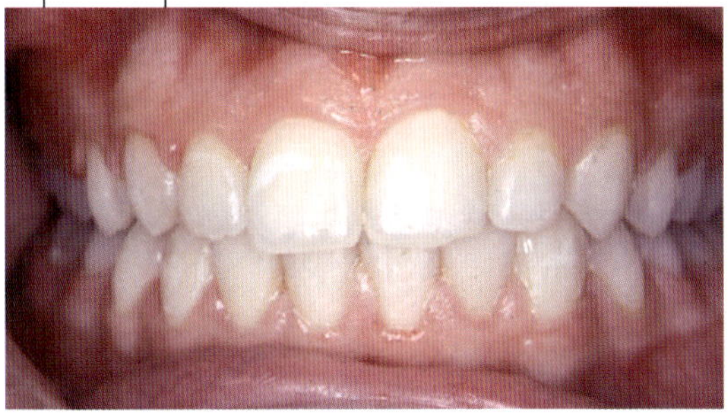

3-88

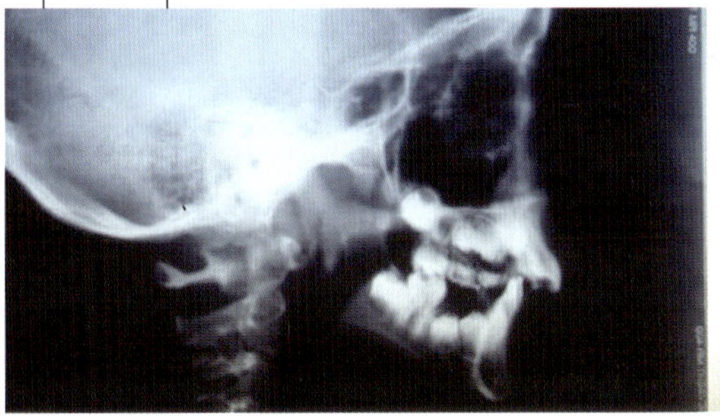

Figs. 3-86 & 3-87
Post-treatment occlusion.

3-89

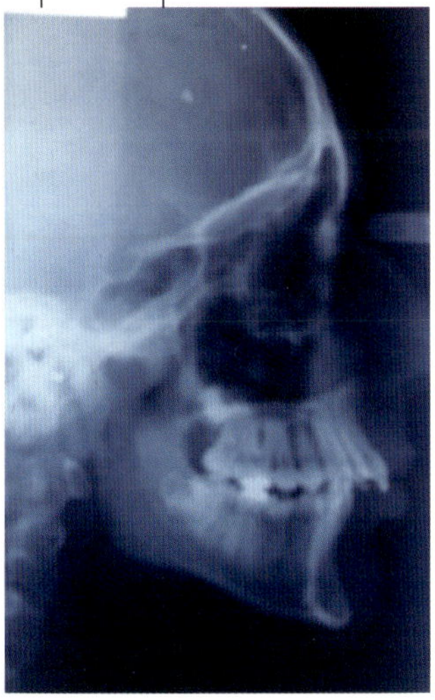

3-90

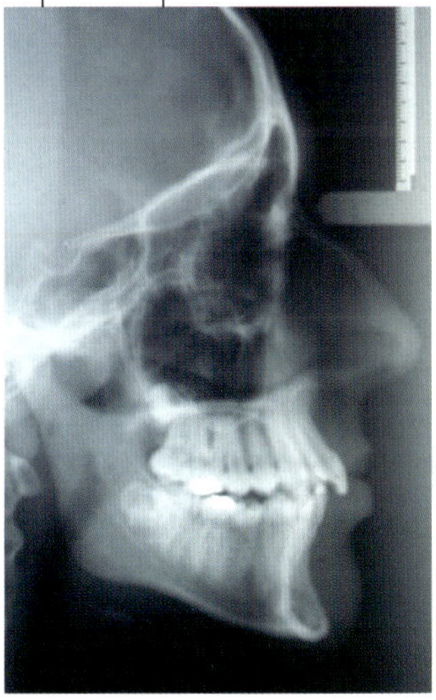

3-91

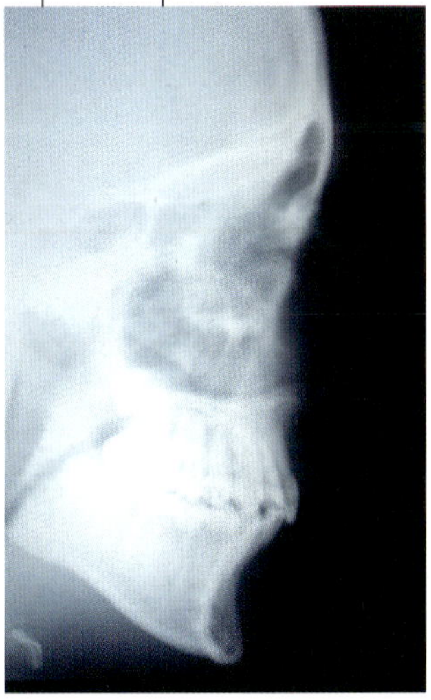

Figs. 3-88 to 3-91
Lateral cephalogram from the beginning to the end of treatment (almost 3 years).

	Age 9	Age 10	Age 13	Age 14
SNA	78°	77°	77°	77°
SNB	72°	72°	73°	75°
ANB	6°	5°	4°	2°
1/GoGn	87°			103°

CASE NUMBER 10

This case is a Class II in a dolicofacial patient. To make the correction, vertical control of the growth is necessary. By controlling the growth, anticlockwise rotation of the mandible is possible, advancing the point B and reducing the ANB angle. A good result is obtained with an RV1 connected to a high pull headgear.

3-92

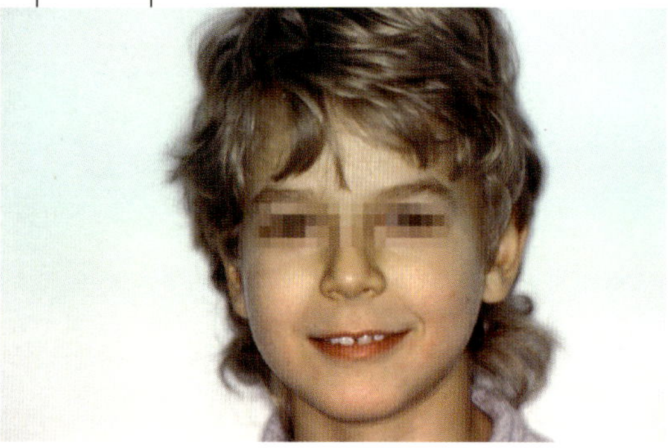

Fig. 3-92
Face before treatment.

3-93

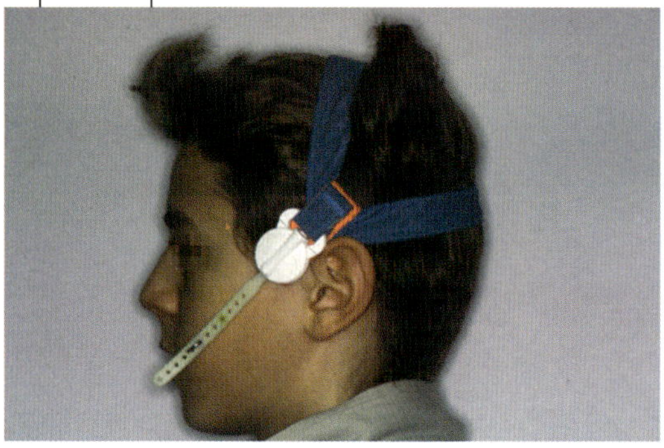

Fig. 3-93
RV 1 and high pull.

3-94

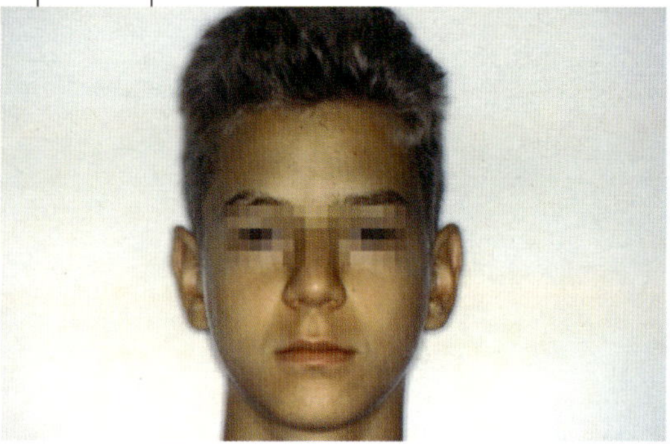

Fig. 3-94
Face at the end of treatment.

3-95

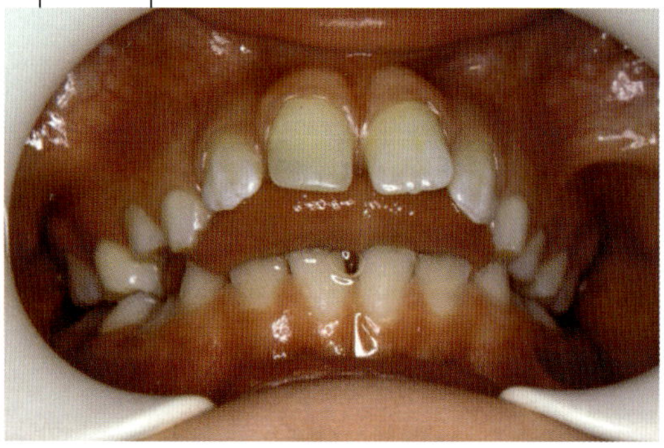

3-96

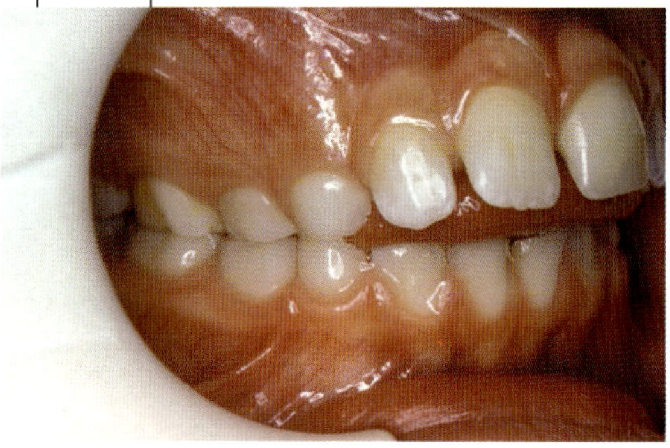

Figs. 3-95 & 3-96
Pre-treatment occlusion.

3-97

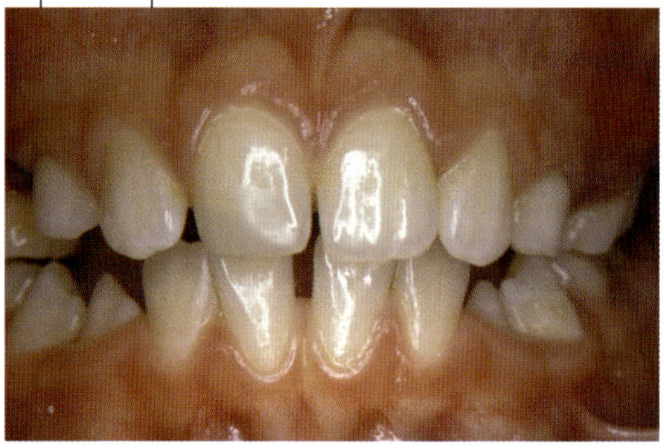

3-98

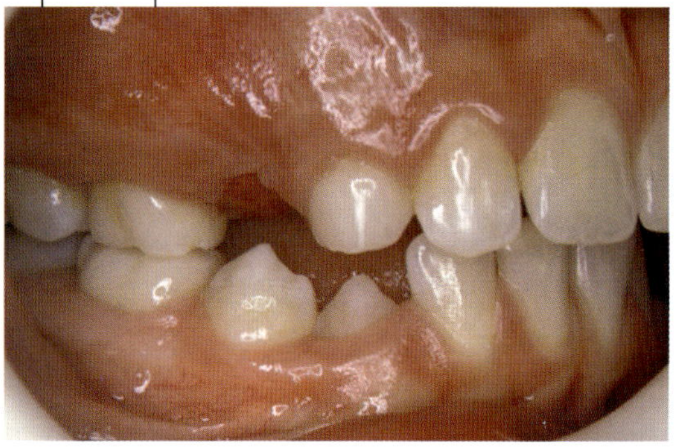

Figs. 3-97 & 3-98
Occlusion after 18 months with RV1 and high pull.

3-99

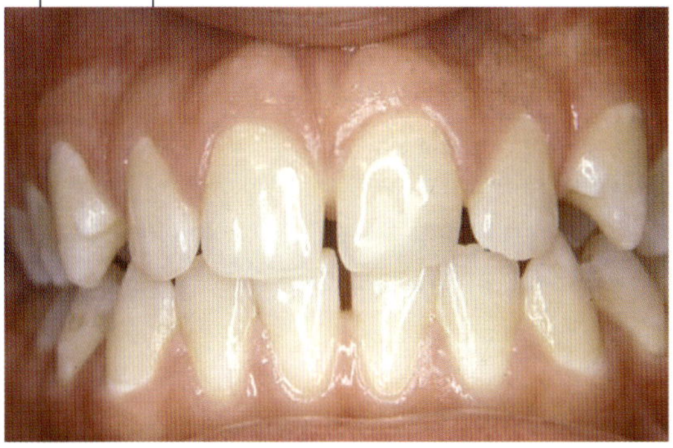

3-100

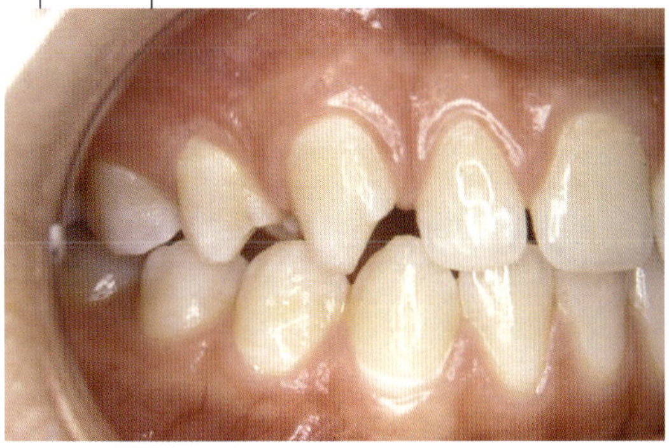

3-101

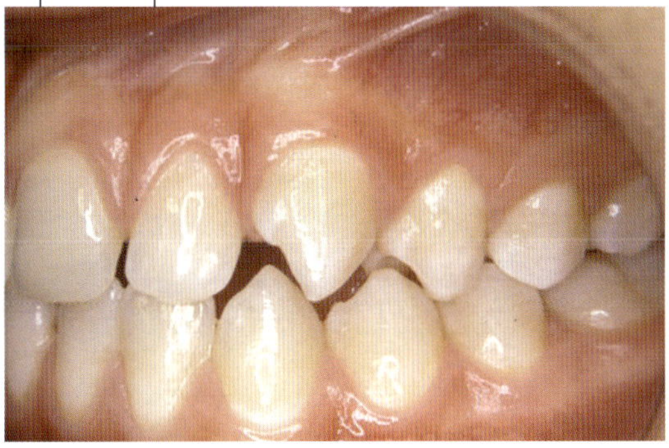

Figs. 3-99 to 3-101
Occlusion 12 months later.

3-102

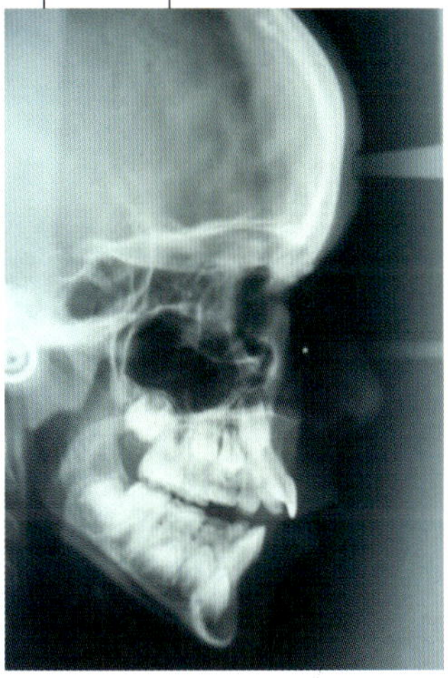

3-103

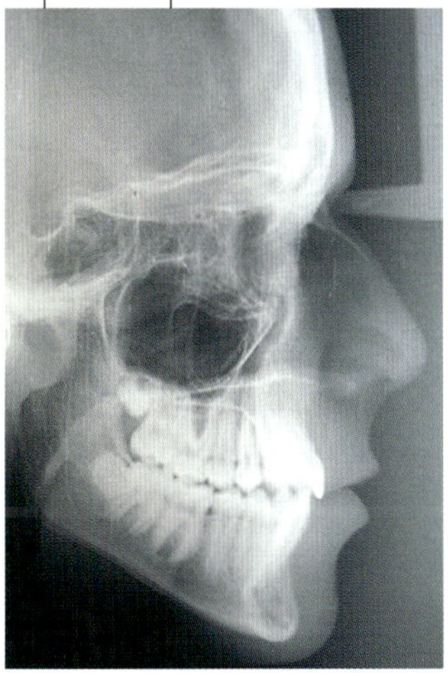

Fig. 3-102
Pre-treatment lateral cephalogram. ANB = 6°.

Fig. 3-103
Post-treatment lateral cephalogram. ANB = 2°.

CAN HEADGEARS BE DANGEROUS?

It is hard to believe but the answer is **YES!** In research published in the USA in 1982, 217 accidents with the use of headgears were described[23] (133 intra-oral wounds, 31 extra-oral wounds in the lower part of the face, 5 in the upper part of the face and the remaining ones occurred around the eyes, 5 causing complete blindness).
Holland Arch Ophthalmology 1985 May ; 103 (5): 649 -51 described cases of serious eye wounds following the unexpected opening of the hooks holding the headgear in place. Booth, Mason and Birnie Eur.J Orthod 1988 May; 10 (2) : 111- 4 reported the case of a young girl who suffered irreversible damage and lost an eye while she turned over during sleep. In 1991 in France, a boy took his headgear off without removing the elastics. The arch sprang back sharply and as a consequence the boy also lost an eye.
Thus I strongly recommend the use of headgear with certified safety – where the removal of the headgear can be done without the need for excessive force - to prevent violent recoil.

ORTHODONTIC FIXED APPLIANCES IN CONSERVATIVE TREATMENT OF CLASS II

The main part of conservative (no extraction) functional orthopedic treatment of Class II is carried out with the appliances described previously. However, in the USA there are many orthodontists who do not believe in functional orthopedic philosophies and utilize fixed appliances only.

Using the bi-dimensional arch technique, Gianelly [103] distalized the first upper molars into a first class relationship. This is possible in 90% of cases before second upper molar eruption.

Such an orthodontic result is accompanied by an orthopedic effect determined by the Class II elastics that are usually applied. The research of Petrovic and Stutzmann showed that Class II elastics in an edgewise appliance can increase the length of the mandible (condylion – gnathion).[196] N.B It is important that the treatment coincides with the pubertal growth spurt.

The increase of the condylion – gnathion length depends essentially on an extra condylar growth suggested by an increase of blood flow in the retrodiscal tissue. Other research carried out by the same authors documented the important role of retrodiscal tissue and the external pterygoid muscle in the condylar cartilage growth increase.

CASE NUMBER 11 (EDGEWISE WITH CLASS II ELASTICS + HEADGEAR)

In this Class II division 2 the upper canines are palatally displaced (Fig. 3-104).

The preference is for a fixed appliance to align the canines using headgear and Class II elastics to correct the skeletal Class II.

Note in the pre-treatment lateral cephalogram the displaced canines and the vertically positioned upper incisors. Compare this cephalogram with the post-treatment one where the good torque of the upper frontal teeth and the mandibular advancement is evident.

3-104

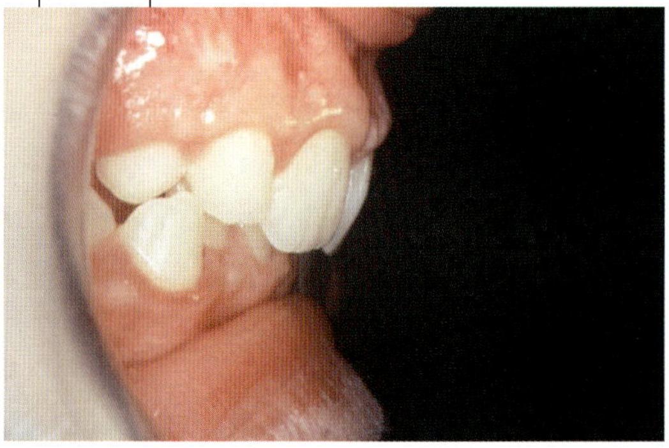

3-105

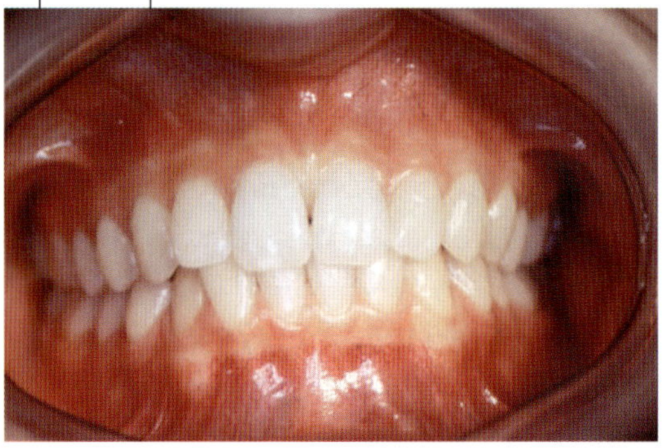

3-106

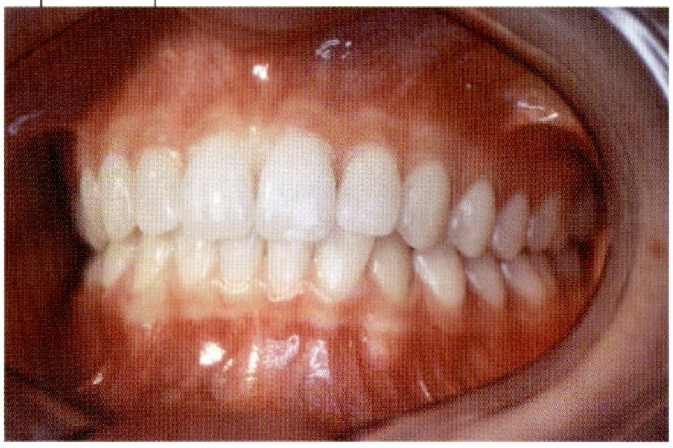

Figs. 3-105 & 3-106 Occlusion at the end of treatment (24 months).

3-107

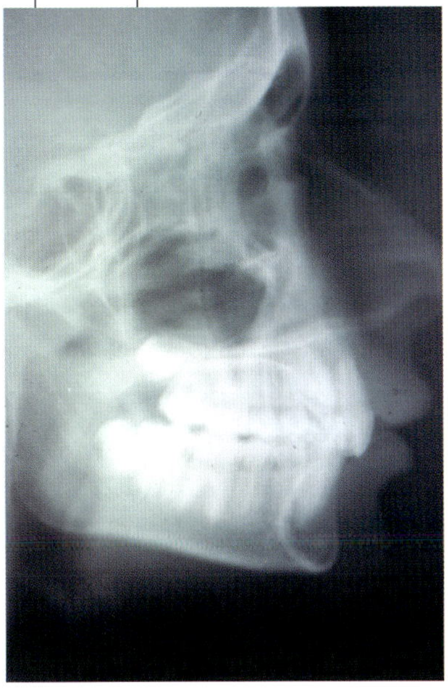

3-108

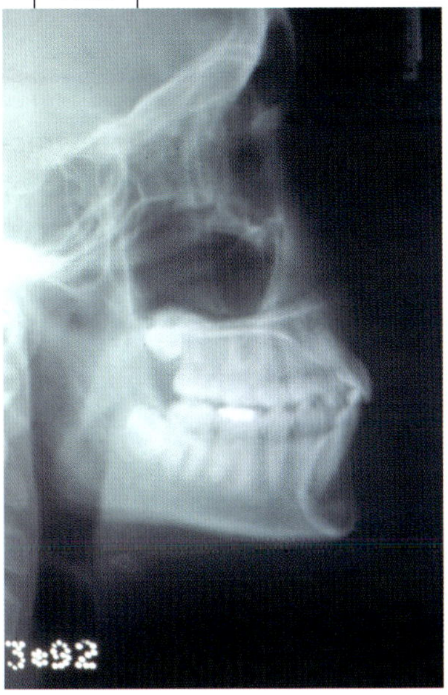

Fig. 3-107
Pre-treatment cephalogram.

Fig. 3-108
Post-treatment cephalogram.

	Before	After		Before	After
SNA	*86°*	*86°*	*lower incisors inclination*		
SNB	*79°*	*83°*	*on mandibular plane*	*88°*	*89°*
ANB	*7°*	*3°*			

CLASS II: ONE PHASE OR TWO PHASE TREATMENT?

There is great discussion in the USA about one phase or two phase treatments of Class II.

Is an early treatment (first phase) better, followed eventually by a second phase with fixed appliances? Or is it better to wait and reach the goal by using a fixed appliance only (one phase)?

In the *American Journal of Orthodontics and Dentofacial Orthopedics*, January 1998, there is an article where Dr. Gianelly says that 90% of Class II can be easily treated in one phase at the end of mixed dentition before missing the second milk premolars. In the same article, drawing on their own specific research, Lund and Sandler demonstrated that functional appliances can enhance mandibular growth even if the effects from the treatment are due to a combination of skeletal and dental change.

Dugani and others Am J Orthod Dentofacial Orthop 1998 ; 113 : 75 – 84 point out the advantages following an early treatment:

- fewer extractions of permanent teeth
- easier second phase or no need of it at all
- fewer cases of orthodontic surgery
- lower incisors have more long term stability
- less root resorption
- fewer gingival problems
- less canine displacement
- better patient cooperation

Ghafari et al Am J Orthod Dentofacial Orthop 1998 ; 113:51-61 remind us that an early correction of an excessive overjet reduces the risks of trauma and increases the self esteem of very young patients.

CONCLUSIONS

What are the conclusions? We can say that the discussion is still open. Critics state that the influence of functional orthopedic treatments on natural human growth has not been clearly demonstrated. Most experiments are performed on animals that do not have malocclusions. Therefore, their results are not reliable. Finally, many studies show contradictory data.

While discussion continues, what should a good and honest orthodontist do? What should he offer to his patient? The first element that can help the clinician is the knowledge that a **Class II does not correct itself.** Bobic criticized Mills' presentation of a correction of Class IIs with Twin Block appliances, saying that the mandibular growth would have been the same without the Twin Block. Mills replied, noting that she had never seen the self correction of a Class II, and she invited Bobic to demonstrate the contrary. (*AJO*, Nov. 98)

It is also difficult to believe that many wonderful results obtained with functional orthopedic treatments are not true. If they somehow have the desired effect, why shouldn't they be used?

The choice of appliance depends on the doctor. Some fall in love with the "guru" of the time, others follow the trend, while a big group is always seeking the "best".

Melsen wrote an amusing article on the discovery of the secrets of haute cuisine: a famous cook told his students to bake a simple pie. The students asked many questions about the different procedures. How should the butter be mixed? What about the flour? When should the eggs be added? Some of them made a note of the muscles used to beat the eggs and the flour whilst others were very careful about the speed of work. All the pies were good, but no student was able to say what made each of them unique. - B.Melsen " Recenti controversie in ortodonzia " SIDO (Sorrento 1991) pag.121 - 123

This could be a paradigm to explain the small differences in the design of the functional appliances. Remember that it is possible to obtain good results with all of them, but only if the diagnosis and the indications are correct.

Gianelly et al.[105] and Petrovic and Stutzmann[196] say that it is possible to obtain good results not only with functional appliances but also with fixed appliances and headgear or Class II elastics. Personally I have had many satisfying results using the appliances described earlier, mainly with my RV, of course.

I have always said that the best outcome is reached after a good functional result (phase one). However, we are not able to guarantee the outcome because the biological response and the patient's compliance are not always optimal.

When, after a phase one if the result is not satisfactory at the end of growth, there are two ways to improve a Class II malocclusion - (i) treatment with fixed appliances and extractions of permanent teeth, or (ii) orthognathic surgery.

CLASS II TREATMENT AT THE END OF GROWTH (ADULT PATIENTS)

Is it possible to correct a Class II at the end of growth without reducing the distance between the maxilla and the mandible? It is possible to move the teeth to obtain a "camouflage" of the malocclusion (Fig. 3-109). There could also be a possible "gnathologic" movement of the mandible which we will discuss later.

CLASS II DIVISION 1

A) 2 upper premolar extractions and fixed appliances when the lower arch is well aligned or potentially well aligned.

B) 4 premolar extractions and fixed appliances when the lower arch is crowded

C) Combination of A and B with upper incisor retroclination and lower incisor proclination.

D) Combination of A-B-C and small mandibular advancement (gnathologic skid).

There are questions that need to be asked:

WHEN IS IT BETTER TO AVOID EXTRACTION OF THE UPPER PREMOLARS?

In cases of retropositioned mandible because the facial profile would worsen.

WHEN CAN ONLY TWO UPPER PREMOLARS BE EXTRACTED?

When the lower teeth are well aligned.

3-107

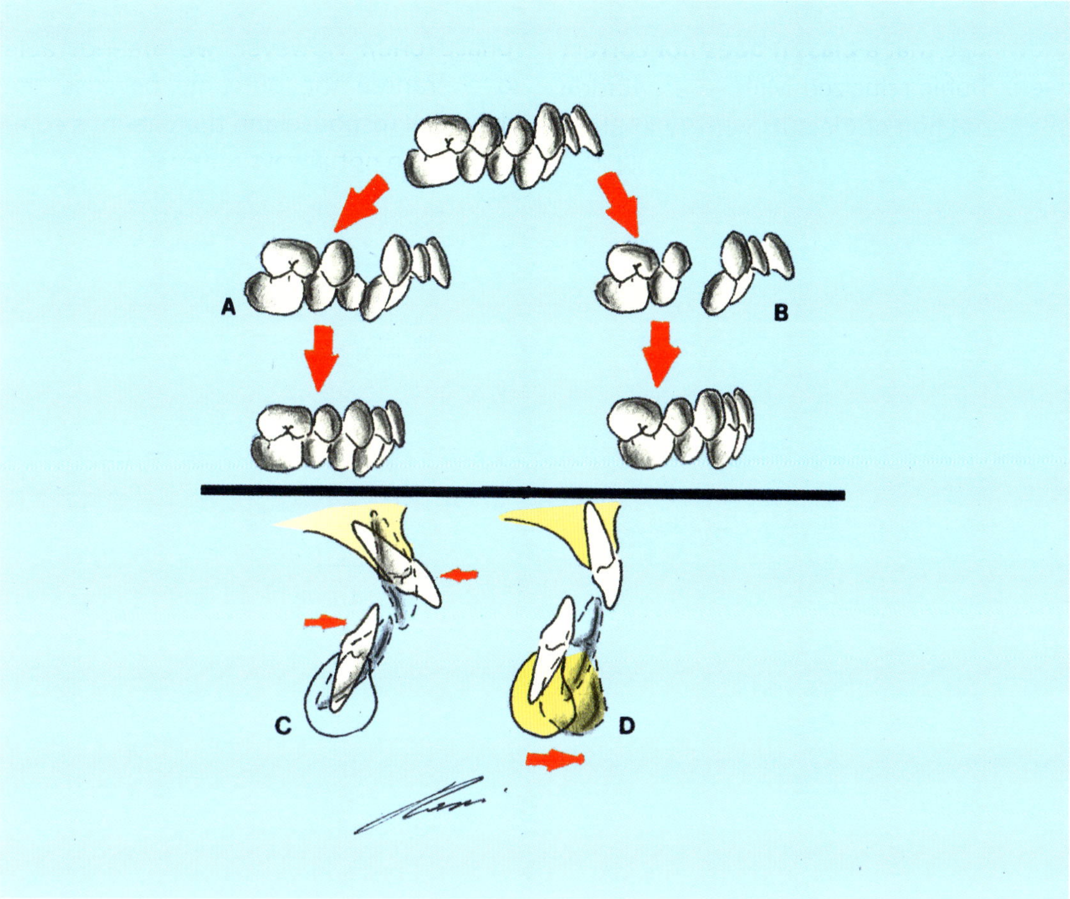

Fig. 3-109
Schematic representation of possible "camouflage":

WHEN DO FOUR UPPER PREMOLARS NEED TO BE EXTRACTED?

When the lower arch is crowded and its alignment without extraction is possible with an excessive lower incisor proclination (C).

WHAT ARE THE LIMITS OF LOWER INCISOR PROCLINATION?

The most tolerant "guru" still remains R. Ricketts with the lower incisors at 1 ± 2 mm on A/Po.

HOW MANY MILLIMETRES CAN A "GNATHOLOGIC SKID" BE?

2-3 mm (D), supposing that the condyle is in the rear of the glenoid fossa. The distance corresponds to its advancement within the fossa. The protrusion of the mandible at the end of the growth can determine a dual bite. During growth, the dual bite might present at the beginning, and disappear later, since a remodelling of tissues is supposed to happen. However, it is not clear whether the dual bite can be acceptable (if always, or only when there are no symptoms, etc.).

Many orthodontists believe that a lower jaw advances, more often than not, during the correction of a Class II division 2 where a mandible rear position is determined by the vertical upper incisors.

This is not always true (see the following case).

CASE NUMBER 12

There are Class II division 2 cases which Langlade[151] defines as "difficult". I understood what he meant while I was treating a case (Fig. 3-110) similar to one observed on a course.

On the typodont a similar case was corrected without extractions and an excellent result obtained, but in the mouth of the patient the result was not as had been observed on the typodont wax.

With high vertical angles, increased values of the sellar angle, the articular angle and the gonial angle, the use of Class II elastics is dangerous. They can open the bite and worsen the sagittal relationship of the jaws. When the bone is thin it is not possible to move teeth out of cortical bone to reach a Class I.

Due to the poor cooperation of the patient regarding an alternative like a high pull headgear, after 8 months of treatment I did not know how to move forward. That was when I met Dr. Langlade and followed his suggestion of performing an extraction of the first upper premolars. The procedure allowed me to find a good solution (figs. 3-112 & 3-113).

In other situations with low vertical angles a "forward skid" improves the result. But is such mandibular advancement acceptable from a gnathological point of view?

In the 1970s gnathologists believed that the condyle had to occupy a rear, upper, medial position in the glenoid fossa. An advanced position was considered wrong and a cause of TMJ problems. In the 1980s Ricketts expounded his view on the centric relationship, that the condyle should be located centrally in the fossa, and stated that 93% of TMJ problems were present with the condyle rearward in the fossa, and only 7% of TMJ problems were with a forward condyle. His theory was the complete opposite of what had been said until that time!

Since then there has been more tolerance about mandibular forward dislocation. However, the limits are not well defined. According to common sense rather than scientific evidence, the condyle anterior limit is the articular eminence.

Therefore, can mandible advancement in adult patients correct a Class II even when causing a dual bite? Korn[138] answered yes to that question! In a surgical Class II with a retropositioned mandible, he applied a fixed appliance and Class II elastics for some months in order to prepare the neuromuscolar complex to the new relationship following surgery. After this phase, many patients were satisfied with their occlusion (dual bite) and the aesthetic change, and refused surgery. As a result, Korn wondered whether a dual bite was completely unacceptable.

Personally I would be careful and limit a mandibular protrusion in adults to no more than 1.5 mm. However, the choice is based more on common sense than on scientific evidence.

3-110

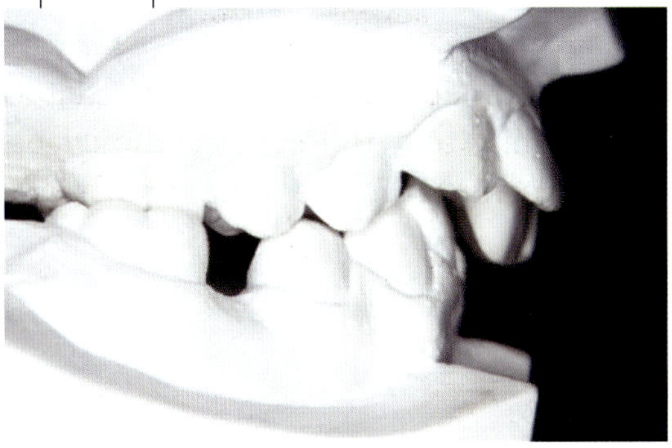

3-111

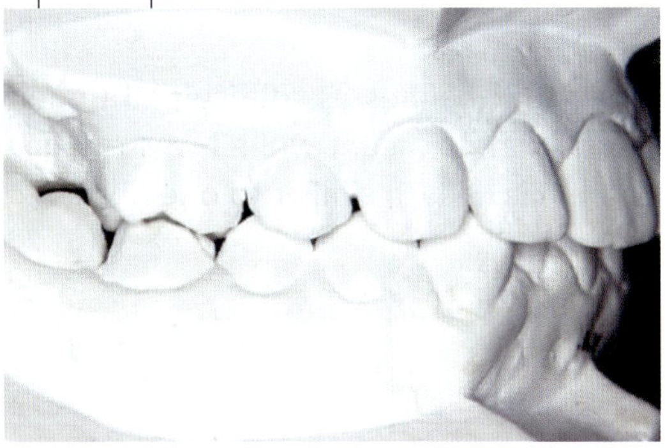

Fig. 3-110
Pre-treatment dental casts.

Fig. 3-111
Post-treatment dental casts.

3-112

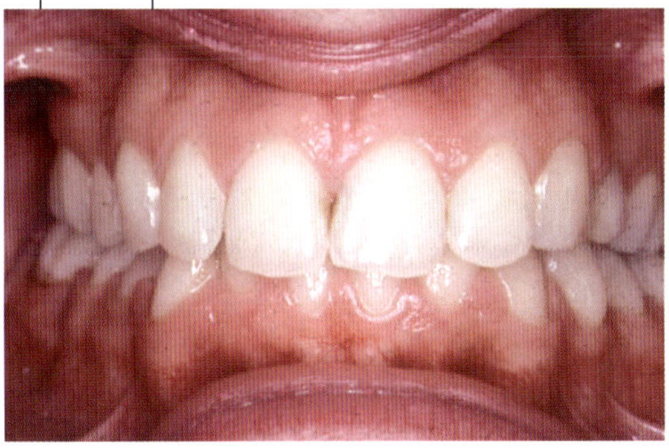

3-113

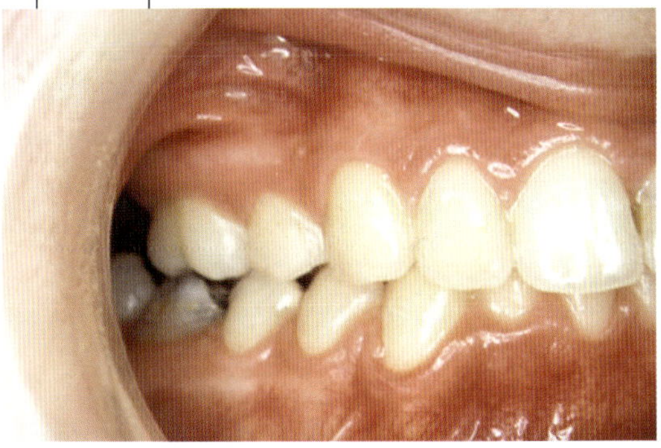

Fig. 3-112 & 3-113
Intraoral view after treatment based mainly on the upper frontal teeth distalization (retraction) after the extraction of the two first upper premolars

3-115

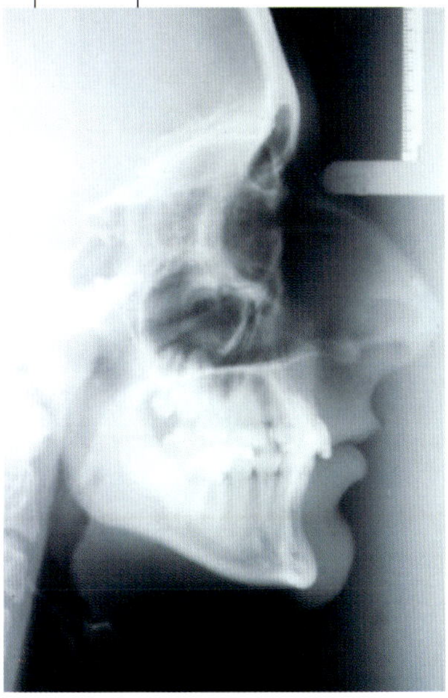

3-114

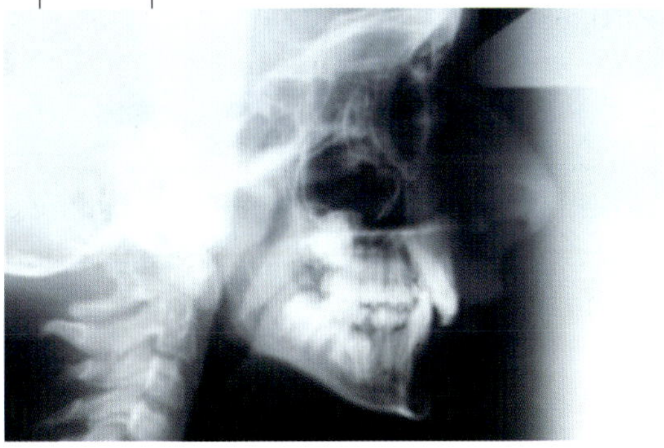

Fig. 3-114
Pre-treatment lateral cephalogram.

Fig. 3-115
Post-treatment lateral cephalogram

CASE NUMBER 13

Case 13 is a Class II division 1 in a 20 year old female patient.

After the extraction of the upper first molar roots, a treatment with fixed appliance followed, allowing a good relationship between the upper and lower arches. With the closure of the extraction spaces there was no need for a prosthetic and a functional improvement of the second and third upper molars. The patient was happy to no longer have rabbit teeth even without the chin advancement that would have made the treatment perfect. Twenty years later a good occlusion can still be observed.

Fig. 3-116
Pre-treatment panoramic X-ray.

Fig. 3-117
Post-treatment panoramic X-ray.

3-116

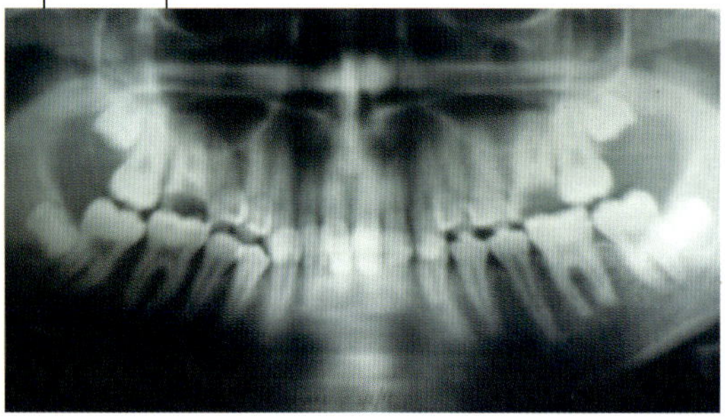

3-117

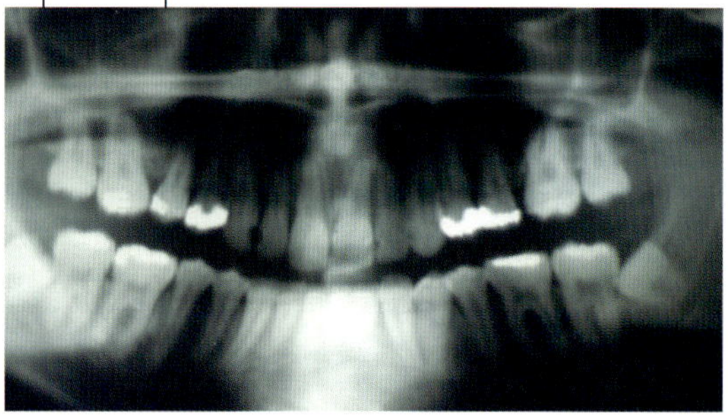

Fig. 3-118
Pre-treatment lateral cephalogram.

Fig. 3-119
Post-treatment lateral cephalogram.

3-118

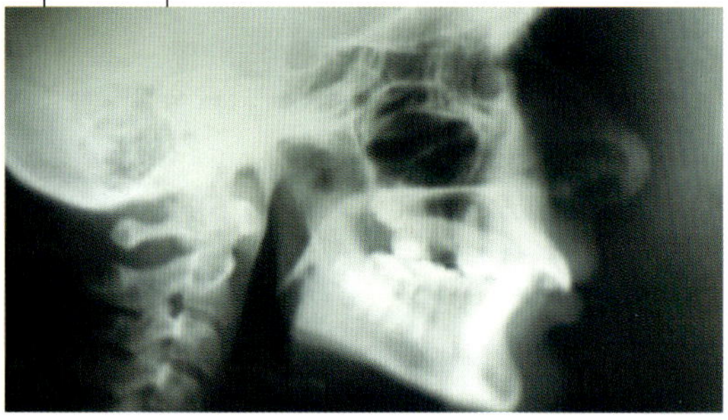

3-119

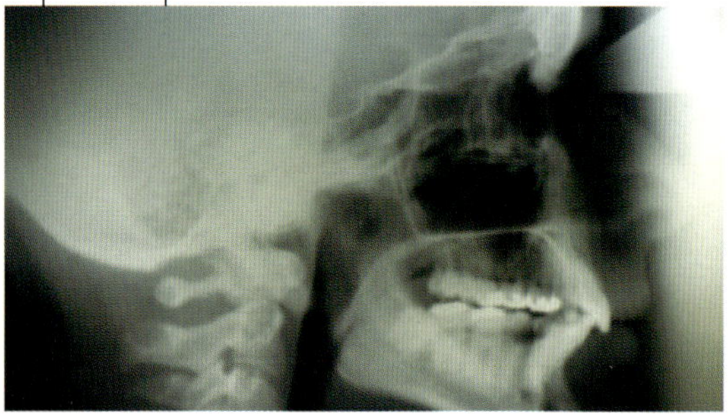

Fig. 3-120
Pre-treatment dental casts.

Fig. 3-121
Post-treatment dental casts.

3-120

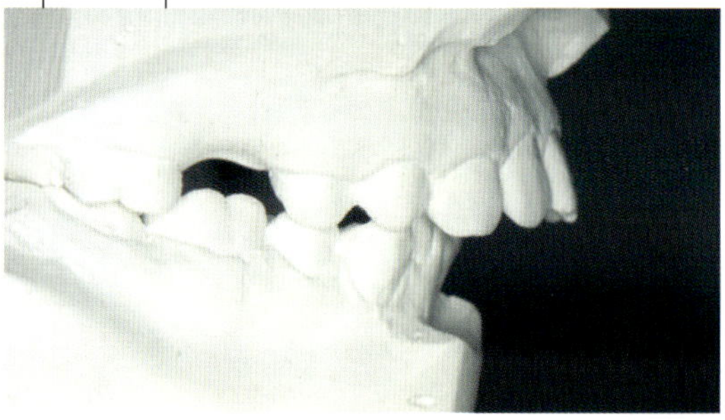

3-121

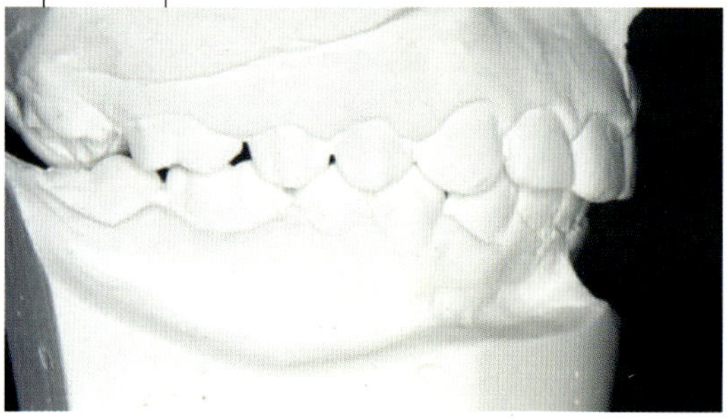

Fig. 3-122
Pre-treatment upper arch.

Fig. 3-123
Post-treatment upper arch.

3-122

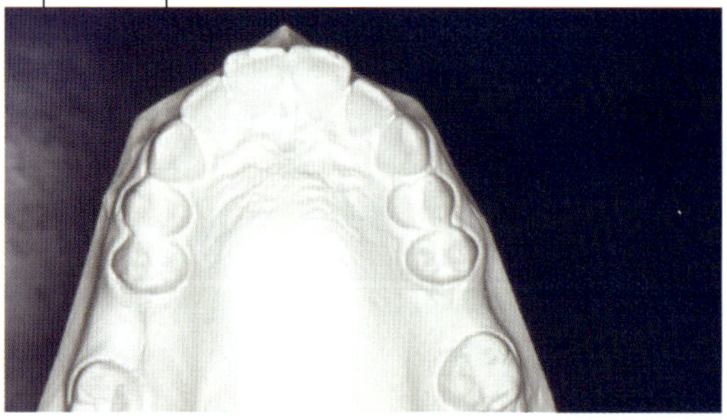

3-123

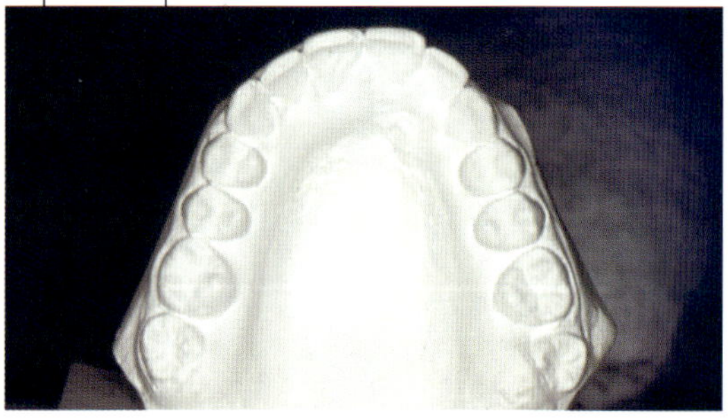

Figs. 3-124 & 3-125
Occlusion, 20 years later. The modest upper incisor gum retraction is due to over brushing.

3-124

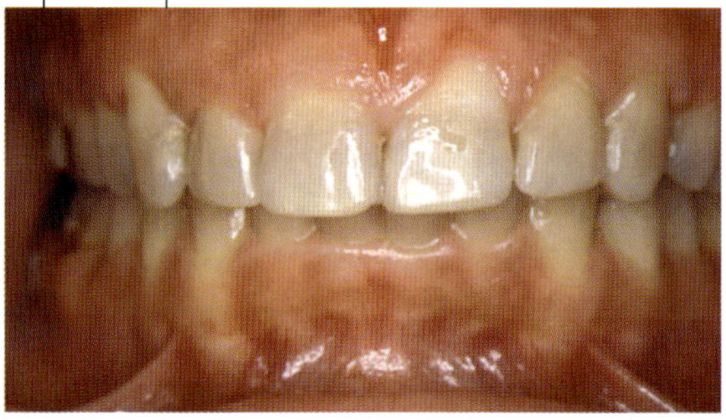

3-125

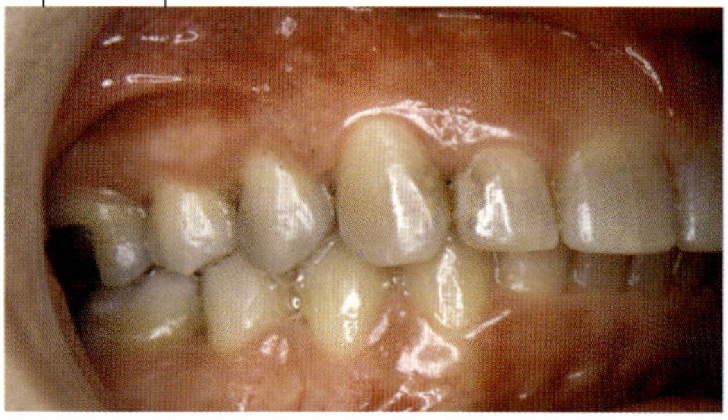

CASE NUMBER 14

The case is a Class II division 1 in a 16 year old male patient. Orthodontic treatment was given with a fixed appliance, without extractions. The good result is achieved by closure of the spaces with retroclination of the upper incisors, a slight proclination of the lower incisors, a mandibular advancement as a combination of residual growth and gnathologic skid. Note the improvement of the facial profile.

3-126

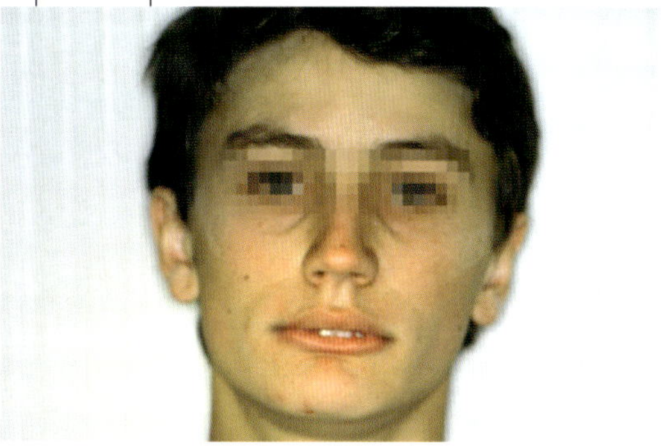

Fig. 3-126
Face of the patient before treatment.

3-127

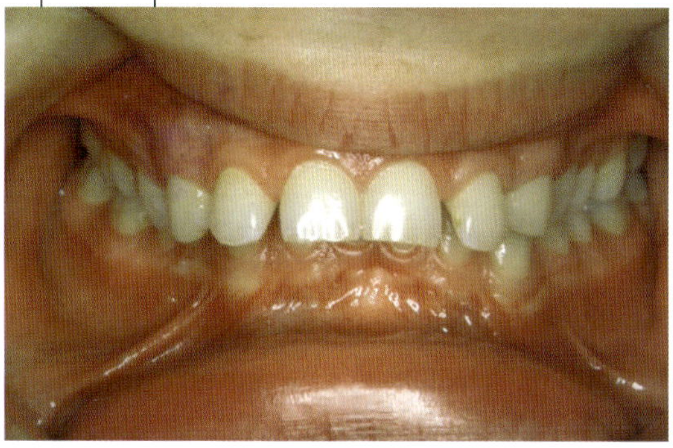

3-128

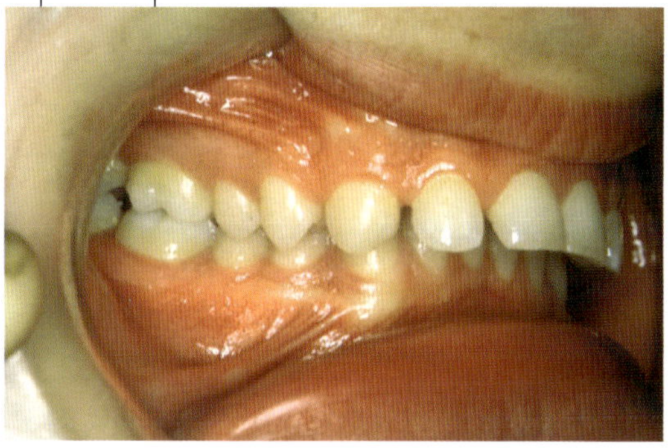

Figs. 3-127 & 3-128
Pre-treatment occlusion.

3-129

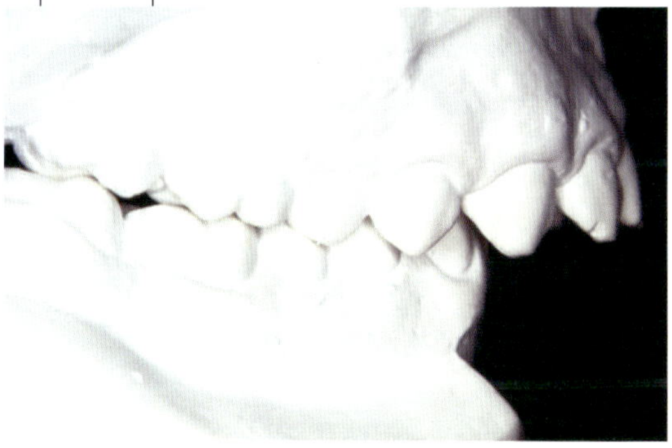

Fig. 3-129
Pre-treatment dental cast.

3-130

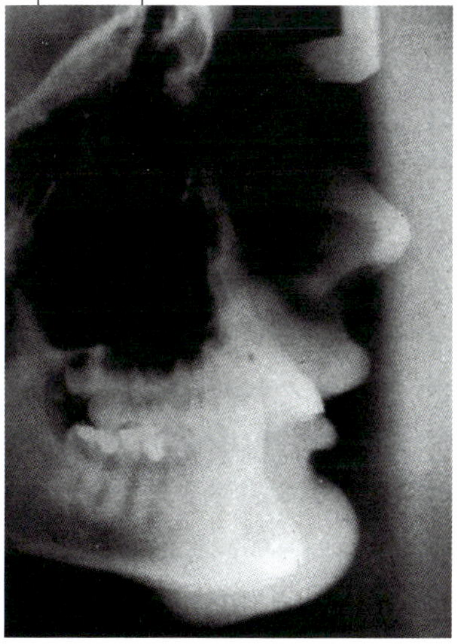

3-131

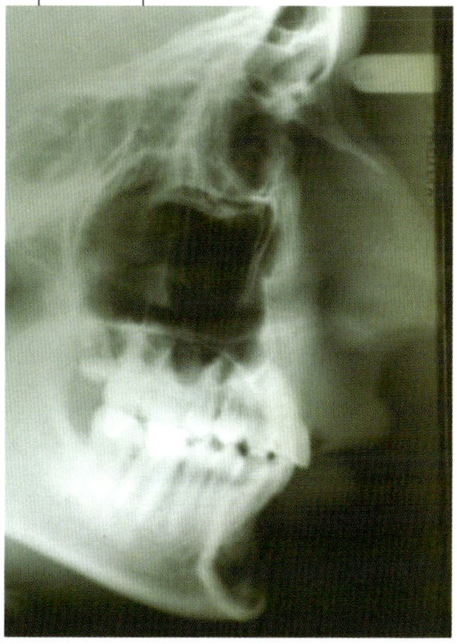

3-132

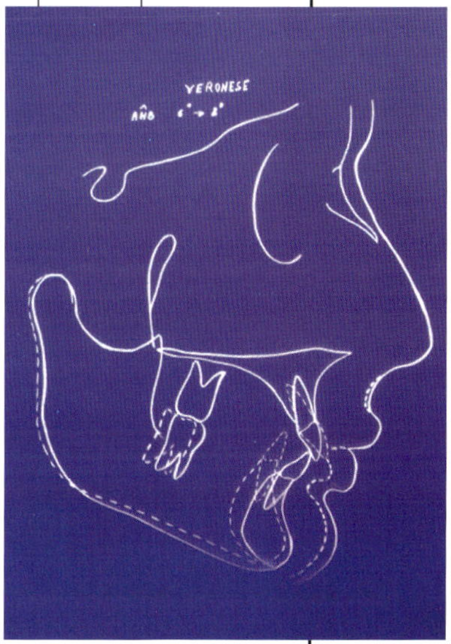

Fig. 3-130
Pre-treatment lateral cephalogram.
Fig. 3-131
Post-treatment lateral cephalogram.

Fig. 3-132
Tracing superimpositions.
Dotted line: pre-treatment.
Regular line: post-treatment.

3-133

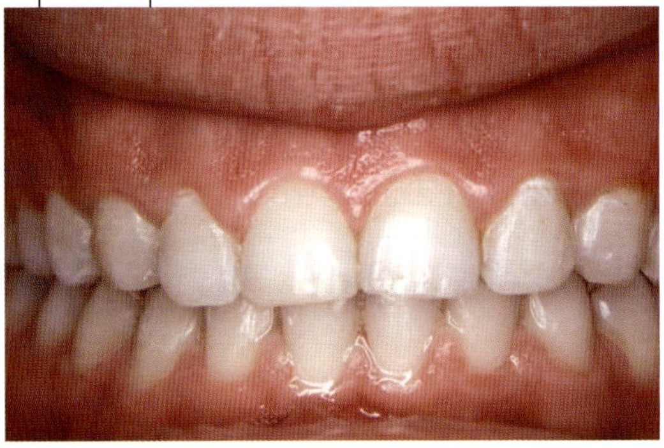

3-134

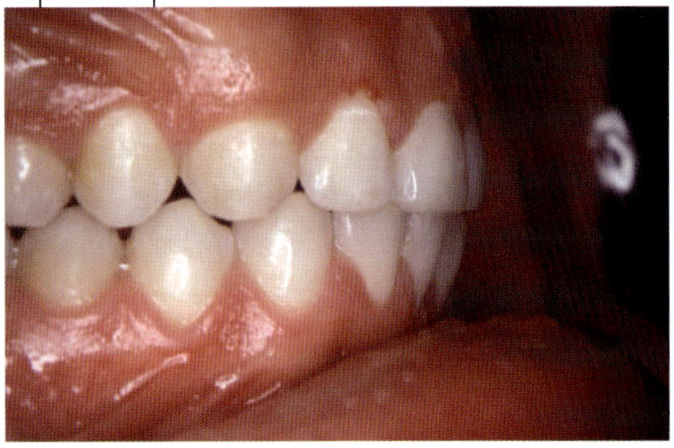

Figs. 3-133 & 3-134
Post-treatment occlusion.

3-135

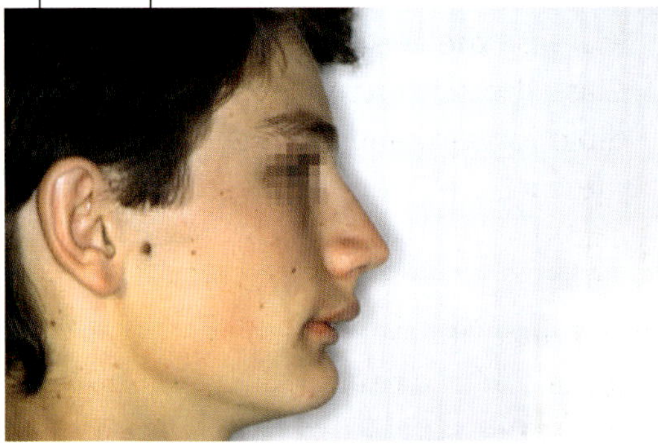

3-136

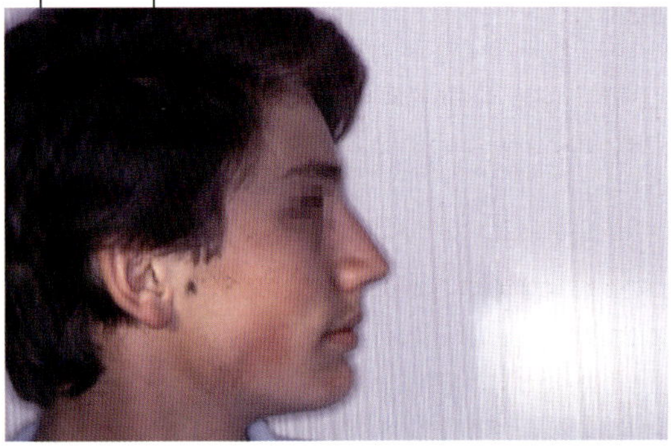

Fig. 3-135
Pre-treatment profile.

Fig. 3-136
Post-treatment profile. The improvement is evident!

FOUR EXTRACTION TREATMENTS IN CLASS II MALOCCLUSIONS

Many orthodontists and dentists believe that a four extraction treatment of a Class II, deepening the bite and distally entrapping the mandible, causes TMJ problems. This is not true and, in order to prove it, I will provide two Class II cases: one with low vertical angles, the other with high vertical angles. Both of them showed TMJ internal derangement before the treatment. (For more details see chapter VI.)

3-137

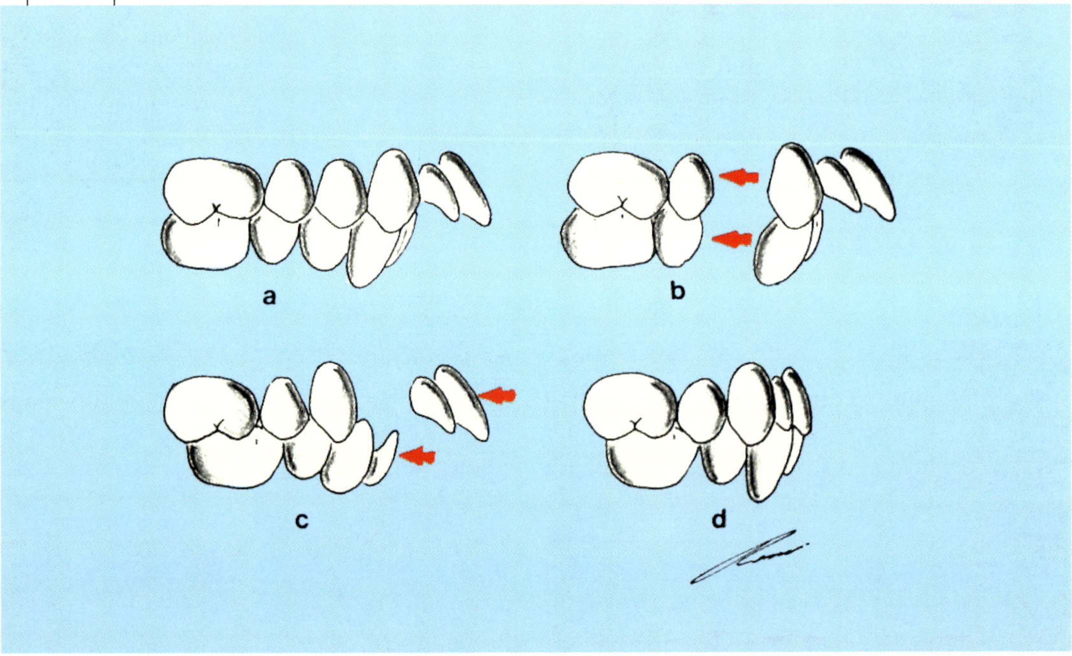

Fig. 3-137
Scheme of treatment. After extractions, from A to B the canines are moved distally. After the canines' distal movement, in C the incisors are distalized. D shows the final occlusion.

CASE NUMBER 15

The case is a Class II division 1 in a female patient at the end of her growth (15 years old), after five years of treatment with a removable appliance: a simple acrylic plate with a median screw. The negative result is evident. It is also evident that good orthodontics entails more than just turning a screw.

TMJ clicking sounds are present. Are they caused by the treatment? Was it bad treatment? Or could the sounds happen even with a better treatment? Do not forget that most clicking sounds are observed in patients who have never seen a brace before.

The occlusion shows a bilateral scissor bite due to excessive transverse upper arch expansion.

For an orthodontic correction of the overjet and good alignment of the lower arch, first premolar extractions are necessary. However, this case presents a deep bite, which, for many, would worsen and cause TMJ problems.

But this is not exactly true.

- A deep bite worsens when the molars which maintain the vertical dimension are extracted. When the *first premolars are extracted* and spaces are closed without moving the molars forward, the *vertical dimension is maintained*.
- Sometimes the use of Class II elastics can increase the vertical dimension.
- Class II elastics tend to move the mandible forward and this could improve an Internal Derangement condition (TMJ clicks).

In this case, the extraction of the first premolars has been followed up by the application of a fixed appliance. There is a good result after 18 months of treatment and the clicks have disappeared.

3-138

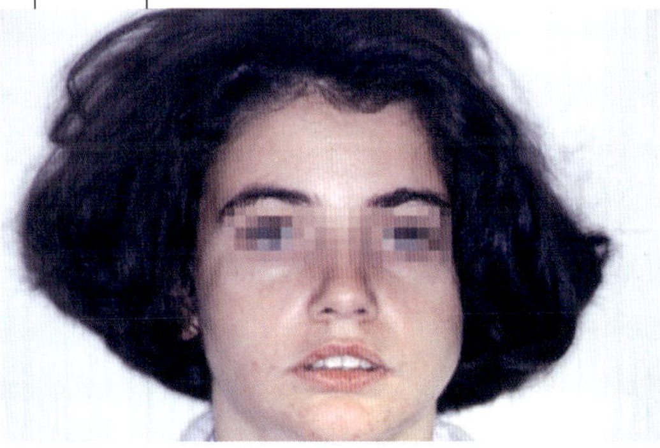

3-139

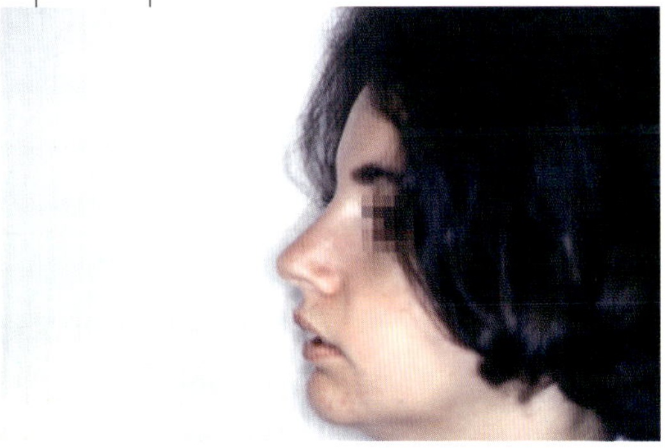

Figs. 3-138 & 3-139 Pre-treatment face and profile.

3-140

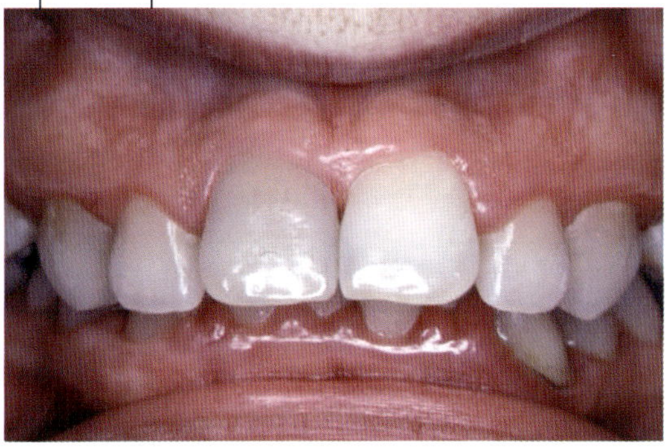

3-141

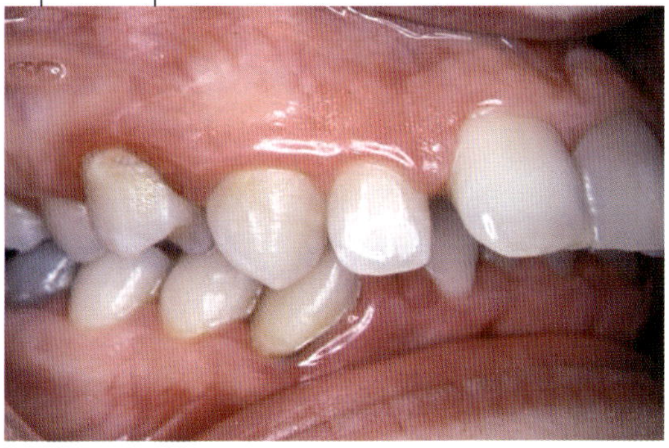

Figs. 3-140 & 3-141 Pre-treatment clinical view.

Figs. 3-142 & 3-143 Dental casts after the first "treatment". Note the exaggerated upper arch expansion.

3-142

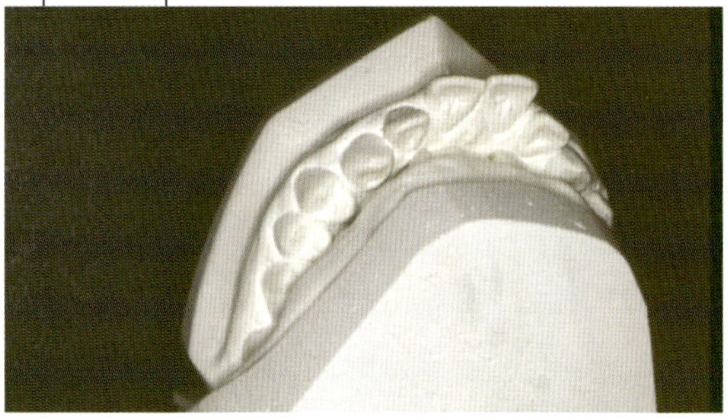

3-143

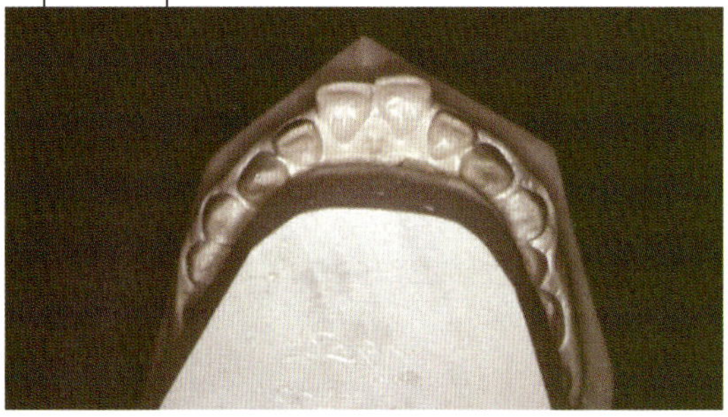

Fig. 3-144 Dental casts. Pre-treatment upper arch.

Fig. 3-145 Dental casts. Post-treatment upper arch.

3-144

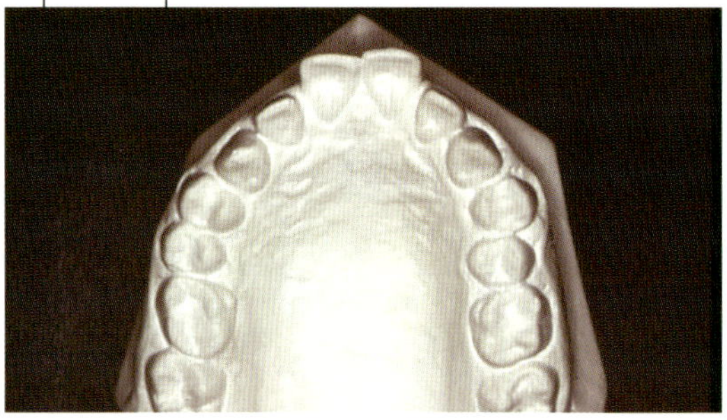

3-145

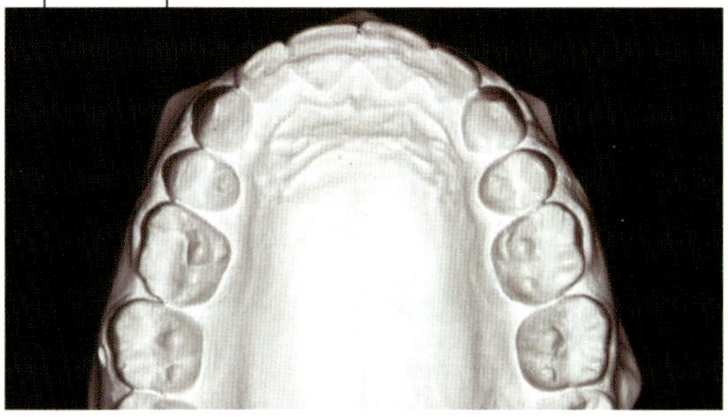

Fig. 3-146 Pre-treatment lower arch.

Fig. 3-147 Dental casts. Post-treatment lower arch.

3-146

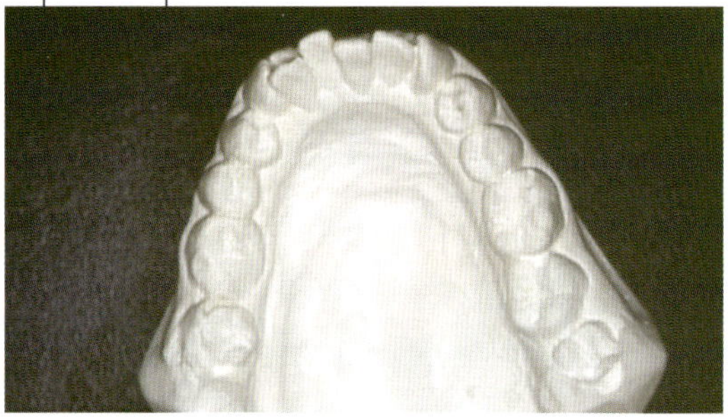

3-147

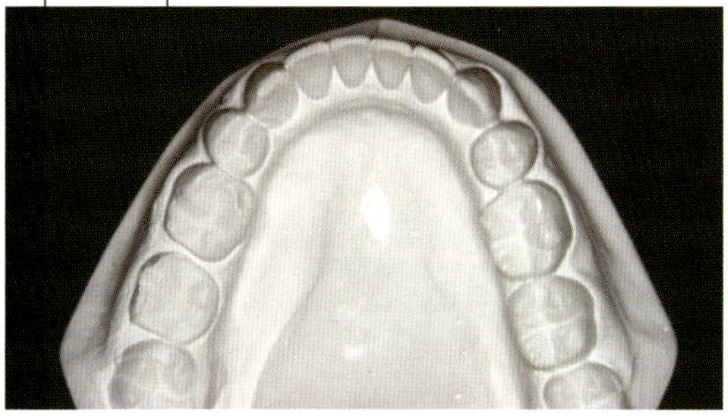

Fig. 3-148 Pre-treatment dental casts. Frontal view.

Fig. 3-149 Post-treatment dental casts. Frontal view.

3-148

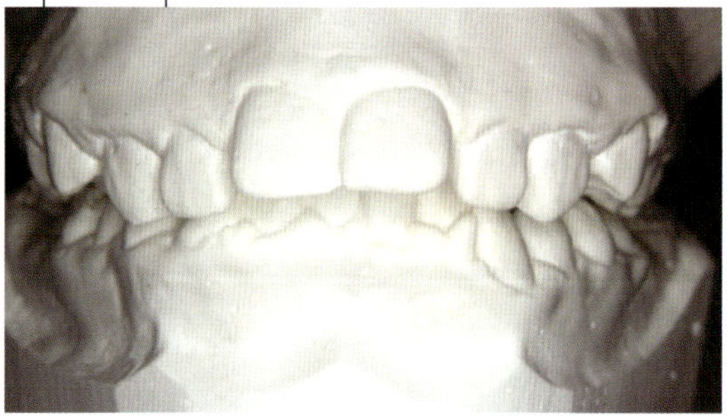

3-149

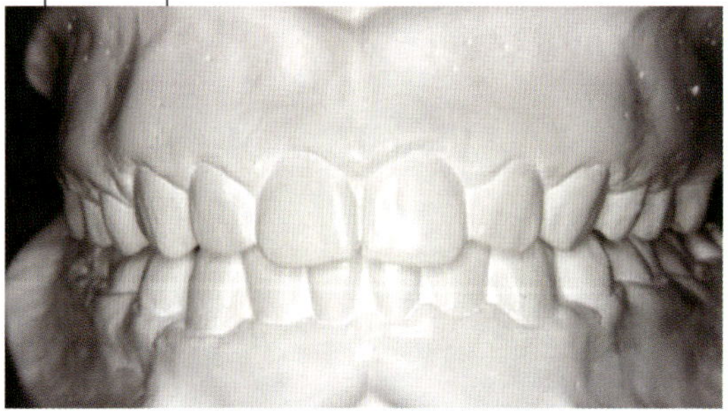

Fig. 3-150 Pre-treatment dental casts. Lateral view.

Fig. 3-151 Post-treatment dental casts. Lateral view.

3-150

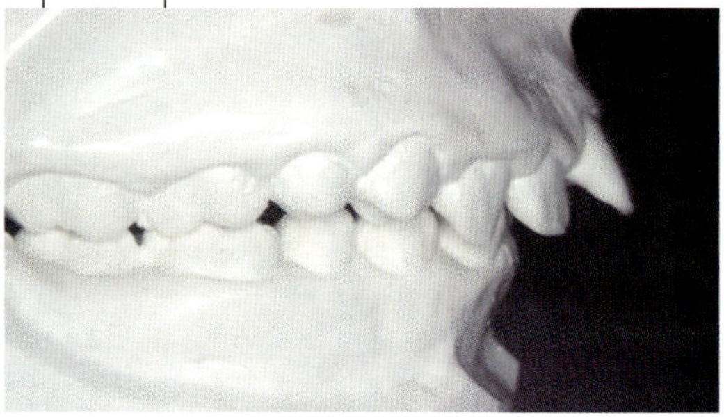

3-150

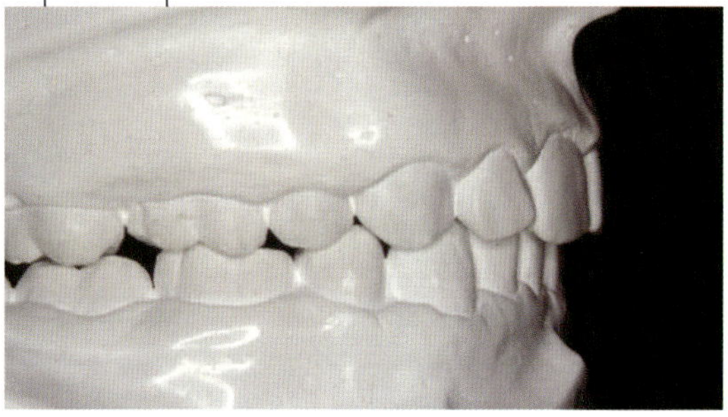

3-152

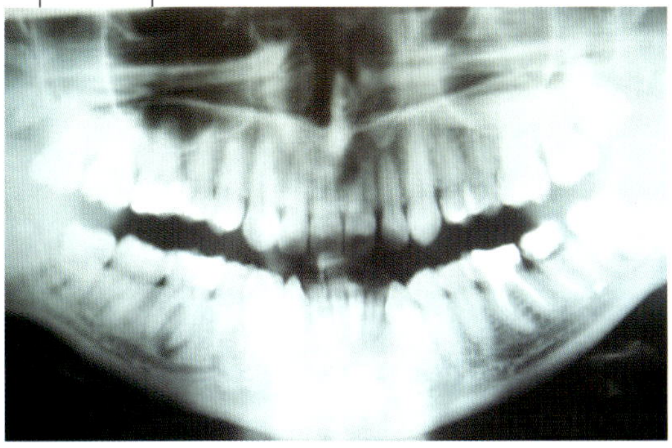

3-153

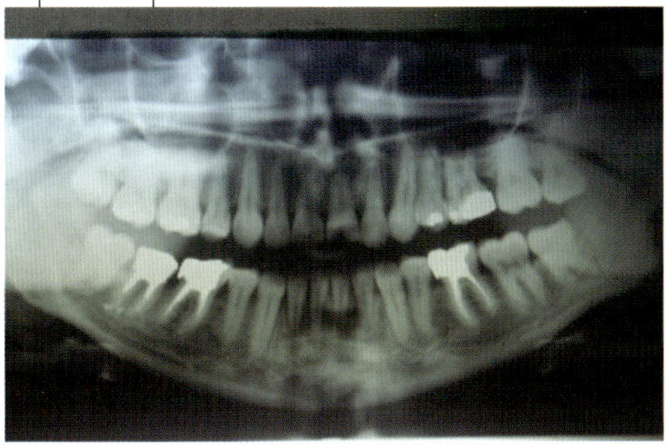

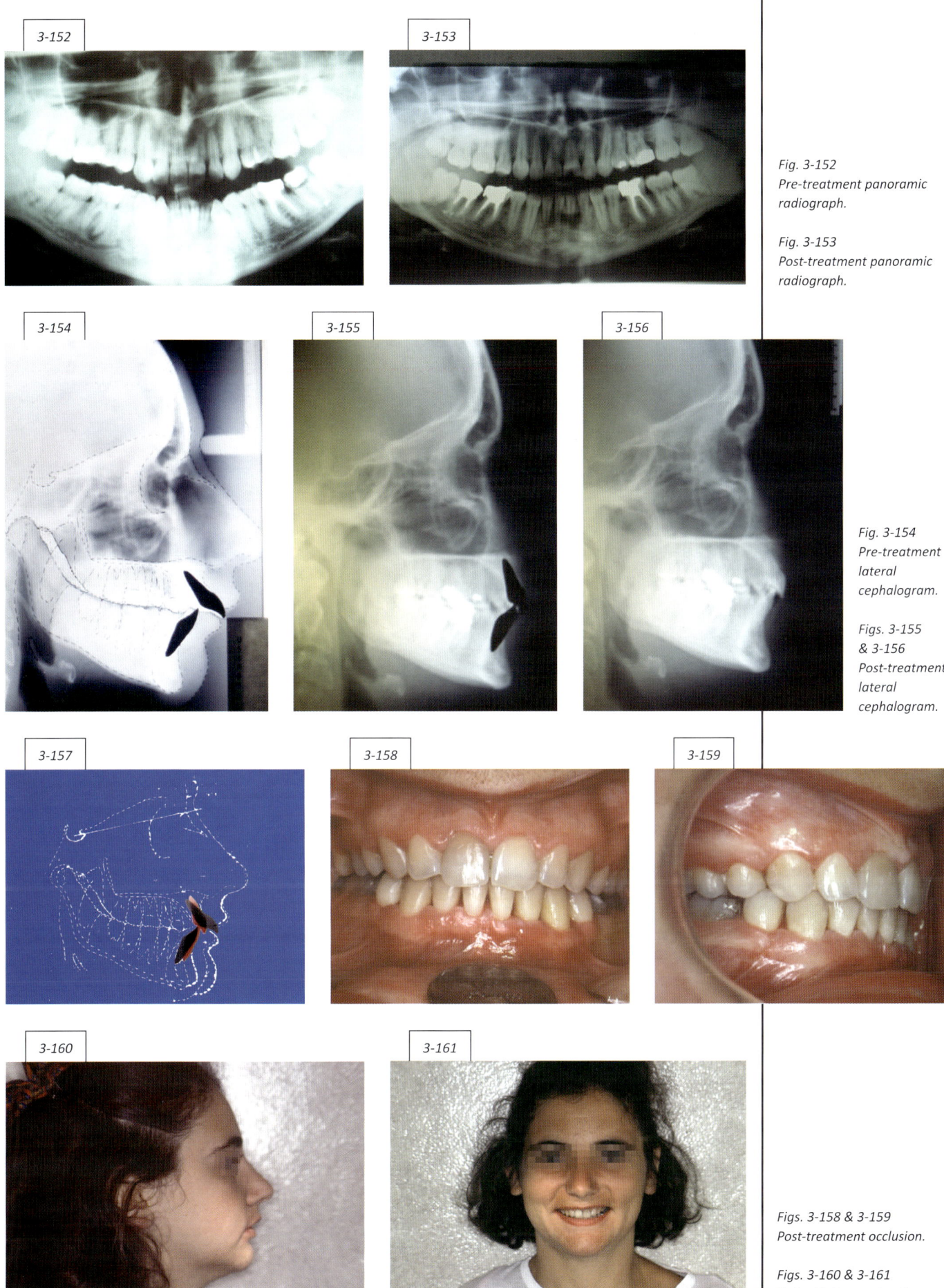

Fig. 3-152
Pre-treatment panoramic radiograph.

Fig. 3-153
Post-treatment panoramic radiograph.

3-154

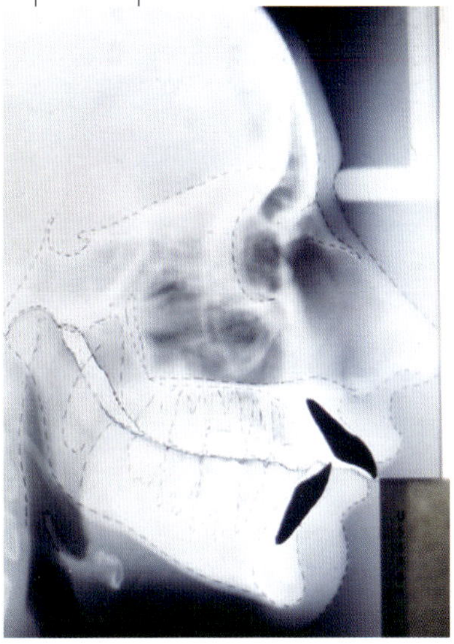

3-155

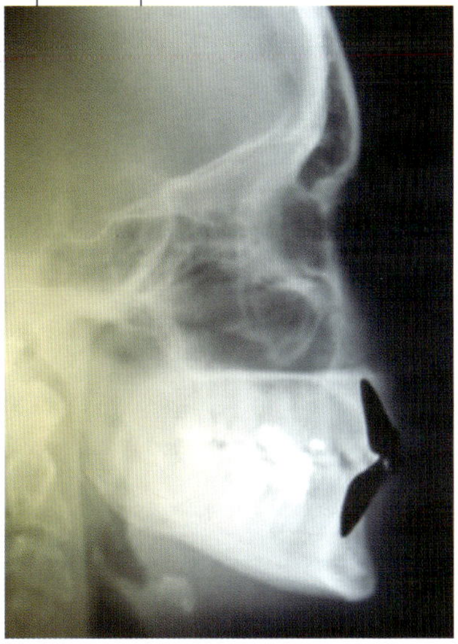

3-156

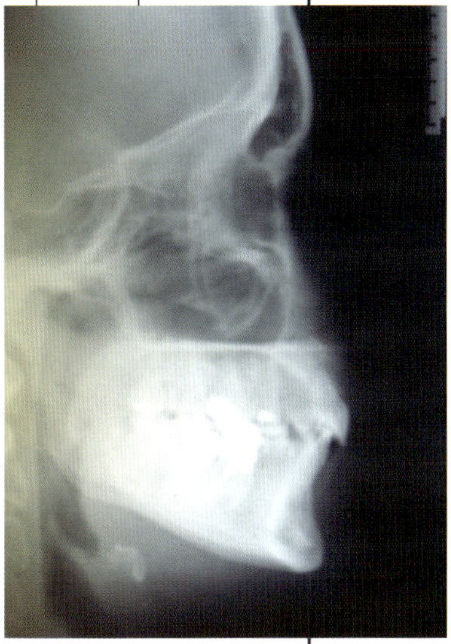

Fig. 3-154
Pre-treatment lateral cephalogram.

Figs. 3-155 & 3-156
Post-treatment lateral cephalogram.

3-157

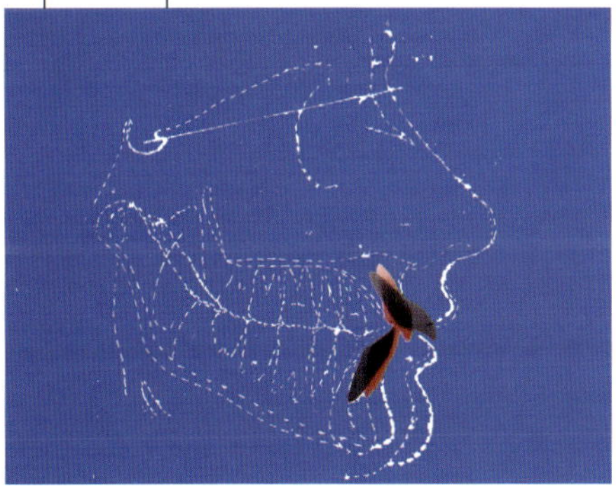

3-158

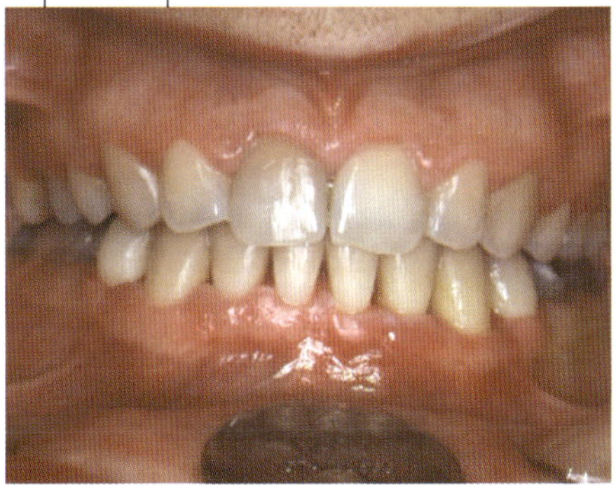

3-159

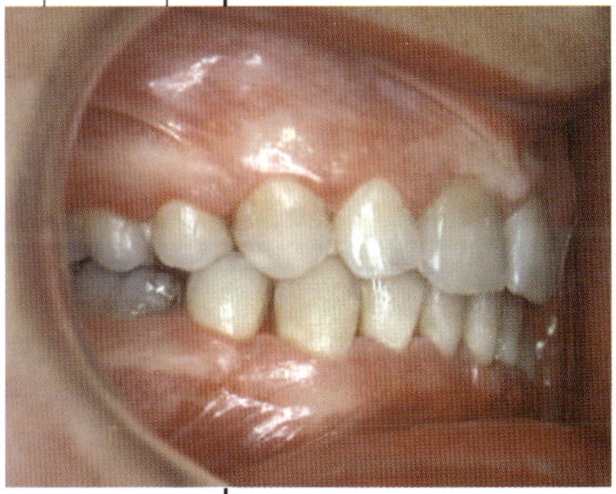

3-160

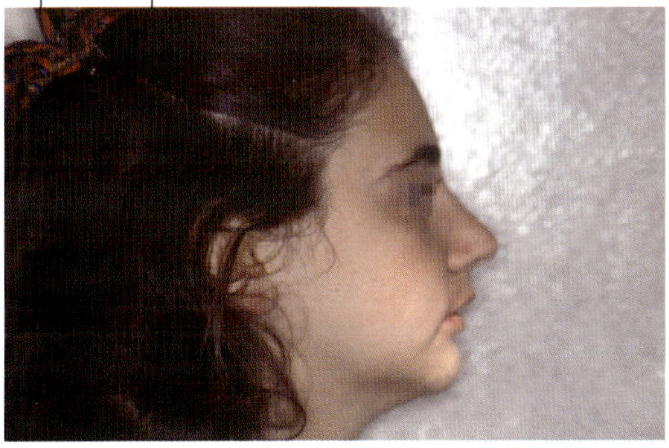

3-161

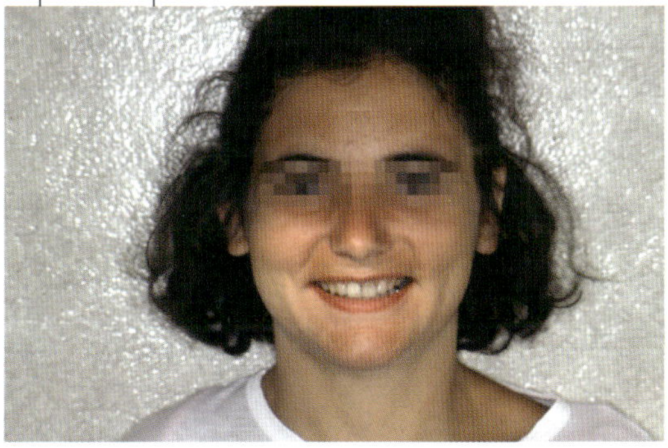

Figs. 3-158 & 3-159
Post-treatment occlusion.

Figs. 3-160 & 3-161
Patient's face and smile.

CASE NUMBER 16

The case is a severe Class II division 1 (ANB: 10°), dolico, in a 15 year old patient with facial asymmetry and TMJ clicks. After extraction of the first upper and the second lower premolars, treatment with an edgewise appliance follows for 18 months. The result is good: ANB 3°, TMJ clicks disappear and there is aesthetic and facial profile improvement.

3-162

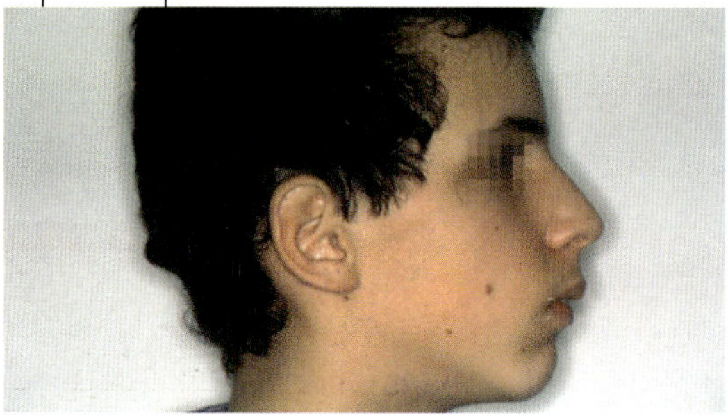

Fig. 3-162
Pre-treatment profile.

3-163

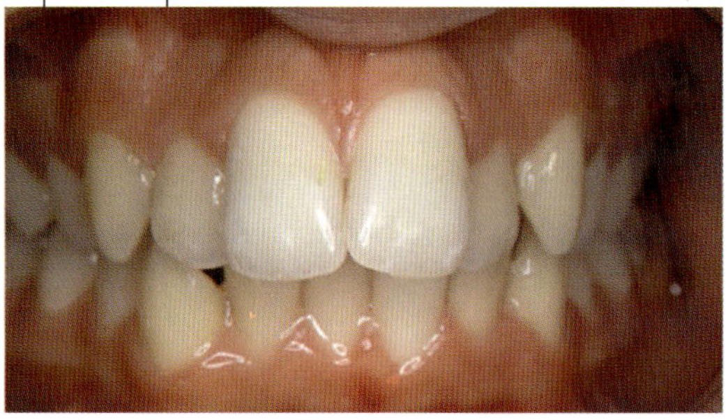

3-164

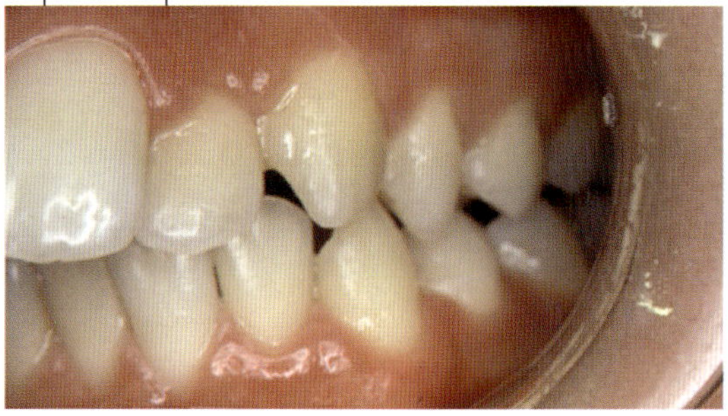

3-165

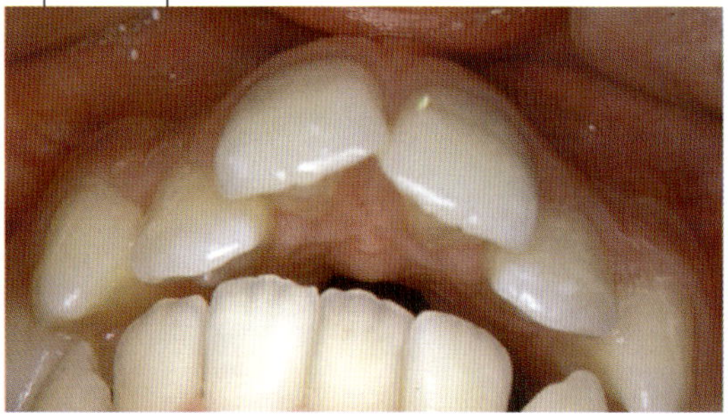

3-166

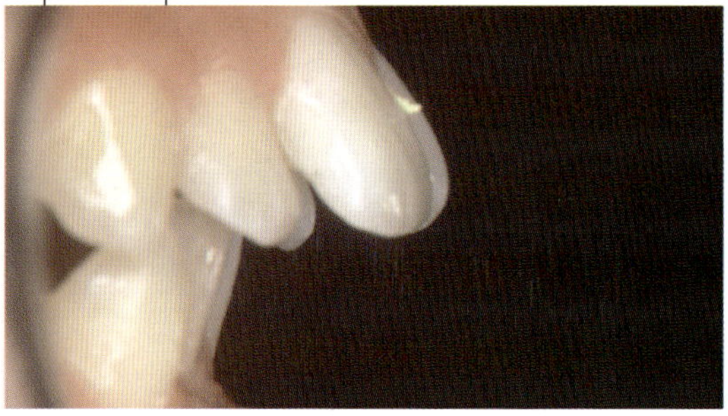

Figs. 3-163 to 3-166
Pre-treatment occlusion. The laterally positioned mandible causes the asymmetry and explains the canine Class I on one side while it is a Class II one on the other side.

3-167

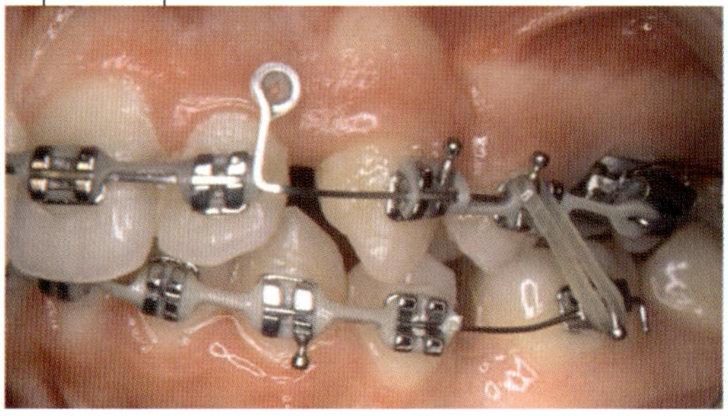

Fig. 3-167
Treatment with edgewise appliance and Class II elastics.

3-168

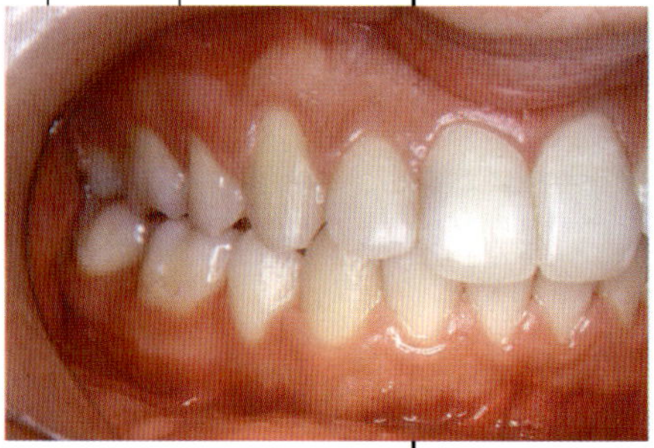

3-169

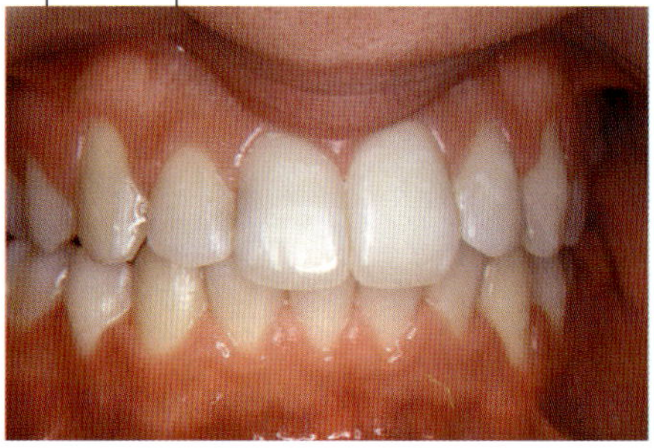

3-170

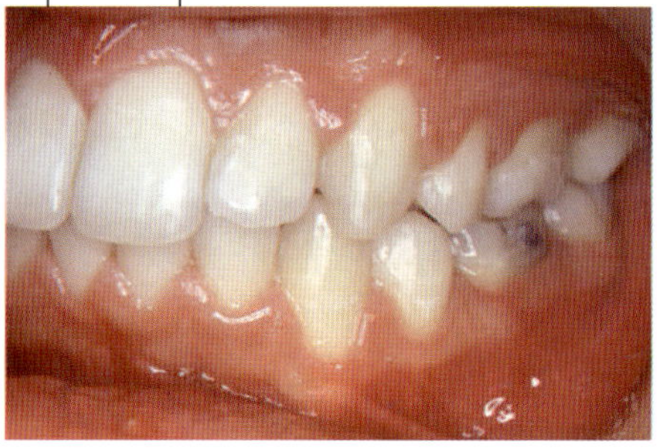

Fig. 3-168 to 3-170
Post-treatment occlusion.

3-171

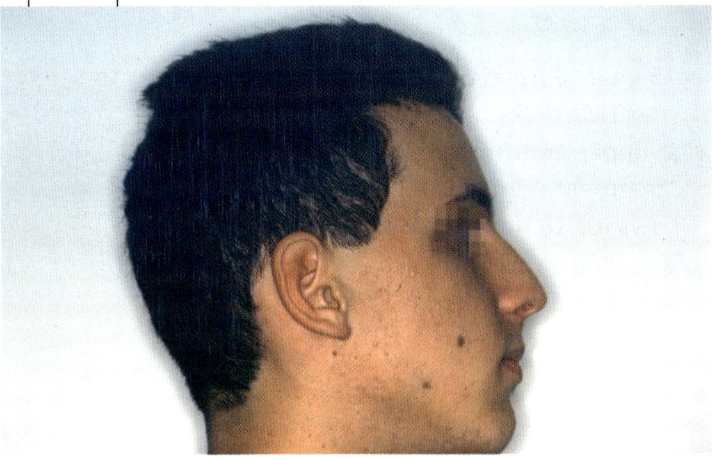

Fig. 3-171
Post-treatment profile.

3-172

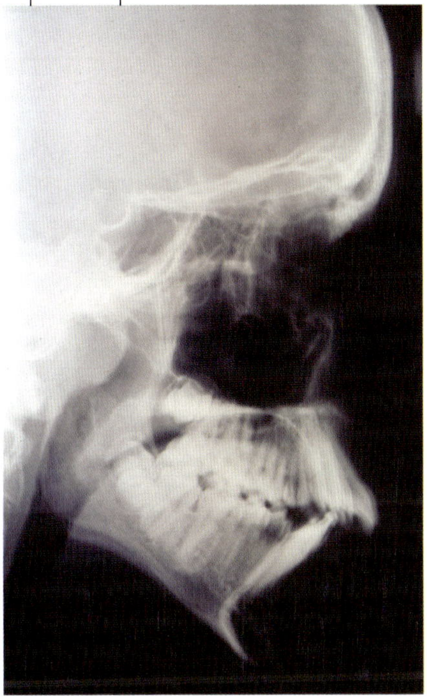

3-173

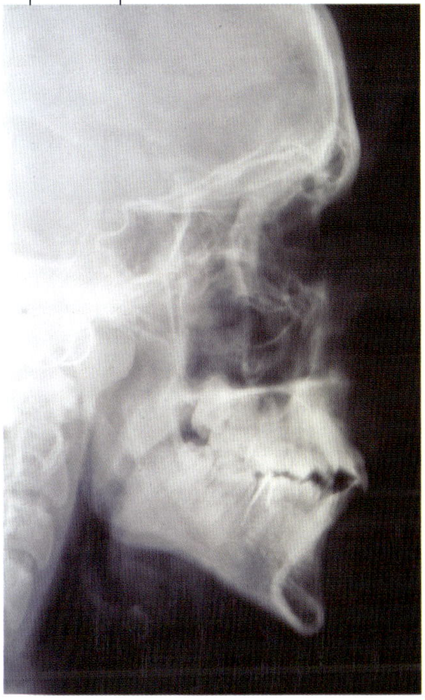

Fig. 3-172
Pre-treatment lateral cephalogram.

Fig. 3-173
Post-treatment lateral cephalogram.

CLASS II TREATMENTS WITH TWO EXTRACTIONS

There are many cases of Class II at the end of growth which can be treated with the extraction of two first upper premolars. These are the ones where the upper arch needs to be retracted while the lower arch is (or can be) well aligned and the mandible is not too retrusive.

In the last cases, the facial aesthetic profile requires mandibular advancement surgery.

At the end the results can be very satisfactory. There is a Class I canine relationship with the molars in Class II.

TREATMENT OF A CLASS II WITH TWO UPPER FIRST PREMOLAR EXTRACTIONS (A SCHEMATIC REPRESENTATION OF A SLIDING MECHANICAL APPLIANCE) (FIG. 3-174)

Treatment of a Class II with two upper first premolar extractions: (a schematic representation of a sliding mechanical appliance) (Fig. 3-174)
Usual procedure:-

- alignment and levelling of the arches
- opens the bite when necessary
- canine distalisation to a Class I relationship with sliding appliance: 200 g of traction with elastic chain or coil spring on a round arch
- be careful with the anchorage because it can be easily lost
- distalisation of four incisors with elastic chain or coil spring on a rectangular arch
- start by preparing the lower arch. It can be useful to apply Class II elastics
- start with the upper arch in Class II division 2, otherwise it would not be possible to apply a fixed appliance on the lower one.

3-174

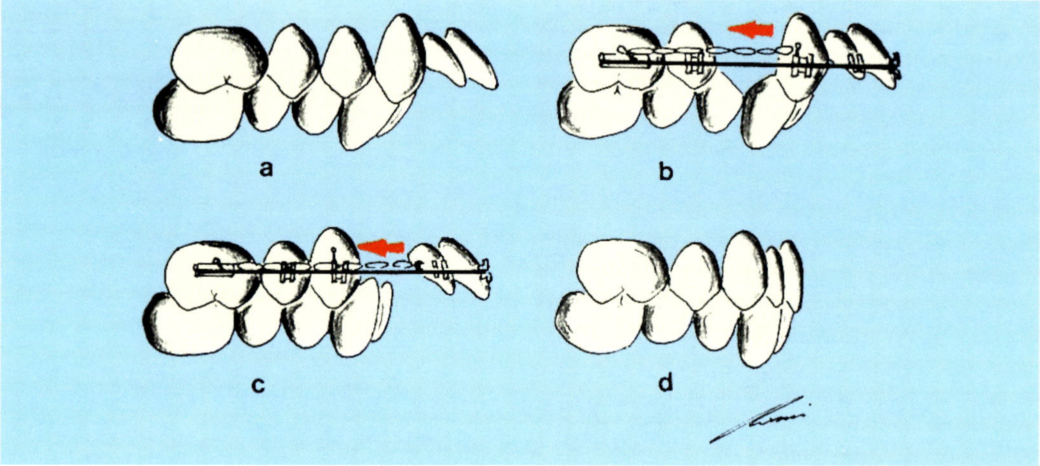

Many believe that this treatment will cause TMJ problems because the frontal teeth retraction entraps the mandible distally and leads to Internal Derangement (clicks). But remember that at the end of a correct treatment there is no contact between the upper and lower incisors.

In this and other aspects there is no evidence of negative gnathologic results (see Chapter VI).

The treatment represents what is also known as "camouflage" of a Class II. Mihalik, Proffit and Phillips report (in AJO-DO 2003;123: 266-78) that the patients in a camouflage group were very satisfied with their treatment overall and they had fewer functional and TMJ problems than the patients in the surgical group. D.L. Turpin comments in the same article "it is good news to hear that camouflage treatment might be a successful alternative to surgery".

Looking at the result of this study I personally think that a camouflage treatment should not be regarded as minor treatment if the stability is comparable to that of surgery and if the patients' perceptions of outcomes are also highly positive.

CASE NUMBER 17

The case is a Class II division 1 in a 12 year old female patient with a notable overjet.

After years of unsuccessful treatments with removable appliances she wants to reduce the overjet orthodontically as quickly as possible. As she is close to the end of her period of growth and the mandible is well positioned (not retruded), the best choice of action is the retraction of upper incisors and canines after the extraction of two upper first premolars. The treatment took 15 months.

3-175

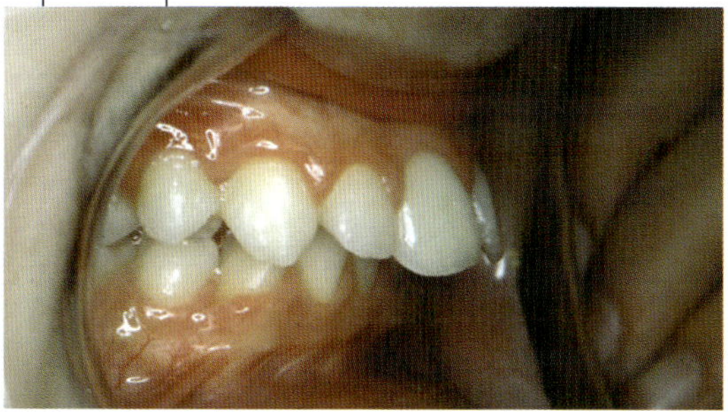

Fig. 3-175
Pre-treatment occlusion.

3-176

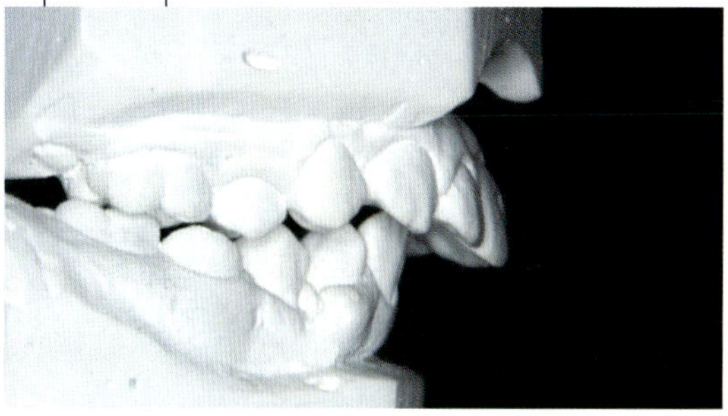

3-177

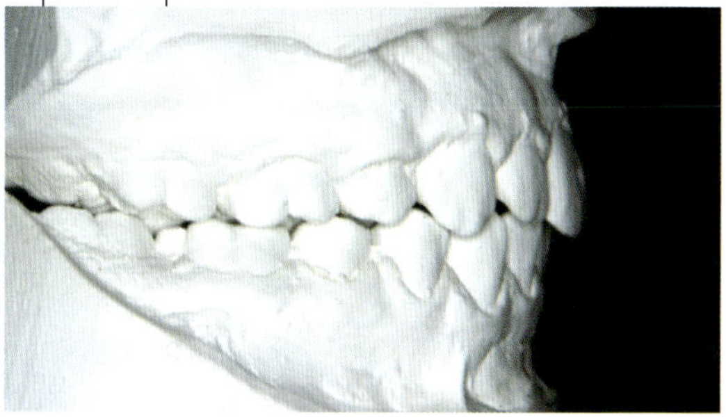

Fig. 3-176
Pre-treatment dental casts. Note the accentuated overjet, typical of Class II division I.

Fig. 3-177
Post-treatment dental casts. The overjet is corrected.

3-178

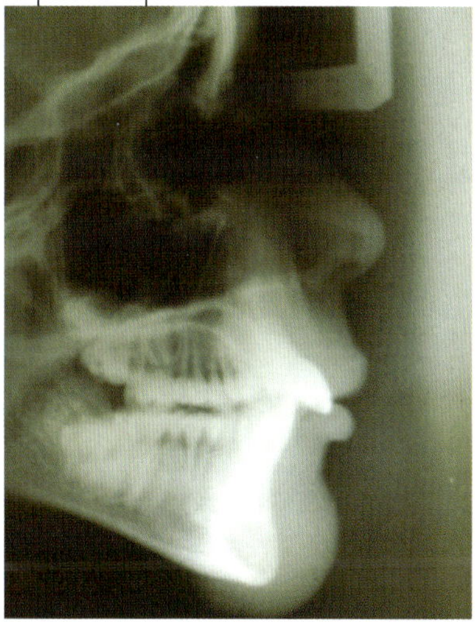

3-179

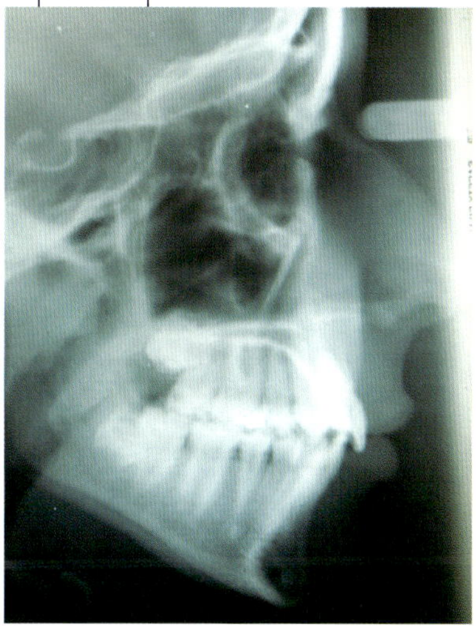

Fig. 3-178
Pre-treatment lateral cephalogram.

Fig. 3-179
Post-treatment lateral cephalogram.

3-180

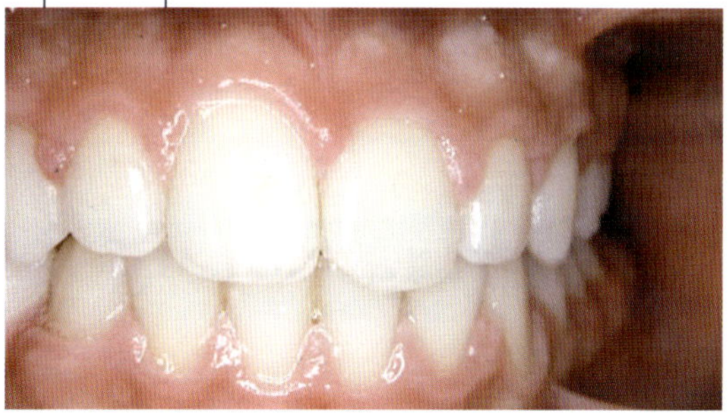

3-181

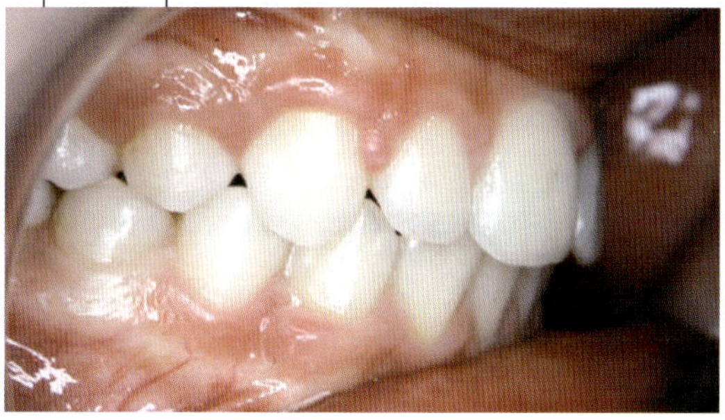

Figs. 3-180 & 3-181
Post-treatment occlusion.

CASES WITH TWO UNUSUAL EXTRACTIONS

There are cases (18 and 19) where extracting teeth other than the first upper premolars can be convenient.

CASE NUMBER 18

3-182

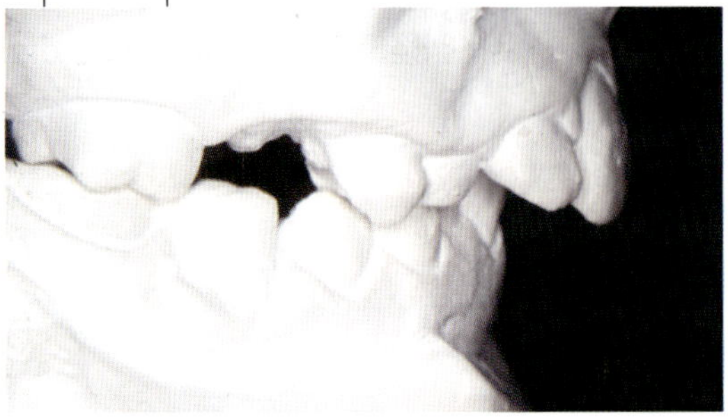

Fig. 3-182
Pre-treatment dental casts.

3-183

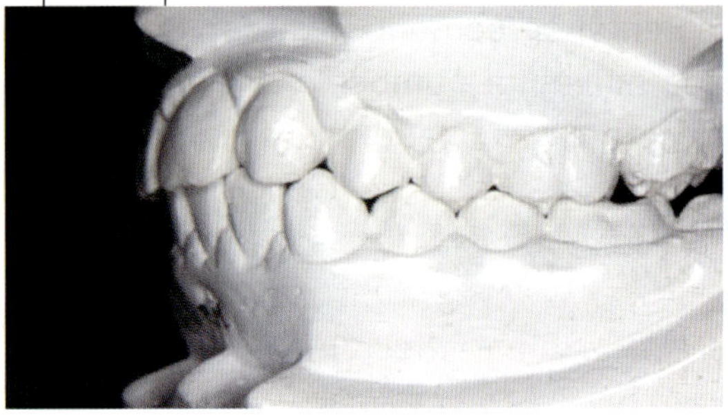

Fig. 3-183
Post-treatment dental casts.

3-184

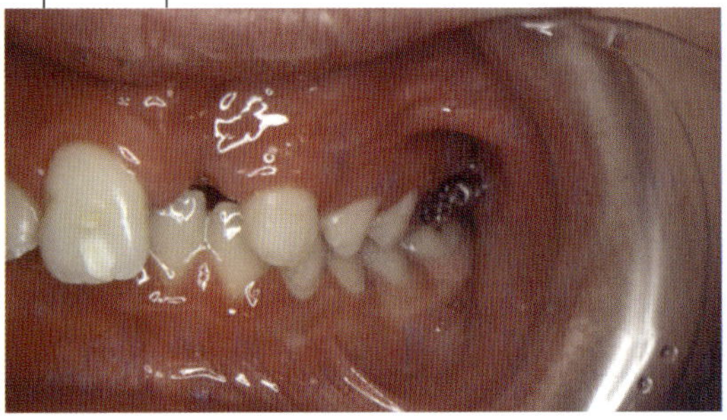

Fig. 3-184
Pre-treatment occlusion.

3-185

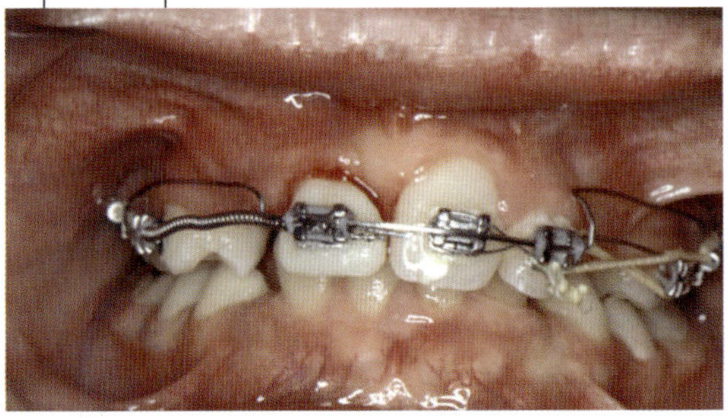

Fig. 3-185
Phase of treatment. Notice the temporary remodelling of the upper left lateral incisor like a central incisor.

3-186

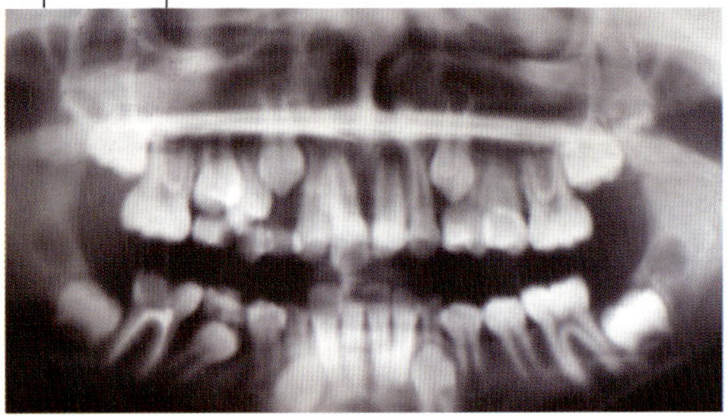

Fig. 3-186
Pre-treatment panoramic radiograph. Notice the crown fracture of the upper central left incisor and the radiolucent periapical zone as sign of endodontic infection.

3-187

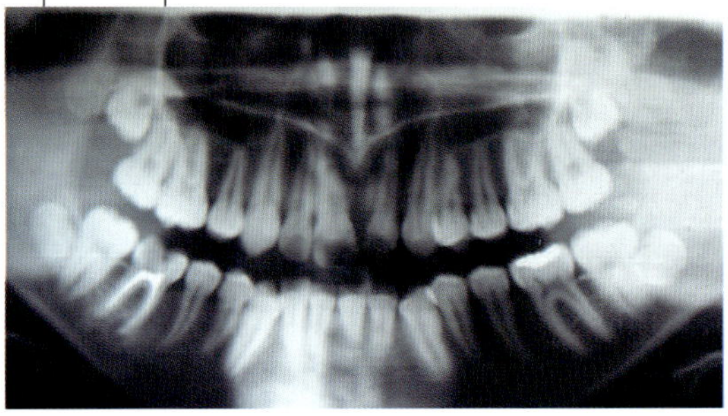

Fig. 3-187
Post-treatment panoramic radiograph. Upper left lateral incisor has been moved to occupy the place of the upper left central incisor, while the upper left canine is in place of the lateral incisor.

3-188

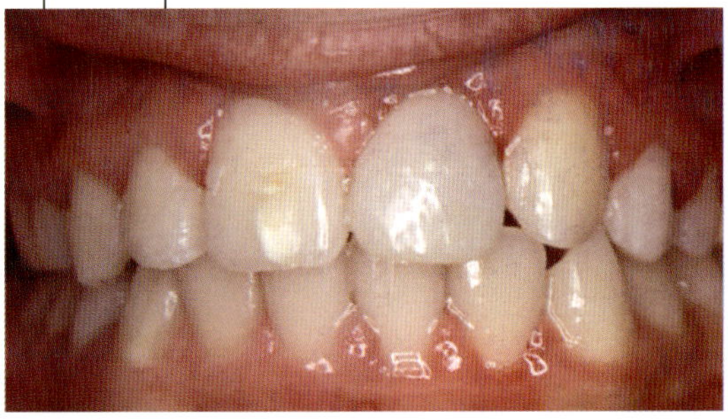

3-189

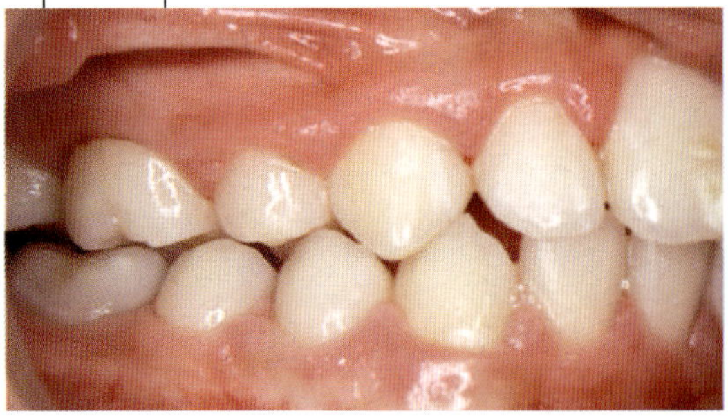

Figs. 3-188 & 3-189
Post-treatment occlusion. It illustrates the description above - the lateral incisor crown, has been modified with composite in order to be the new left central incisor. -The upper left canine shifted to the left lateral incisor's place.

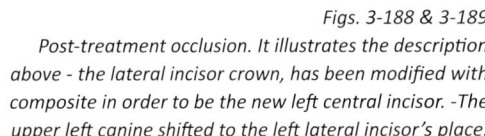

3-191

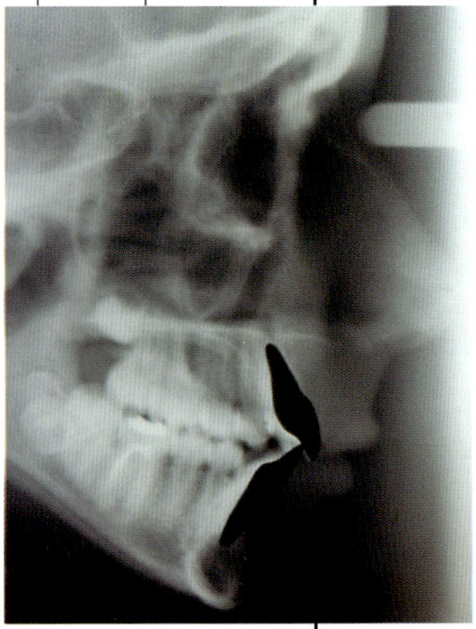

Fig. 3-191
Post-treatment lateral cephalogram.

3-190

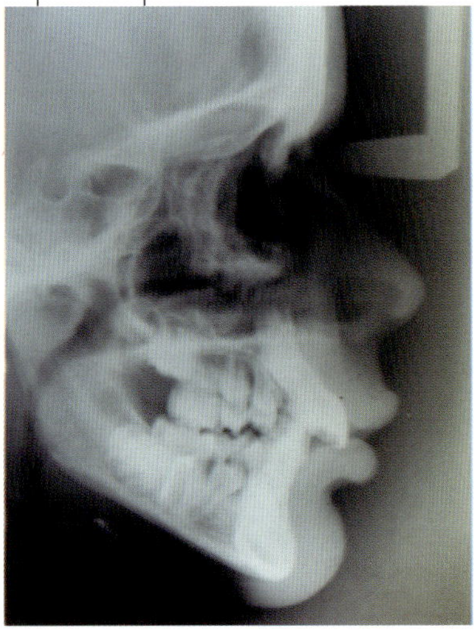

Fig. 3-190
Pre-treatment lateral cephalogram.

The extraction after a traumatic fracture of the upper left central incisor offers an alternative, less common treatment. With parental agreement, in order to perform the minimum number of extractions, the decision was made to remove the first upper right premolar only. To reduce the overjet we extracted only one premolar rather than two. Then the upper left lateral incisor and the upper left canine were shifted towards the median line.

During the treatment, the crown of the upper left lateral incisor was remodelled with composite to make it look like an upper central incisor. The aesthetic result was satisfactory and the functional criteria were respected.

Critics would say that on one side there is no canine tooth guidance. I remind them that instead there is a good group disclusion, which is as beneficial as a canine disclusion.

On the other hand, how many times do dentists see patients of all ages with displaced canines? Do they cause a calamity? If yes, how?

I have been working for 35 years and I am still waiting for some precise answers on the subject. However, I'm sure of one thing: for psychological reasons I would prefer not to have a prosthetic upper central incisor in my mouth.

CASE NUMBER 19

This case is a Class II division 1 in a 13 year old boy with left upper canine displacement.

What should be done? Should we extract the two upper first premolars and try the alignment of the displaced canine after surgery, or extract the canine and the right first upper premolar?

The parents and the patient chose the second course of action. In my opinion, after 18 months of treatment the result is good with an excellent aesthetic balance.

3-192

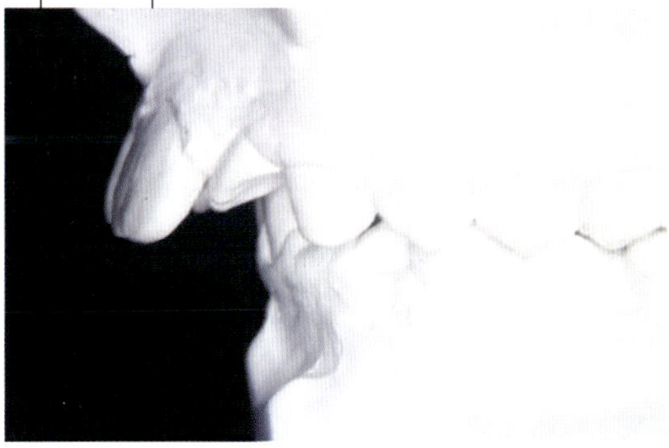

3-193

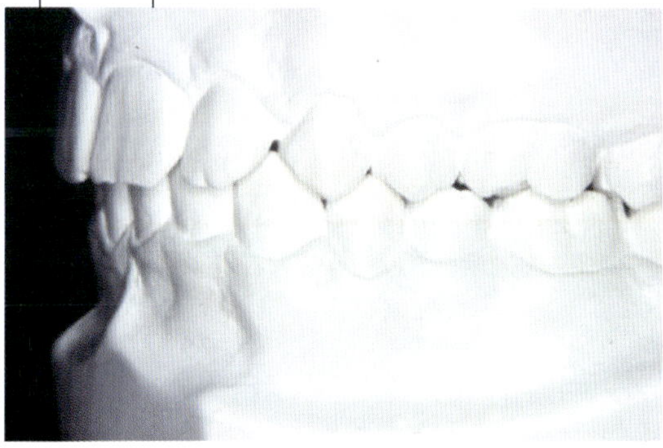

Fig. 3-192
Pre-treatment dental casts.

Fig. 3-193
Post-treatment dental casts.

3-194

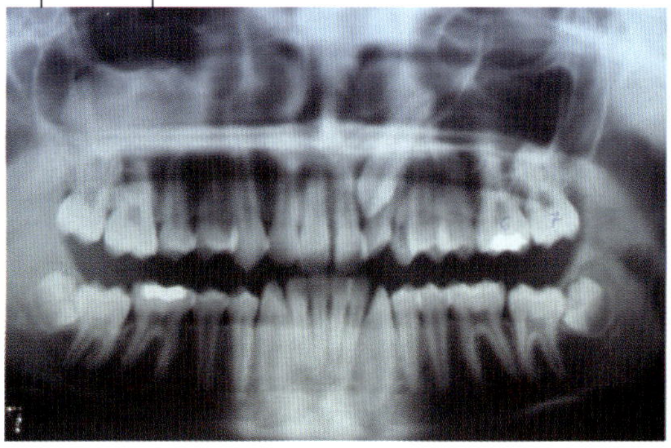

3-195

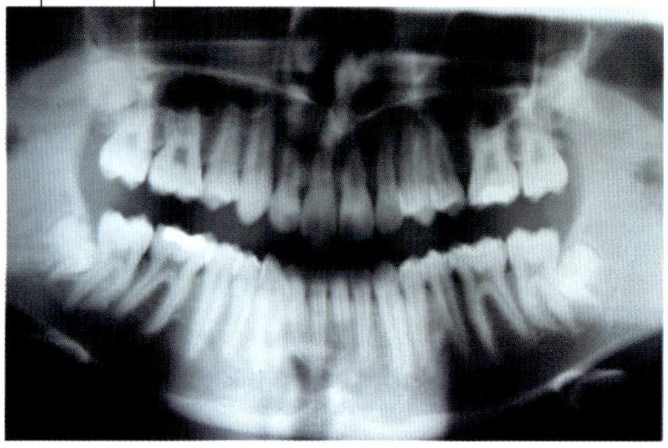

Fig. 3-194
Pre-treatment panoramic radiograph.

Fig. 3-195
Post-treatment panoramic radiograph.

3-196

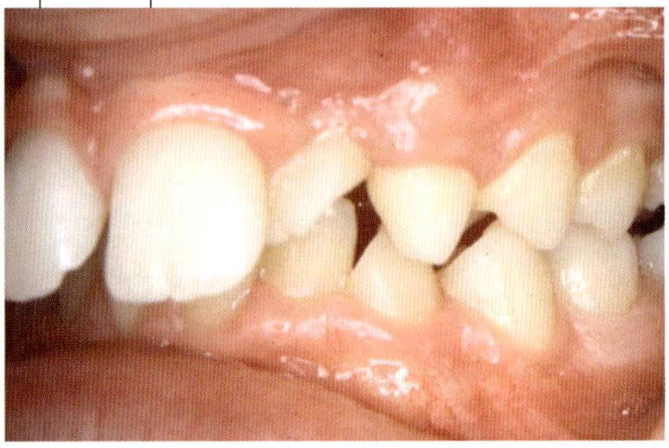

Fig. 3-196
Pre-treatment occlusion.

3-197

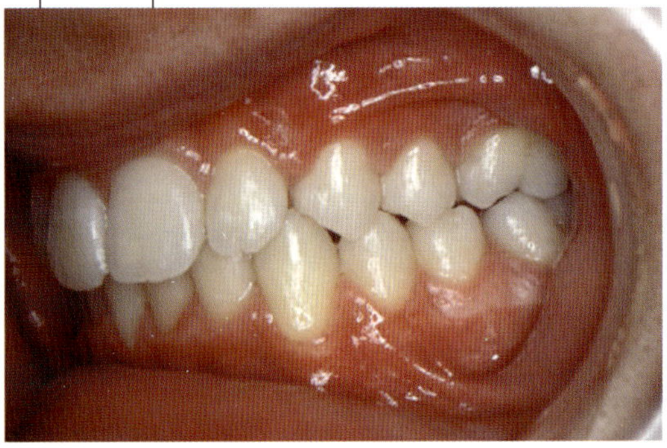

3-198

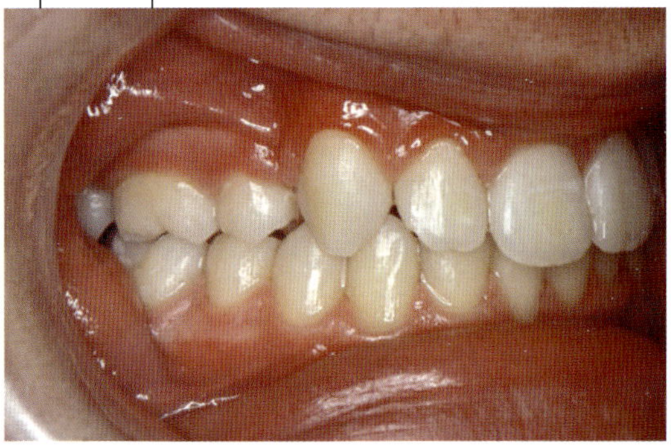

Figs. 3-197 & 3-198
Post-treatment occlusion.

3-199

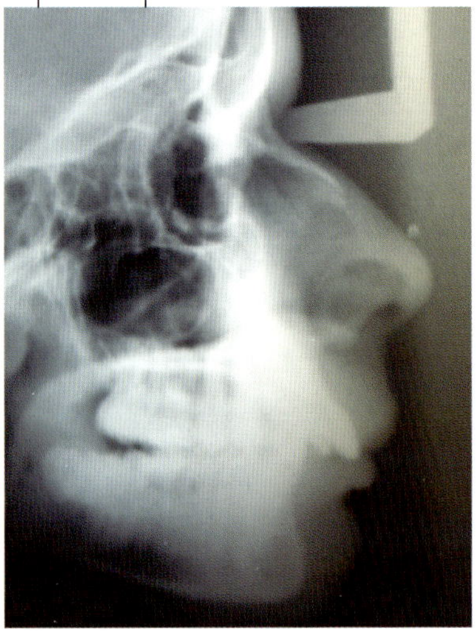

3-200

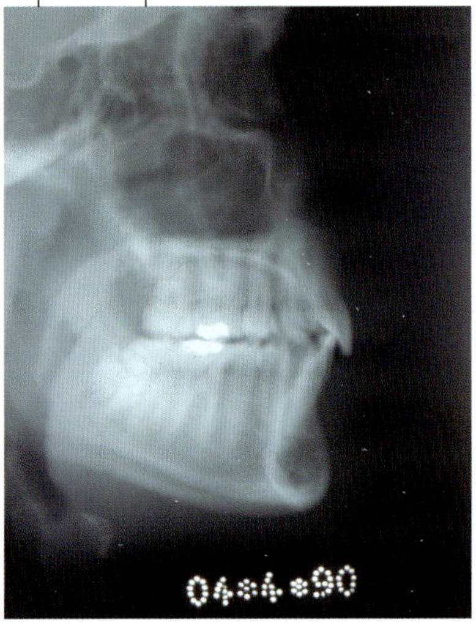

Fig. 3-199
Pre-treatment lateral cephalogram.

Fig. 3-200
Post-treatment lateral cephalogram.

3-201

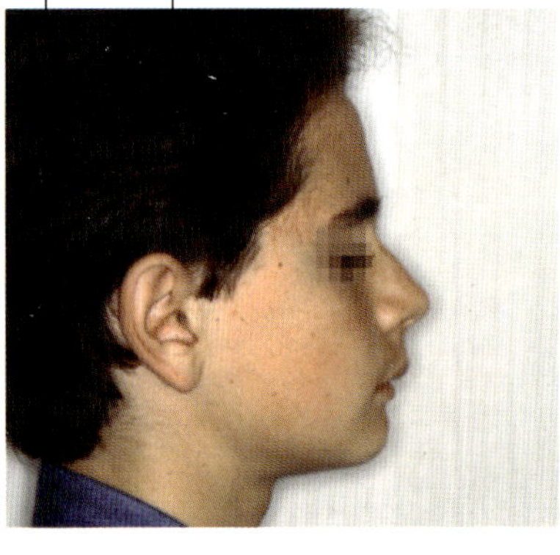

3-202

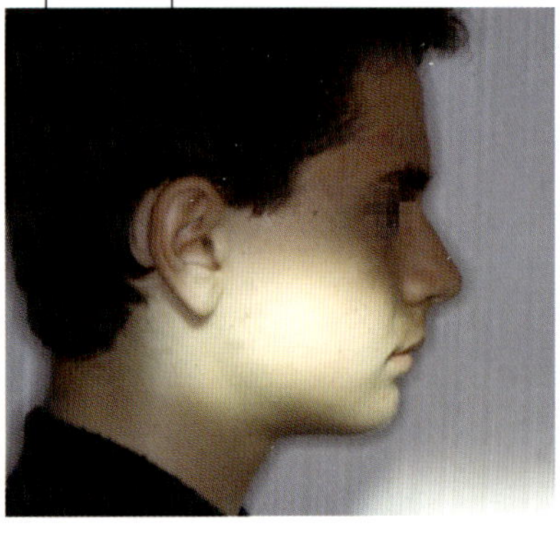

Fig. 3-201
Pre-treatment profile.

Fig. 3-202
Post-treatment profile.

Orthodontics in Clinical Practice

Chapter IV:

Class III

DESCRIPTION AND ETIOLOGY

4-1

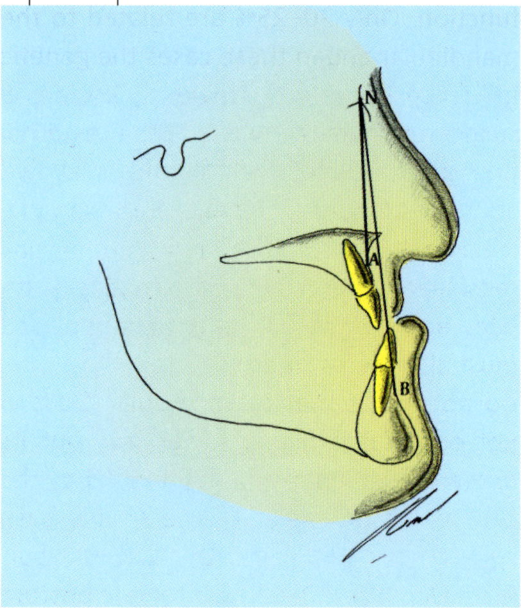

Fig. 4-1
Skeletal Class III:
ANB < O.

Skeletal Class III malocclusions make up about 5% of malocclusion cases in the Caucasian population. The profile (Fig. 4-1) shows the upper jaw (maxillary) behind the lower jaw (mandible). In cephalometric analysis, which uses the ANB angle, the angle is negative.

The value of the SNA angle indicates the extent of the maxilla while the SNB value indicates the extent of the mandible.

Aesthetically in such a case the chin is prominent, there is a flatness of paranasal areas and an increased nasolabial angle with apparent prominence of the nose and upper lip retrusion.

Remember also that the mandibular profile depends on the vertical dimension. Therefore, in a dolicofacial patient, the mandible is less protruded because of its clockwise growth. The ANB angle is less negative and as a result, such a Class III can improve even though there is a skeletal open bite.

According to most authors a Class III has a genetic base that is polygenically transmitted. A malocclusion can occur when inherited factors combine with environmental ones, but sometimes environmental factors alone can lead to the onset of a genetically determined malocclusion. In particular followers of the French school of thought of Jean Delaire firmly believe that facial growth is induced by functional activities.

THE MAXILLA

In a Class III the maxilla grows forward, pushed by the development of the brain and of the ethmoid, while its vertical growth follows the development of the eyes, dental occlusion, expansion of the sinus and muscle activity (lingual muscles, velum pendulum and superficial muscles of the face).

The transversal increase is provoked by the functional forces applied to the sutures. The role of the tongue is fundamental. The act of swallowing (at least 600 times a day) stimulates the palatal vault.

According to Delaire[67] the tongue remodels the premaxillary-maxillary suture inducing advancement, although not all authors recognise the activity of this suture after birth[106]. The increased volume of teeth buds, activities of the nasal complex, the upper lip and occlusal forces also play a role.

For Delaire,[66, 68, 69] (one of the world's foremost experts on the functional orthopedic treatment of Class III), the management of the maxilla is extremely important since it is deficient in many cases, whereas the mandible is usually of normal dimension. Any excessive mandibulary growth is caused by a lingual dysfunction.

Once again, the negative role of mouth breathing caused by anatomical alterations (e.g traumatic nasal septum deviation, amygdala hypertrophy as a consequence of infections, allergy etc.) must be pointed out. Mouth breathing is characterized by a low tongue posture (with the hyoid bone), which stimulates the mandible forward instead of the maxilla. Yet it is important to also bear in mind the genetic influence, otherwise mouth breathing would be synonymous only with Class III and its role in a Class II could not be explained.

THE MANDIBLE

Most Class IIIs are caused by a maxillary deficiency as a consequence of a dysfunction. Only 20–25% are related to the mandibular and in these cases the genetic influence is evident. However, besides a suspected hyperactivity of the external pterygoid muscle, only a little is known about other causal factors. For example, it has yet to be determined whether any muscular hyperactivity is genetically related and the role of the growth hormone must also be considered.

Do not forget that a mandibular Class III not only has a bigger lower jaw, but its forward position can be influenced by the cephalometric angles of the cranial base such as the sellar and the articular surfaces (Jarabak [130]). A lower tongue posture is sometimes present with a short lingual frenum.

It must be remembered that a maxillary deficiency can be determined by other factors such as upper lateral incisor agenesia and impacted canines. Moreover, special attention has to be paid to the cleft palate. In the past especially, this was treated too early with surgery and the resulting scars inhibited maxillary growth.

TREATMENT

Fundamental for treatment and prognosis is the distinction based on verticality of the malocclusion into one of two groups: brachi-mesio Class III (Fig. 2: A) and dolico Class III (Fig. 2: B).

The first group also includes the pseudo-Class III where a large negative bite is usually evident. With a gentle manipulation of the mandible, pushing it back, we can impose an edge-to-edge incisors relationship. The lower incisors have a normal or slightly protruded inclination while the upper incisors are upright or slightly retruded. The centric relation has an ANB angle of a Class I.

FUNCTIONAL APPLIANCES

The treatment of a pseudo Class III case is relatively easy. Usually, functional removable appliances like the Bimler III, Frankel III or Bionator III give good results. They enable the remodelling capability of the tongue and, by changing the inclination of the incisors, there is the correction of the anterior negative bite together with the repositioning of the mandible.

To change the inclination of the incisors, the appliance usually has an anterior metallic archwire and an acrylic component. On the upper arch the acrylic is in contact with the palatal surface of the incisors, labially positioned, while the metallic archwire doesn't touch the teeth, allowing their advancement by removing lip pressure. Incisor advancement can also be

4-2

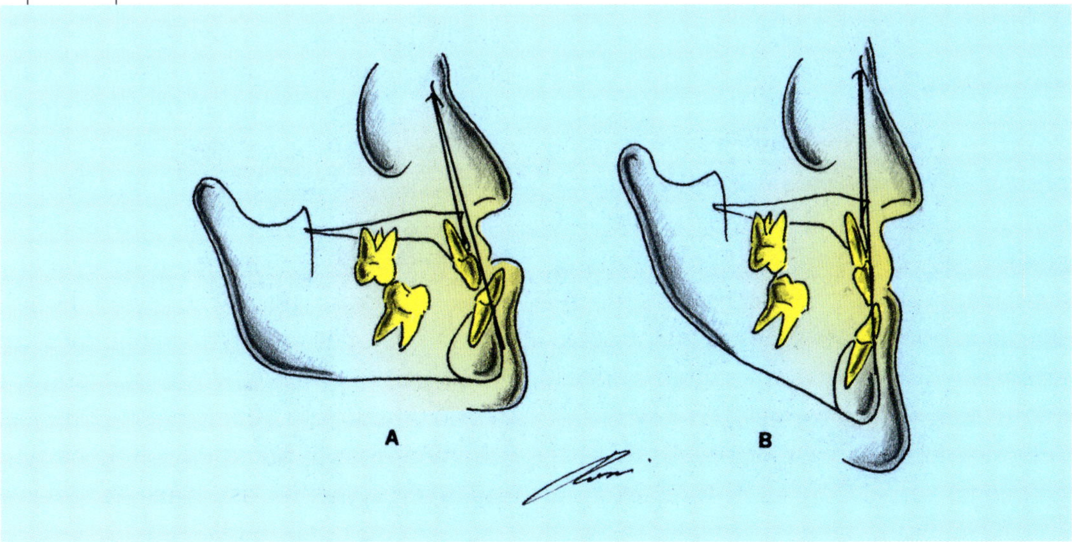

helped by springs positioned in the acrylic (fig.4-4), or a 3 way screw (fig. 1-101).
On the contrary on the lower arch, when the incisors need to move lingually, the acrylic doesn't touch the lingual surface, whereas a metallic archwire in contact with the labial surface sometimes can be useful.

In such cases there are usually good results with a good long-term prognosis.
It is better to begin the treatment as soon as possible, usually between 6 and 8 years of age. As a matter of fact, many believe that in this way we avoid the malocclusion evolving from positional to structural.

CASE NUMBER 1

Dramatic clinical cases can be very easy to treat. In this instance of a pseudo Class III, through the use of a removable appliance it was possible to obtain a good dentoskeletal relationship in a few months. However, even when cases are easy to treat there is no time to waste because, from starting out as positional, they can become structural.

4-3

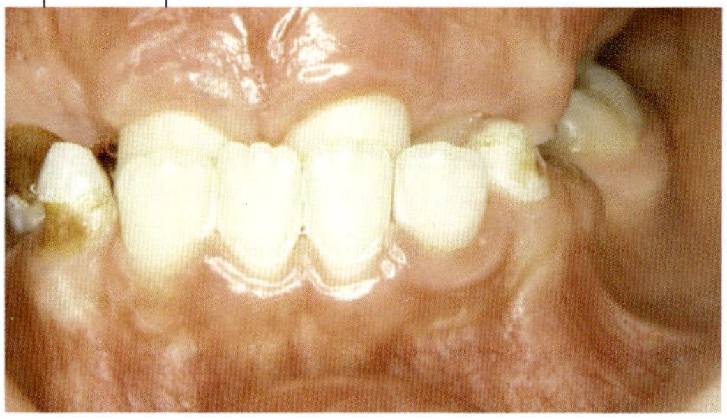

Fig. 4-3
Pre-treatment occlusion.

4-4

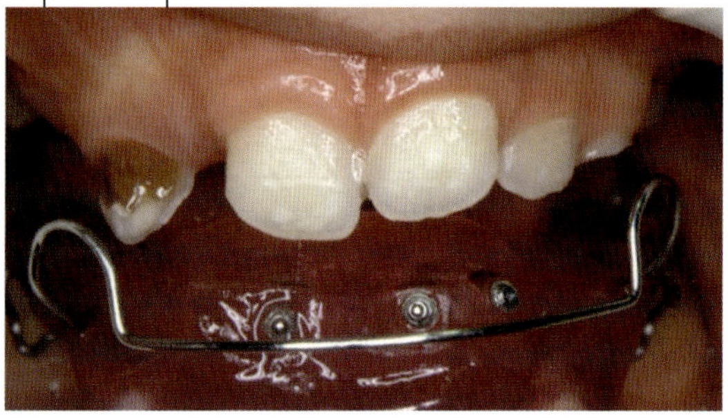

Fig. 4-4
Removable appliance.

4-5

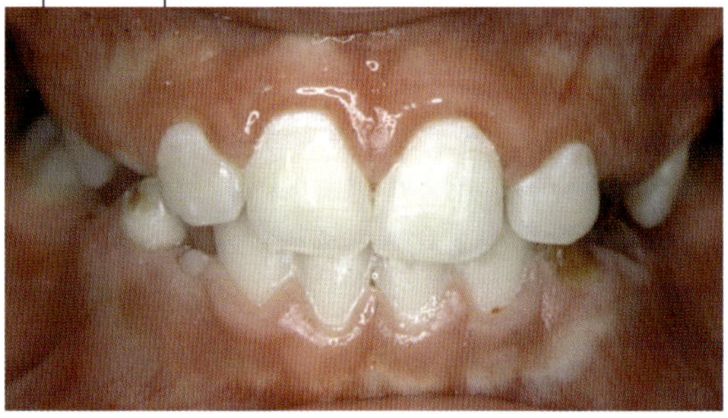

Fig. 4-5
Occlusion after a few months.

4-6

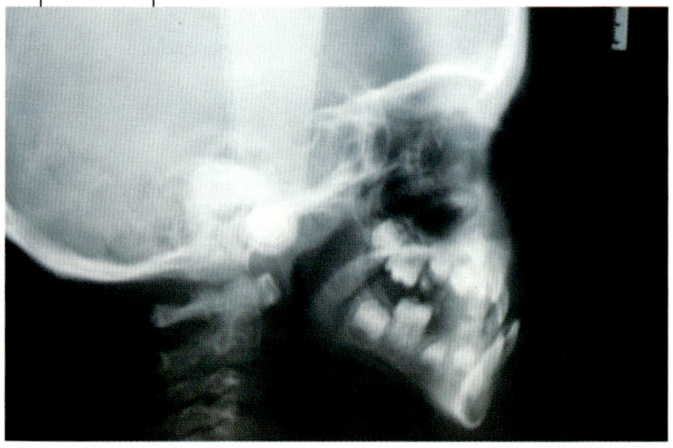

Fig. 4-6
Pre-treatment lateral cephalogram.

4-7

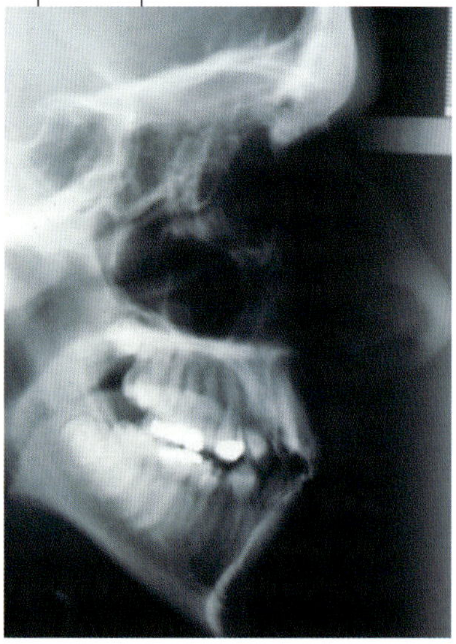

Fig. 4-7
Post-treatment lateral cephalogram. The ANB angle now is positive.

CASE NUMBER 2

4-8

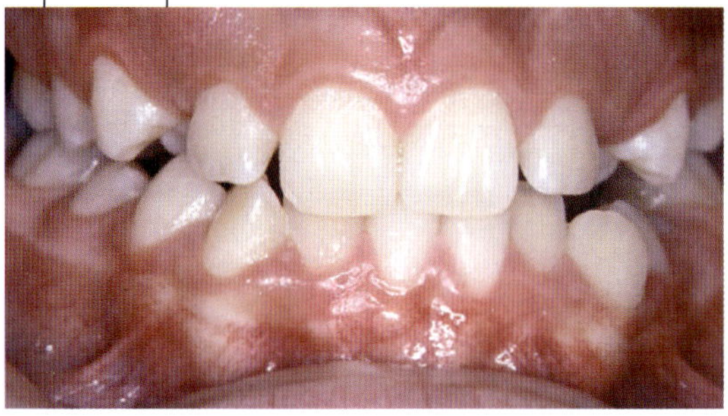

4-9

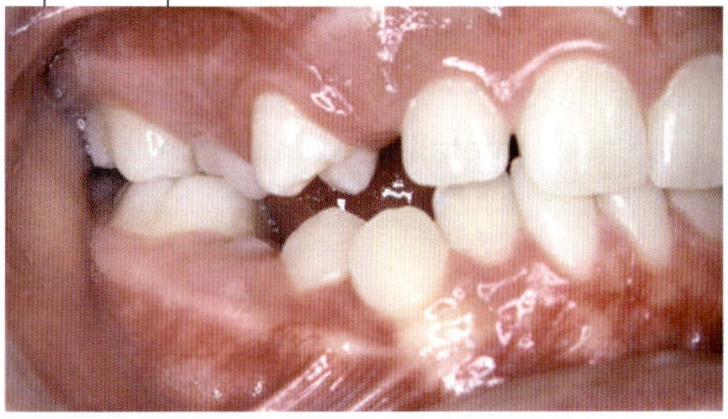

Figs. 4-8 & 4-9
Pre-treatment occlusion.

4-10

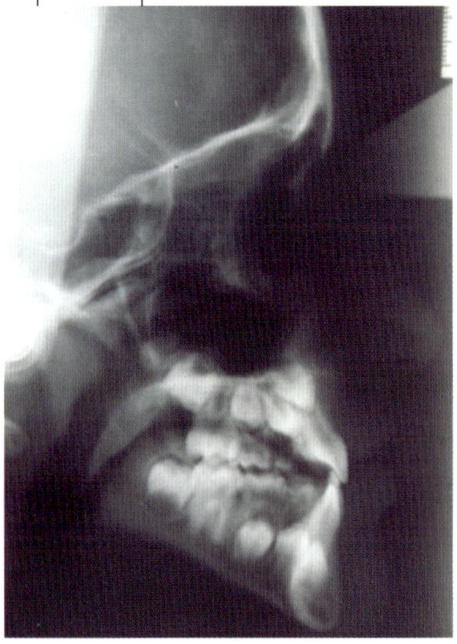

4-11

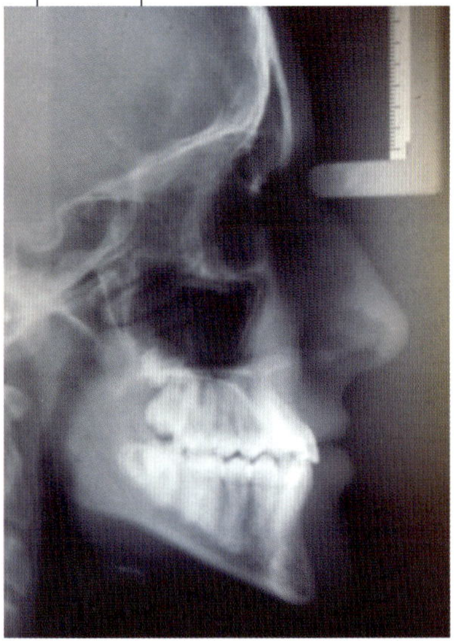

Fig. 4-10
X-ray which confirms the clinical suspicion. SNA 76.5, SNB 78, ANB -1.5°.

Fig. 4-11
X-ray at the end of treatment. The angle values are the same.

4-12

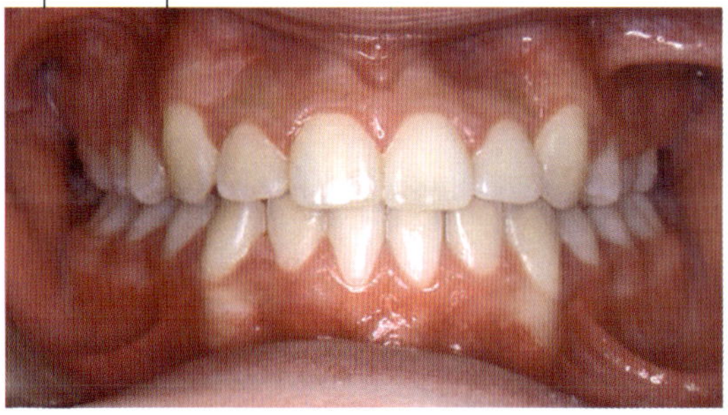

4-13

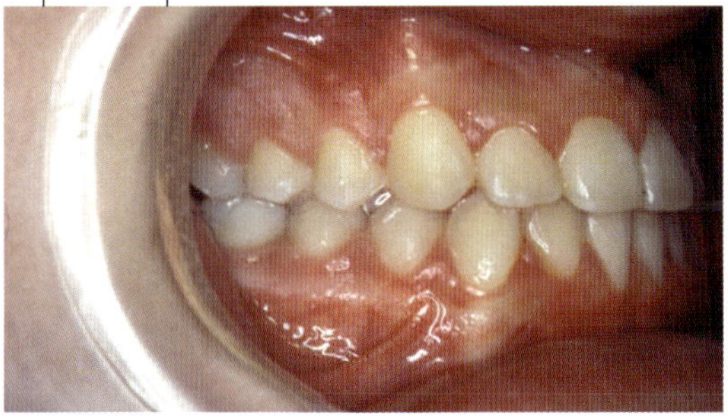

Figs. 4-12 & 4-13
There is an acceptable balance between the teeth and the jaws.

4-14

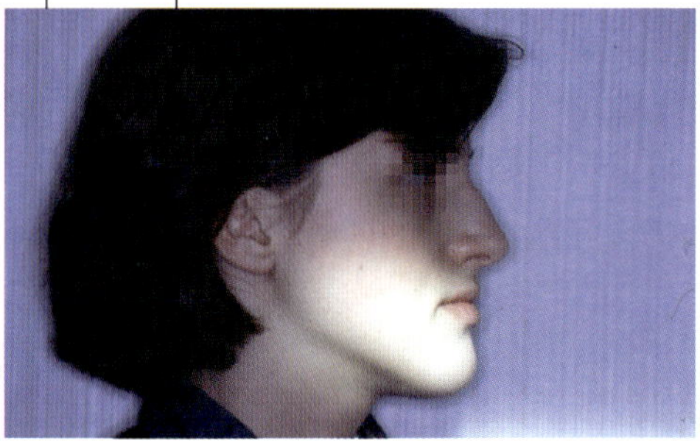

Fig. 4-14
Profile at the end of the treatment.

In the beginning this case had a positive dental anterior relationship but one that was more severe than the previous case. The suspicion that it was a true Class III was based on the lingual inclination of the lower incisors which compensate the negative distance between the jaws. The final occlusion and face profile represent an acceptable functional aesthetical compromise.

By considering the vertical dimension it is easier to treat a brachi or mesio Class III rather than a dolico one. This happens because, as we will later observe, many improvements during the treatment of a Class III are determined by increased verticality, which when combined with the maxillary advancement, allows a correction of any present negative overjet. For these reasons we must be careful in a Class III dolico because by performing a clockwise rotation of the mandible we can induce a skeletal open bite that goes beyond certain aesthetic limits.

4-15

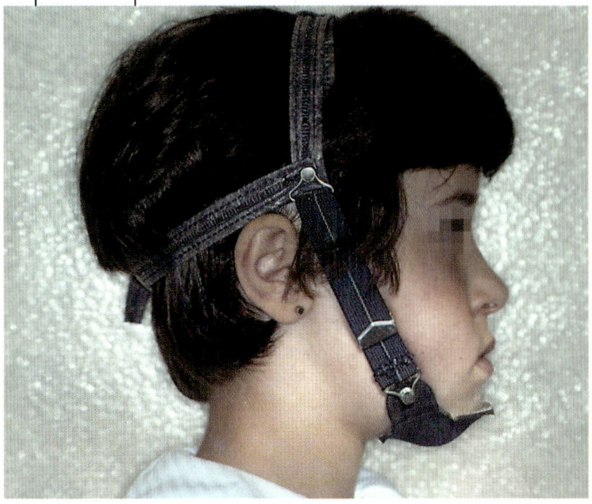

Fig. 4-15 Chin Cup

CHIN CUP

A well-known appliance used for the treatment of a Class III since the early 19th century is the chin cup. In theory it works by transmitting a force from the chin to the condyle, thus inhibiting the sagittal growth of the mandible. Sugawara et al.[237] summarise the chin cup "problem" from a Japanese clinical realm where there are many Class III patients:

As a matter of fact, in the last twenty years many studies have demonstrated that numerous orthopedic effects can be obtained by using a chin cup. Particularly, it is possible to change the direction of mandibular growth by inducing its remodelling and back positioning. These effects can determine permanent skeletal changes and modify the prognathic profile especially when the treatment takes place at a young age. However, there are also some limits.

In fact, they say that even though with a chin cup it is possible to influence somehow the vertical position, the same influence does not always apply to the anteroposterior position.

While at the beginning of the quotation it seemed possible to gain full control of the mandibular growth, reading on it begins to appear less likely. Later we will also learn that *"it is difficult with the chin cup to obtain a good profile on patients with severe mandibular protrusion".* When it comes to long-term results it is better not to overestimate the effects of the chin cup. That is why I personally suggest PRUDENCE.

According to my clinical experience, with a chin cup it is possible to influence the vertical position of the mandible inducing its clockwise rotation and ANB angle improvement.

By keeping the mouth closed, nasal breathing can also improve. However, I would not expect to gain full control of mandibular growth because, when it comes to male patients, they would have to wear the chin cup until they turn 18–19 years old and this is a very unlikely scenario.

PROTRACTION FACEMASK

Having explained the indications and limits of the chin cup, let us consider, in my opinion, the main orthopedic appliance for the treatment of a Class III: the protraction facemask, also known as the Delaire mask (Fig. 4-16).

The mask is an extra-oral appliance that is in contact with the chin and the forehead. It is fixed by two elastics to an intra-oral structure which consists of a double arch – buccal/labial and palatal – welded to molar bands.

According to Verdon[250] the tractions are to be applied during the night only. In his opinion a nightly application gives a more physiological stimulation of the suture followed by better reorganization and little chance of relapse. Others, always respecting the concept of intermittent forces

described by Reitan,[205] suggest an application of 10–12 hours per day.
Proffit[201] talks about 14 hours a day with a force of 450 g each side (12 oz). The Delaire school classically indicates heavy forces, from 600 g to 1000 g on each side. More recently orthodontists like Verdon[250] have suggested a reduction to 450 g on each side or less, and about 250 g on each side in younger patients (4–5 years old). Verdon also suggests continuing with the traction beyond a Class I relationship if possible. But for how long? The answer is - until there is an advancement. In order to reduce the risk of relapse after traction, Verdon applies a removable brace, the lingual ramp of Salagnac,[216] to correct the low posture of the tongue.
The action of an anteroposterior traction occurs, not only on the nasal-frontal-maxillary, palatal-maxillary and other sutures, but also on the dento-alveolar processes, inducing their draw-sliding on the basal bone.
When a cross-bite is present it is better to correct it before the traction is applied. In those cases preceded by a rapid palatal expansion with a Haas appliance, the maxillary moves down and forward. We can observe an advancement of point A. That is good in a Class III. Moreover, when an anteroposterior traction is needed the mask can be hooked to the expander.
In a Class III dolico, orthopedic control is considered more difficult because together with the traction there is usually an increase of the vertical dimension. If the Class III improves sagittally showing a less negative ANB angle, then there is a skeletal open bite with mandibular clockwise rotation, which can be acceptable in a brachi-mesio Class III, but not in a dolico. Verdon et al. say that by using an intra-oral double arch with a SPEE concavity it is possible not only to control the clockwise rotation of the mandible but sometimes to counteract it.

4-16

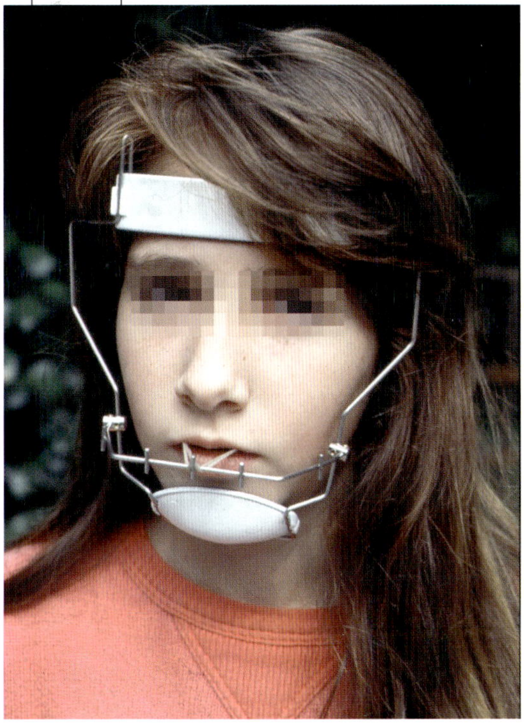

Fig. 4-16
Protraction mask

CASE NUMBER 3

In this case, the great dental-skeletal and facial-aesthetic improvement that can be obtained with anteroposterior traction is evident. The treatment turned the patient from an ugly duckling into a young swan. In my opinion, without the treatment it would have evolved into a surgical case. *Indeed, how many cases labelled as "surgical" just did not receive good orthodontic treatment at the right time?*

4-17

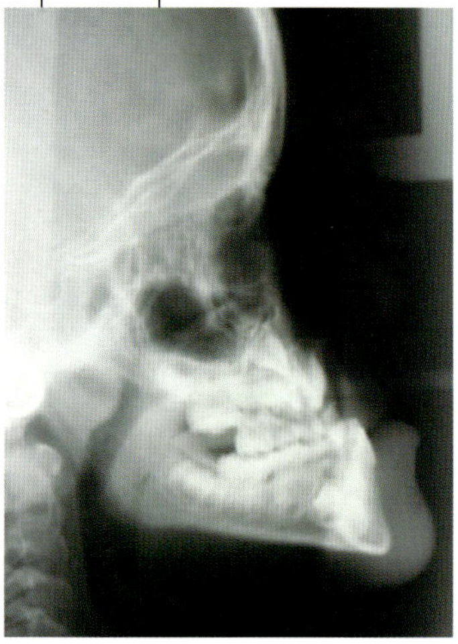

4-18

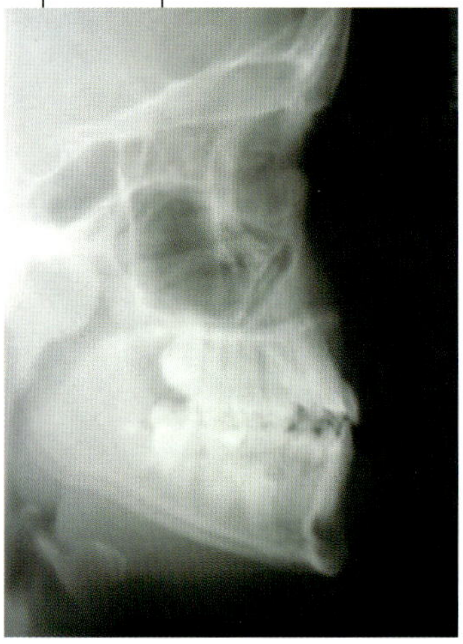

Fig. 4-17 Pre-treatment lateral cephalogram.

Fig. 4-18 Post-treatment lateral cephalogram.

4-19

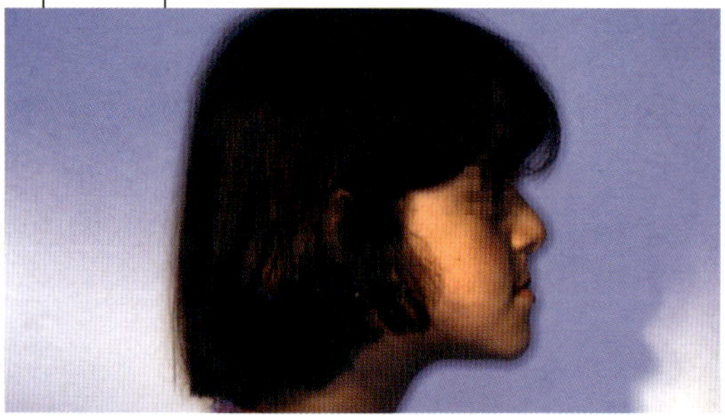

4-20

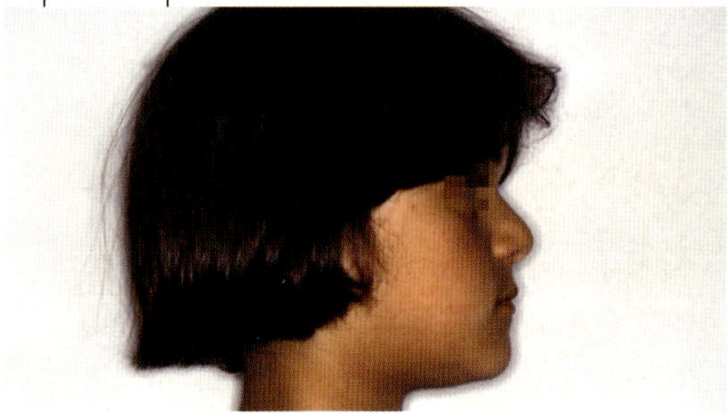

Fig. 4-19 Pre-treatment profile.

Fig. 4-20 Post-treatment profile.

CASE NUMBER 4

Even if the ANB angle is slightly negative, don't be fooled, from the skeletal point of view it is an important Class III. The angle is only -1.5° because point N is back positioned. This is due to the fact that in a well-proportioned male or female 12 year old patient, SN

4-21

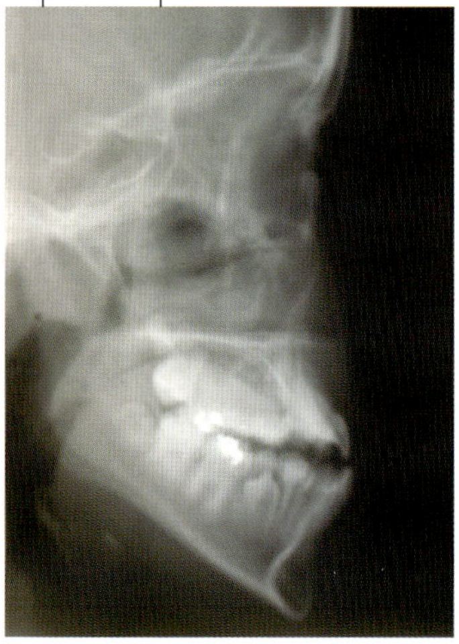

4-22

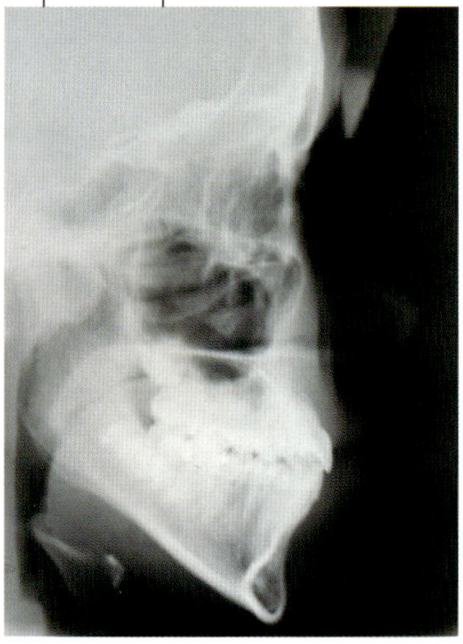

Fig. 4-21 Pretreatment lateral cephalogram (SNA : 83° SNB : 84° ANB : -1°)

Fig. 4-22 Posttreatment lateral cephalogram (SNA : 85° SNB : 83° ANB : + 2°)

4-23

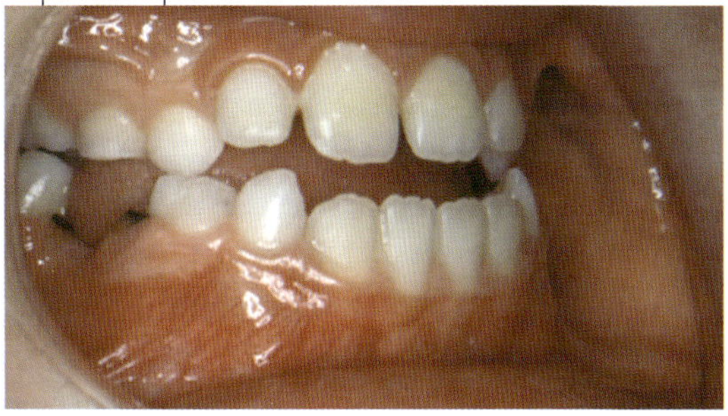

4-24

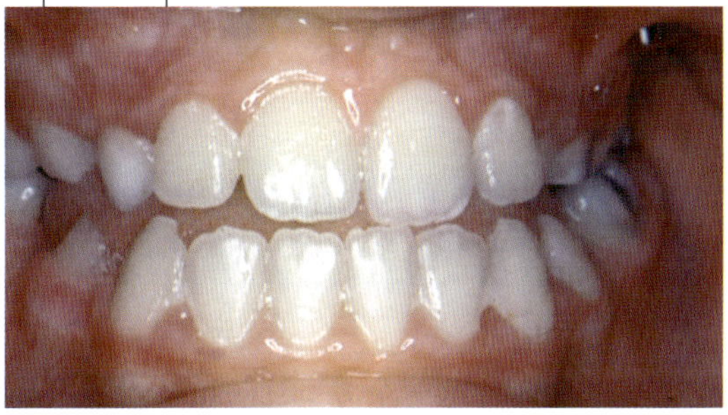

4-25

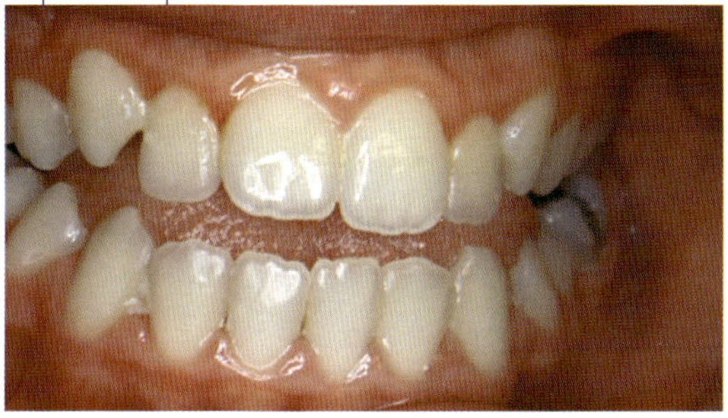

4-26

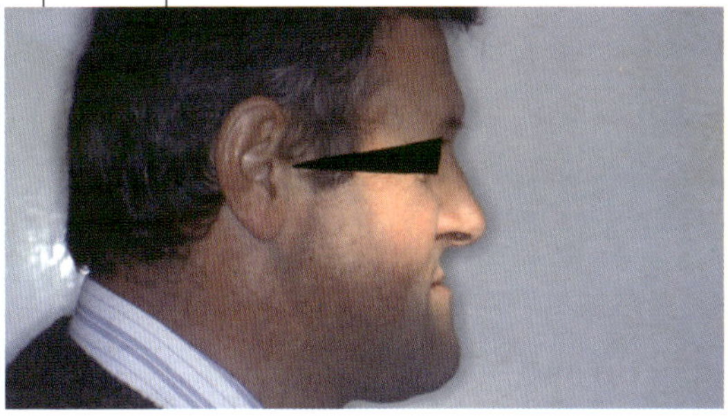

4-27

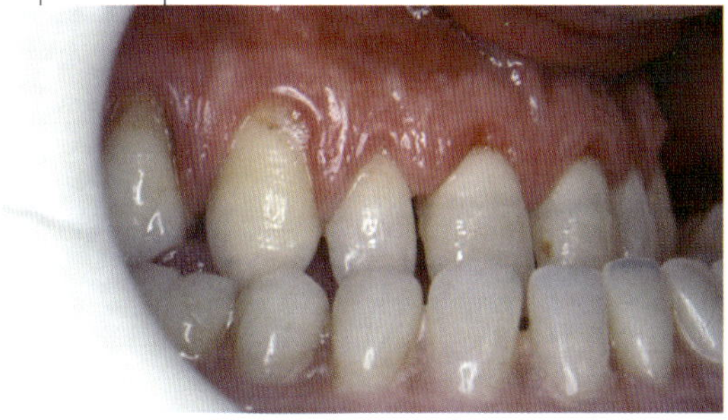

4-28

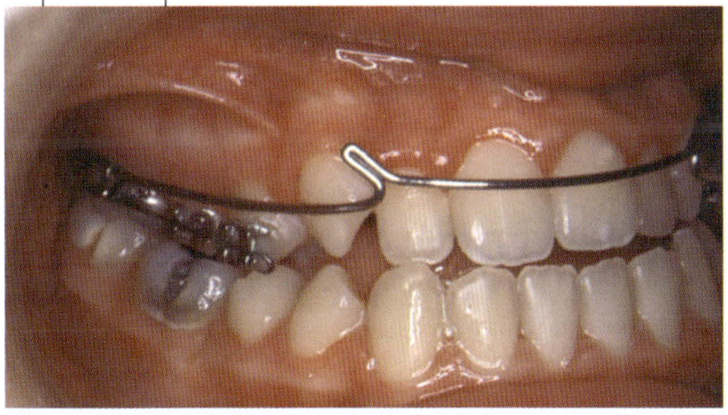

4-29

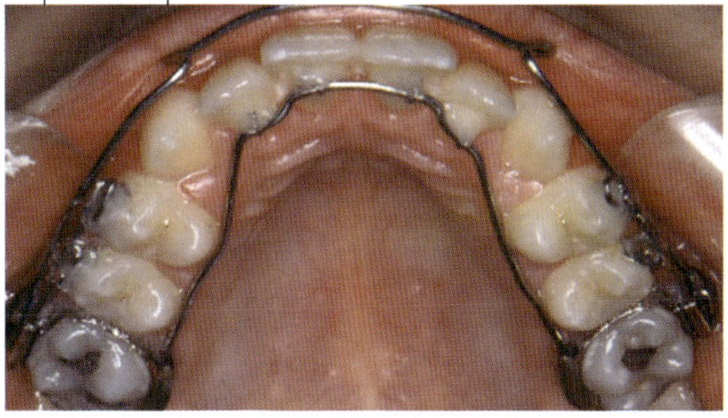

4-30

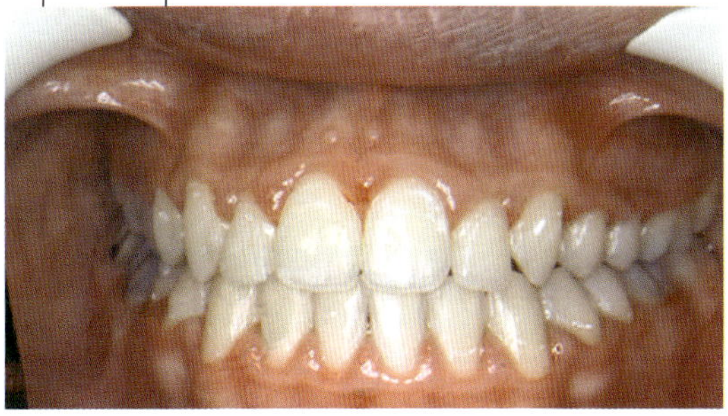

4-31

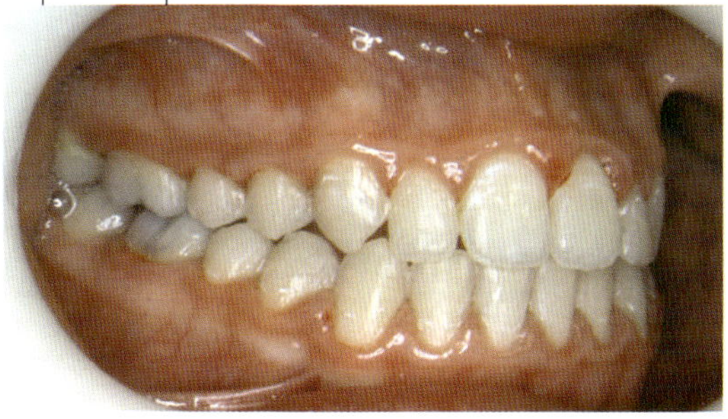

Fig. 4-23 to 4-31
Explanation overleaf

has the same measurement as GoMe.[130] In this case, SN is 65 mm and GoMe is 73 mm (we therefore have an 8 mm difference). If we imagine to push point N 8 mm forward with an harmonic relationship between the anterior cranial base and mandible, the ANB angle would be -4°.

Do not forget to keep all the data in mind. An early treatment does not always mean major stability, especially if there is not a good occlusion and, worse, if the patient has bad habits.

Fig. 4-23 shows the case at the beginning. There is a Class III dental relationship and an anterior open bite due to lower tongue posture. Fig. 4-24 shows the improvement obtained after 16 months of treatment with functional appliances and a chin cup: closure of the anterior open bite and edge-to-edge incisor contact. At which point the parents interrupted the treatment.

They came back to the office 12 months later when an almost total relapse was evident. (Fig. 4-25.) They are convinced that now in order to avoid surgery – which would be necessary to correct her father's problem (Figs. 4-26 & 4-27) – the girl must undergo an active treatment and be regularly checked until the end of her growth.

In order to obtain a better dento-skeletal relationship, a protraction facemask with an intra-oral double arch was applied, as suggested by Verdon. In this case the original prescription was modified by fixing the lingual arch to the incisors with composite. (However, it was not very helpful in my opinion.) There are also two lateral sectionals to close the lateral open bite (Figs. 4-28 & 4-29). The post-treatment occlusion is shown in Figs. 4-30 and 4-31.

CASE NUMBER 5

It is true that a Class III dolico is more difficult to treat, but it is also true that we cannot deny the possibility of a good result occurring. Case number 5 is such an example.

A protraction facemask as indicated by Verdon (an intra-oral double arch with SPEE-like curve combined with an elastic pull pointing down) has been applied. To combat the over crowding teeth, the first upper and the second lower premolars have been extracted.

Twelve months of treatment with a fixed appliance followed.

Figs. 4-32 to 4-34 Lateral cephalograms 1985 / 1988 / 1992 with angular values.

	1985	1988	1992
SNA	78º	78.5º	79º
SNB	81º	79º	78º
ANB	-3º	-0.5º	+1º

4-32

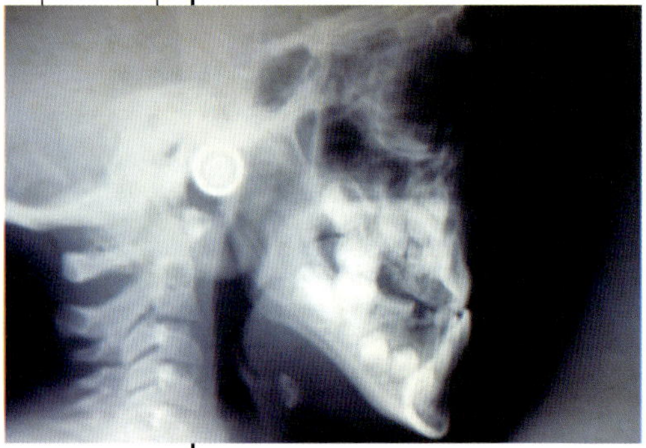

4-33

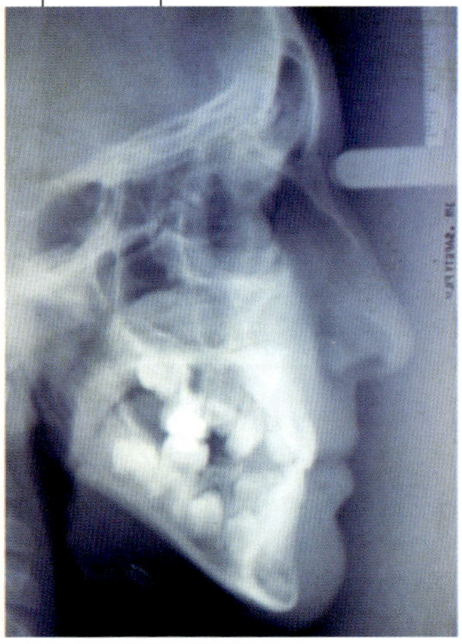

4-34

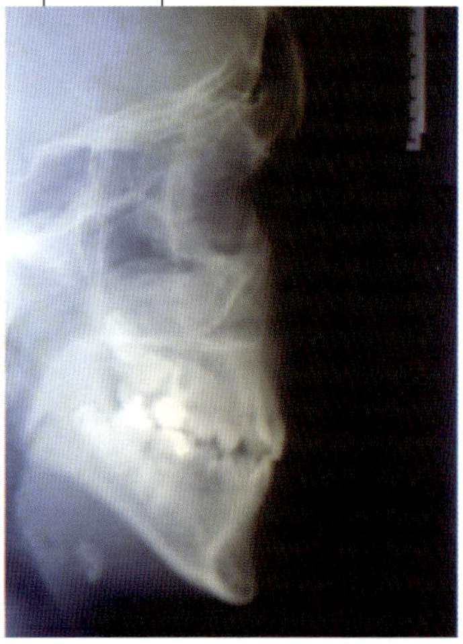

4-35

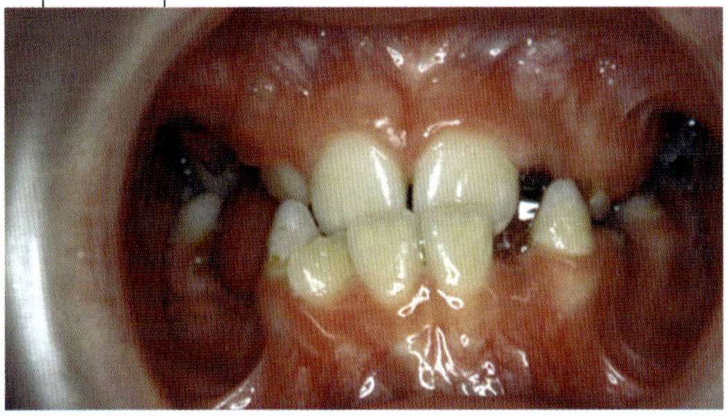

4-36

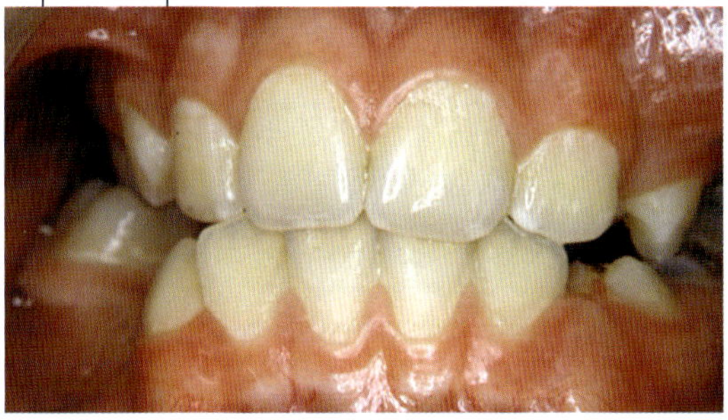

Fig. 4-35
Pre-treatment occlusion.

Fig. 4-36
After wearing a protraction facemask.

4-37

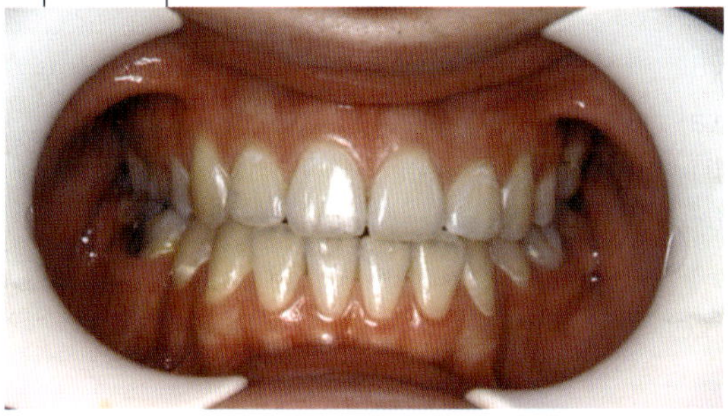

4-38

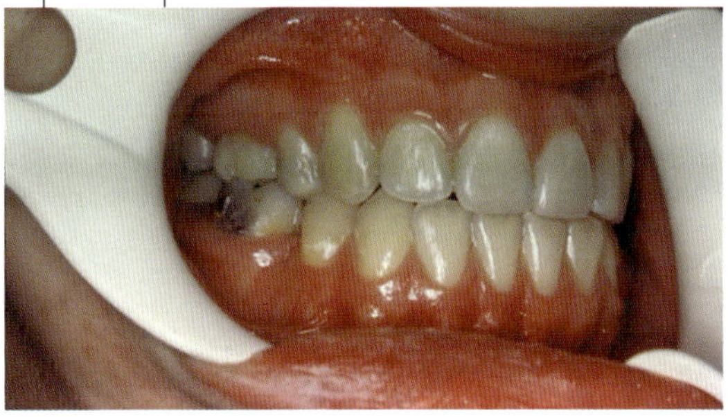

4-39

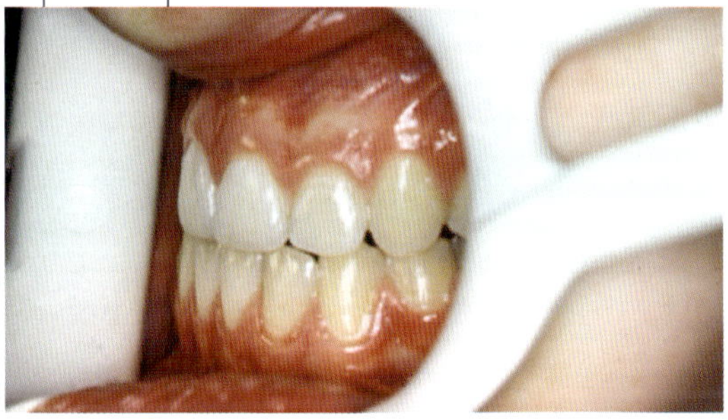

Figs. 4-37 to 4-39
Final result.

4-40

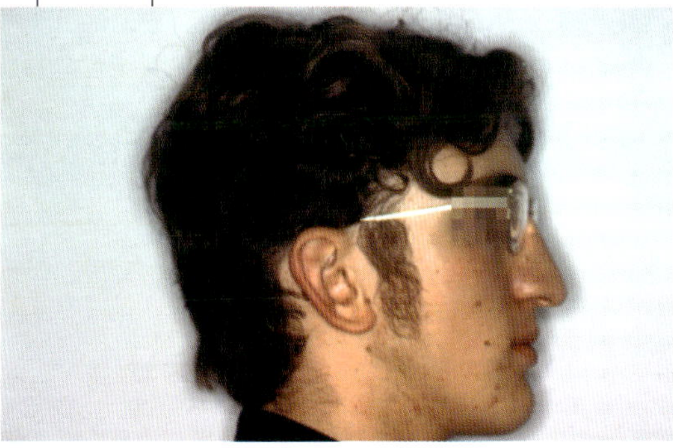

Fig. 4-40
Post-treatment profile.

CASE NUMBER 6

After attending to the vertical and sagittal aspects we must take care of the transverse situation. In this case, the Class III is worsened by the upper right lateral incisor agenesia and by an evident laterodeviation of the mandible which, if not corrected, may evolve from positional to structural with a clear facial asymmetry. In the absence of a lateral cross-bite, correction of the asymmetry is obtained using the anteroposterior traction only.

4-41

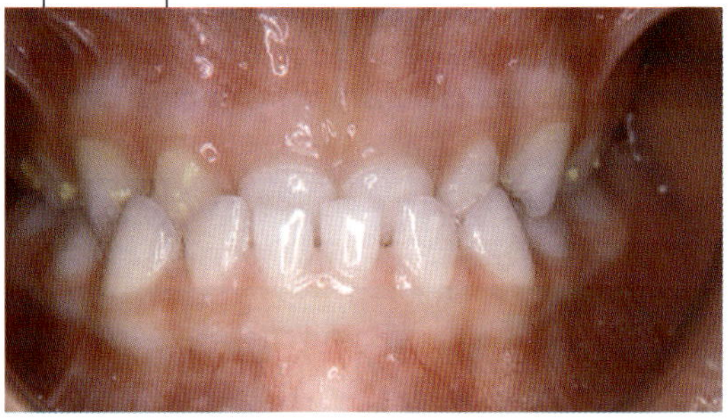

4-42

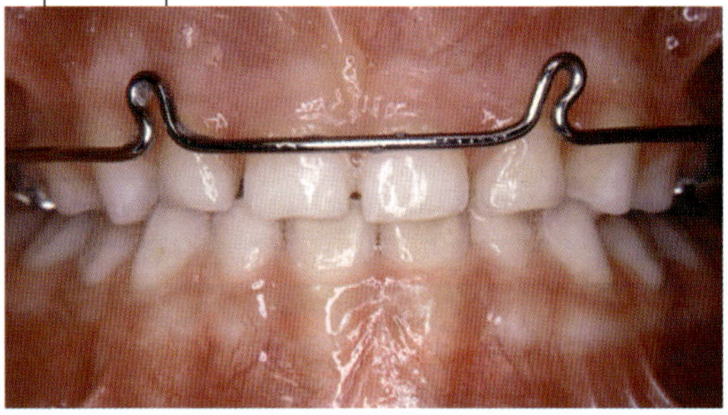

Fig.4- 41
Pre-treatment occlusion.

Fig. 4-42
After protraction mask.

4-43

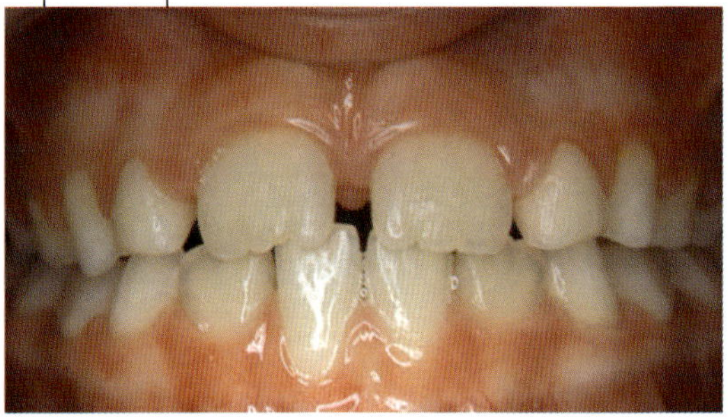

4-44

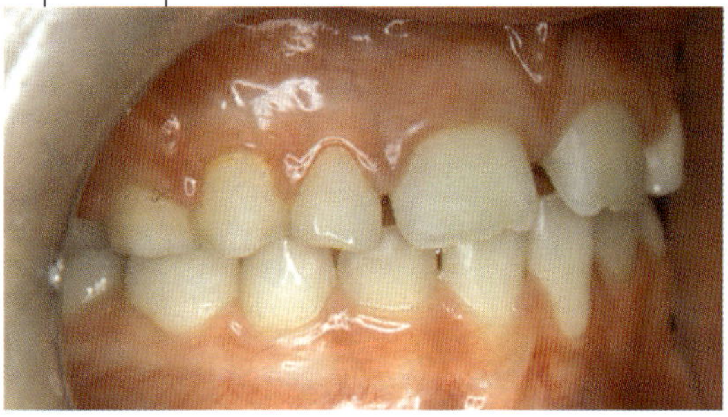

Figs. 4-43 & 44
After protraction mask, later.

4-45

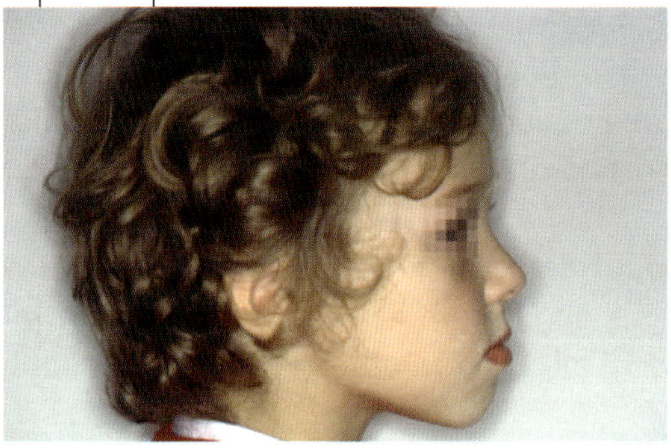

4-46

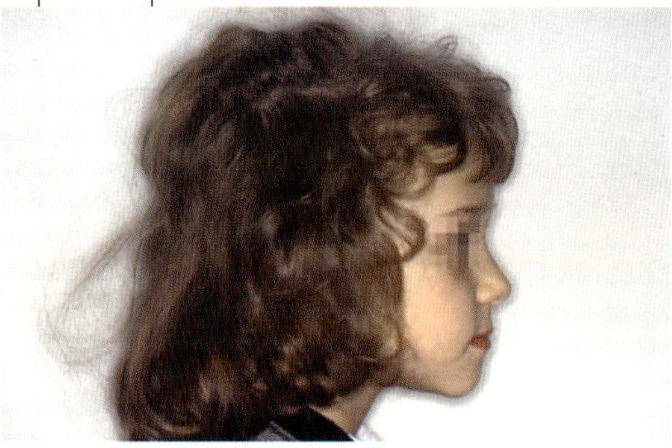

Figs. 4-45 & 46
Patient's profile before and after traction.

4-47

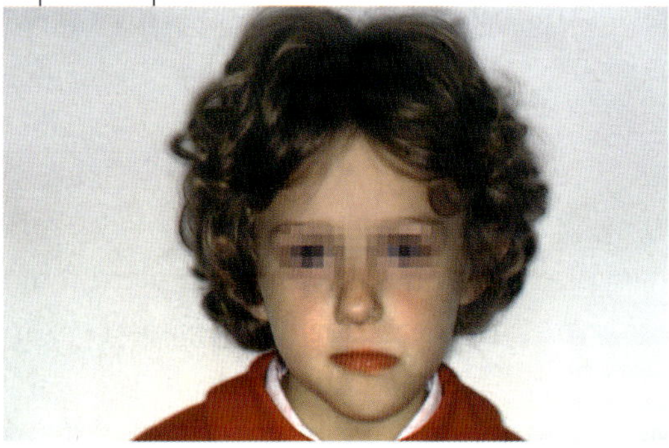

4-48

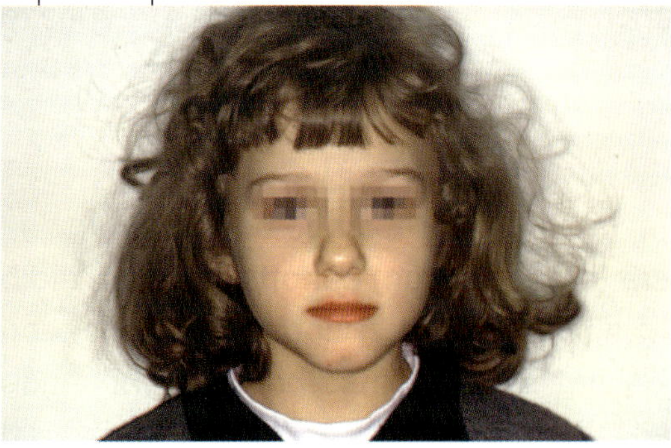

Figs. 4-47 & 48
Frontal view before and after traction.

CASE NUMBER 7

The case is a skeletal Class III dolico with a dental open bite, a laterodeviation of the mandible and a monolateral cross bite in a 15 year old boy.

4-49

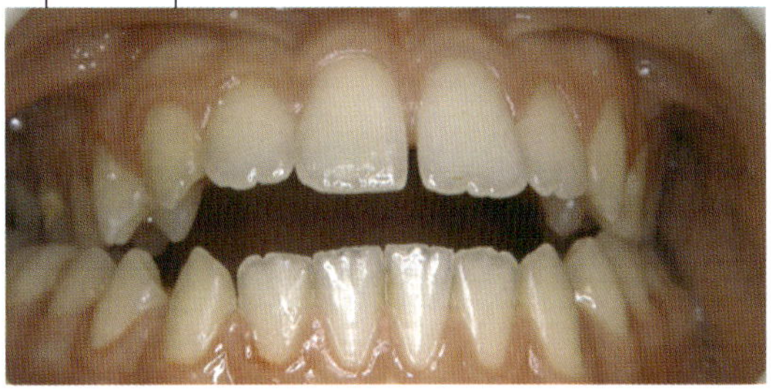

4-50

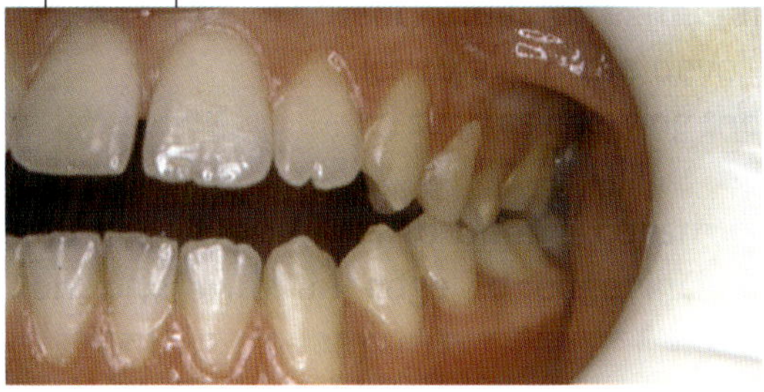

Figs. 4-49 & 4-50
Pre-treatment occlusion.

4-51

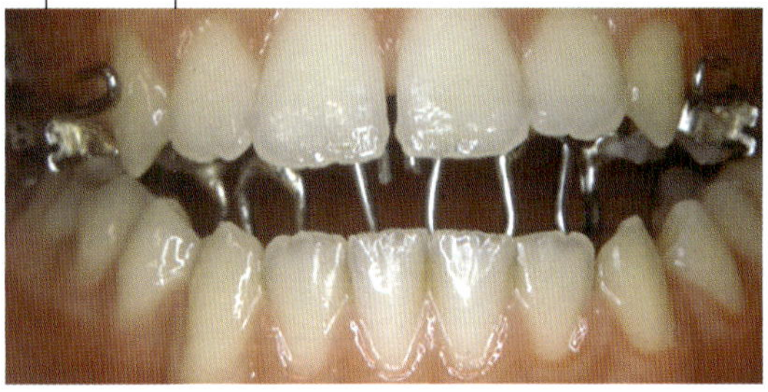

4-52

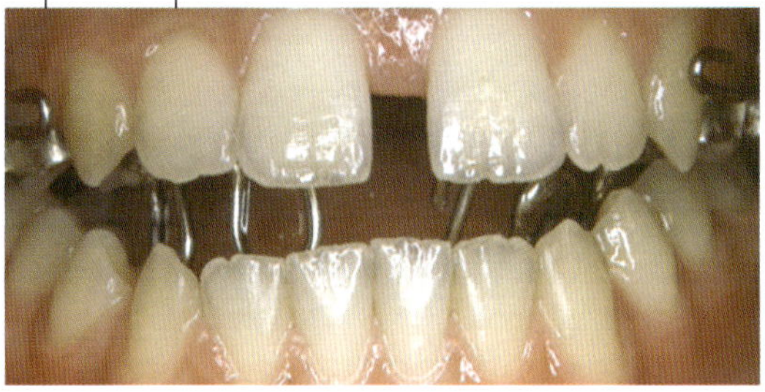

Fig. 4-51
Application of rapid palatal expander with vertical crib. Notice the hooks for the protraction facemask.

Fig. 4-52
With the expansion a central upper incisors diastema appears.

4-53

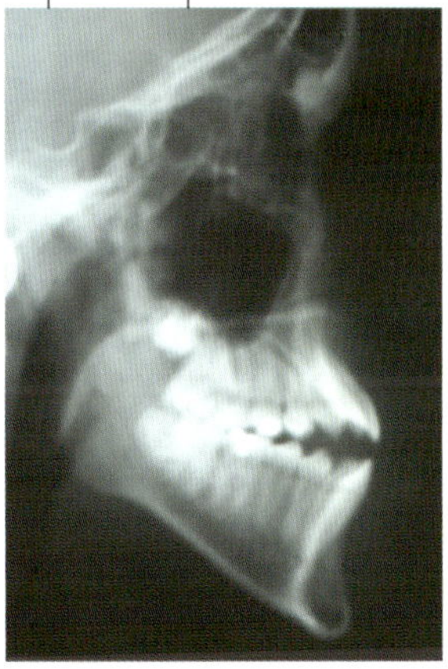

4-54

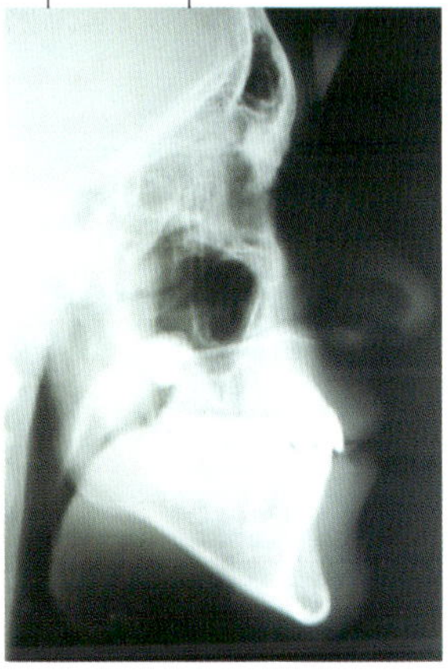

Fig. 4-53
Pre-treatment lateral cephalogram: ANB -1°.

Fig. 4-54
Post-treatment lateral cephalogram: ANB¬ +1.5°.

4-55

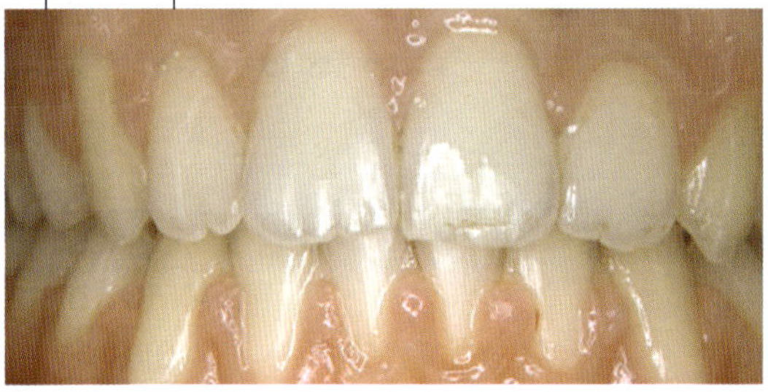

4-56

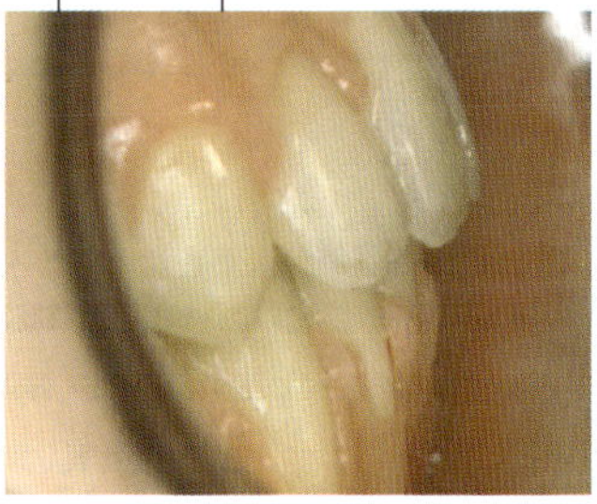

4-57

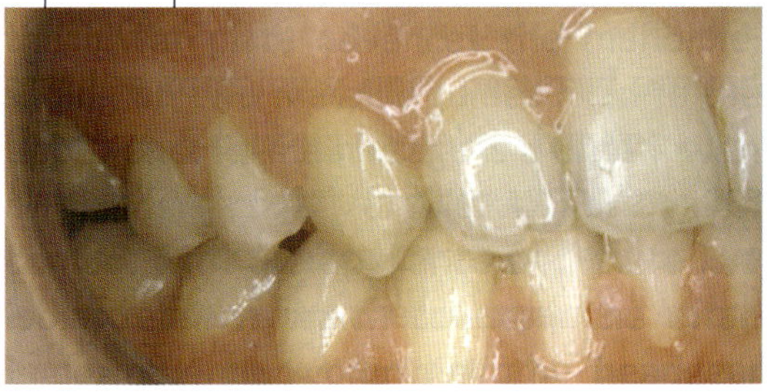

4-58

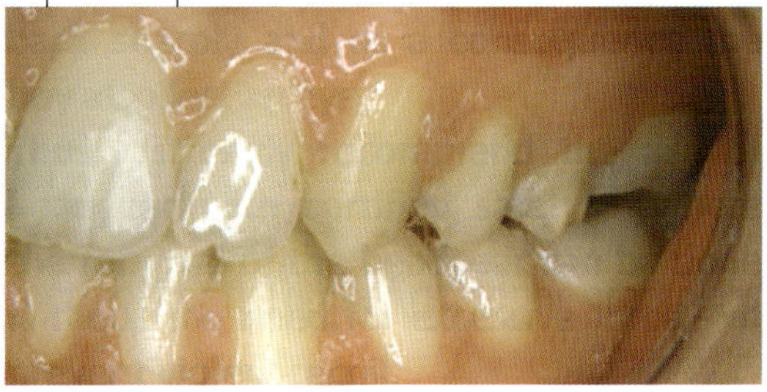

Figs. 4-55 to 4-58
Post-treatment occlusion. After the expansion and the protraction facemask, an orthodontic fixed appliance (straight wire) followed.

AT THE END OF GROWTH

At the end of growth we should think of performing dentoalveolar compensation or surgery without a protraction mask. I say "we should" because there is an expert on orthopedic treatment of Class III, Di Malta[74], who states that it is possible to also obtain good results in adults with maxillary deficiency.

Of course, when it comes to adults, the appliance must be personalised, for example, with a specially made chin cup that has perforations in it at the points of maximum pressure. Theoretically, it could work with a back mandibular rotation, with a sliding of the teeth on the basal bone (just like the sliding of a drawer) and without complete ossification of the sutures.

The limitations of the treatment are not clear. Looking at the cases showed by Di Malta, the amount of anterior discrepancy is no more than 2–3 mm.

Personally I am not sure about Di Malta's positive approach. (I would suggest applying a facial mask from the end of the growth onwards only in well-selected cases accompanied by a detailed informed consent.) The cases presented are interesting but not comparable to more important "surgical" case studies. Di Malta's critics focus on potential TMJ problems, which can lead to pushing back the condyle. To counter the criticism, if there is some articular discomfort Di Malta suggests changing the direction of the pull in order to avoid a distal condylar compression.

CEPHALOMETRIC VALUES IN A "SURGICAL" CLASS III (by Ricketts)

A Cranial deflection angle more than 27°

B Short anterior cranial base

C Distance between porion and PTV less than 39 mm

D Xi Pc/PTV angle less than 15º

E Obtuse condylar – mandibular angle

F Facial angle more than 90°

In a patient with:

- a long mandibular body (more than 65 mm) a long and narrow condyle neck
- concave profile with Class III dental relationship

4-59

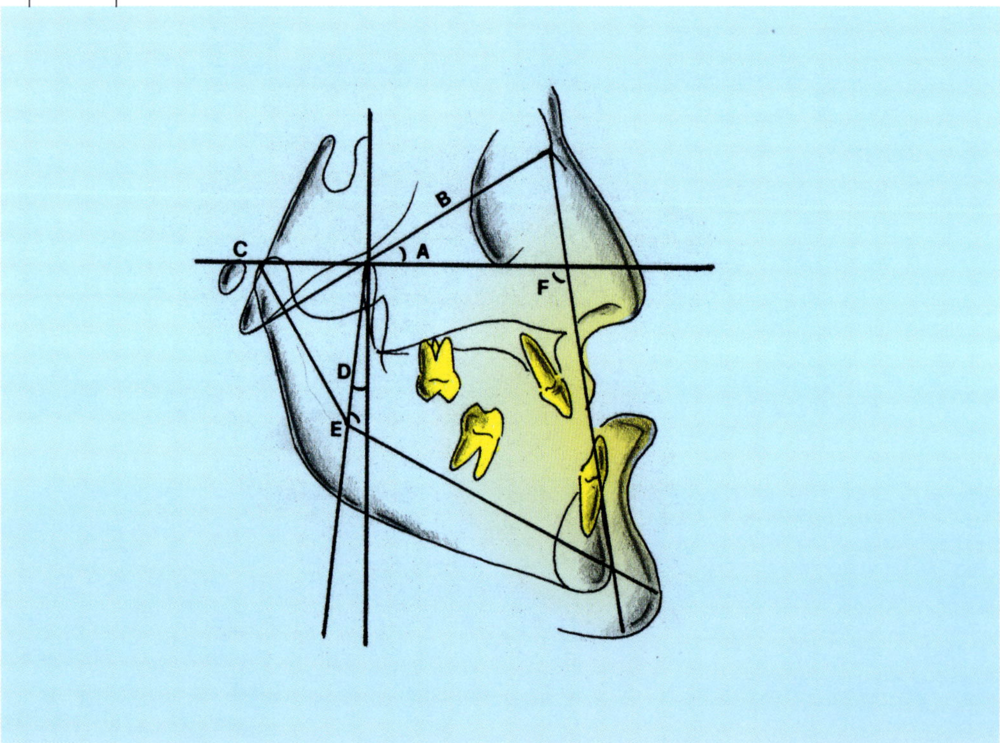

TREATMENT WITH FIXED APPLIANCES

The treatment of a "true" (skeletal) Class III with fixed appliances is limited to minor discrepancies. (For the pre-surgical preparation of the occlusal arches see Chapter 7.)

With orthodontic treatment we basically obtain a dentoalveolar compensation of the bone discrepancy in a similar but inverted way to that of a Class II after the growth (fig. 4-60).

Depending on the overcrowding situation we can make no extractions, four extractions (classically two upper and two lower premolars), two lower extractions (first premolar) or only one (lower incisor).

Most orthodontics' prescriptions increase a positive torque on the upper frontal teeth and a negative one on the correspondent lower frontals, with or without the use of Class III elastics.

For correction of the anterior cross-bite some space distally in the mandible is needed.

We extract the first lower premolars in order to move the canines distally and gain space to put lingually the lower incisors.

The following can be useful for the treatment:

- facemask protraction
- Class III elastics to reinforce the anchorage distally or to move back the frontal lower teeth
- lip bumper (distal anchorage)
- lingual arch (distal anchorage).

In any case, beware of TMJ! As a matter of fact, very often the condyle can be pushed distally (see the chapter on ortho-TMJ).

Some orthodontists suggest moving point A forward in order to apply a reverse torque on the maxillary arch. In my opinion, pushing the roots of upper incisors against the cortical bone can cause root resorption or bone damage (dehiscences and fenestrations). I do not see any advantage to this practice. We cannot expect a significant facial change and the smile is not necessarily better. Indeed, there are many cases where the upper incisors are slightly protruded and look very pleasant.

DISCUSSION

Most surgeons criticise functional orthopedic treatments by stating that they are unsuccessful on young patients and sooner or later, in order to obtain a good result,

4-60

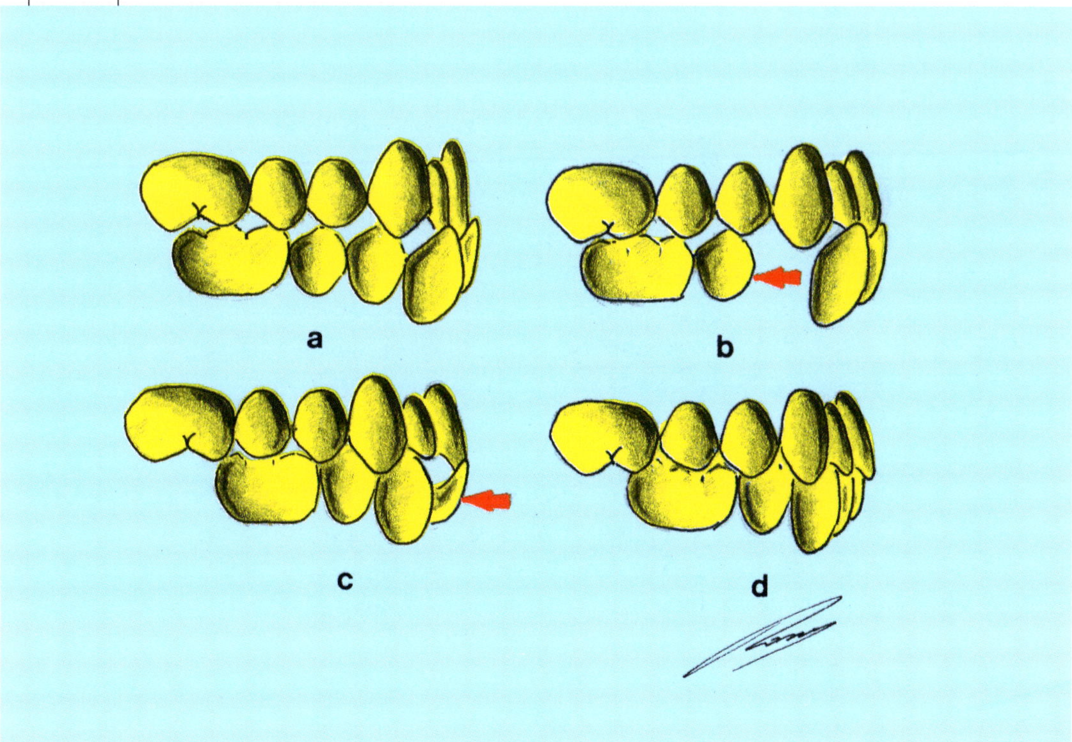

patients have to undergo surgery. This particularly relates to the Class III dolico and where mandibular cases are genetically determined. Any dental compensation must be eliminated before surgery.

Others believe that maxillary deficiency can always be controlled by the consequent prognathism, while it is impossible to recognize in advance a pure mandibular Class III.

It is also impossible to predict the amount of mandibular growth, so even when we are supposedly dealing with a pure mandibular Class III, we cannot exclude the possibility that a maxillary advancement can positively influence mandible growth.

Some say that treatment performed at a young age reduces at least the jaw discrepancy, improves the facial aesthetic of the patient and offers psychological benefits during growth.

Then there are those who believe that a reduction of the bone discrepancy is always useful even if followed by surgery. In those cases the surgery will be more easily performed and provide more stability. Surgeons, however, do not agree with that.

CONCLUSIONS

Orthodontists are worried about Class III for rational and irrational reasons. On the basis of what was written until now, it is irrational to think that young patients (4–5 years old) cannot avoid surgical treatment at the end of their growth.

It is rational to worry about the unpredictability of the amount of a mandibular increase, especially in male patients who continue to grow up to 18 or19 years. How is it possible to control growth for a long time? How is it possible to obtain the patient's cooperation for so many years? It is also understandable to be concerned about the genetically-based hypermandible and the Class III dolico that are more difficult to treat.

Clinically, during growth there is a prevalence of functional orthopedic treatments ending in failure and thus requiring surgery, but not everybody agrees. As a result, the patient is often "stuck in the middle", having to decide between the surgical and non-surgical approach. There are surgeons who ridicule the dentoskeletal compensation and the protraction mask at the end of growth, while there are orthodontists who discourage surgery. Unfortunately I have got the impression that very often the advice given is not exactly in the patient's best interest.

In order to avoid those situations I think it is absolutely necessary to obtain consent from the patient. That is why a good doctor should inform patients or the parents of underage patients about all the treatment possibilities and their indications, contraindications, limits and side effects, pointing out what is certain and what is uncertain, so that everybody can decide for themselves.

Those orthodontists who, at the end of growth, propose an orthodontic treatment or a protraction mask while failing to suggest or ridiculing surgery are not honest in my opinion. The same applies to those surgeons who deny or ridicule an orthopedic treatment, instead suggesting surgery at the end of growth. Remember that it is extremely rare but there is also the possibility of surgical mortality, and the patient must be informed of it.

Orthodontics in Clinical Practice

Chapter V:
Issues Common to the Three Classes

SERIAL EXTRACTIONS[72]

In selected cases, particularly Class Is with crowding, the extraction of permanent teeth at the right moment can offer an easy and stable solution. Usually the extraction of the first premolars as soon as they erupt is followed by a subsequent alignment of the other teeth. If an orthodontic treatment with fixed appliances is used, the realignment is easy and fast.

It may be that after the extractions the occlusion is very good and consequently the patient and his relatives refuse to opt for the finishing touch achieved with a brace (case number 1).

In order to avoid this, Dale[60] suggests removing the teeth after pre-payment of the full orthodontic program (including the cost of the braces).

In a maxillary Class II division 1, the extraction of the upper first premolars can improve the anterior dental protrusion.

It is important to remember that:

A) There is a normal sequence of permanent teeth eruption (Figs. 5-1 & 5-2).

B) When a deciduous tooth is extracted too early, a delay in the eruption of the correspondent permanent tooth may follow. So, do not extract premolars or canines until their root is at least ½ of the final length.

C) A tooth erupts when the root is ¾ of the final length.

D) The canine root takes 2½ years to increase its length from ¼ to ½. It takes 1 year to go from ½ to ¾ in length.

E) The first premolar root takes 1 year and 9 months to increase its length from ¼ to ½.

   It takes 1½ years to go from ½ to ¾.

With a serial extraction plan, the first premolars are extracted as soon as they erupt. Usually the eruptive sequence in the maxillary is favourable, while in the mandible it needs to be guided with the extraction of the first deciduous molars. In this way the first permanent premolars can erupt before the canines.

USUAL SEQUENCE OF ERUPTION OF PERMANENT TEETH

MAXILLARY	MANDIBLE
first molar	first molar
central incisors	central incisors
lateral incisors	lateral incisors
first premolar	canine
second premolar	first premolar
canine	second premolar
second molar	second molar

5-1

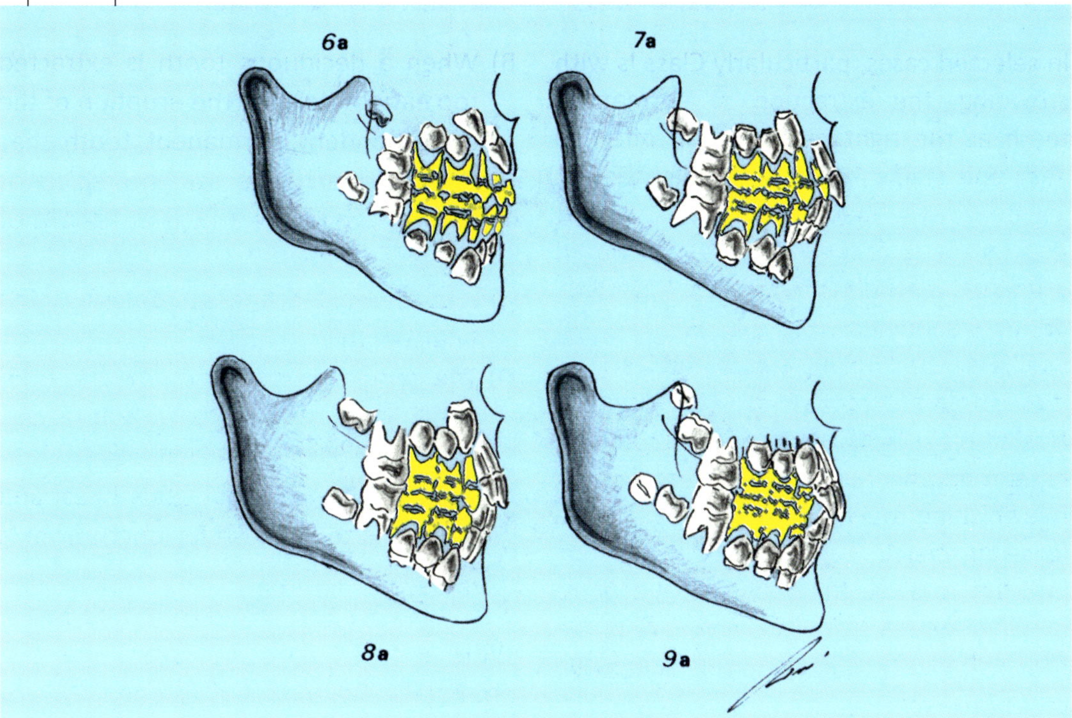

5-2

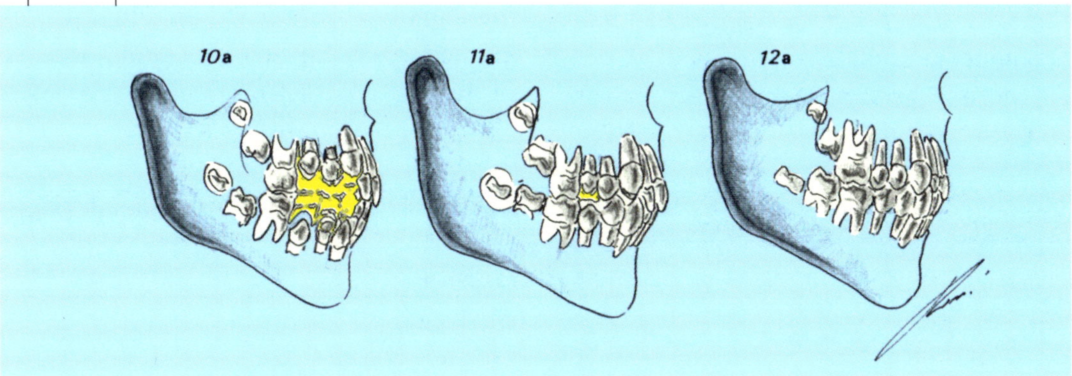

Fig. 5-1 & 5-2
Permanent teeth eruption

Fig. 5-1
Age: 6–7–8–9

Fig. 5-2
Age: 10–11–12.

CASE NUMBER 1

The case features a Class I with an anterior dentoalveolar open bite and protrusion (Fig. 5-9). After the open bite correction another orthodontist applied a palatal bar (upper) and a lip bumper (lower) (Figs. 5-3 & 5-6). At this point the patient came to my office.

If you look at the dental casts the lack of space for canine eruption is evident.

I explained to the patient and his relatives the possible treatments and they agreed on an extraction program. The first premolars were extracted with a delay of a few months compared to a more usual, slower serial extraction program, but the evolution and the results are the same. Note the final occlusion is obtained **without** braces (Figs. 5-7 & 5-8).

5-3

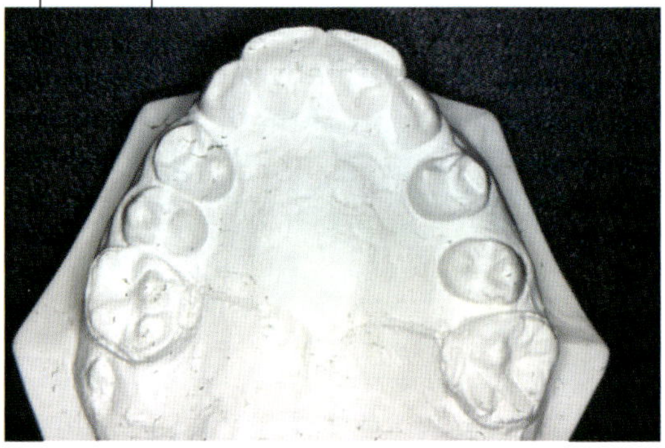

5-4

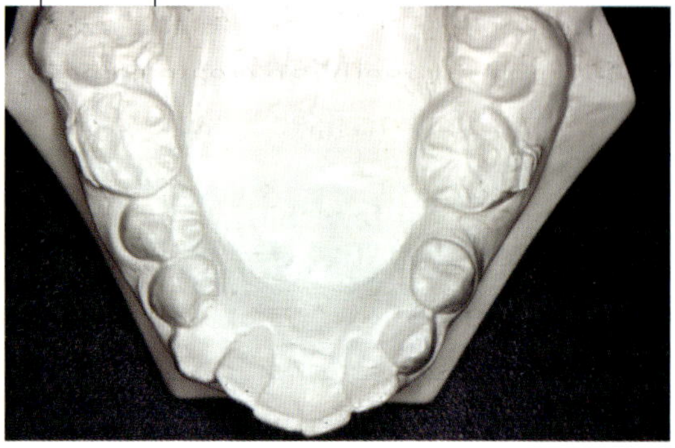

5-5

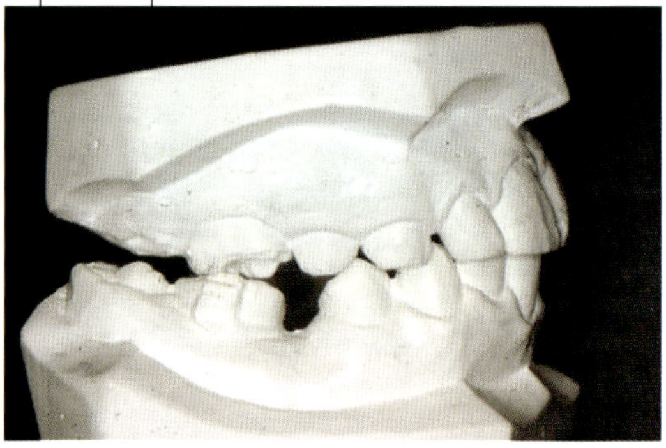

5-6

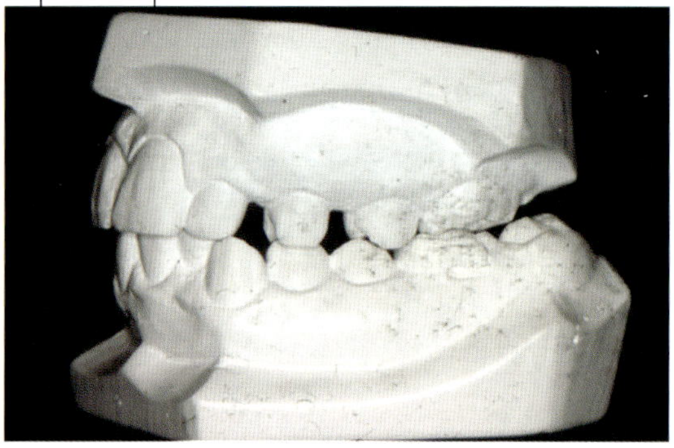

Figs. 5-3 to 5-6
Dental casts. The lack of space for teeth eruption is evident.

5-7

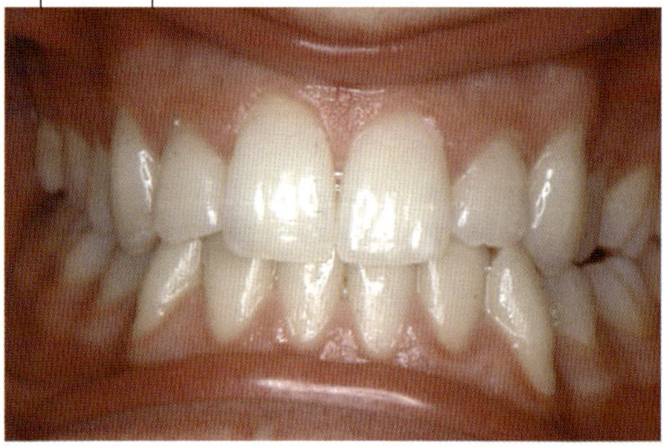

5-8

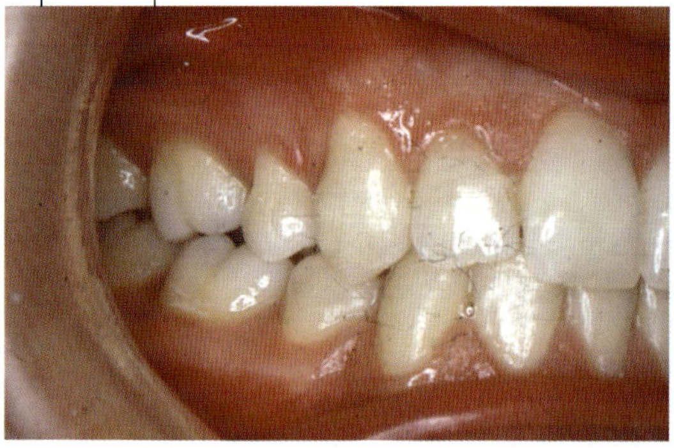

Figs. 5-7 & 5-8
Final occlusion. No braces have been applied.

5-9

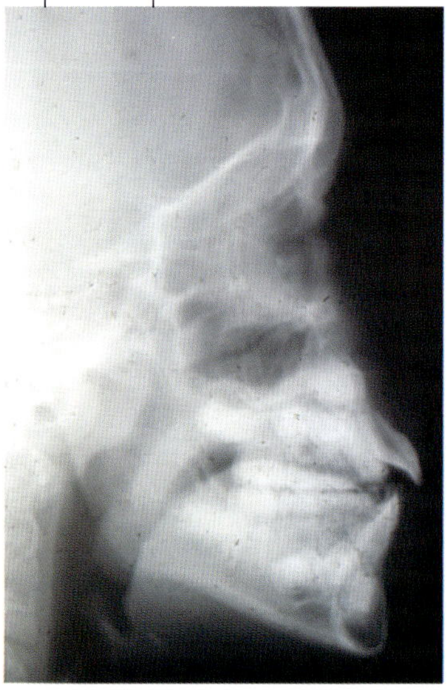

5-10

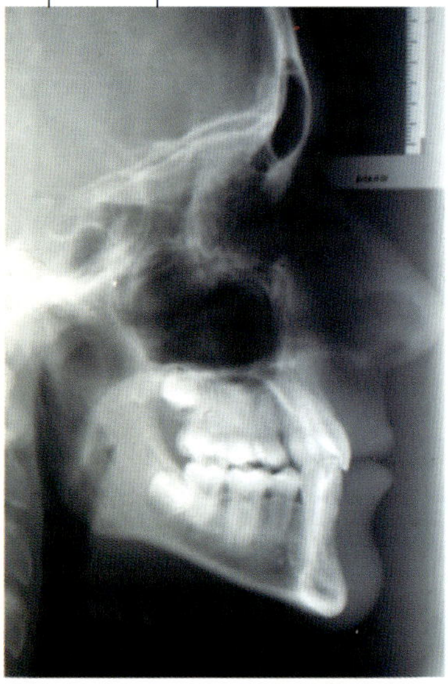

Fig. 5-9
Pre-treatment lateral cephalogram. The alveolodental biprotrusion is evident.

Fig. 5-10
Post-treatment lateral cephalogram. A harmonious result.

DENTAL ANOMALIES (SUPERNUMERARY AND AGENESIS)

Supernumerary teeth can create some orthodontic problems (see Chapter I, Figs. 1-37 to 45).

There are only a few things to note and treatment usually consists of their extraction.

However, when it comes to tooth agenesis there are numerous aspects to analyse.

Hrdlicka (in Anthropology and Medicine 1927) suggests that 3% of lateral maxillary incisors are missing because of congenital reasons.

According to many studies, missing teeth are (in order of prevalence): third molars, lateral incisors, second maxillary premolars, lower central incisors, first maxillary premolars. The first molars, canines and maxillary central incisors agenesis are rare. Genetics has a primary role, even when the parents are not missing teeth. Tooth agenesis can be isolated or may be part of more complex syndromes. When it comes to treatment, case analysis makes a difference.

In a Class I or Class II dolico the extraction of the deciduous molars could work better as the consequent mesialization of the first permanent molars improves the vertical and the sagittal relationship. When the second premolars are missing, for example in a Class I brachi or mesio, it may be better to keep the deciduous teeth as much as possible as they can last for decades. So, early X-ray screening is important to prevent decays and avoid what happened to one unlucky child (Figs. 5-11 to 5-15).

An interesting treatment is offered by the autotransplantation of teeth. More than a century ago badly positioned canines were extracted and transplanted into a more convenient position. Apfel and Miller in 1950, Fong in 1953, Nordenram in 1963, Agnew in 1966, and Andreasen in 1970 put third molar buds in the site of first/second molar extractions. In 1967 and 1970 Slagsvold and Biercke[229, 230] published interesting works about premolar transplantation.

The ideal time for an autotransplantation is when the root of the tooth is between ½ and ¾ of the final length. Before then there can be a delay in development. Afterwards there is a high risk of root resorption.

The success of an autotransplantation also depends on correct surgical technique using low speed burs and abundant irrigation. Great attention has to be paid to tooth removal in order not to damage the periodontal ligament. Once the element is in the new site, the suture keeps it in place. If the tooth crown is emerging it can be fixed to the adjacent elements with a splint and ground to avoid contact with the antagonistic dental arch.

When a cephalometric analysis and the treatment plan indicate the substitution of missing teeth, prosthesis and implantology can offer solutions. There are cases where the orthodontic closure of spaces is convenient. In some others, like the following one, a mixed treatment is more suitable (Figs. 5-11 to 5-15).

5-11

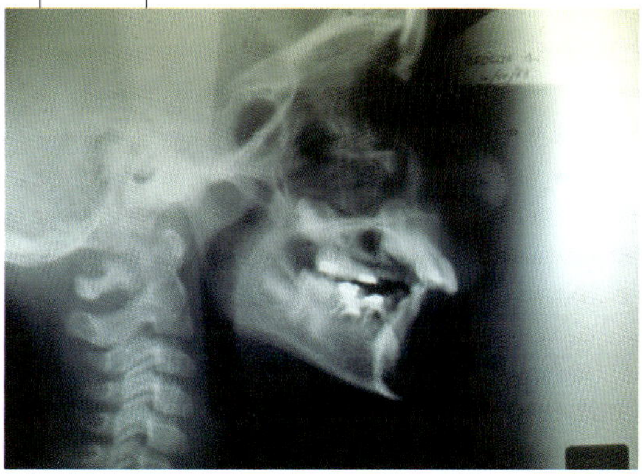

5-12

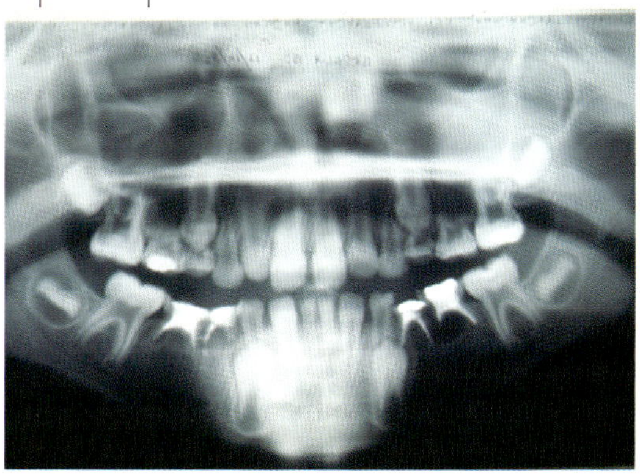

Fig. 5-11 & 5-12 Pre-treatment lateral cephalogram and panoramic radiograph. Class II division 1. Multiple ageneses are evident. They were discovered late when many deciduous teeth were heavily compromised by decay. The endodontic treatments were followed by an increased root resorption causing the premature loss of the teeth involved in a matter of just a few years.

5-14

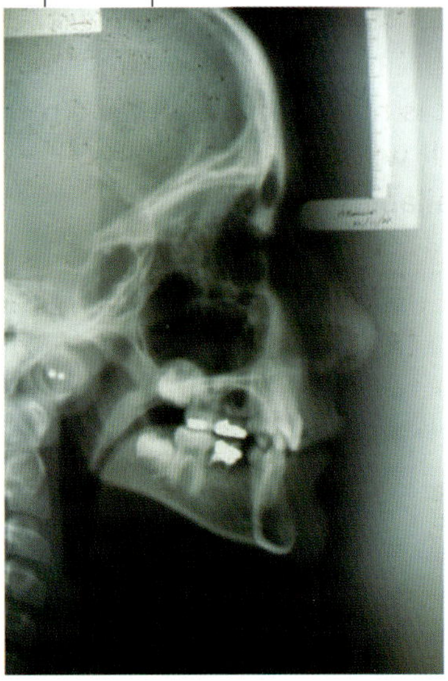

5-13

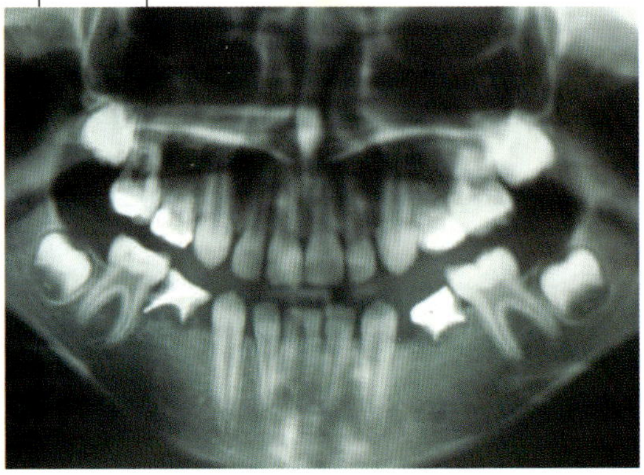

Figs. 5-13 & 5-14
Post-treatment panoramic radiograph and lateral cephalogram.
The orthodontic treatment correcting the excessive overjet closed the space of missing upper first premolars. A removable prosthesis was applied to the lower jaw.

5-15

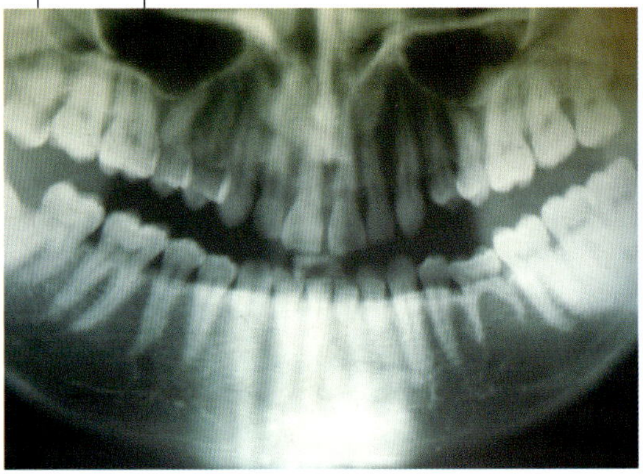

Fig. 5-15
Second lower left premolar congenitally missing in a 36 year old patient. Notice the excellent condition of the deciduous molar. Without the endodontic treatment there can be root resorption with a slower progression. Imagine what different dental future the young patient of figures 11 to 14 could have had if his multiple agenesis had been discovered earlier, thus avoiding all the decay.

PROBLEMS (AND MISTAKES) IN ORTHODONTICS

The list of problems and mistakes in a difficult discipline like orthodontics is very long. I would like to point out those that are, in my opinion, the most important.

The most serious problem that can probably occur is to actually make worse the initial situation (case number 2). This can be done by a wrong diagnosis or by misuse of appliances. A good appliance badly used can lead to negative results, just like a bad appliance.

Performing a treatment at the wrong time can lead to a negative outcome. For example, think of a removable appliance used for an orthopedic purpose: even the best one does not work without the inherent function of growth.

A fundamental principle of physics is that to every action corresponds a reaction, but unfortunately this is ignored far too often. As a consequence it can happen that when we want to move one tooth we move other teeth in an undesirable way. Good anchorage is therefore very important.

What should a relapse be considered as? There are situations where the final occlusion is unstable and a relapse will definitely occur without artificial retention. Is that a problem, a mistake, or both? I personally consider these to be mistakes that become problems.

However, there are also situations where even if the occlusion is good at the end of treatment a retainer must be applied. Such is the case when you have to deal with an unpredictable overcrowding of the lower incisors.

That is one problem. Another problem could be, for example, an upper molar distalization. If the use of headgear in a young patient is normal, it becomes a mistake in an adult when no-compliance alternatives are available.

Root resorption is a phenomenon well-known to all orthodontists.[14, 107, 114, 157] Instances of apical resorptions of 1.5–2.5 mm are common. The type of orthodontic tooth movement, the intensity of the applied forces and the duration of treatment are some of the most studied factors. But resorption still remains a problem with an unclear etiology. We do know that the process of resorption stops when the active treatment is interrupted by fixed appliances. Therefore, before and during treatment it is important to monitor the root conditions with frequent X-rays. If we do not do that, a problem can turn into a mistake (Fig. 5-16).

5-16

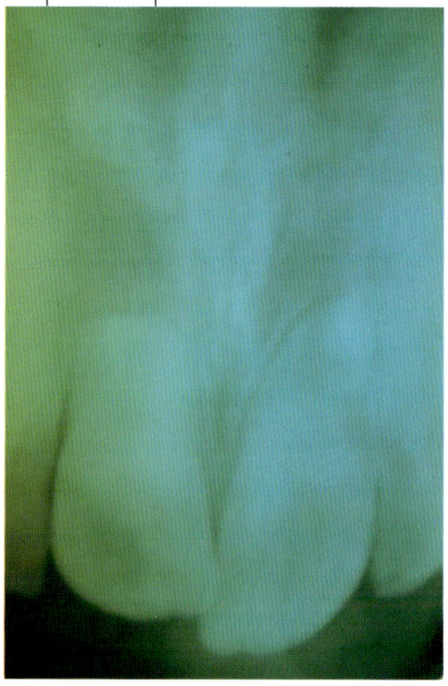

Fig. 5-16
X-ray of upper central incisors after 24 months of treatment with fixed appliances. There was a half root resorption, which was a mistake because it was discovered at the end of treatment. It is true that these teeth can last very long but it is also true that a periodontal disease can have greater consequences than usual.

CASE NUMBER 2

A case starting with a normal vertical relationship suddenly becomes “difficult”. What happened? Diagnostic error? Unexpected growth ? TMJ problems?

5-17

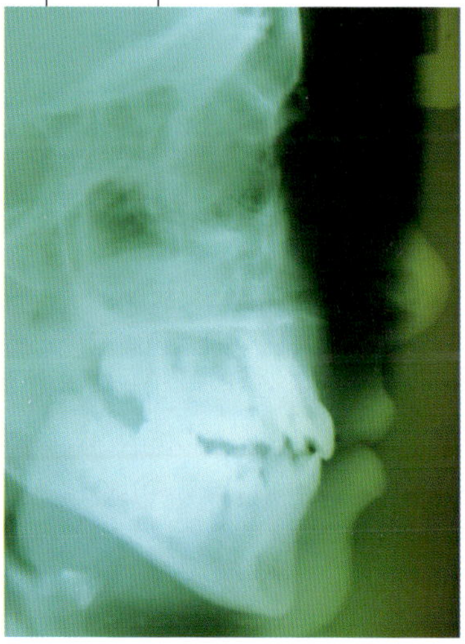

5-18

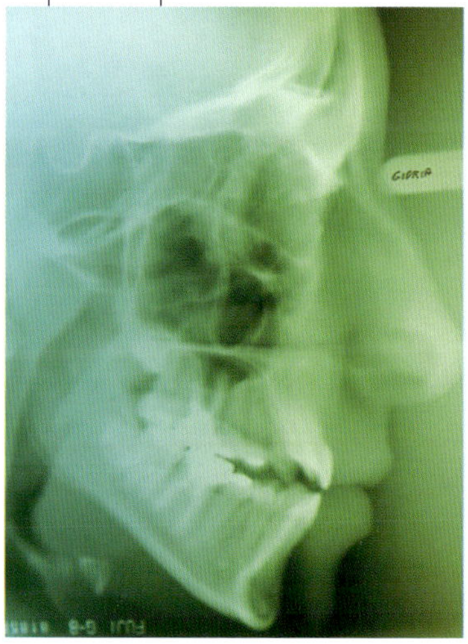

5-19

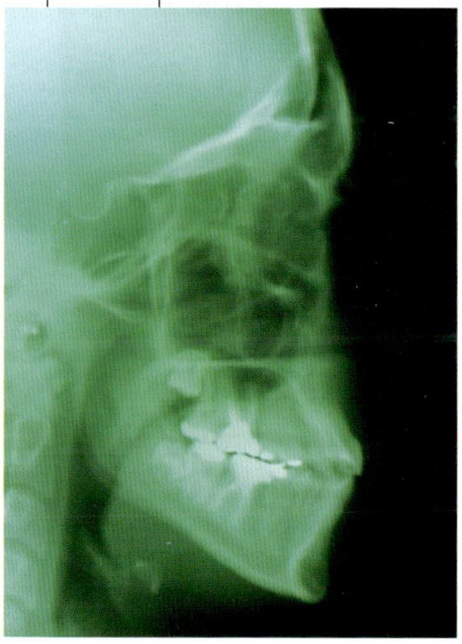

Fig. 5-17
Pre-treatment lateral cephalogram.

Fig. 5-18
Lateral cephalogram after 6 months of treatment with a removable appliance. The patient came to my office worried by the worsening of the situation. An inadequate control of the appliance caused prematurity with the unwanted opening of the bite.

Fig. 5-19
With a fixed appliance and the coordination of dental arches it was possible to correct the occlusion.

5-20

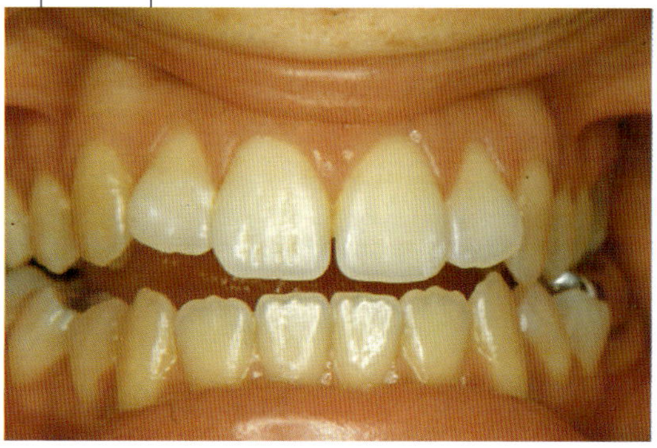

5-21

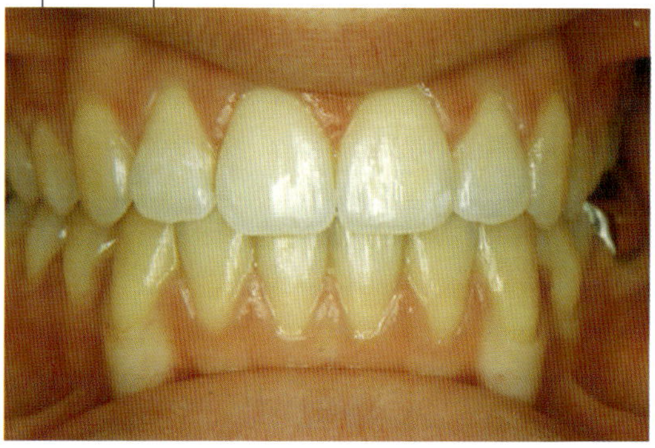

Fig. 5-20
Occlusion after the wrong treatment.

Fig. 5 – 21
Occlusion after the correction with a fixed appliance.

THE VERTICAL DIMENSION

When classifying a malocclusion, many orthodontists place a lot of importance on the sagittal relationship of the jaws. In my opinion they must also make the effort to remember the influence of the vertical dimension on the anteroposterior situation. Wylie (in *Overbite and Vertical Facial Dimension in terms of Muscle Balance, Angle Orthod Jan 1944 Vol 14 no. 1 pp13-17)* suggested a division of the face into two parts, where the upper facial height (N – SNA) corresponds to 45%, while the lower facial height (SNA – Me) corresponds to 55% (see also Chapter I).

5-22

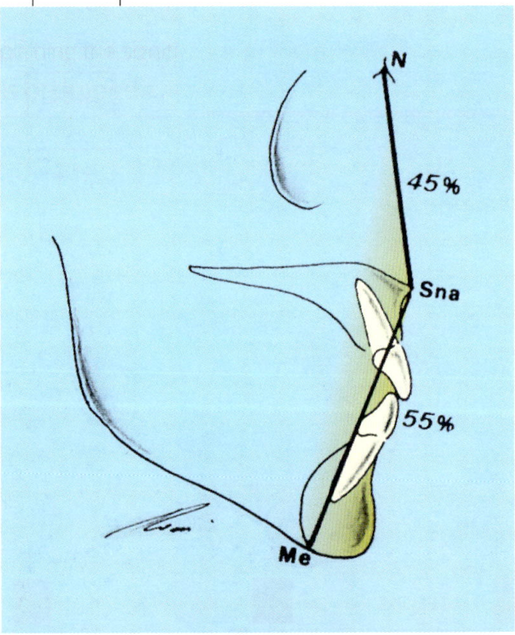

INCREASED VERTICAL DIMENSION

Regarding increased vertical dimension, according to Ricketts we speak of dolico[208] , Sassouni discussed the literal term open bite[219] and Schudy came up with hyperdivergence.[222]

Radiologically, the anterior facial height is increased while the posterior height is decreased.

There is a prevalence of clockwise mandibular growth expressed in Class I and in Class III with an elongated face. In a Class II the extreme case is a "bird face". Facial and masticatory muscles are generally hypotonic. The distinction between the skeletal and dental aspects is very important.

It is true that an anterior dental open bite is usually associated with increased skeletal verticality. However, sometimes a skeletal open bite presents a dental deep bite. This happens when there is dentoalveolar growth which is compensating for the jaw verticality.

Regarding its etiology, Hunter et al.[127] point out that genetics has an important role in skeletal open bites. And in a study of 70 twins, Wahnick[251] concluded that genetics influence the vertical dimension far more than the sagittal one. Also, don't forget that hereditariness includes functional aspects which can influence the relationship between bones and teeth.

PROBLEMATIC ASPECTS OF FUNCTION

Respiratory problems are a major factor when considering the circumstances of open bite. Ricketts[208] describes the "obstructive respiratory syndrome" as characterised by:

- mouth breathing
- anterior dental open bite with increased verticality and mandibular clockwise rotation growth
- posterior cross bite
- tonsil and adenoidal hypertrophy
- tongue thrust during swallowing.

Others (e.g. Harvold[116], Paradise and Bluestone[189] and Gundlach[112]) confirm the influence of obstructive respiratory syndrome in a skeletal open bite malocclusion.

It is very interesting to observe how this syndrome could cause the malocclusion. With mouth breathing there is a low tongue posture which reduces normal stimulation of the transverse palatal expansion provoked by the tongue during swallowing. With a narrow upper dental

arch there is often a cross bite situation and a clockwise mandibular rotation.
A forward tongue posture or a forward swallow explains the dental anterior open bite.
Dental open bites are also caused by oral habits: nail biting, thumb sucking, lip biting...
These habits may be present not only in cases with increased verticality, but even in those with normal or decreased verticality.
The lack of overjet–overbite induces an incorrect articulation of lingual alveolar speech sounds "t", "d", "s" and "z". A skeletal open bite can be worsened by bad functional aspects which cause dentoalveolar malocclusion.

TREATMENT

Why should we treat an open bite? Once more remember the difference between skeletal and dental aspects. An increased verticality per se does not need any treatment and there are many people with a long well-balanced face with a good occlusion.
We try to reduce the jaw verticality in a skeletal Class II. The aim is to control the mandibular advancement following its anticlockwise rotation. For opposite reasons a reduction of maxillary / mandibular verticality in a Class III is usually not indicated as it worsens the sagittal jaw relationship. In Class I verticality reduction can sometimes be useful (usually when bordering on Class II).
When it comes to the dental aspects, compared to skeletal aspects, they are easier to control. Even though for some gnathologists an anterior dental open bite could lead to TMJ disorders, the main indications for treatment are speech problems and dental aesthetics.
Many treatments of skeletal open bites during growth have been described in earlier chapters. All are based on diverse attempts to reduce the maxillary / mandible divergence through vertical control of the molars.....

CLASS II

- High pull tractions.
- Removable appliances.
- Combination of both (see also Chapter III).

CLASS I

- Chin cup with vertical pull.
- Combination of chin cup, vertical pull and positioner.

CLASS I – CLASS II

- Molar extractions.

Even though it may be controversial, I really believe in the validity of the procedure of molar extractions in selected cases (see particularly the following case number 6). The extractions must be done at the right time before the second molar eruption. In this way, the second molars will have a bodily mesial movement and there can be a reduction of the vertical dimension with good stability.
At the end of growth we can reduce the vertical maxillary /mandible relationship above all with surgery. The reduction of excessive verticality is mainly indicated in a skeletal Class II (see the chapter on ortho-surgery. Case n.1 - 3) where the surgical maxillary elevation is followed by the anti clockwise rotation of the mandible. Thus there is also a reduction of sagittal jaw discrepancy with a facial aesthetic improvement.

TREATING THE PROBLEMS OF DISFUNCTION

When it comes to dental matters, we must control any relevant negative circumstances:

- by removing what might disturb physiologic nasal respiration (adenoidectomy, tonsillectomy, etc.)
- by removing habits – theoretically, by training the tongue it is possible to correct an anterior open bite
- by using appliances to prevent the tongue's interpositioning between the dental arches

- by using fixed appliance and elastics to close the vertical spaces
- by using mini screws to intrude posterior teeth
- by performing a partial glossectomy (relevant in Down's syndrome patients).

CONCLUSIONS

In the *AJO* September 2006 edition, the editor David L. Turpin commented:

"I have seen the preferred method of correcting anterior open bite change regularly over the past 40 years. I was initially taught to refer these patients to a speech therapist familiar with the elimination of tongue thrust. Then I learned to obtain more direct results by using a crib with spurs to enforce immediate compliance by the tongue. Of course, fixed appliances with various combinations of vertical elastics were used more often than any orthodontist wanted to admit. Then maxillary surgery to impact the posterior portion of the maxilla achieved success and was thought to be the final answer. With the advent of rigid screw fixation in surgery, it became possible to close open bites with mandibular surgery alone, and this is now seen by many as a good solution. Despite our best intentions with these techniques, long-term stability of open bite closure is no better than 80%. With increasing time out of appliances, too many corrected bites tend to open after retention is stopped."

I agree with Turpin. Open bites are challenging to treat and a relapse after treatment is common. In my personal experience the distinction between skeletal and dental aspects is very important. I consider it to be much more difficult to control and change the vertical jaw relationship than the dental one. It is particularly difficult to obtain a stable result.

When it comes to dental open bites I achieve good results with removable appliances. They allow control of the tongue, increase the transverse palatal expansion in the presence of a cross bite and influence molar eruption. And as mentioned before, I believe that first molar extractions lead to good and stable outcomes. In all cases, orofacial myofunctional therapy improves the reliability of results.

CASE NUMBER 3

The patient is a 16 year old with an anterior dental open bite and a posterior cross bite. Lingual bad habits are evident. A quadhelix with an anterior vertical crib to stop the tongue forward swallow is used.

5-23

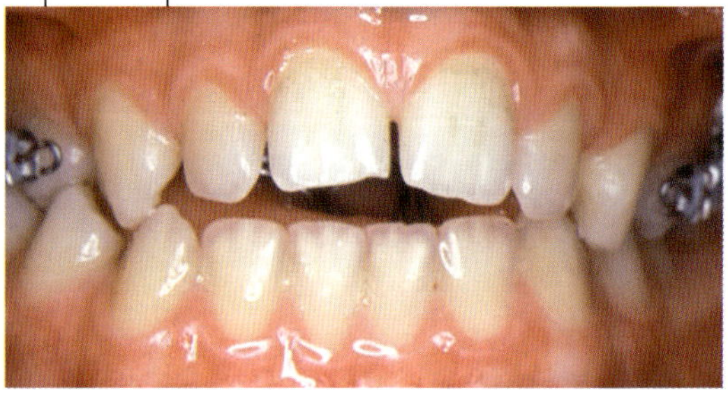

Fig. 5-23
Pre-treatment occlusion. A dentoalveolar open bite is present caused mainly by forward swallow.

5-24

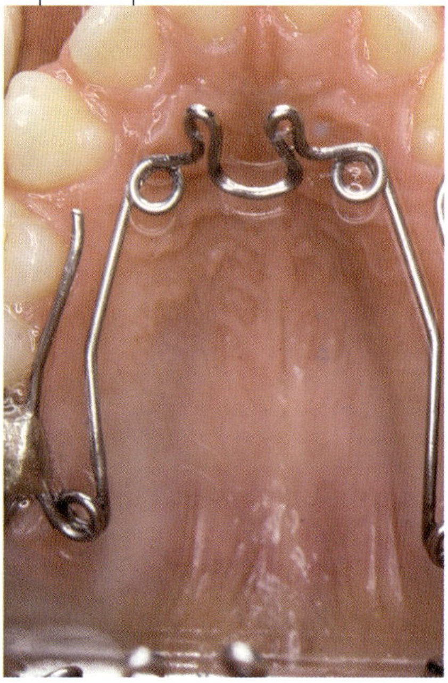

Fig. 5-24
Quadhelix with vertical crib.

5-25

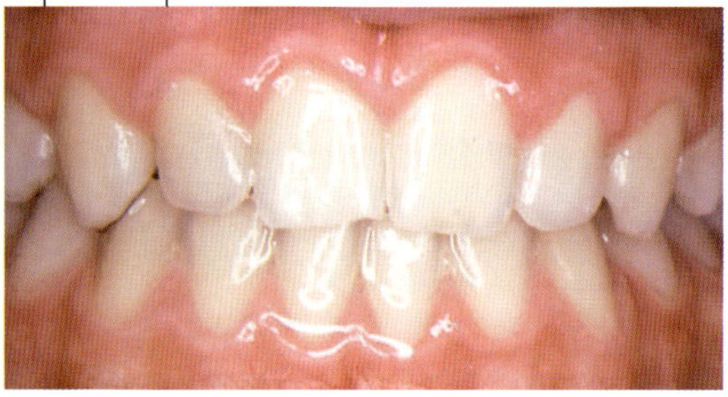

Fig. 5-25
Occlusion 6 months later.

CASE NUMBER 4

Lateral dental open bite cases are not so common. In this case, a palatal bar with vertical shields to stop the tongue was applied. To use vertical elastics, some hooks were bonded to the upper and lower posterior teeth (first molars and deciduous molars).

5-26

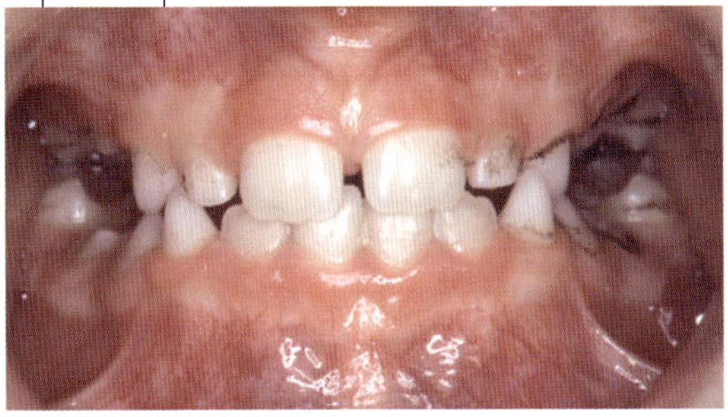

5-27

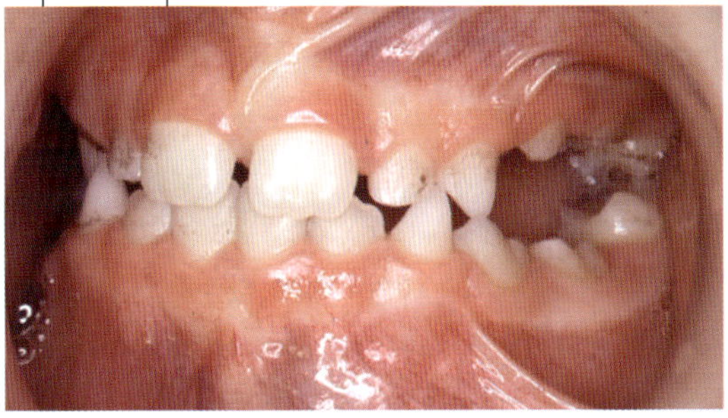

Figs. 5-26 & 5-27
Pre-treatment occlusion. The wide lateral gaps are evident.

5-28

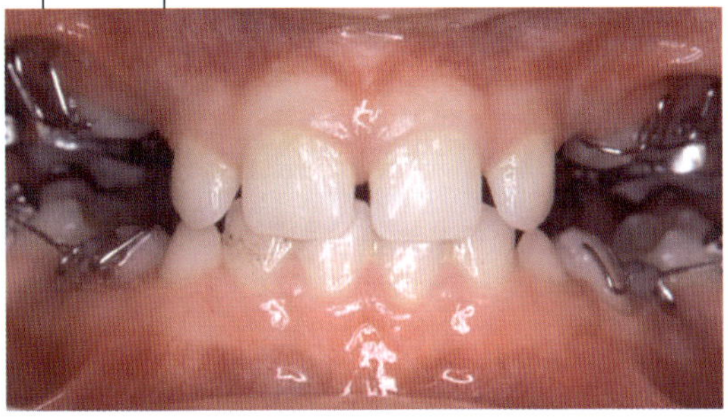

5-29

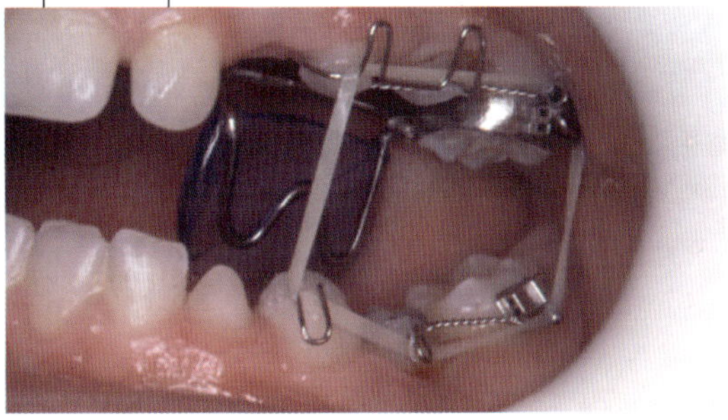

Figs. 5-28 & 5-29
Palatal bar with lingual vertical shields and hooks for vertical elastics.

5-30

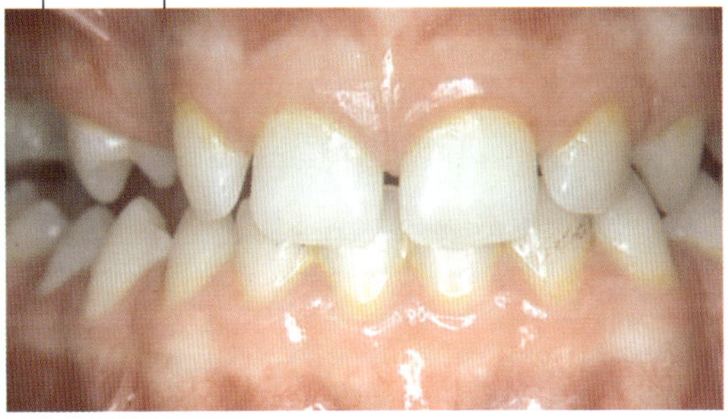

5-31

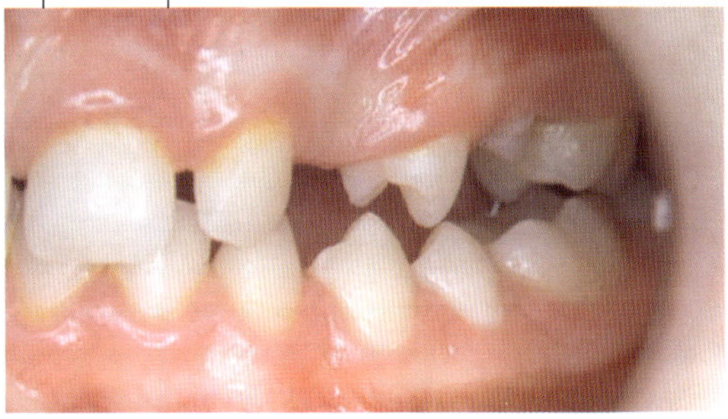

Figs. 5-30 & 5-31
Intermediate stage. Premolars are erupting.

5-32

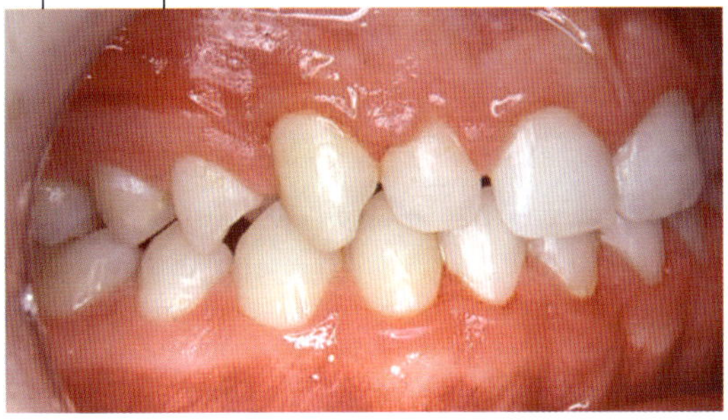

5-33

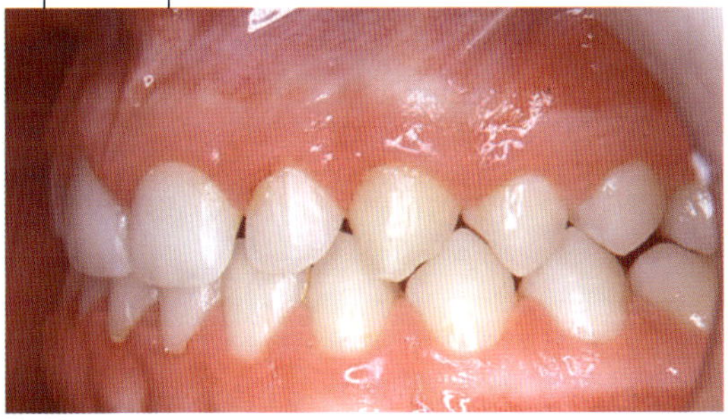

Figs. 5-32 & 5-33
Post-treatment occlusion.

CASE NUMBER 5

The case is an 11 year old patient with "obstructive respiratory syndrome", aggravated by the habit of thumb sucking. Class II division 1 anterior open bite, a posterior cross bite and increased jaw verticality. It has been treated by slow maxillary expansion using a removable appliance (RV1 – see Chapter III) with buccal tubes for high pull traction to control the vertical growth, followed by extraction of the upper first premolars and lower second premolars when they have erupted. Finally a fixed appliance has been applied.

5-34

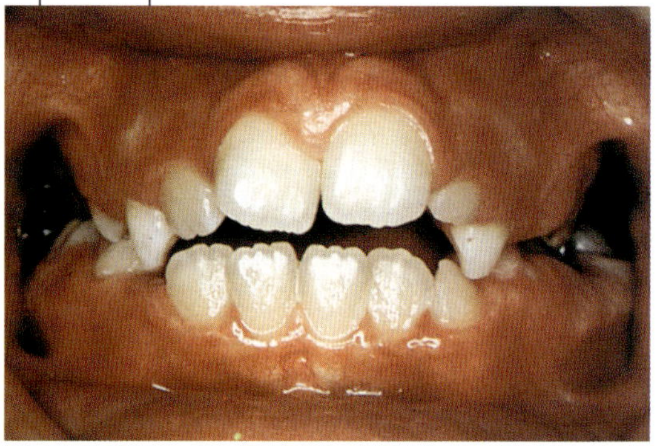

5-35

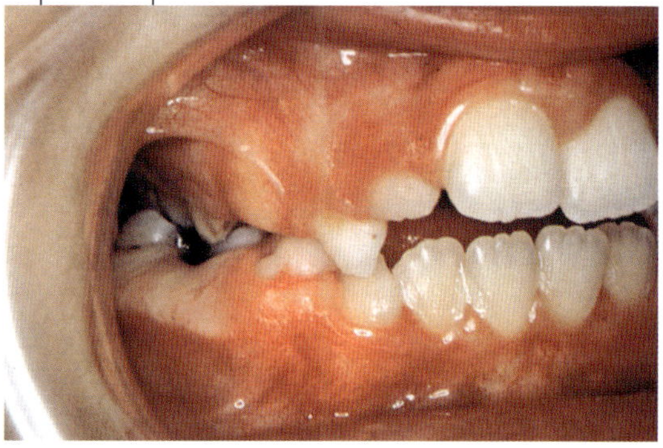

Figs. 5-34 & 5-35
Pre-treatment occlusion.

5-36

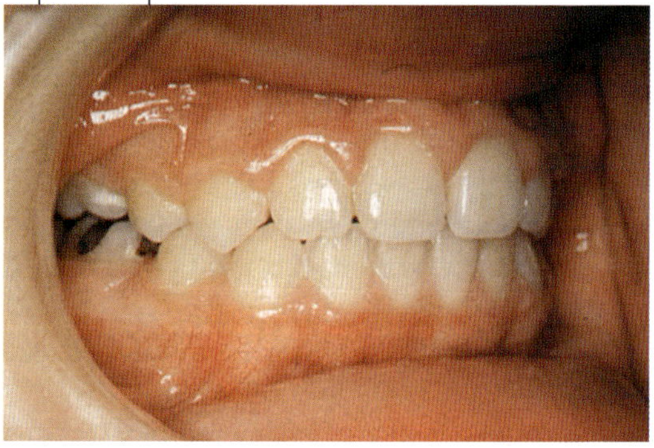

5-37

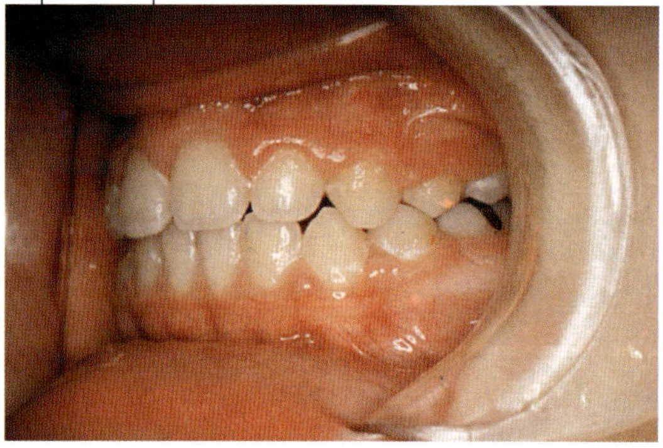

Figs. 5-36 & 5-37
Post-treatment occlusion.

5-38

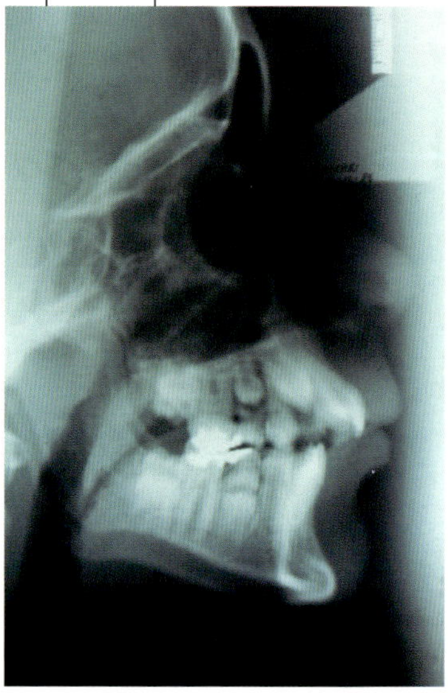

5-39

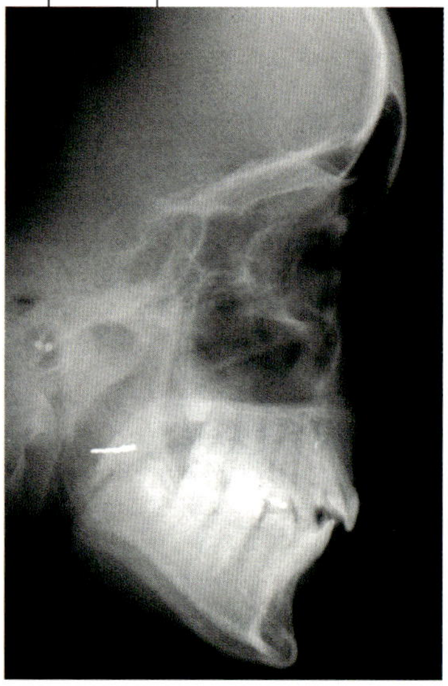

Fig. 5-38
Pre-treatment lateral cephalogram.

Fig. 5-39
Post-treatment lateral cephalogram.

CASE NUMBER 6

The case is a 10 year old with a dental and skeletal open bite.
After receiving a detailed informed consent concerning the various treatments, the relatives chose extraction of the first molars. The excellent result without braces and its stability are an example of what can be obtained with simple and inexpensive procedures.

5-40

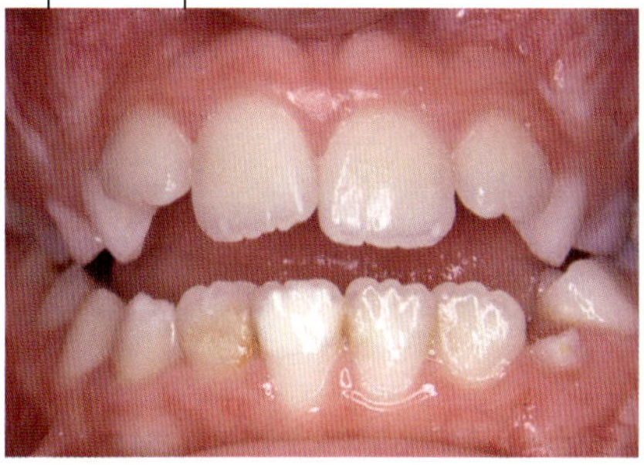

5-41

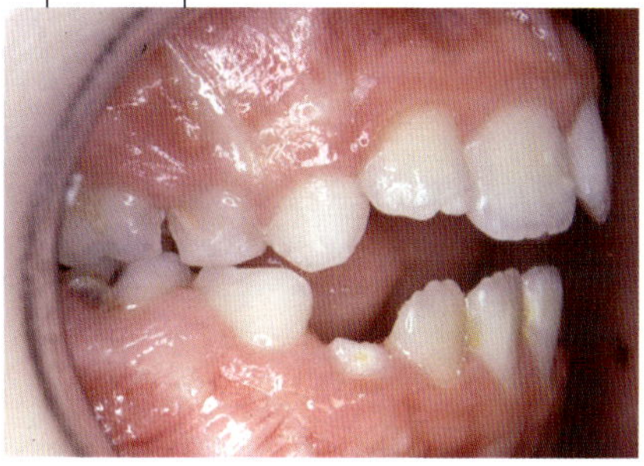

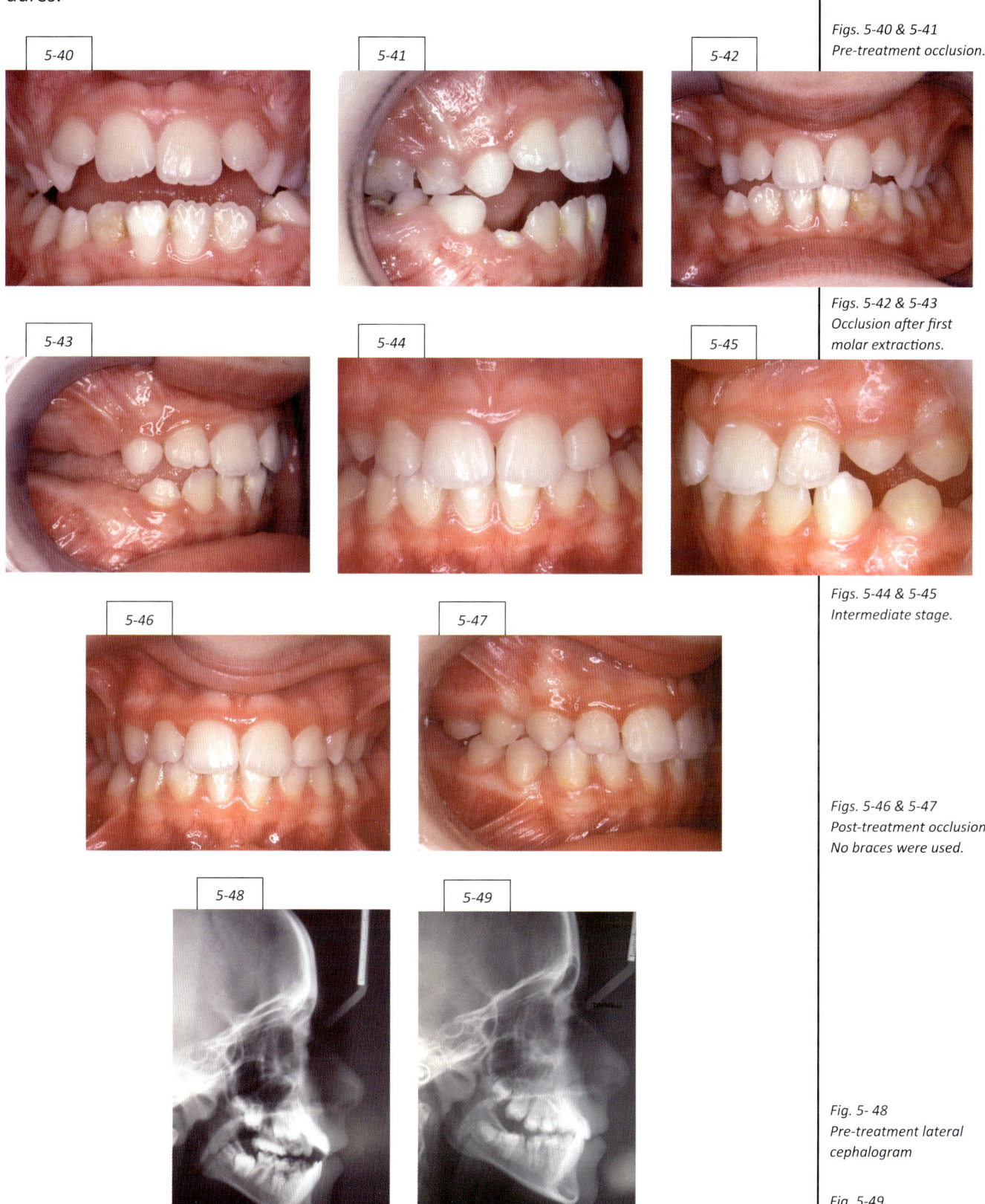

Figs. 5-40 & 5-41
Pre-treatment occlusion.

5-42

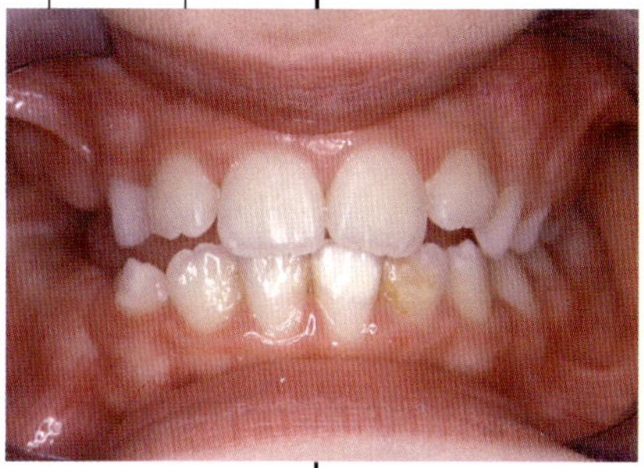

5-43

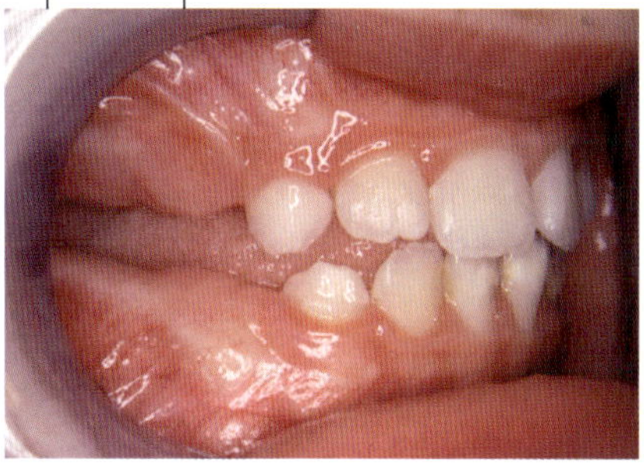

Figs. 5-42 & 5-43
Occlusion after first molar extractions.

5-44

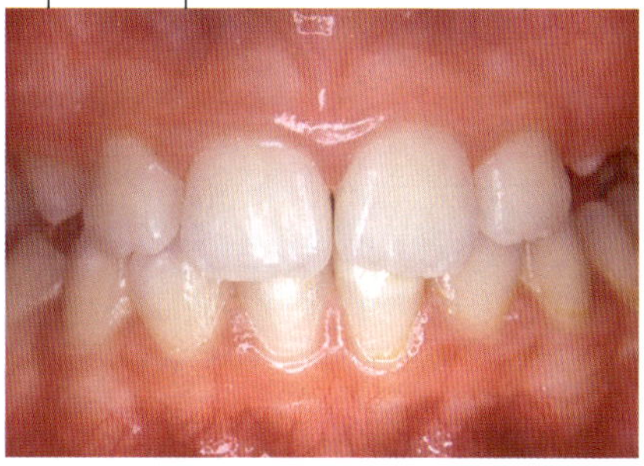

5-45

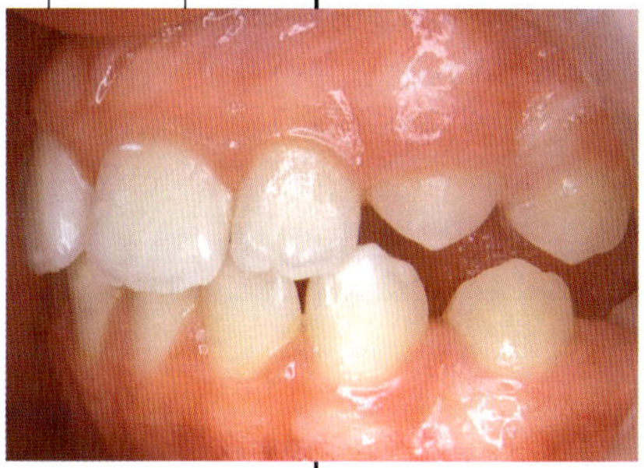

Figs. 5-44 & 5-45
Intermediate stage.

5-46

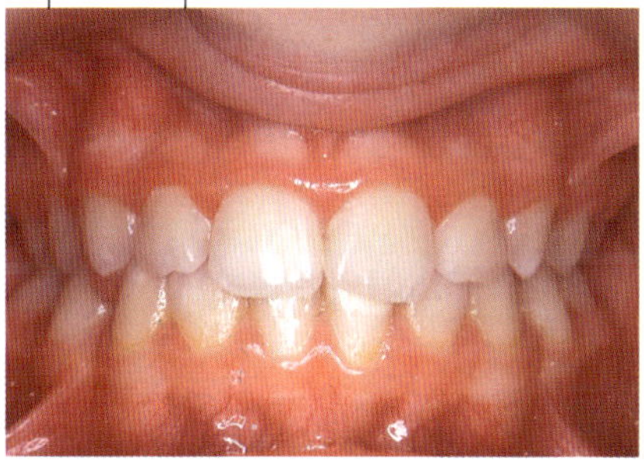

5-47

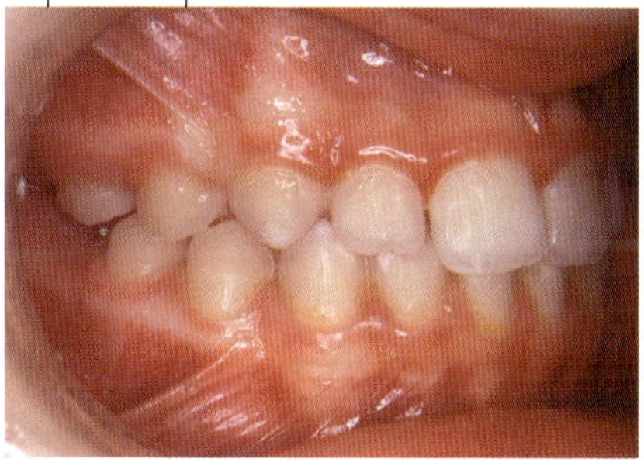

Figs. 5-46 & 5-47
Post-treatment occlusion.
No braces were used.

5-48

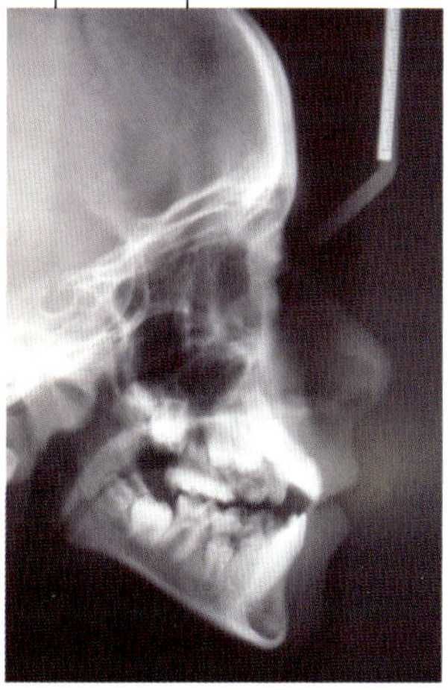

Fig. 5- 48
Pre-treatment lateral cephalogram

5-49

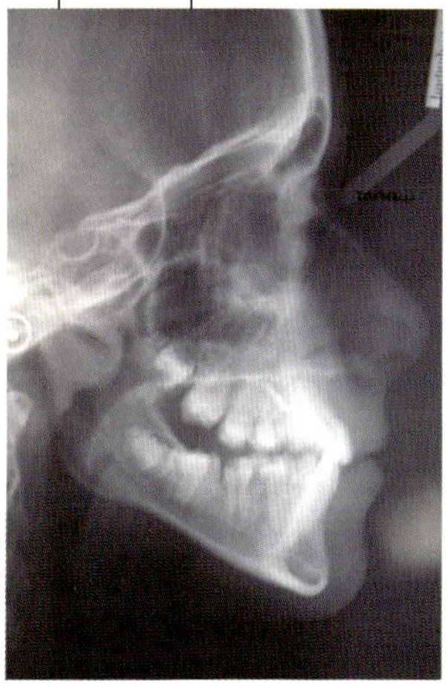

Fig. 5-49
Lateral cephalogram after the first molar extractions.

CASE NUMBER 7

The case is a 20 year old patient with a skeletal open bite and dental open bite. She complained about her bad smile and speech problems, but refused surgery. The case is a dental and skeletal Class II relationship with proclination of the upper incisors. Accepting this verticality, extraction of the first upper premolars followed by treatment with a fixed appliance brought a satisfactory result, and a happy patient.

5-51

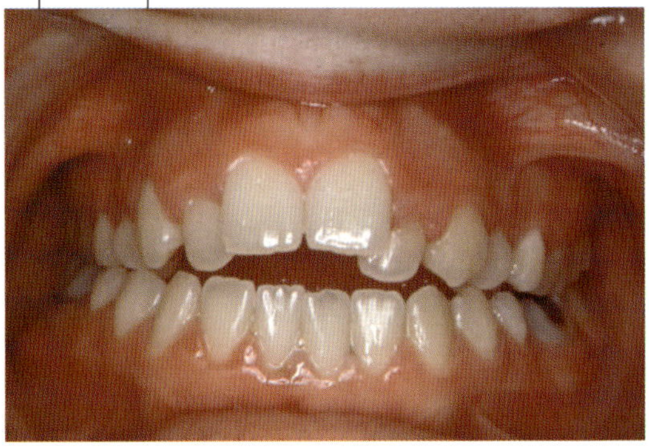

5-52

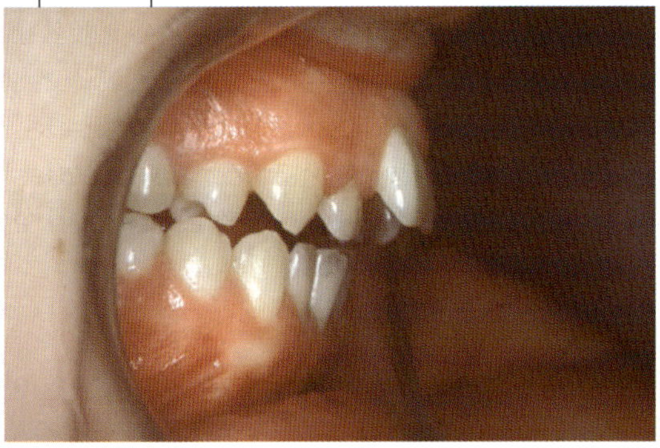

Figs. 5-51 & 5-52
Pre-treatment occlusion.

5-53

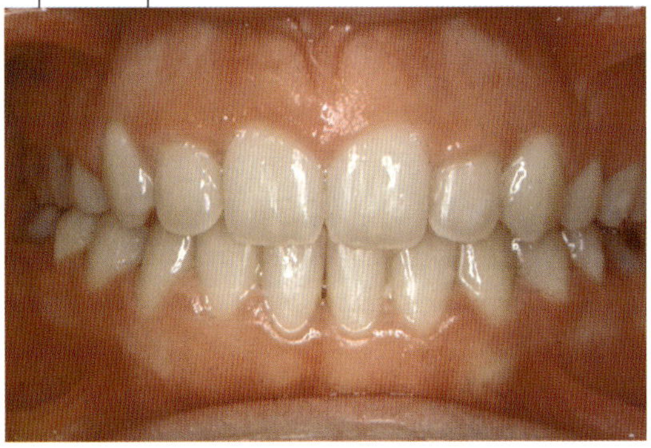

5-54

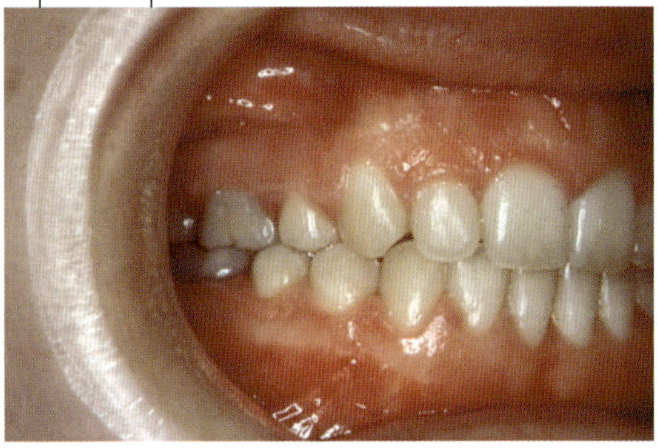

Fig. 5-53 & 5-54
Post-treatment occlusion.

5-55

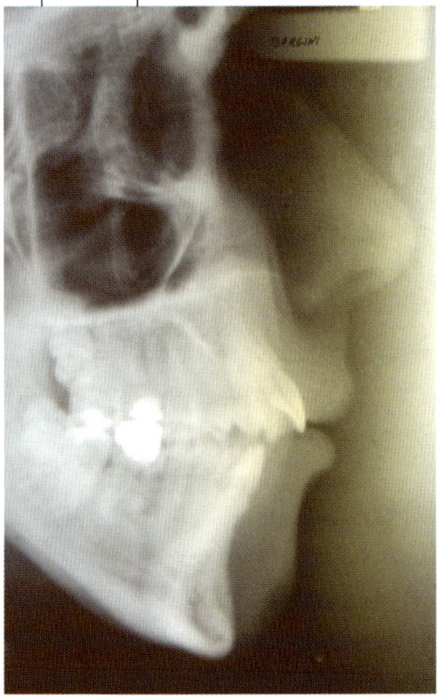

5-56

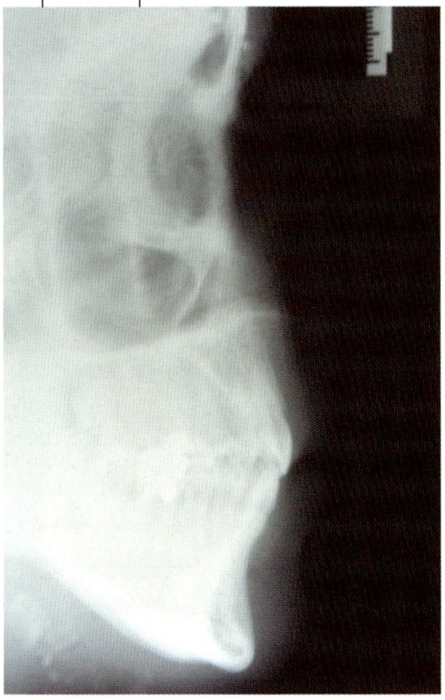

Figs. 5-55
Pre-treatment cephalogram.

Fig. 5-56
Post-treatment lateral cephalogram.

DECREASED VERTICAL DIMENSION

Just as in the earlier discussions of increased vertical dimension, so the same writers coined the terms now in common usage with decreased verticality -
Ricketts: brachi Sassouni: deep bite Schudy: hypodivergent.
Once again, the distinction between skeletal and dental aspects is very important. Skeletal characteristics are the opposite of the features of an open bite. There is a prevalence of transverse measures over the vertical ones. The masticatory muscles are hypertonic, the cephalometric values indicate a reduced jaw verticality and a dental deep bite is often present.

TREATMENT

Just like with open bites, skeletal deep bites do not necessarily need to be treated, there is no evidence of their involvement in TMJ diseases. A dental deep bite can sometimes cause periodontal suffering (case number 8) and an aesthetic motivation is always present.
How do we change a deep bite? (Figs. 5-57 & 5-58) The anterior dental change is the same (Fig. 5-57), but the ways to make it happen are different (Fig. 5-58).
We can open a dental deep bite by intruding the anterior teeth (Fig. 5-58: top) or by increasing the jaw verticality (Fig. 5-58: bottom). The choice depends on the malocclusion.
In a Class III the sagittal aspect improves by increasing the jaw verticality, while it worsens in a Class II. An intrusion of the anterior teeth is better In a Class II, except, in my opinion, when it comes to the Class II deep bite during growth where we try to obtain a mandibular advancement and molar extrusions. In those cases we use Class II elastics and cervical headgear.
Class I is borderline as usually there is a mix of anterior dental intrusion and posterior dental extrusion. That happens particularly during growth when we try to change the verticality and where the incisor intrusion does not come from active biomechanics but instead from passive control of the dentalalveolar vertical growth.
A weak point in deep bite correction is its stability. Just like in open bite treatment, there can be several relapses. These happen because while we are trying to obtain a "new" skeletal and dental balance, the "old" neuromuscular system tends to try to revert to the previous circumstance. For this reason, according to my experience, more stable results are reached during growth when we can expect a reliable progressive adaptation to the new relationship.
There now follow three cases of skeletal / dental reduced verticality (deep bite). Cases 8 and 9 are Class II division 2, so to open the dental bite it is better to intrude the frontal teeth (Fig.57 - upper right) If we achieve it by increasing the verticality (Fig. 57 - lower right) then we sagittally worsen the Class II relationship and the facial aesthetic profile.
Case 10 is also a skeletal/ dental deep bite but with skeletal Class I borderline to a Class III. Here, if we open the dental bite

5-57

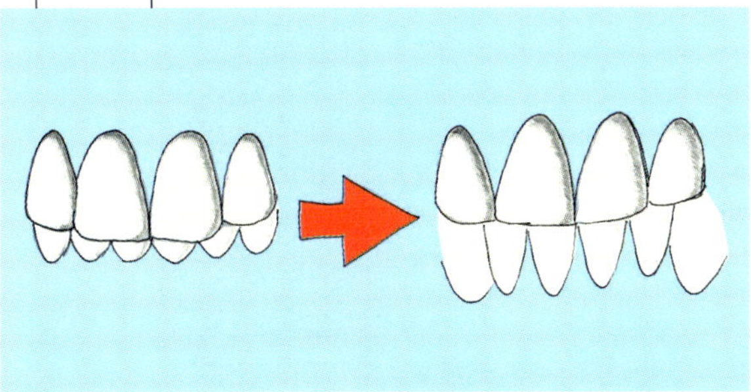

5-58

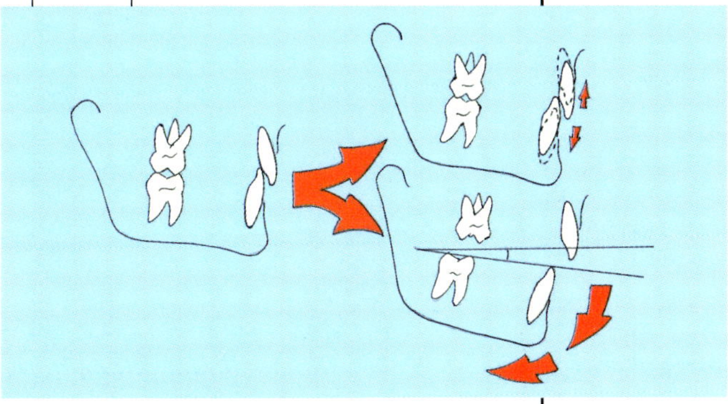

increasing the verticality (Fig. 57 - lower right) we improve the sagittal bones relationship, reaching a full Class I. Also the facial profile improves.

In all three cases it is very important to replace the missing molars with implants or bridges, in order to stabilize the occlusion and mantain the result over time.

CASE NUMBER 8

A 25 year old patient with a skeletal and dental deep bite in a Class II division 2.
There is lower gingival recession and the traumatic origin is evident. With the use of implants, it was possible to upright the lower molars and achieve a better occlusal stability.
In order to prevent relapses an occlusal splint is recommended for life.

5-59

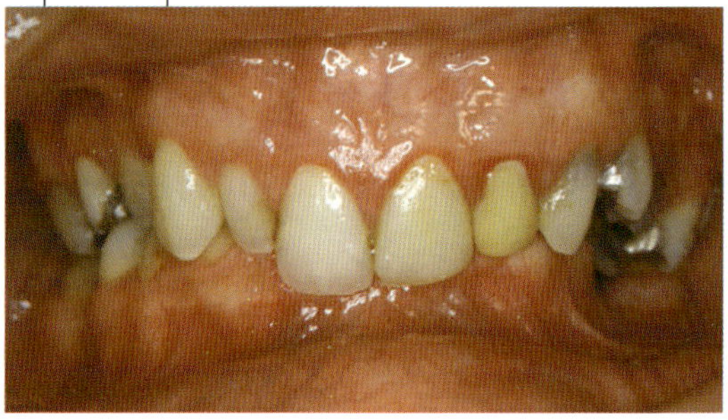

5-60

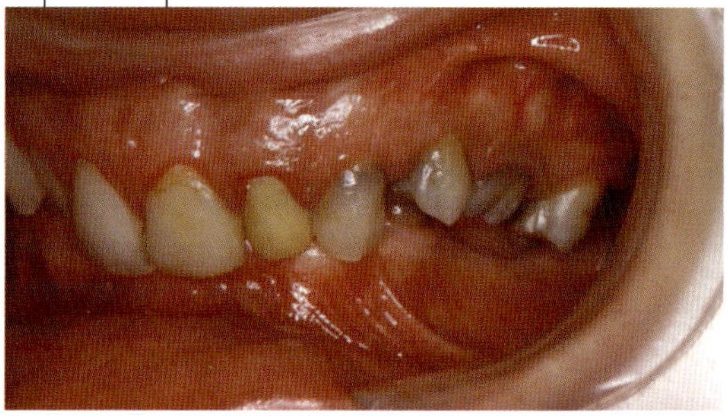

Figs. 5-59 & 5-60
Pre-treatment occlusion.

5-61

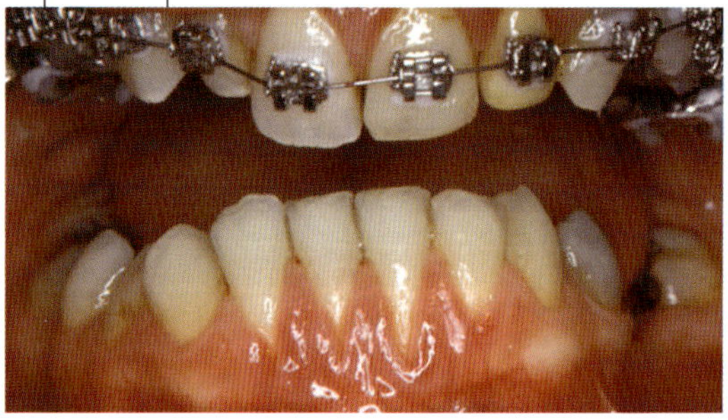

5-62

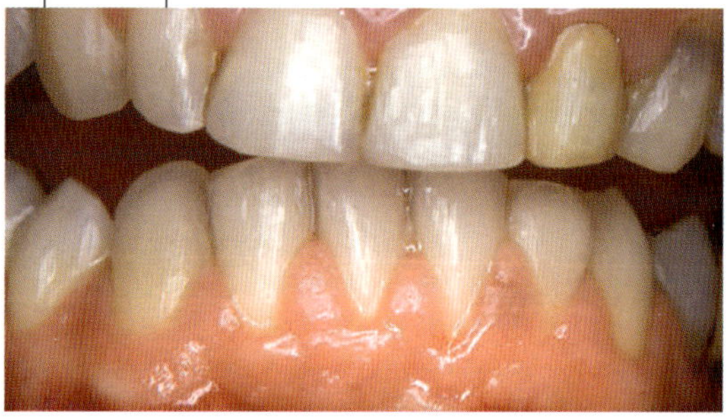

Fig. 5-61
Periodontal situation.

Fig. 5-62
Post-treatment periodontal situation after the orthodontic treatment and a periodontal laterally positioned flap.

5-63

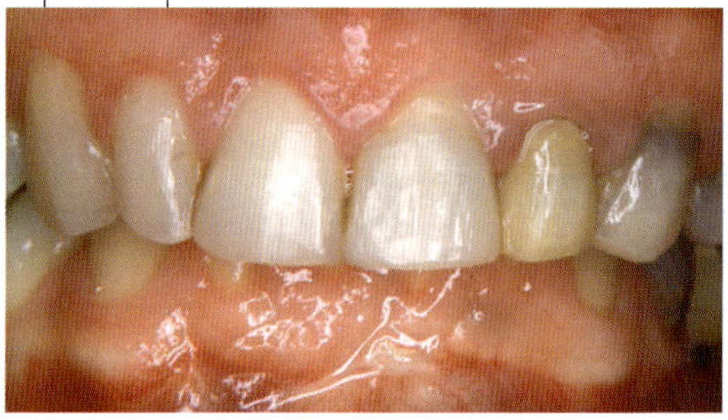

5-64

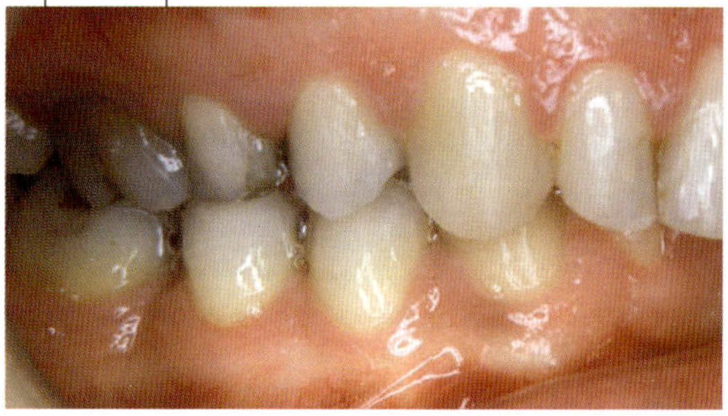

Fig. 5-63 & 5-64
Post-treatment occlusion. A gentle remodelling of the central incisor edge has been made.

5-65

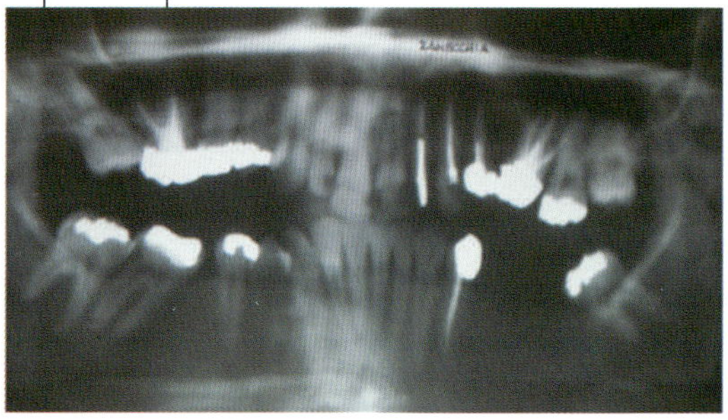

5-66

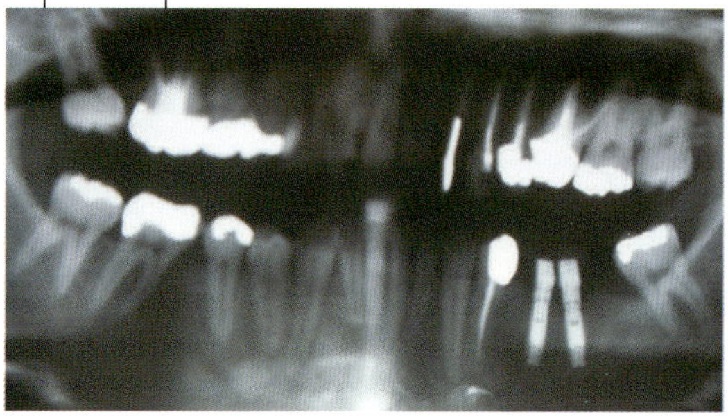

Fig. 5-65
Pre-treatment panoramic radiograph.

Fig. 5-66
Post-treatment panoramic radiograph.

5-67

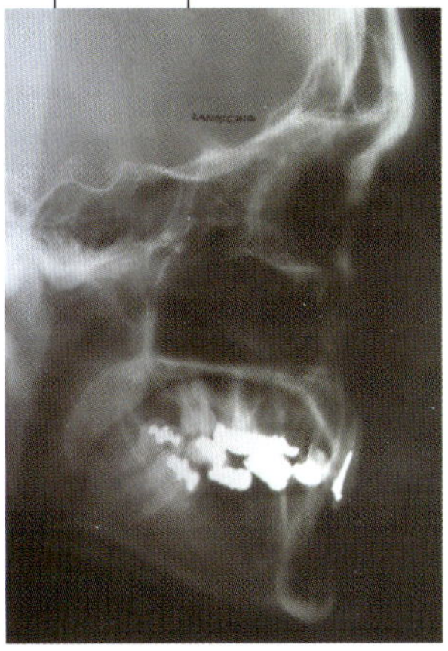

5-68

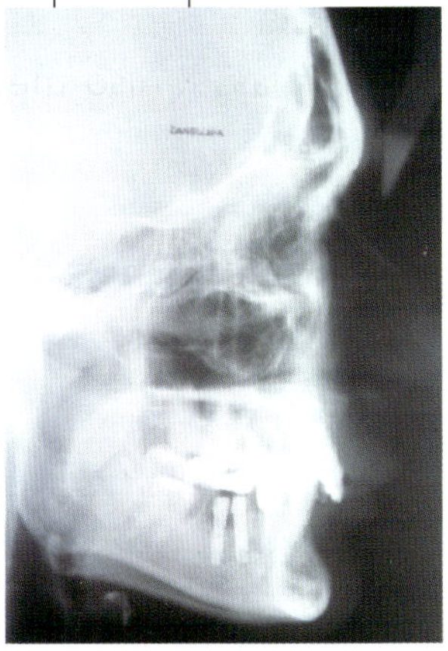

Fig. 5-67
Pre-treatment lateral radiograph.

Fig. 5-68
Post-treatment lateral cephalogram.

CASE NUMBER 9

The main difference between this case and the previous one is the patient's age. Now we have a Class II division 2 in a 63 year old patient. Two implants are important to stabilize the occlusion and a retainer is recommended for life.

5-69

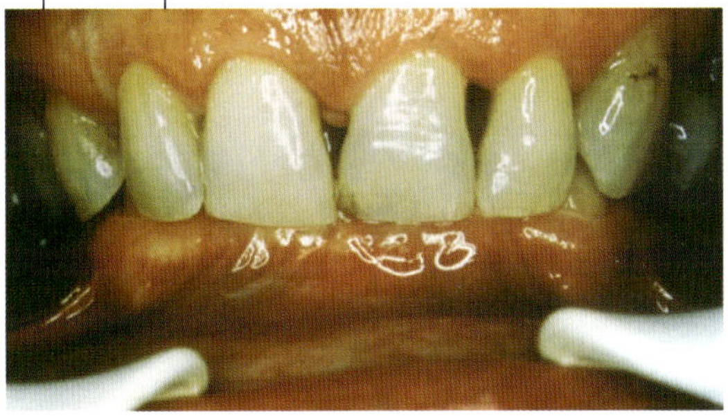

5-70

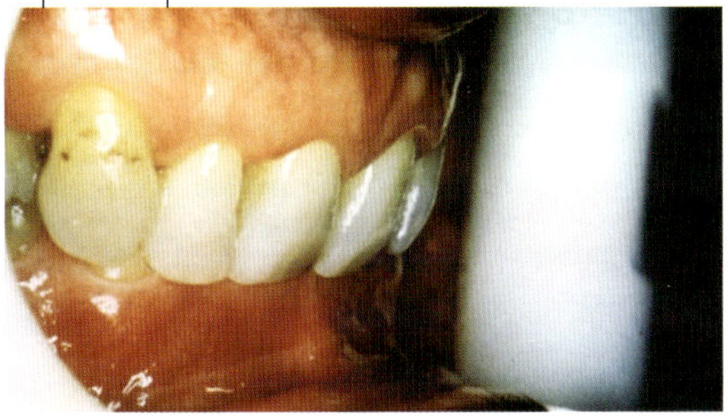

Figs. 5-69 & 5-70
Pre-treatment occlusion.

5-71

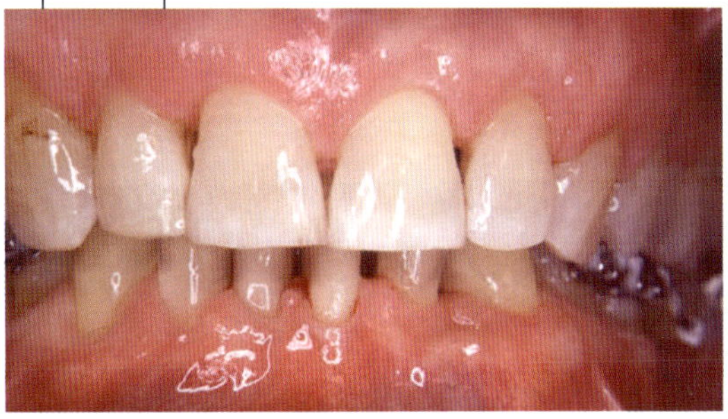

5-72

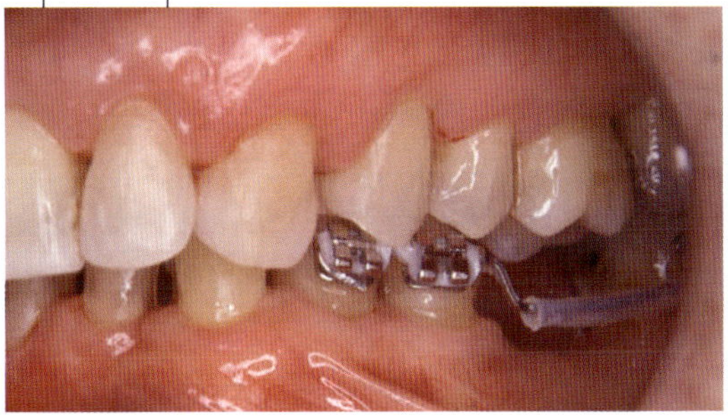

Figs. 5-71 & 5-72
Post-treatment occlusion. Two lower sectionals maintain the space for two implants.

5-73

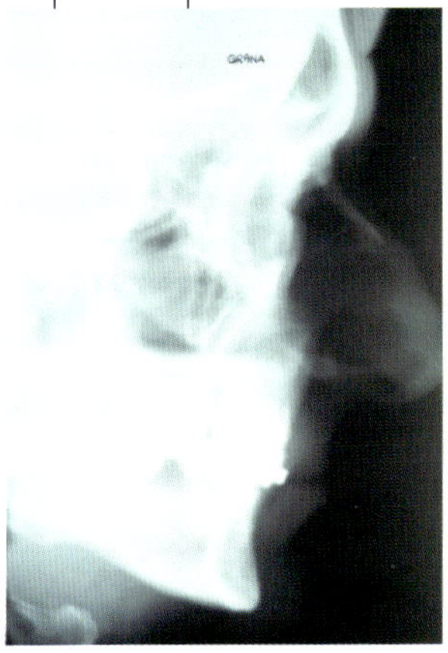

5-74

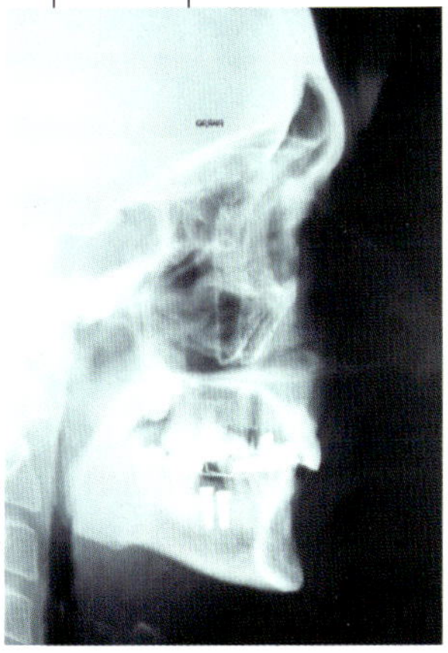

Fig. 5-73
Pre-treatment lateral cephalogram.

Fig. 5-74
Post-treatment lateral cephalogram.

CASE NUMBER 10

In this case there is a skeletal and dental deep bite. The upper right canine has been extracted. There is lower arch crowding with the incisors lingually inclined. The treatment plan was to open the space to replace the missing upper canine with an implant. Then open the bite and replace the missing molars with implants in order to stabilize the occlusion.

5-75

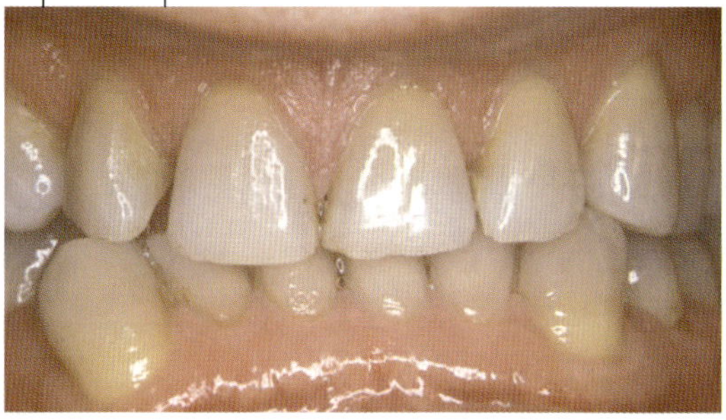

5-76

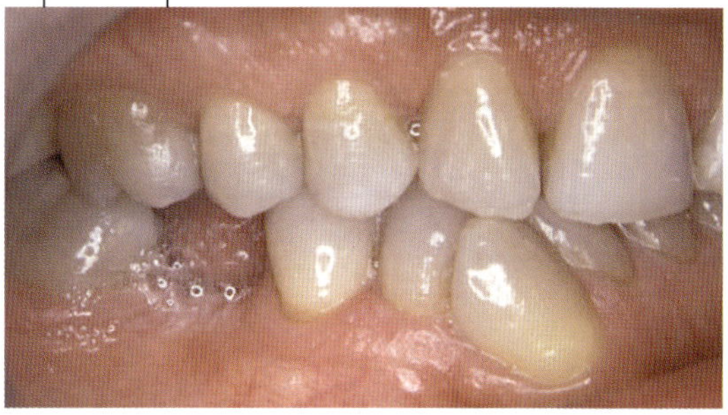

Figs. 5-75 & 5-76
Pre-treatment occlusion.

5-77

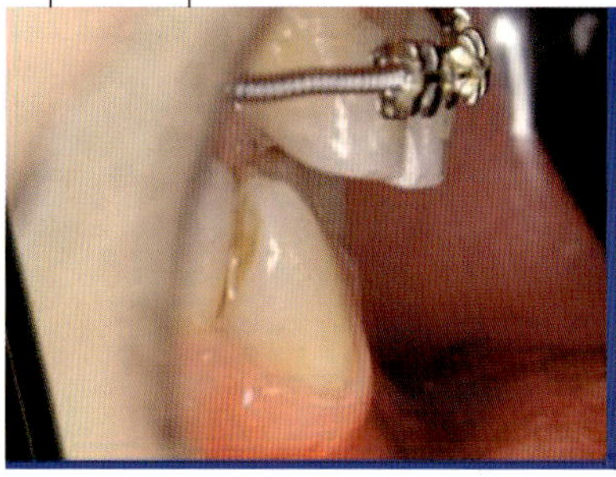

5-78

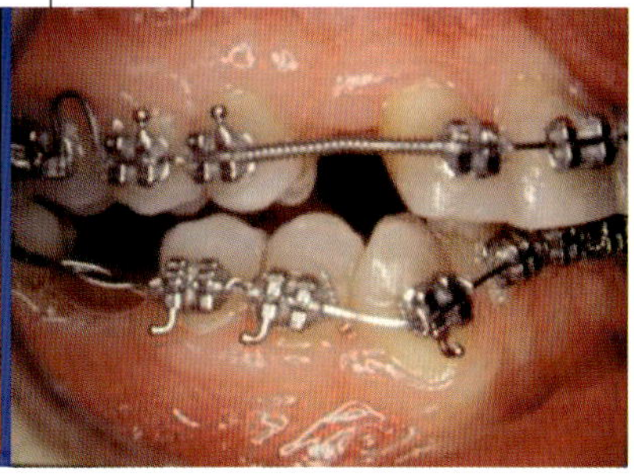

Fig. 5-77
First step: open the space to replace upper right canine.

Fig. 5-78
Second step: the fixed appliance is extended on the lower arch.

5-79

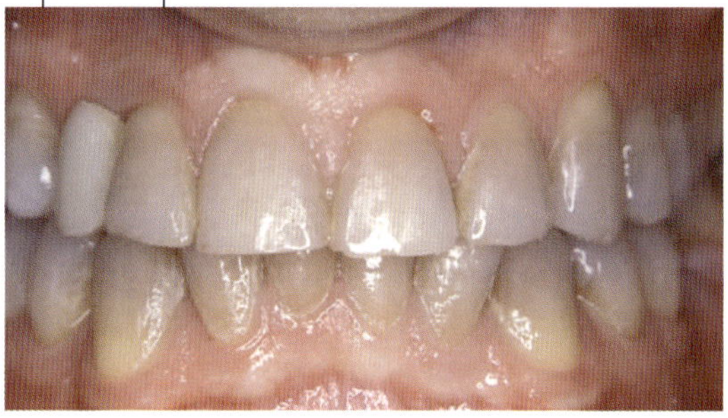

5-80

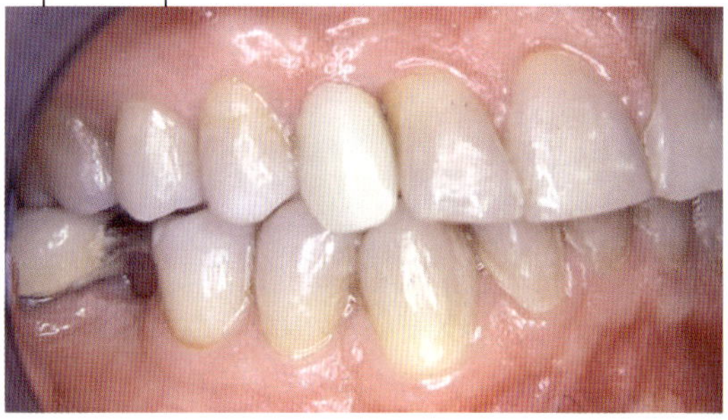

5-81

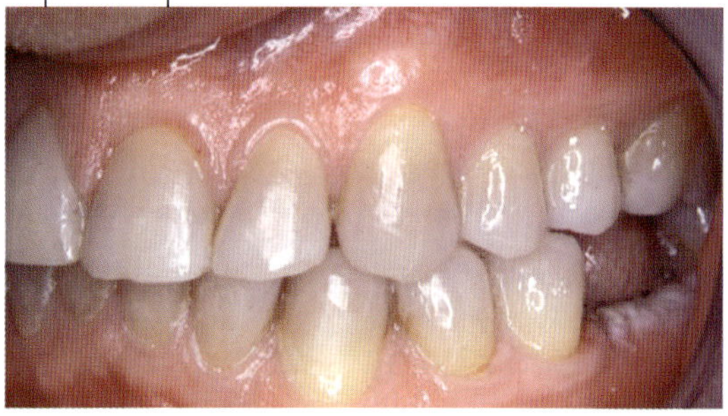

Figs. 5-79 to 5-81
Post-treatment occlusion. An implant and temporary crown replaces the missing canine.

5-82

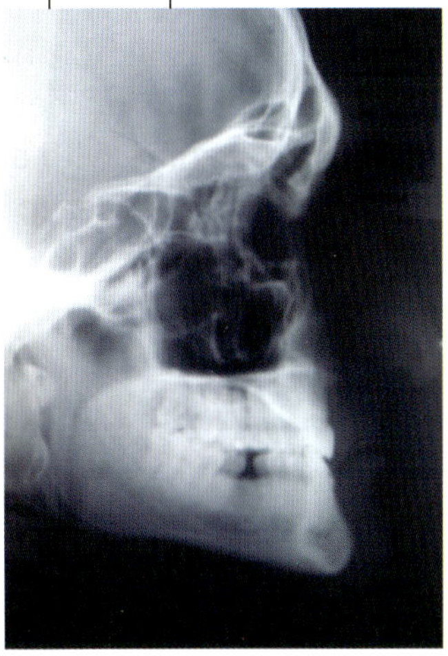

5-83

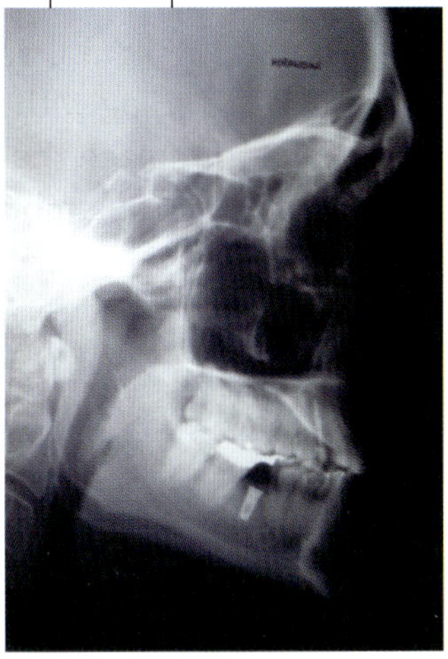

5-84

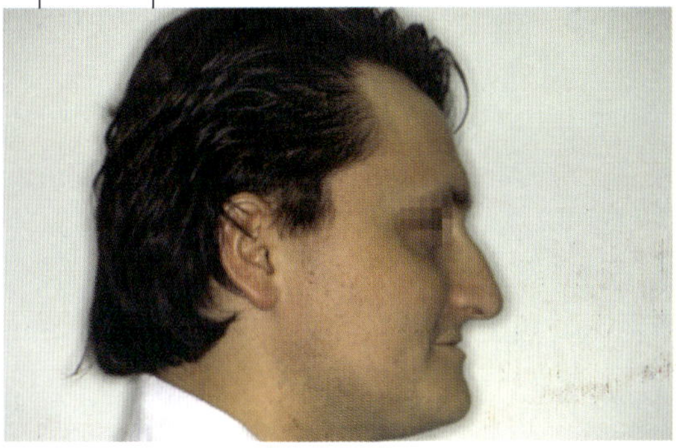

5-85

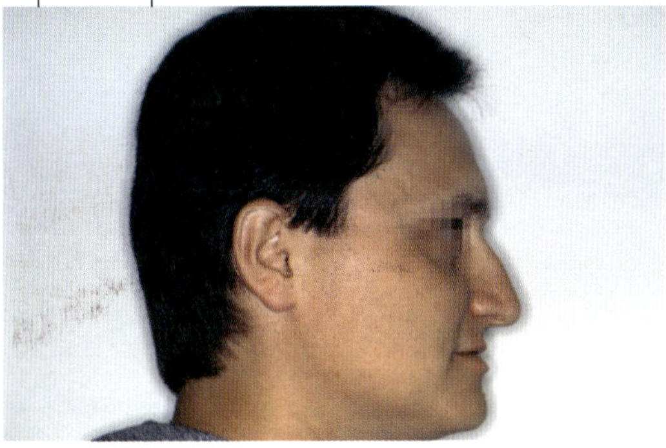

Fig. 5-82
Pre-treatment lateral cephalogram.

Fig. 5- 83
Post-treatment lateral cephalogram.

Fig. 5-84
Pre-treatment facial profile.

Fig. 5-85
Post-treatment facial profile. ***The patient looks younger.***

RETAINERS

The aim of an orthodontic treatment is a good and stable result. However, the tendency of many malocclusions to relapse is clinically well known. We must remember that the better the occlusion, the better its stability because the muscular forces are well distributed on dental arches. The best occlusion is to be had with a correct jaw relationship. Many people ignore this and pretend that after their inadequate "treatments" the teeth won't move. In those cases, the only way to keep teeth aligned is by using retainers, either fixed or removable. Typical removable braces are occlusal splints or the Hawley plate (Fig. 5-86). With some appliances, thanks to their elasticity or to the application of springs, small corrections of dental positions are possible. I would recommend their application not only during the night but for a few hours during the day too.

This must be done mostly in those cases where growth leads to unpredictable outcomes: skeletal open/deep bites, Class III, presence of habits...

When it comes to a single tooth, rotational correction has a great tendency for relapsing which can be minimised with a circumferential fibreotomy. With this procedure, the cutting of the epithelial attachment and of the transeptal fibres is performed. The latter of which, because of their elastic "memory", are responsible for the relapse. Once cut, the periodontal fibres re-organize in the new position achieved with the orthodontic treatment. The process takes approximately three months.

Lower incisor crowding also deserves to be mentioned. As for its causes, there is no evidence that lower third molars influence anterior crowding. I suspect it is the result of facial and masticatory muscular activity. In what I consider a milestone in orthodontic literature, Little et al.[158] showed that even after four premolar extraction treatments there can be unpredictable lower incisor crowding. The only way to avoid it is by lifelong retention that is usually achieved with a multistrand wire lingually bonded with composite (Fig. 5-87).

In another work, Little[159] concluded:

- The dental arch length diminishes over the course of years in both treated and non-treated patients.
- After a treatment the dental arch tends to return to the original form.
- The inter-canine distance diminishes after treatment, in those cases treated with and without expansion.
- Relapses are minimally influenced by third molars.

5-86

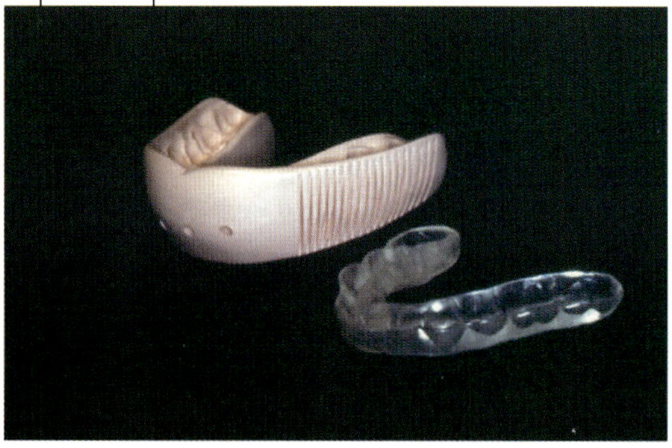

Fig. 5-86 Examples of removable retainers.

5-87

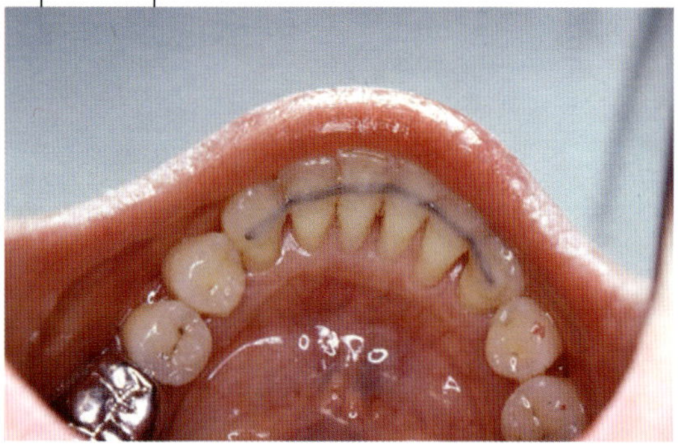

Fig. 5-87 Fixed retention.

DIASTEMAS

The space between teeth is called the diastema. During growth, diastema between the upper central incisors is normal. The space reduces and closes with the mesial pressure determined by upper canine eruption. This does not happen when there is fibrous septum between the incisors. According to the School of Milan, only in those cases is a frenotomy necessary.

However, diastemas are present in other situations also, such as cases of microdontia. Usually they must be corrected without closing the spaces but instead by increasing the crown width with composite, crowns etc.

There can be spaces after tooth extractions. The correct treatment would be to close the spaces and replace the missing teeth.

When labial musculature is hypotonic, the pressure of the tongue can cause diastemas (cases11 & 12 to follow).

In a dental deep bite, the occlusion determines the space between the upper incisors. In other cases the gaps are a sign of a more important problem like periodontal disease, often accompanied by inflammation and unfavourable crown/root ratio.

Teeth weakened by the periodontal situation can easily migrate with the opening of spaces.

Closure of the spaces by widening dental crowns with facets, for example, would be a mistake because there is a risk of hiding a pathology in progress.

CASE NUMBER 11

The case is a 9 year old patient with a posterior cross bite and anterior wide diastemas. Tongue posture was the main cause of this situation (Fig. 5-88). After the cross bite correction (Fig. 5-89) a fixed appliance followed (Fig. 5-90). At the end of treatment a good occlusion was achieved (Fig. 5-91).

5-88

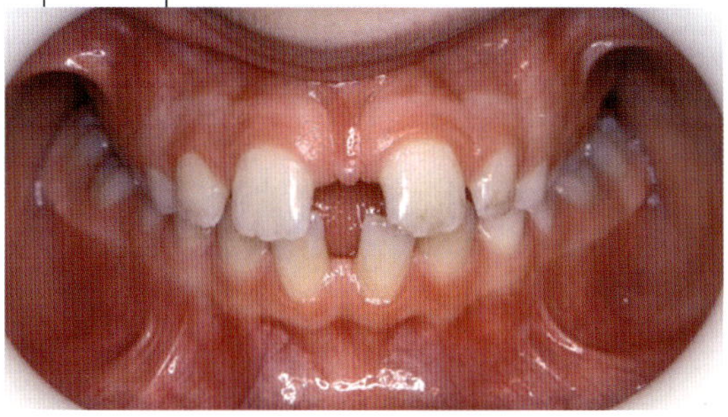

5-89

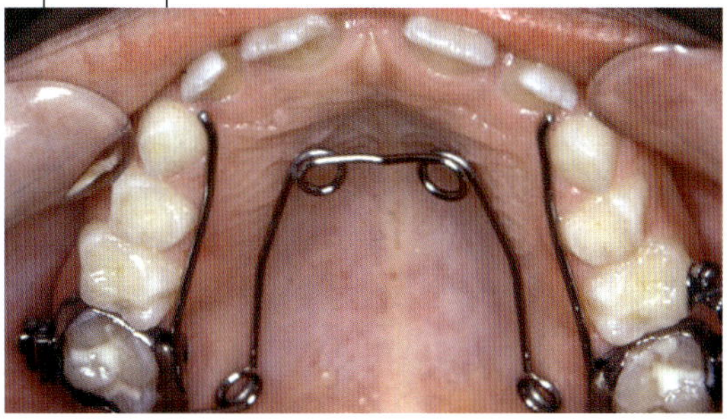

5-90

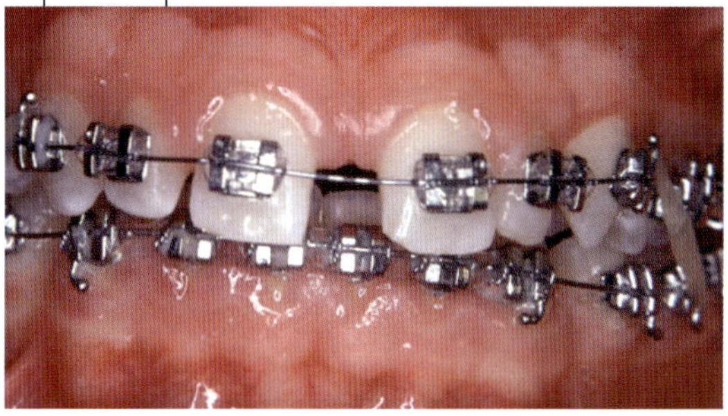

5-91

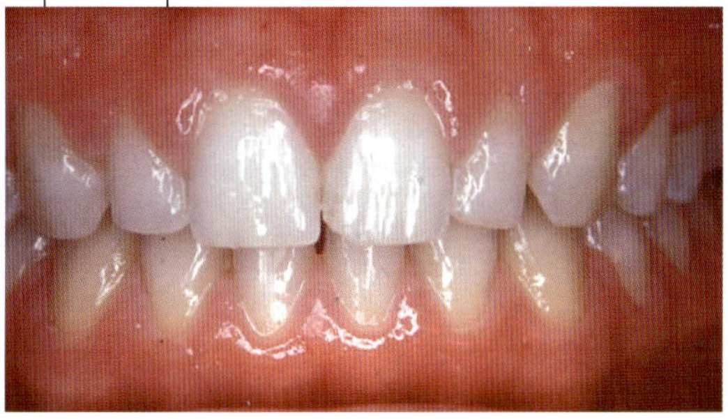

CASE NUMBER 12

The case is a 30 year old patient with a wide diastema. The tongue posture and a lower first molar extraction were the causes of this occlusion (Figs. 5-92 & 5-93). The patient wanted to improve his bad smile and five different dentists proposed to widen the teeth, either by crown, bridge or implant in the gap! In my opinion this was crazy. Only orthodontic treatment could deliver a satisfactory outcome (Fig. 5-94 & 5-95).

5-92

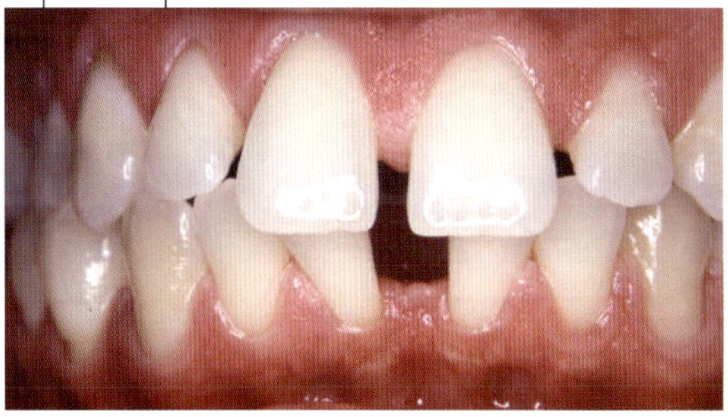

5-93

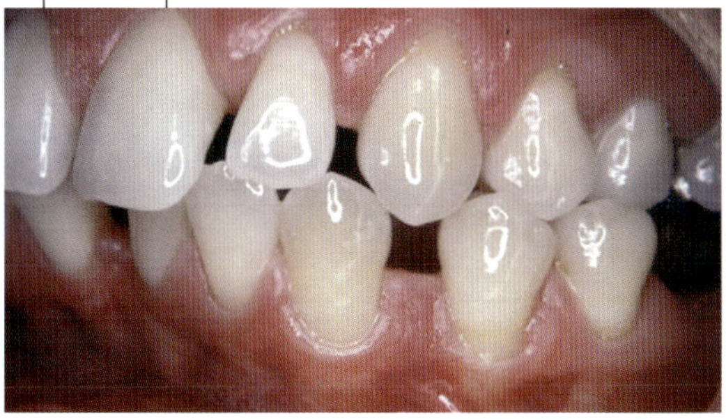

5-94

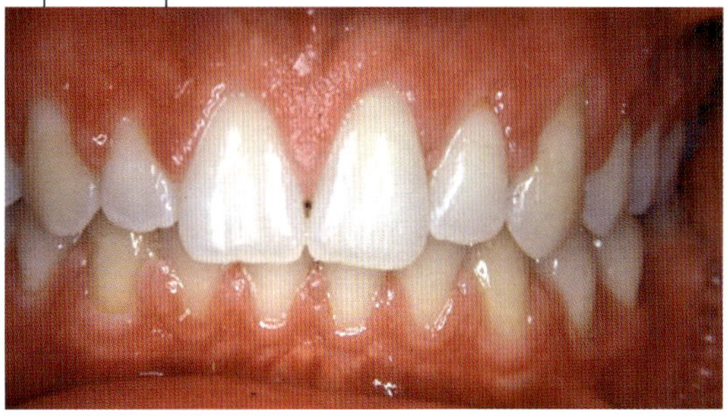

5-95

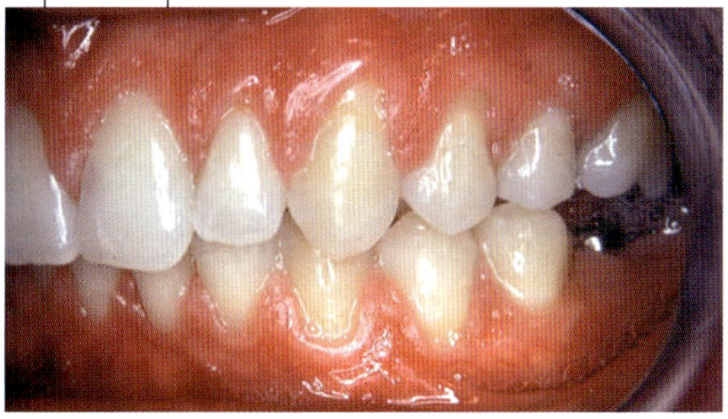

CASE NUMBER 13

5-96

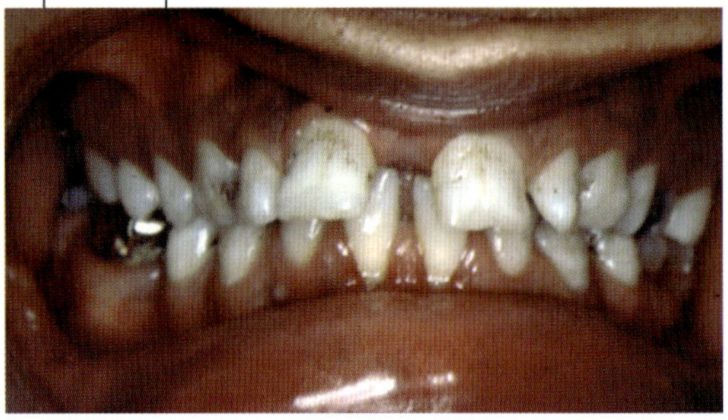

5-97

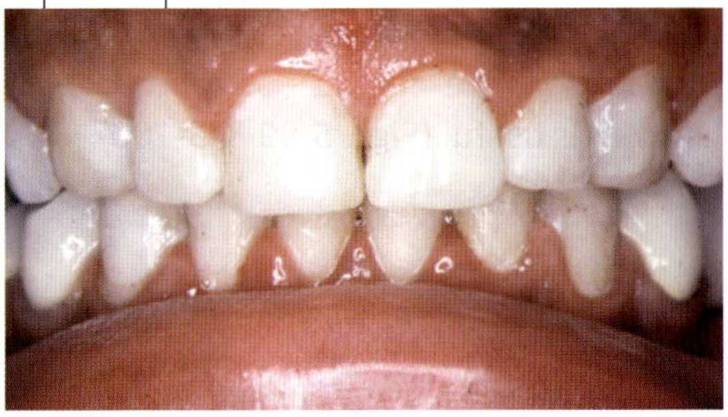

The case is a 33 year old patient with a wide diastema between the upper incisors.

This space is caused by a deep bite occlusion (Fig. 5-96). So to close the diastema it is necessary to open the bite with fixed appliances, and thus obtain a good result (Fig. 5-97).

Notice the bad smile caused not only by the dental relationship but also by enamel dysplasia (fig.5-96). The evident improvement in fig. 5-97 is obtained with both orthodontic treatment and the use of composite on the anterior surface of the frontal teeth.

CANINE DISPLACEMENT

Third lower molars are the most frequently displaced teeth, the maxillary canines are next.

5-98

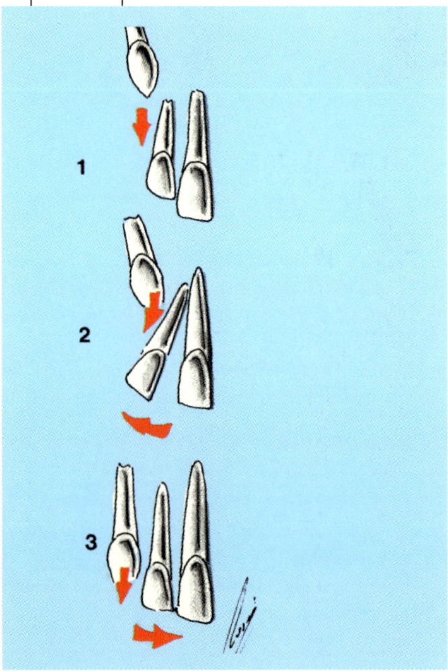

Fig. 5-98
The 3 stages of upper canine eruption:
1) The canine is high positioned, the lateral incisor is straight.
2) The canine moves down. There is a pressure that causes the distal inclination of the lateral incisor (ugly duckling phase).
3) There is canine eruption with lateral incisor uprighting.

Treatment of third molar impaction is usually by extraction, while canines can sometimes be aligned with a surgical-orthodontic treatment. Palatally displaced canines are the most common. As for the causes, many factors can be involved, for example the presence of obstacles, traumas on the corresponding deciduous teeth, inflammatory processes and iatrogenic treatments. There are also cases that do not show an evident cause.

We can identify three steps in upper canine eruption (Fig. 5-98) where the *guidance theory* is expressed. According to this theory, the distal aspect of the lateral incisor root is a guide for canine eruption.

In the presence of crowding there is a prevalence of buccal displacement. With adequate spacing then palatal displacement is prevalent, probably because in this case lateral incisor guidance to a correct eruption is less common.

Clinically, we must anticipate some problems with canine eruption in young patients between 9 and 12 years because at that age the canine bulge is not palpable. At that time we must carefully consider the upper lateral incisor inclination. In fact, lateral incisors can be distally-inclined and also buccally-inclined in cases of buccal displacement.

When a deciduous canine stays too long in the mouth it is time to react and take an X-ray.

Radiologically, the first sign of canine displacement is the overlapping of its crown with the root of the permanent lateral incisor. This is what appears, for example, on a panoramic radiograph. However, we do not know if it is buccally or palatally impacted because the image only shows two dimensions. Therefore to view the teeth with a lateral cephalogram, where most of the time the canine position is clearly shown, is useful (Figs. 5-99 & 5-100).

An alternative is the use of two intra-oral periapical radiographs along with the technique of parallax introduced by Clark (1909) (Fig. 5-101).

5-100

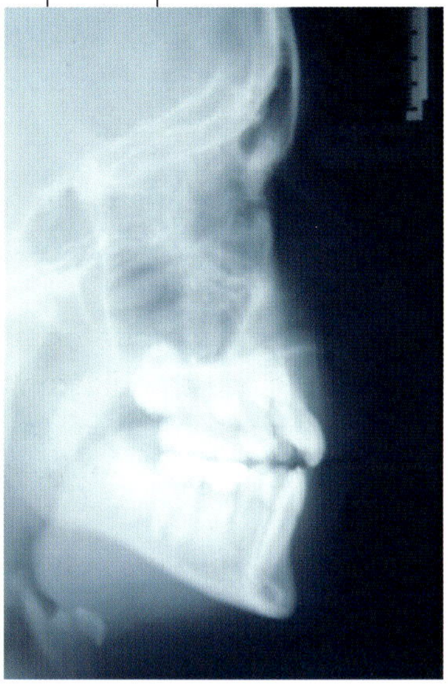

5-99

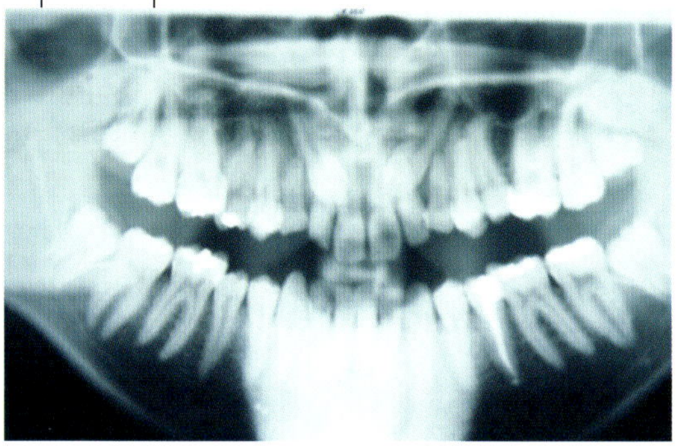

Fig. 5-99
Panoramic radiograph with upper canines overlapping the lateral incisors. It is a sign of canine displacement, but it does not indicate whether they are displaced palatally or buccally.

Fig. 5-100
Lateral cephalogram. The palatal displacement is evident.

5-101

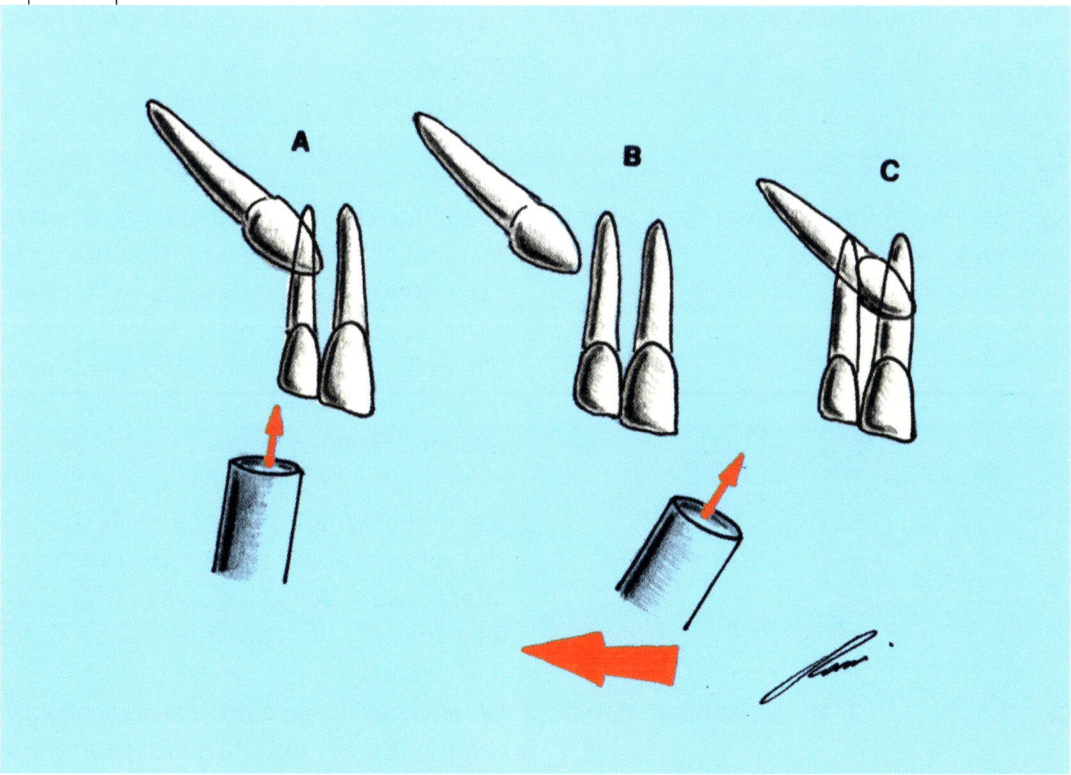

Fig. 5-101
Two radiographs are taken at different horizontal angles with the same vertical angulation. The (A) first radiograph shows the upper canine overlapping the lateral incisor. The second (B), taken by shifting the X-ray tube laterally, shows the canine in a different position. Due to parallax, if the canine appears to move in the same direction of the tube shift it is palatally displaced. When the canine appears to move in the opposite direction of the tube (C), it is buccally displaced.

If some doubts remain they can be cleared with the use of a spiral computed tomography (CT) or cone-beam CT (CBCT) which give 3-dimensional imaging.

TREATMENT

Before beginning treatment for an impacted canine an orthodontist must make sure that the canine was not the reason behind lateral incisor root resorption. Otherwise when resorption is present, the treatment could be indicated as its cause (see Figs. 5-133 to 5-136 further on).

The treatment is based on using a fixed appliance which applies a traction to the impacted canine after its surgical exposure. When there is buccal displacement, a surgical procedure that ensures a good keratinized gingival amount is important. With more frequent palatal displacements the problem does not exist because all the gingival tissue is keratinised.

Once the crown is exposed, a bracket, a button or a hook can be bonded.

We can apply traction mainly when it comes to palatal displacement, in an attempt to avoid a dangerous contact, which could cause root resorption to adjacent teeth. For this reason, in order to move away from the lateral incisor root, the canine crown must be moved down (Fig. 5-108 & 5-117). Afterwards it can be pulled and aligned into the dental arch (Fig. 5-109). It might be rotated and buccally torqued many times.

The use of light force is very important, just like the control of anchorage units. In fact, sometimes we see teeth other than the canines move against our wishes. In my experience, the younger the patient, the easier the treatment.

Treatments are usually successful (the success rate in various published reports is between 70% and 90% with a duration of treatment ranging from 7 to 21 months), but sometimes they can fail. The major causes of failure are poor anchorage, mistaken positional diagnosis and directional traction, and ankylosis. The ankylosis can have an unknown origin or it can result from injuries to the periodontal ligament during surgical exposure, including chemical trauma caused by orthophosphoric acid etchant. In such cases, remedial surgical luxation followed by traction can be successful.

The last resort of impacted canine treatment, before surrendering, is canine extraction and its autotransplantation.

CASE NUMBER 14

In this case the canines are palatally displaced.
After surgical exposure with a fixed appliance:
(i) move down the canine crowns (Fig. 5-104 and Fig. 5-105)
(ii) pull and align the canines (Figs. 5-106 and 5-107).
Fig. 5-105 shows a palatal bar. It has been applied to increase the anchorage.

5-102

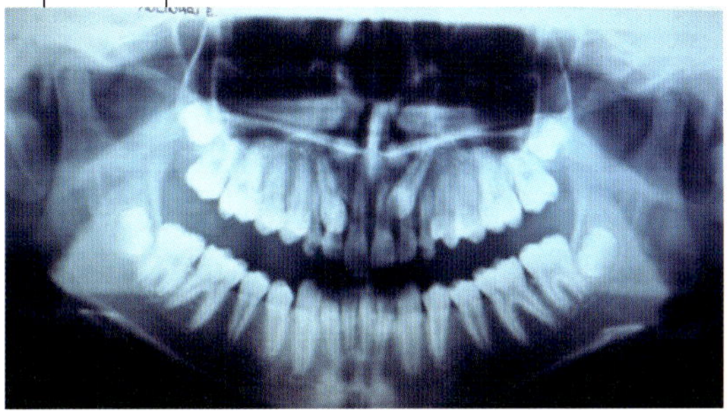

Fig. 5-102 Pre-treatment panoramic radiograph.

5-103

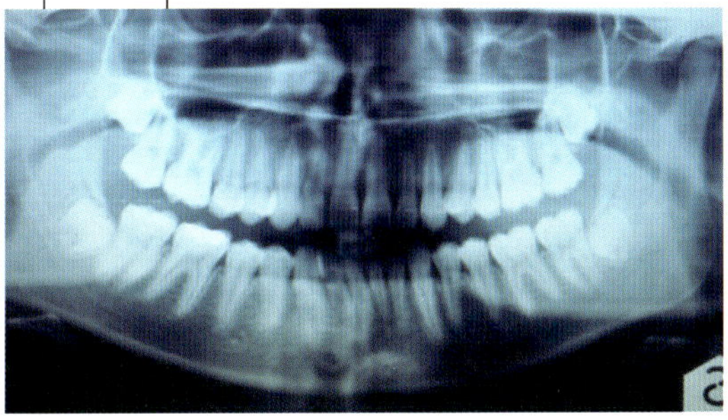

Fig. 5-103 Post-treatment panoramic radiograph.

5-104

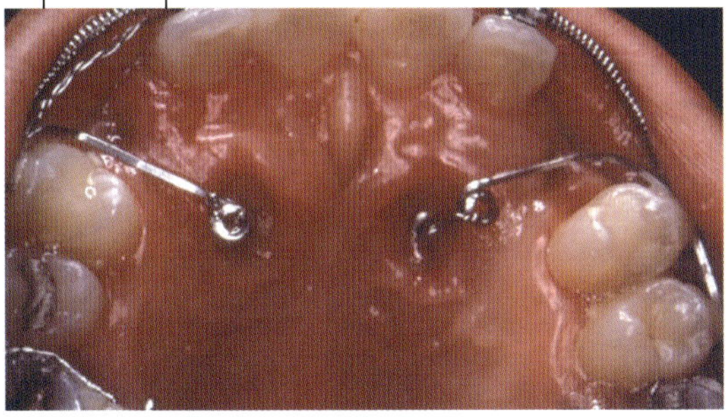

5-105

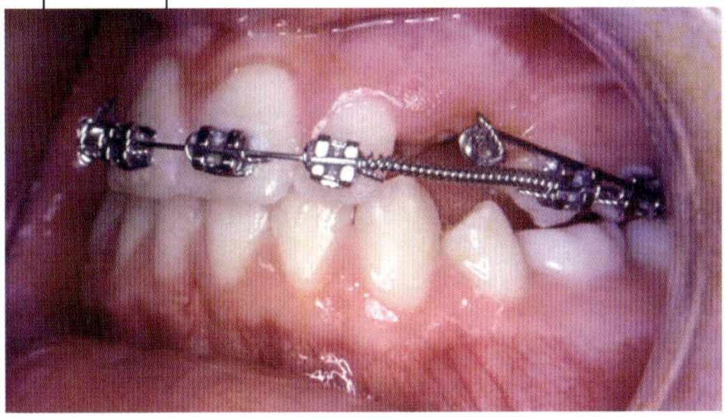

Fig. 5-104 & 105 Move down the canine crowns.

5-106

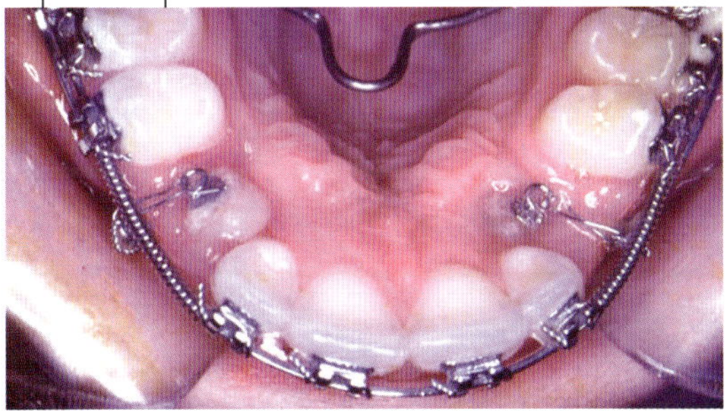

5-107

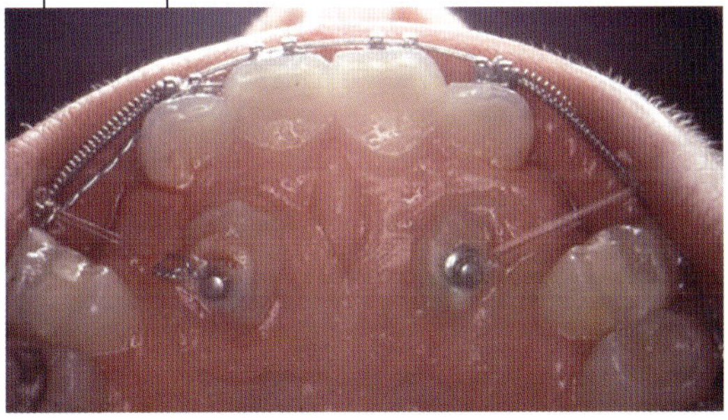

Figs. 5-106 & 107 Pull and align the canines.

5-108

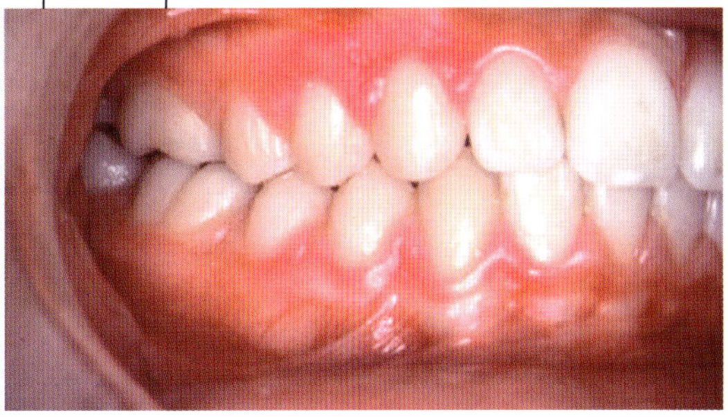

5-109

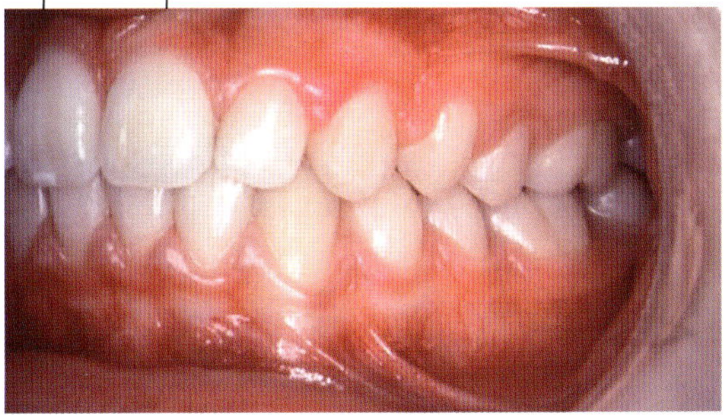

Figs. 5-108 & 109 Post-treatment occlusion.

CASE NUMBER 15

The case is a 33 year old patient. The presence of the upper right deciduous canine and the distal crown inclination of the lateral incisor suggest an upper right canine buccal displacement (Figs. 5-110 & 5-111). During the first phase, a sectional appliance is followed by surgical canine exposure and the bonding of a button used for traction. The surgical flap is apically positioned in order to maintain the keratinized gingival tissue during movement (Figs. 5-112 & 5-113). In the second phase the fixed appliance is extended to the rest of the upper dental arch.

5-110

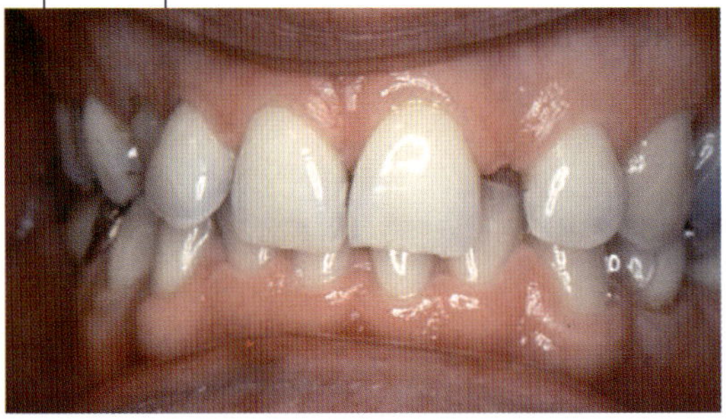

5-111

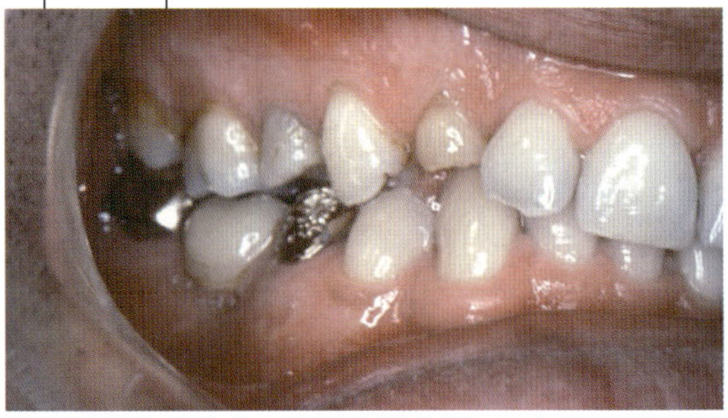

5-112

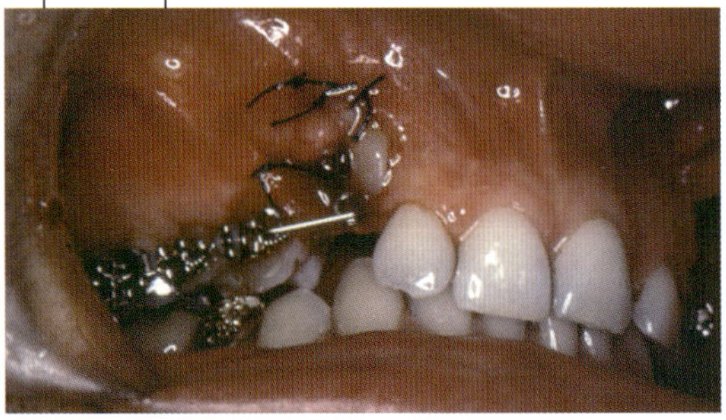

5-113

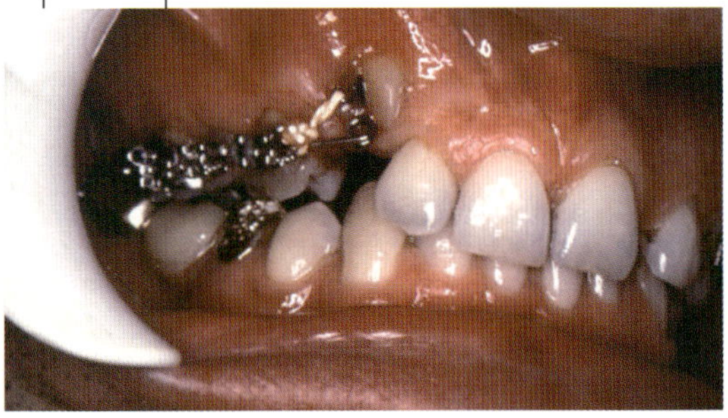

5-114

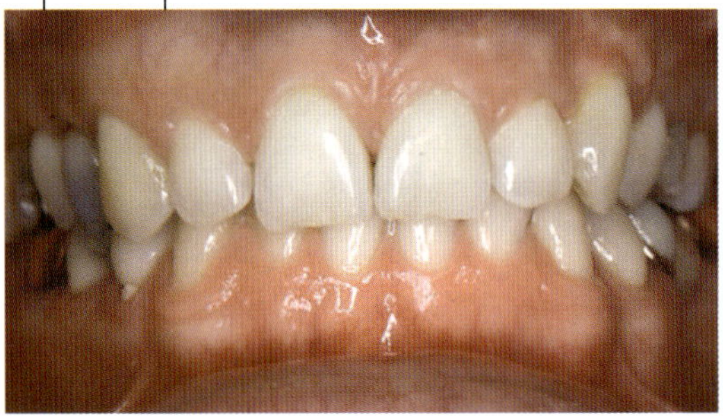

5-115

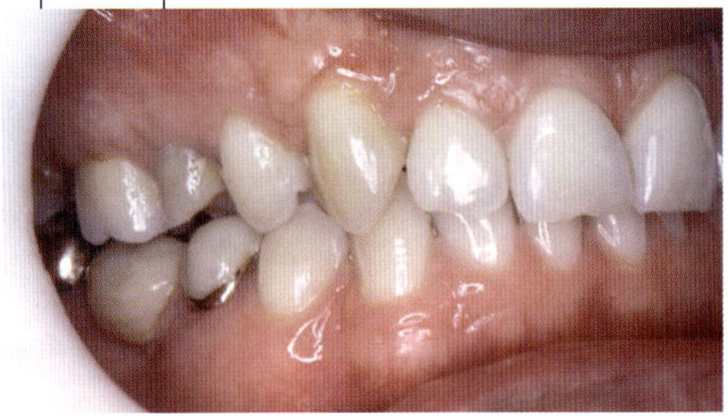

Figs. 5-114 & 5-115
Post-treatment occlusion.

CASE NUMBER 16

The case is one of failure. It concerns a 25 year old patient with upper right impacted canines (Fig. 5-116). A fixed appliance with a palatal bar has been used to increase the anchorage.
The canine crown has been exposed (Fig. 5-117).
The buccal traction caused root resorption of the right lateral incisor and buccal fenestration of the right first premolar. For this reason the arch appliance has been interrupted in order to stop active forces developing (Fig. 5-118). After this phase another attempt at traction followed but it resulted in a negative outcome. Therefore the patient, after being informed of various possibilities, agreed to canine extraction and space closure (Fig. 5-119). The final occlusion was perfectly satisfactory. (Figs. 5-120 & 5-121).

5-116

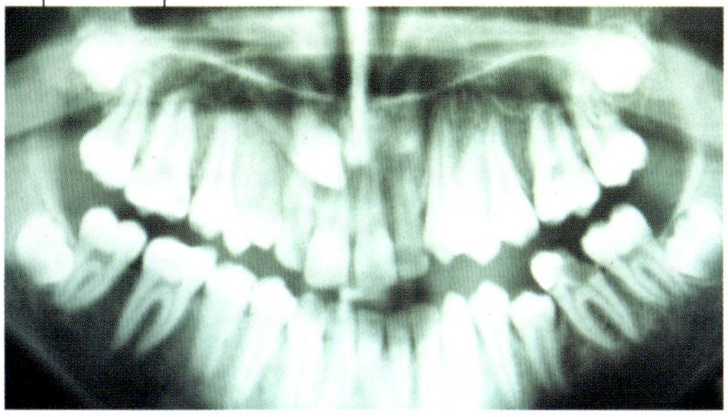

5-117

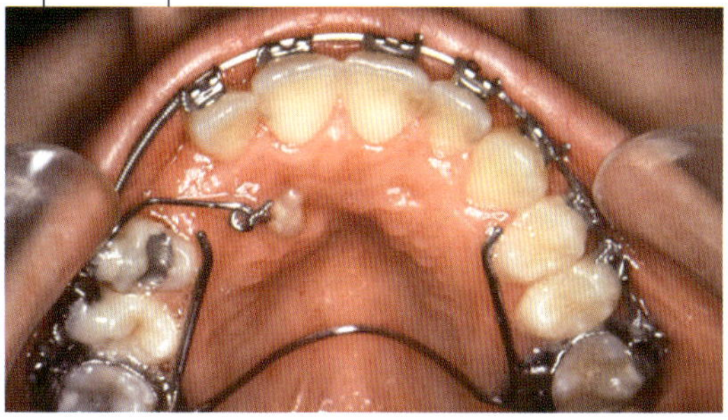

5-118

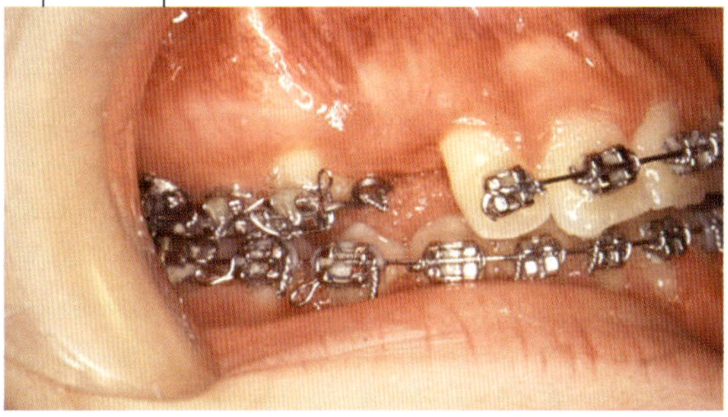

5-119

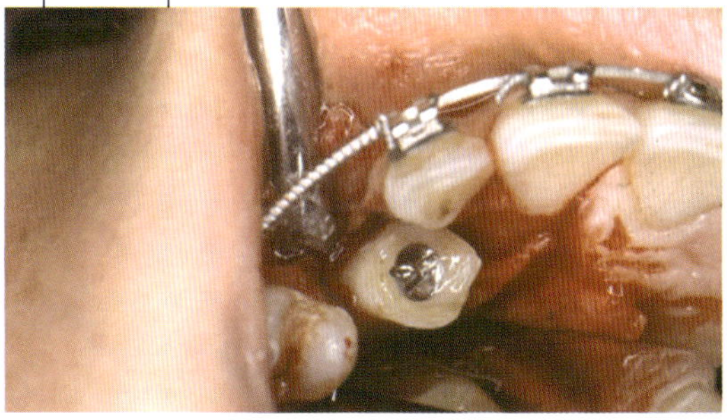

5-120

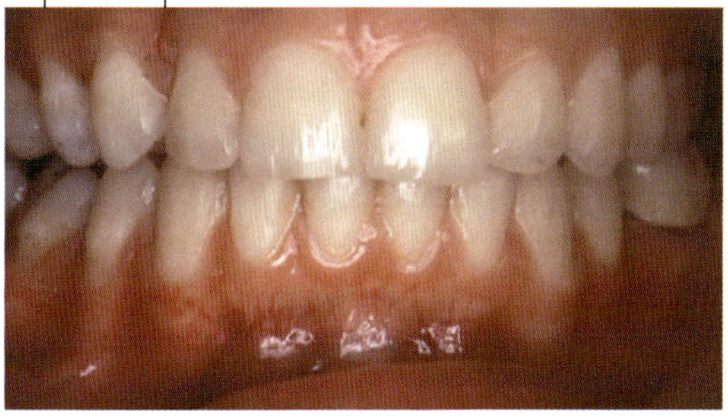

5-121

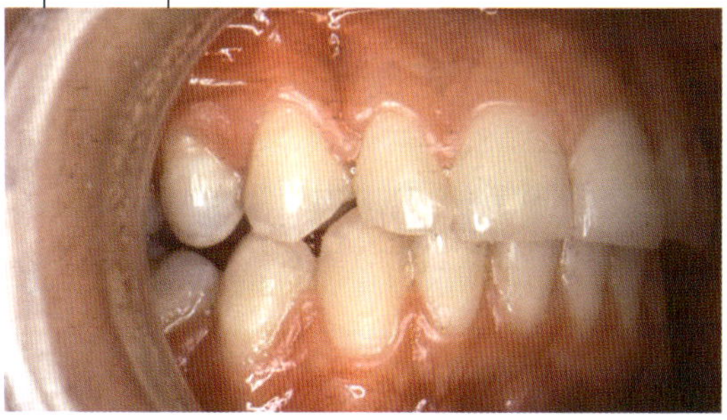

CASE NUMBER 17

The case highlights the importance of clinical observation and preventive procedures. In this 10 year old patient the upper central incisor diastema is suspect. The upper right incisors are shifted to their right. Why is that? (Fig. 5-122) The answer comes from the panoramic radiograph, which shows a good eruptive direction of the upper left canine while the right one is displaced.

The deciduous right canine has been extracted (Fig.5-125). In 80% of cases when the space has been maintained there is a spontaneous correction of the canine eruption pathway (Figs. 5-126 & 5-127).

As indicated by Bonetti et al.[9**] 97% of cases have a successful outcome after extracting the deciduous canine and first deciduous molar. This information is very important and illustrates how, with a simple preventive treatment, it is possible to avoid more complicated solutions.

5-122

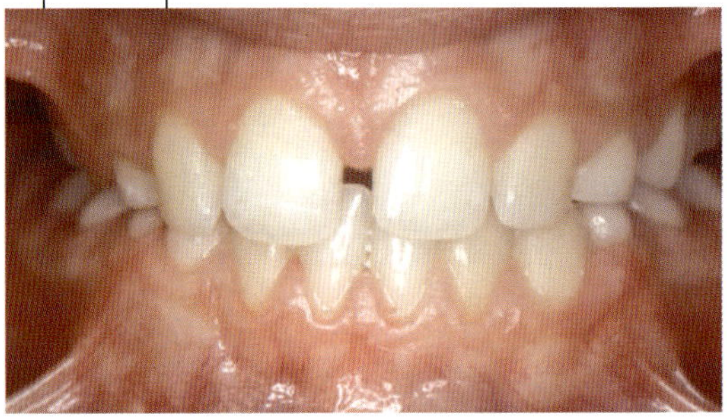

5-123

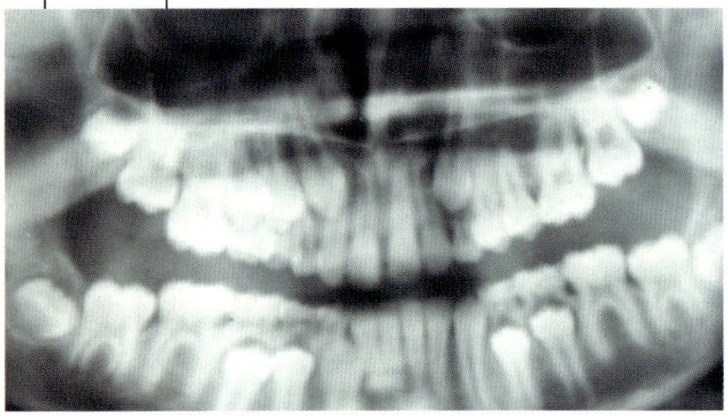

Fig. 5-123 panoramic radiograph showing a good eruptive direction of the left canine while the right one is displaced.

5-124

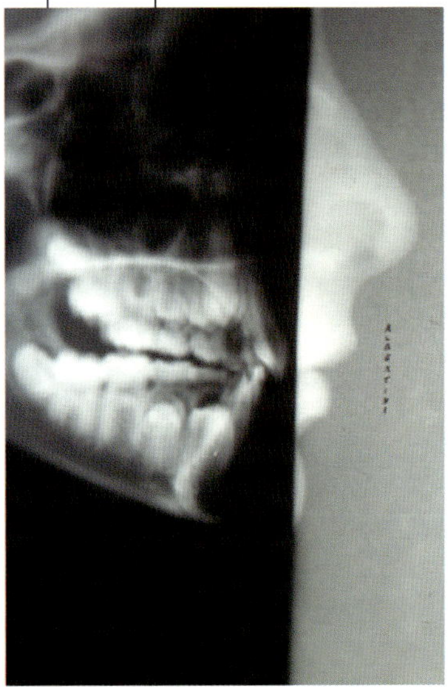

Fig. 5-124 Lateral cephalogram showing the canine palatal displacement.

5-125

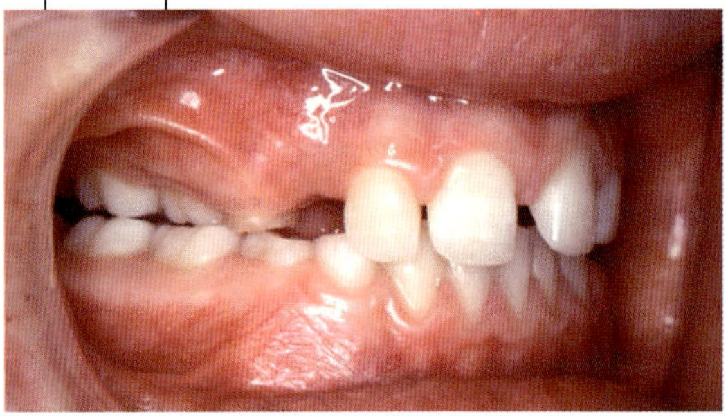

5-126

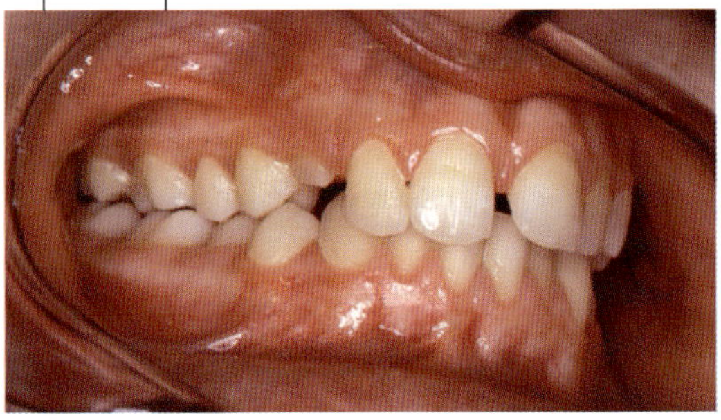

5-127

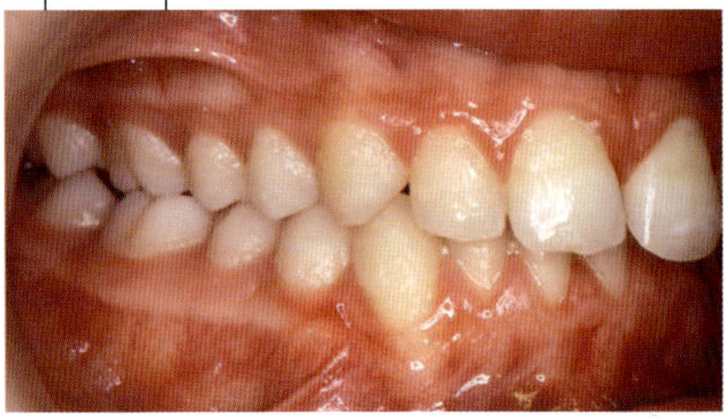

CASE NUMBER 18

IATROGENIC DISPLACEMENT

The previous case showed the importance of deciduous canine extraction in correcting a permanent canine displacement .It is a good example of early treatment. However, early treatment can be irrational and cause iatrogenic outcomes.

Figs. 5-128 and 5-129 show radiographs of a normal situation. But Fig. 5-130 shows that the permanent canines are likely to displace. Just as in the preceding case 17, the deciduous canines were extracted but, instead of keeping the space and waiting for the eruption of the permanent ones, a brace was applied. The lateral incisors have been moved and the anterior spaces closed. The consequence of this procedure is worsening of the canine displacement (Figs. 5-131 & 5-132).

5-128

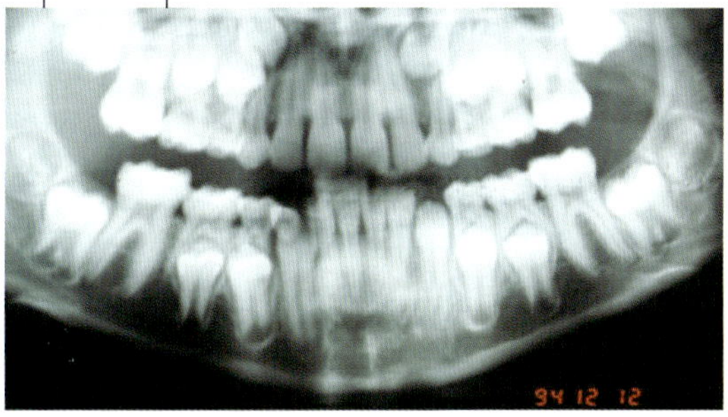

5-129

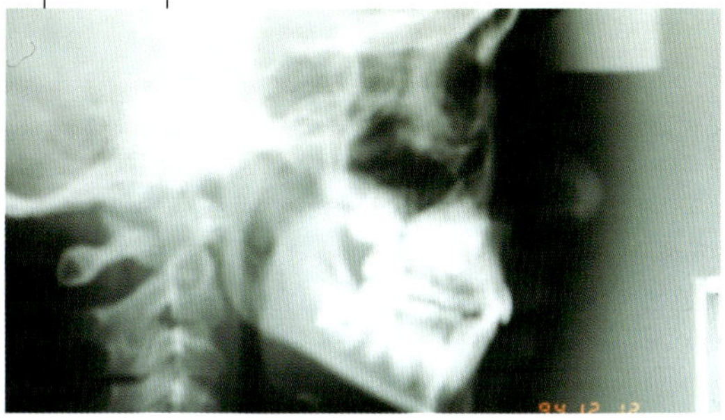

5-130

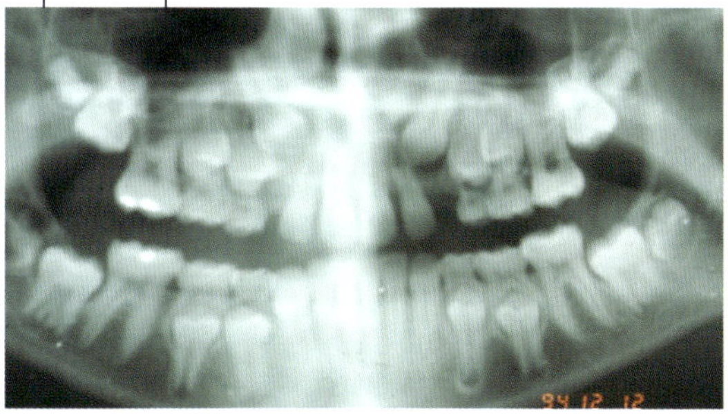

5-131

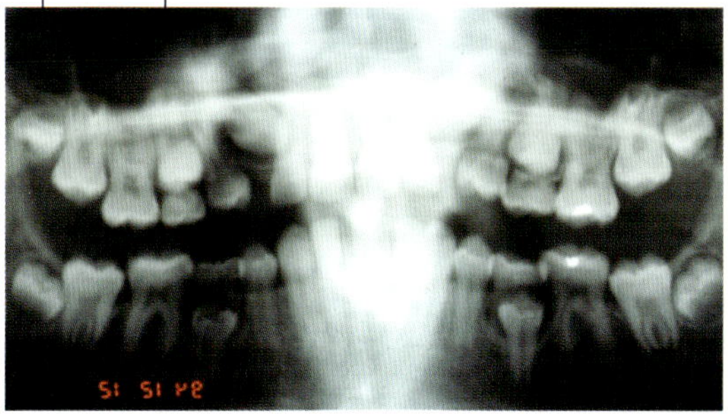

5-132

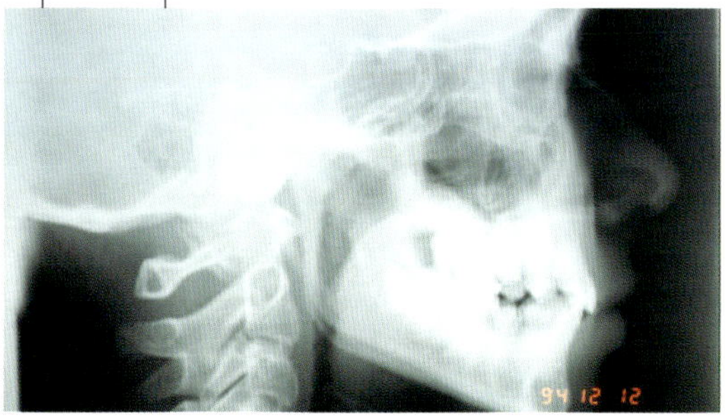

ROOT RESORPTION

We have already seen that the orthodontic movement of impacted canines can cause root resorption in the adjacent teeth, especially of the upper lateral incisors (Figs. 5-133 & 5-134).

Often some mistakes take place during the orthodontic procedure and we have seen how to avoid the main ones.
In the following figures 135 and 136 the upper left lateral incisor shows root resorption which is present prior to the orthodontic treatment.

5-133

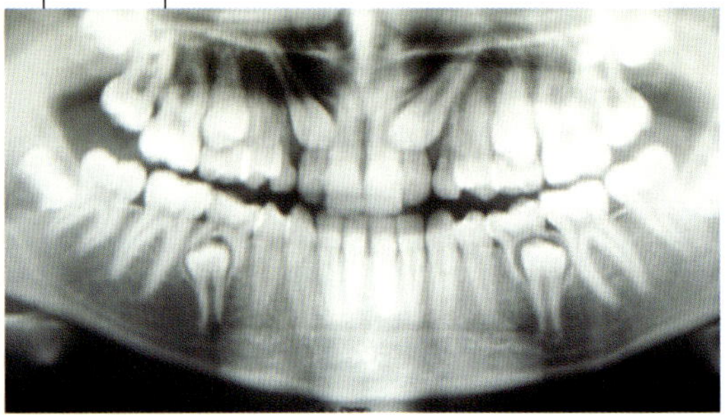

5-134

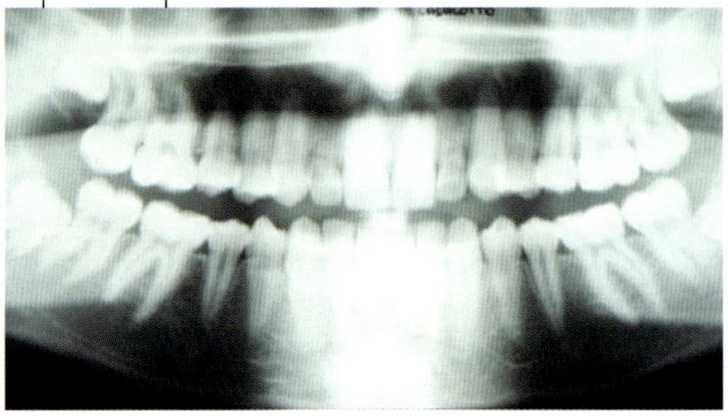

Fig. 5-133 Pre-treatment panoramic radiograph.

Fig. 5-134 Post-treatment panoramic radiograph. Note the upper lateral incisor root resorption.

5-135

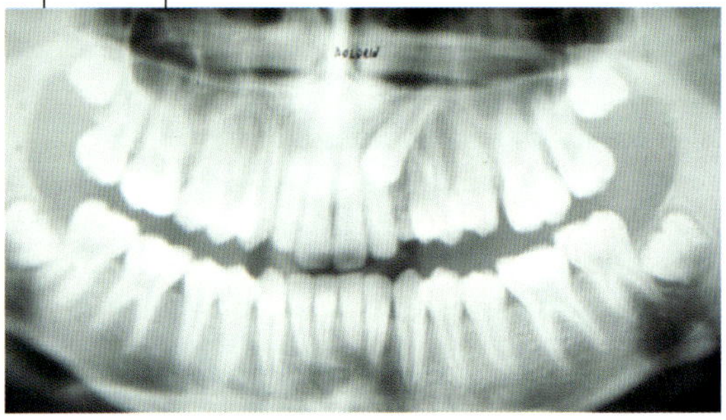

5-136

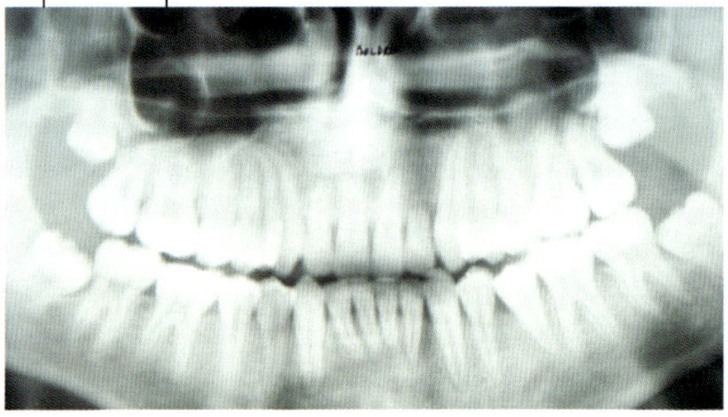

Fig. 5-135 Pre-treatment panoramic radiograph.

Fig. 5-136 Post-treatment panoramic radiograph.

WHAT ARE THE LIMITS OF TREATMENT ON IMPACTED CANINES?

As far as the use of a radiological image is concerned, it has been suggested that when the canine long axis forms an angle of less than 30° with a horizontal plane (for example the palatal plane), there are no chances of success for the treatment.
Considering case 19 it is probably best to say that the treatment was extremely difficult.

5-137

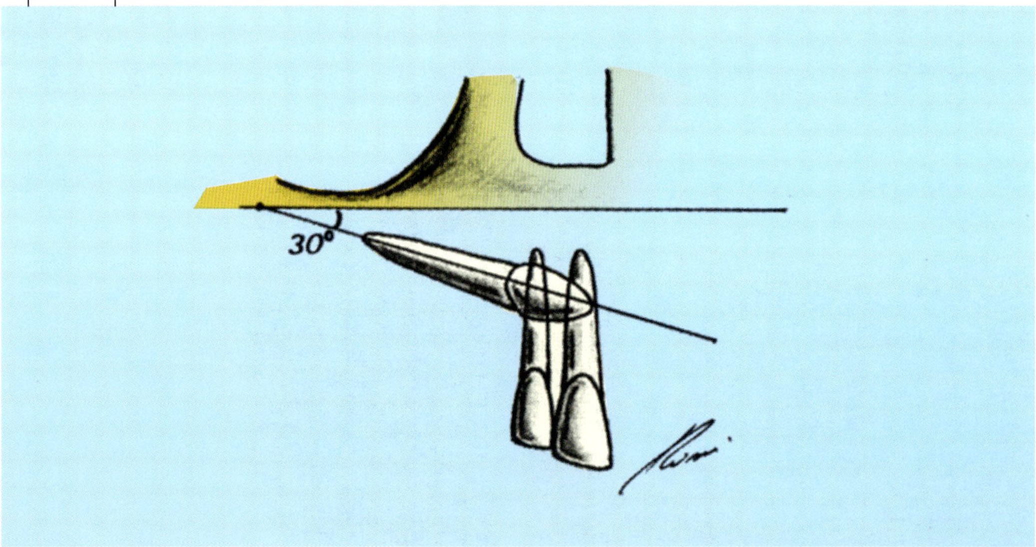

CASE NUMBER 19

The patient is an 11 year old girl. The panoramic radiograph shows a mandibular displacement of the permanent lower canines (Fig. 5-138). Nobody could guarantee their recovery. Firstly the lower left canine was exposed and a button was bonded (Figs. 5-139 & 5-140). A passive metallic ligature was applied (Fig. 5-141) followed by an active traction.

Panoramic radiograph at the end of treatment is shown in Fig. 5-150.

Looking at the final occlusion (Figs. 5-151 & 5-152) makes me ask whether there really are any limits to the treatment of displacements.

5-138

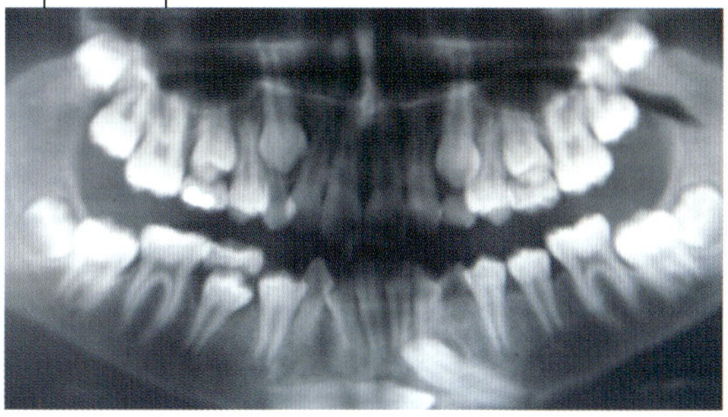

5-139

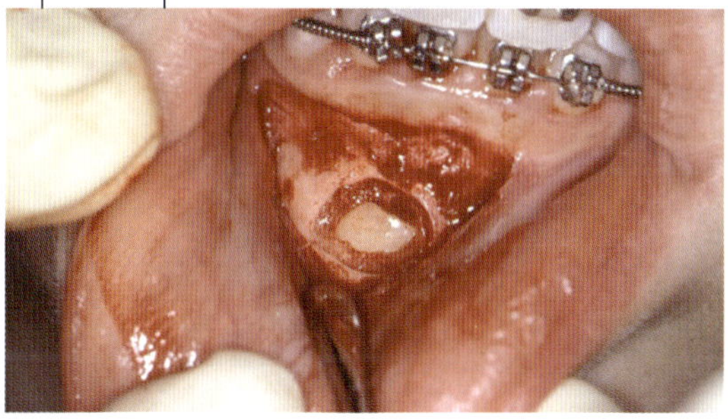

5-140

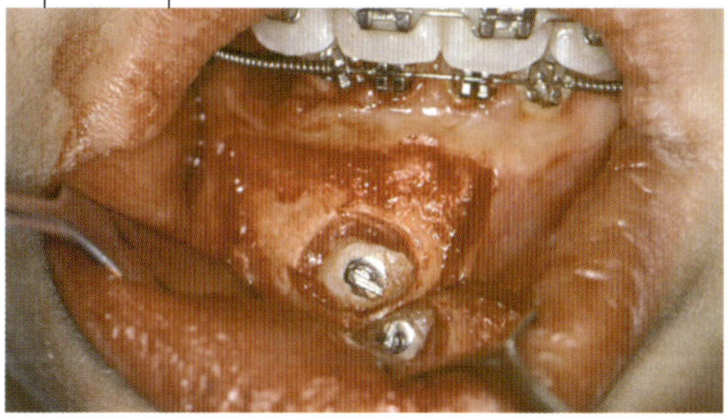

5-141

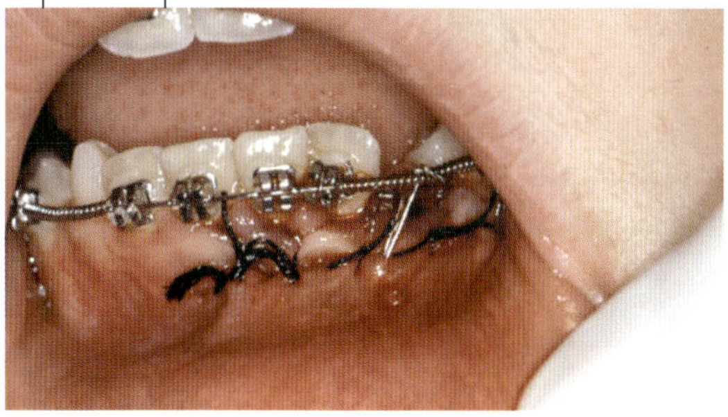

5-142

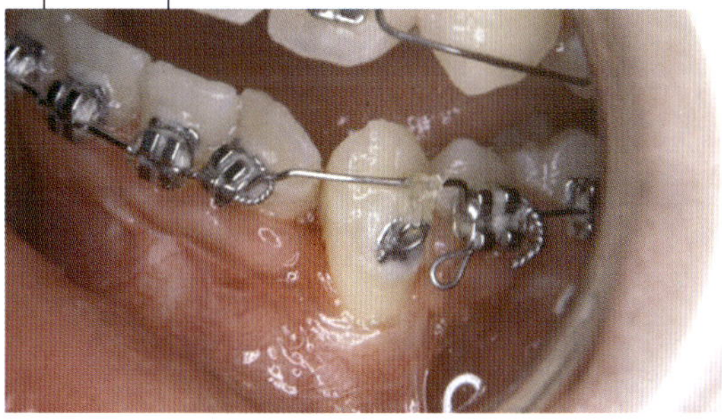

5-143

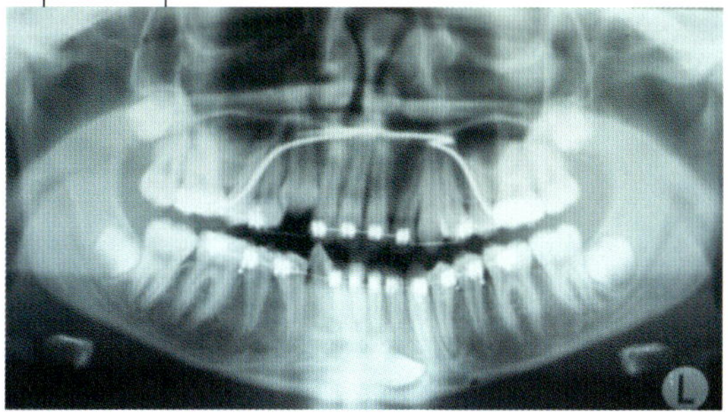

5-144

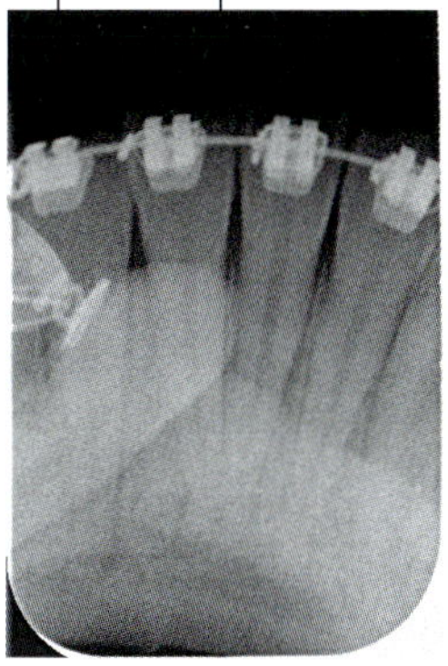

Fig. 5-142 shows the situation after 8 months of elastic traction.

Fig. 5-143 is a panoramic radiograph which shows the lower left canine alignment.

Fig. 5-144 features the same procedure with traction on the lower right canine. The lower right deciduous canine used as an anchorage unit was extraordinary. It offered a wonderful and unexpected resistance to the permanent canine traction (Fig. 5-145). The deciduous canine was extracted before the alignment of the permanent one (Fig. 5-146).

5-145

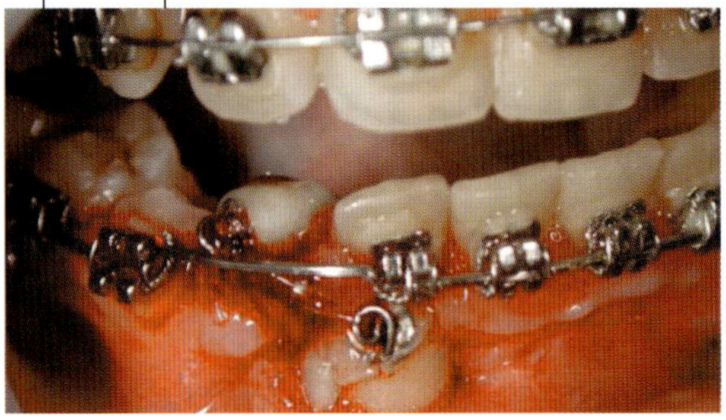

5-146

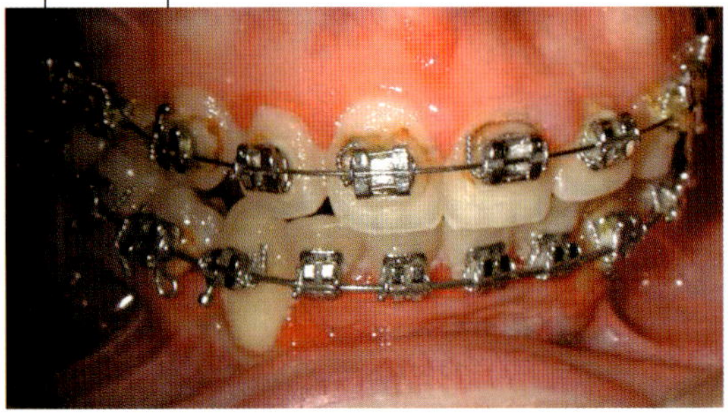

Fig. 5-147 is a radiograph before the deciduous canine extraction. The "heroic" deciduous canine after its extraction is shown in Fig. 5-148.

5-147

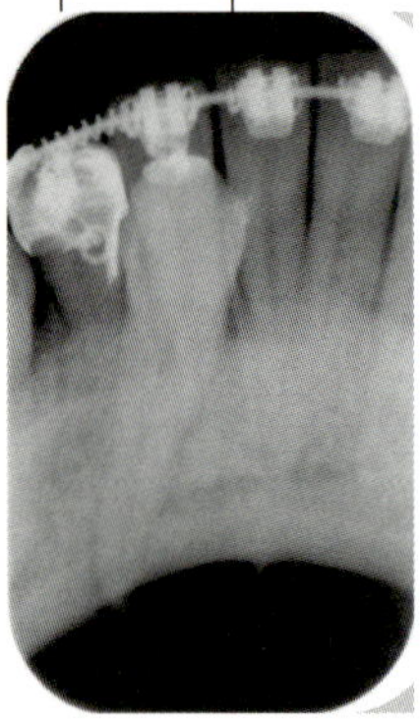

5-148

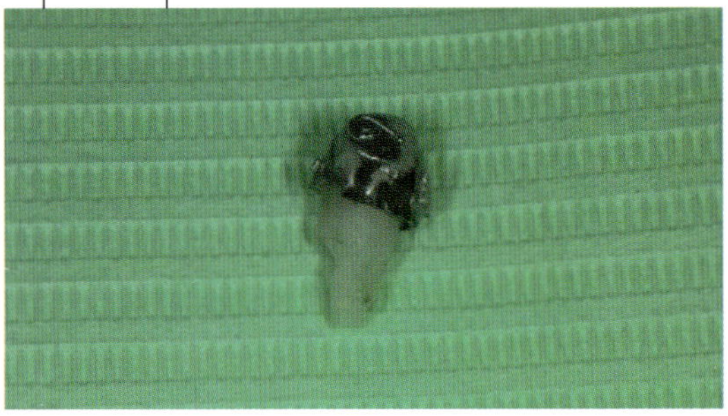

Fig. 5-149 is a radiograph after the deciduous canine extraction (Fig. 5-149).

5-149

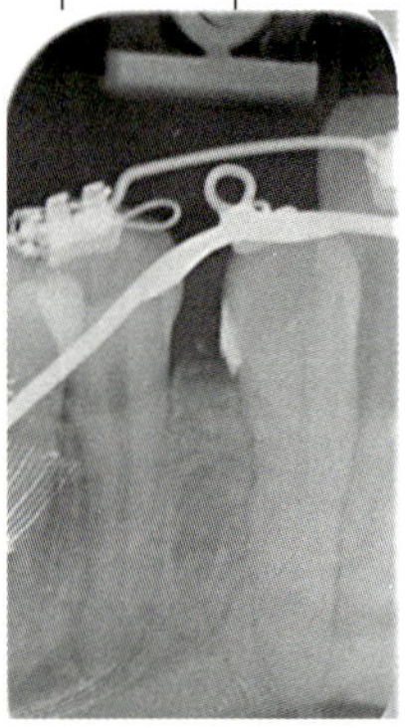

5-150

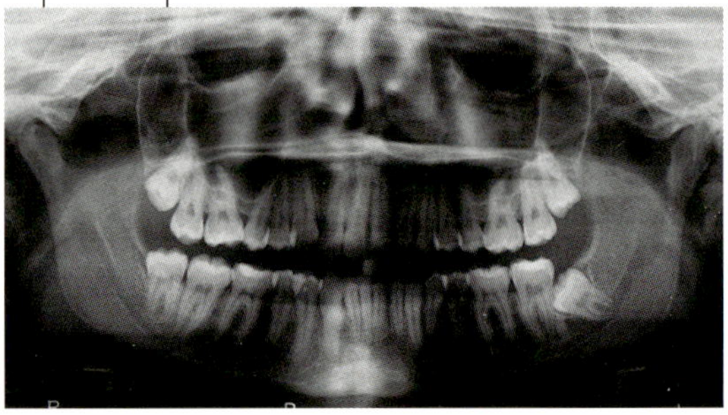

5-151

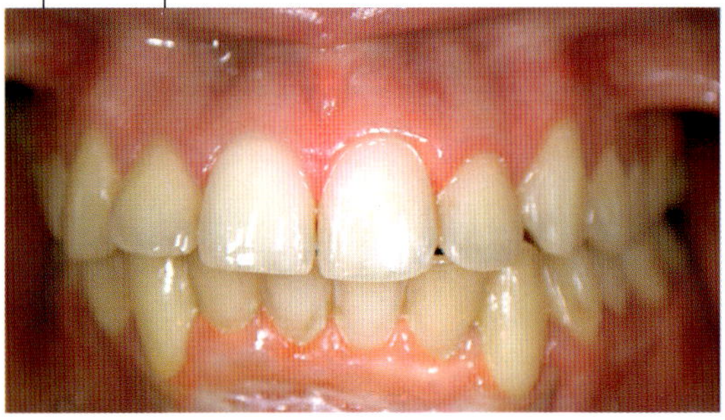

5-152

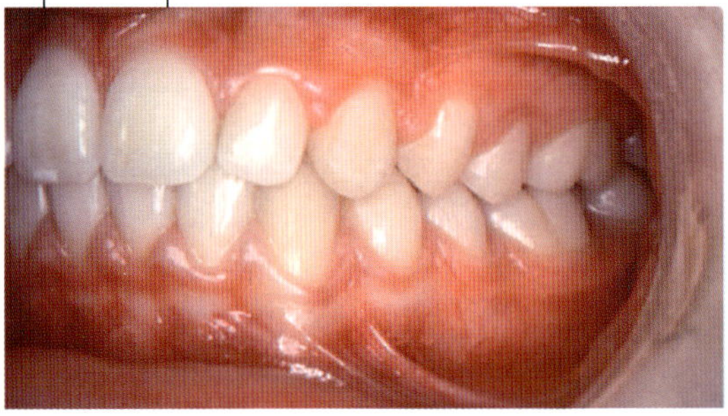

CASE NUMBER 20

This is a 43 year old patient showing a partially erupted upper left canine. After the spontaneous loss of the upper left lateral incisor a fixed brace was applied in order to align the teeth and recover the canine. The real challenge was offered by the anchorage units because all the other teeth were affected by advanced periodontal disease (Fig. 5-153). The teeth withstood the treatment and the canine was aligned (Fig. 5-154).

5-153

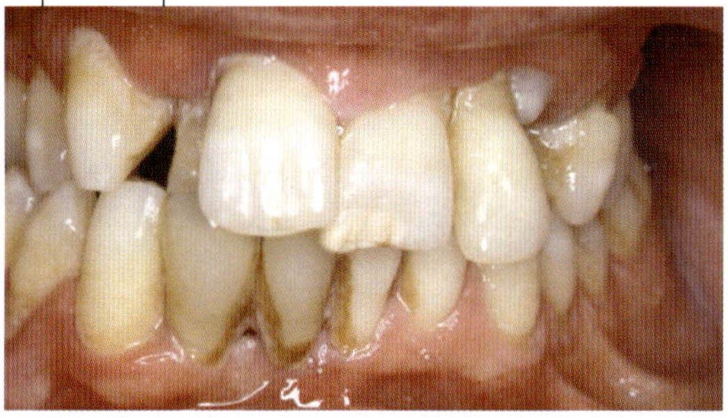

5-154

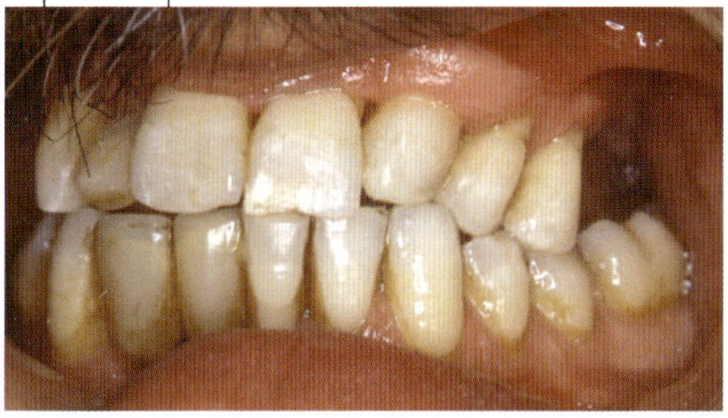

5-155

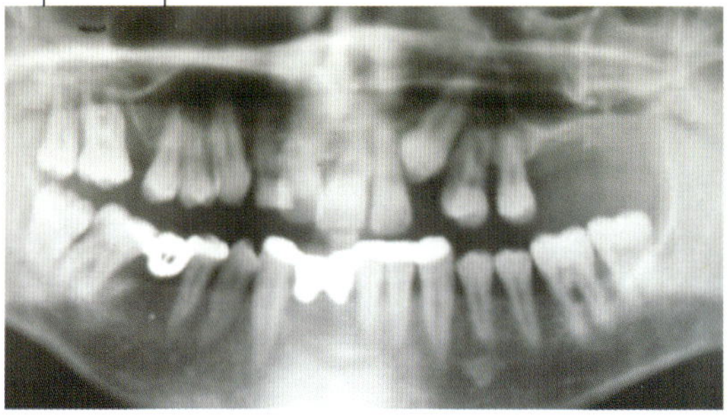

Fig.5-155 Pre-treatment panoramic radiograph.

5-156

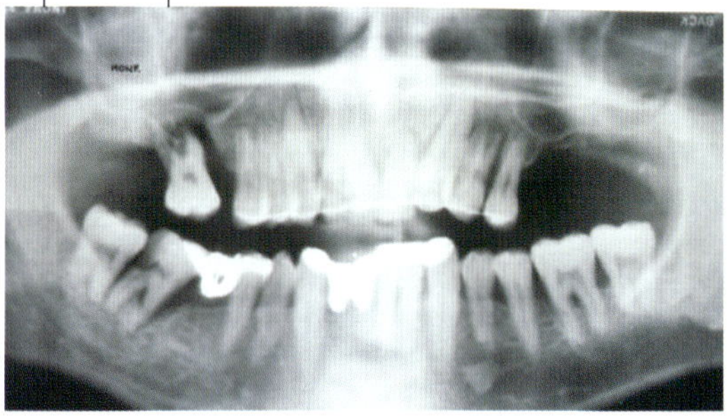

Fig. 5-156 Post-treatment panoramic radiograph.

OTHER TEETH DISPLACEMENT

Lower third molars are more frequently displaced than canines. Usually the only treatment offered is their extraction but the following case shows a very interesting alternative.

CASE NUMBER 21

The panoramic radiograph (Fig. 5-157) shows the pre-treatment situation. After the extraction of the lower right first molar, the space has been orthodontically closed but the third molar is still impacted (Fig. 5-158). Is treatment other than extraction possible?

5-157

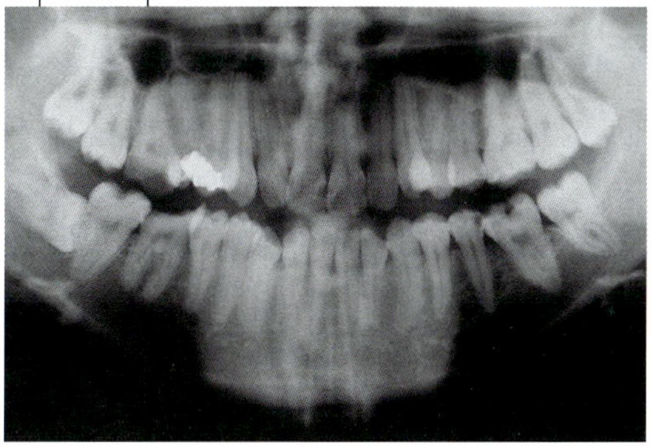

5-158

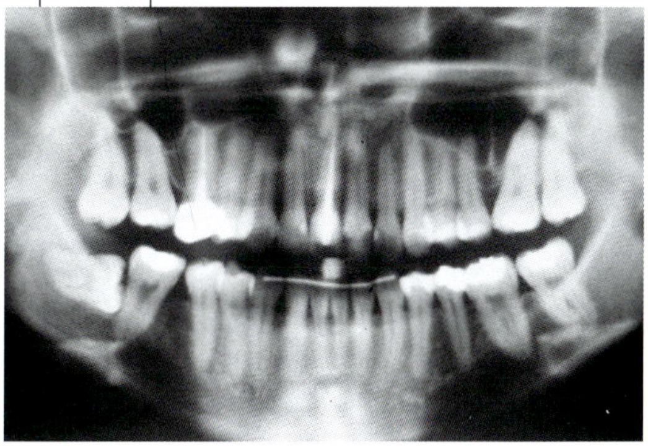

5-159

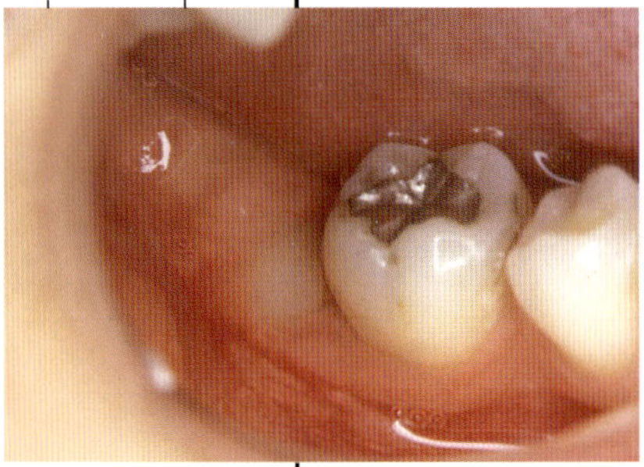

5-160

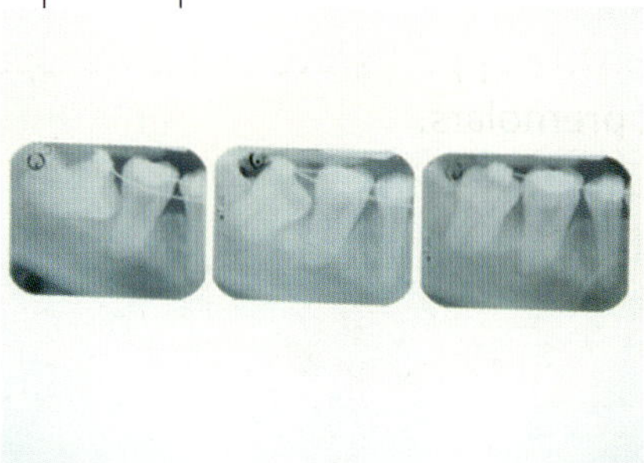

5-161

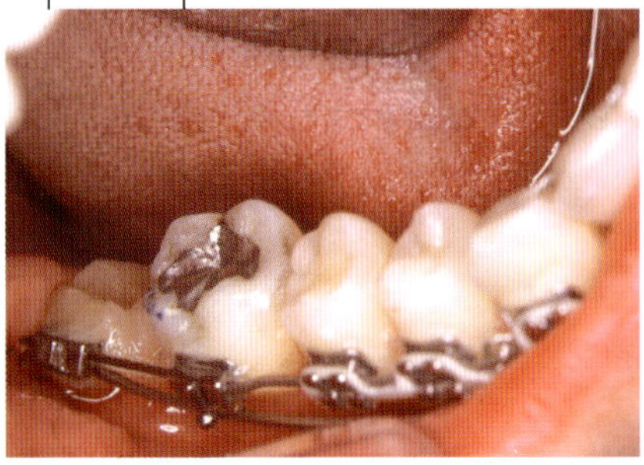

5-162

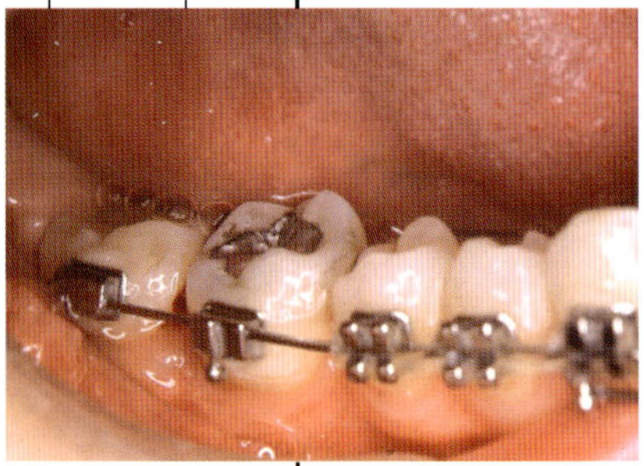

5-163A

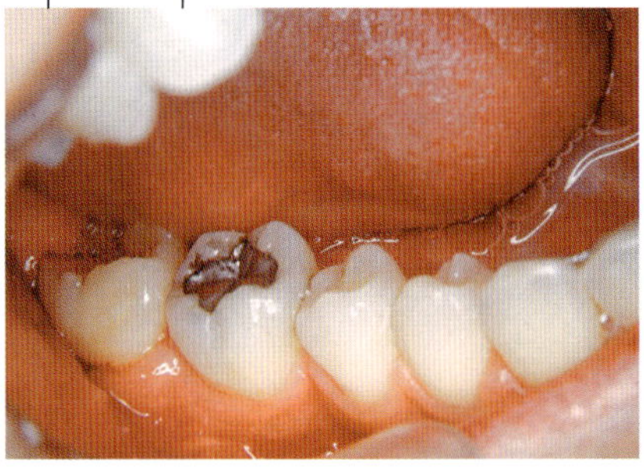

5-163B

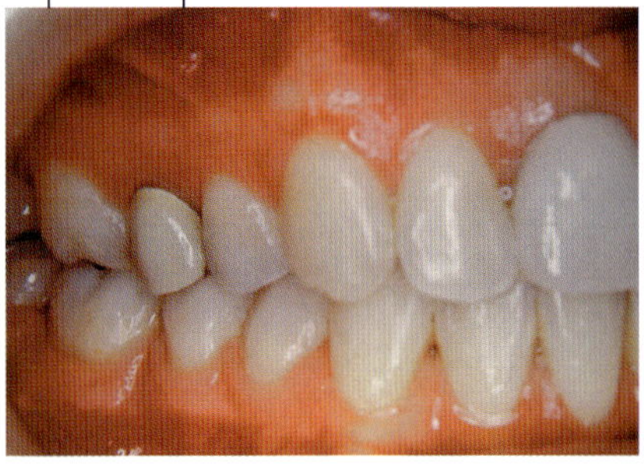

5-164

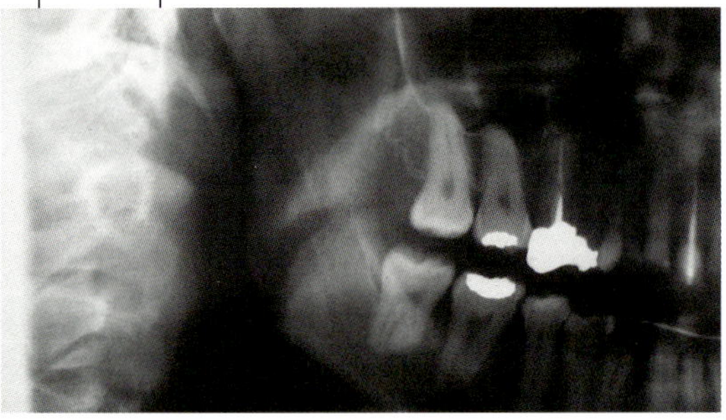

Fig. 5-159 shows the clinical situation before the new orthodontic treatment.

Fig. 5-160 is a series of radiographs showing some steps of the third molar uprighting. Phases of the treatment are visible in Figs. 5-161 to 5-163: B (clinical view).

Fig. 5-164 Final lateral radiograph

TRANSPOSITIONS

Transpositions are less common types of ectopia. They are characterized by situations where one tooth tends to erupt in the place that is normally occupied by another tooth, usually an adjacent one. Maxillary transpositions are more frequent with a prevalence of canines and premolars. Canines and lateral incisors are mainly involved in the mandible.

Transpositions can be:

- complete, when the crowns and roots are transposed
- incomplete, when the crowns are transposed while the apices are in the normal position.

Treatment

There are two possibilities:

- Align the teeth in the transposed order. Usually this treatment is the easier of the two. The occlusion achieved is not ideal but it can be functionally and aesthetically acceptable.
- Align the teeth correcting the transposition. This option is more complex. There can be root interferences and supporting tissue damage, but if it is successful this approach can provide a good occlusion.

The choice of the type of treatment must be absolutely supported by a detailed informed consent.

CASE NUMBER 22

Fig.5-165 is a panoramic radiograph. The upper left canine is transposed and is likely to erupt between the first and second premolars.

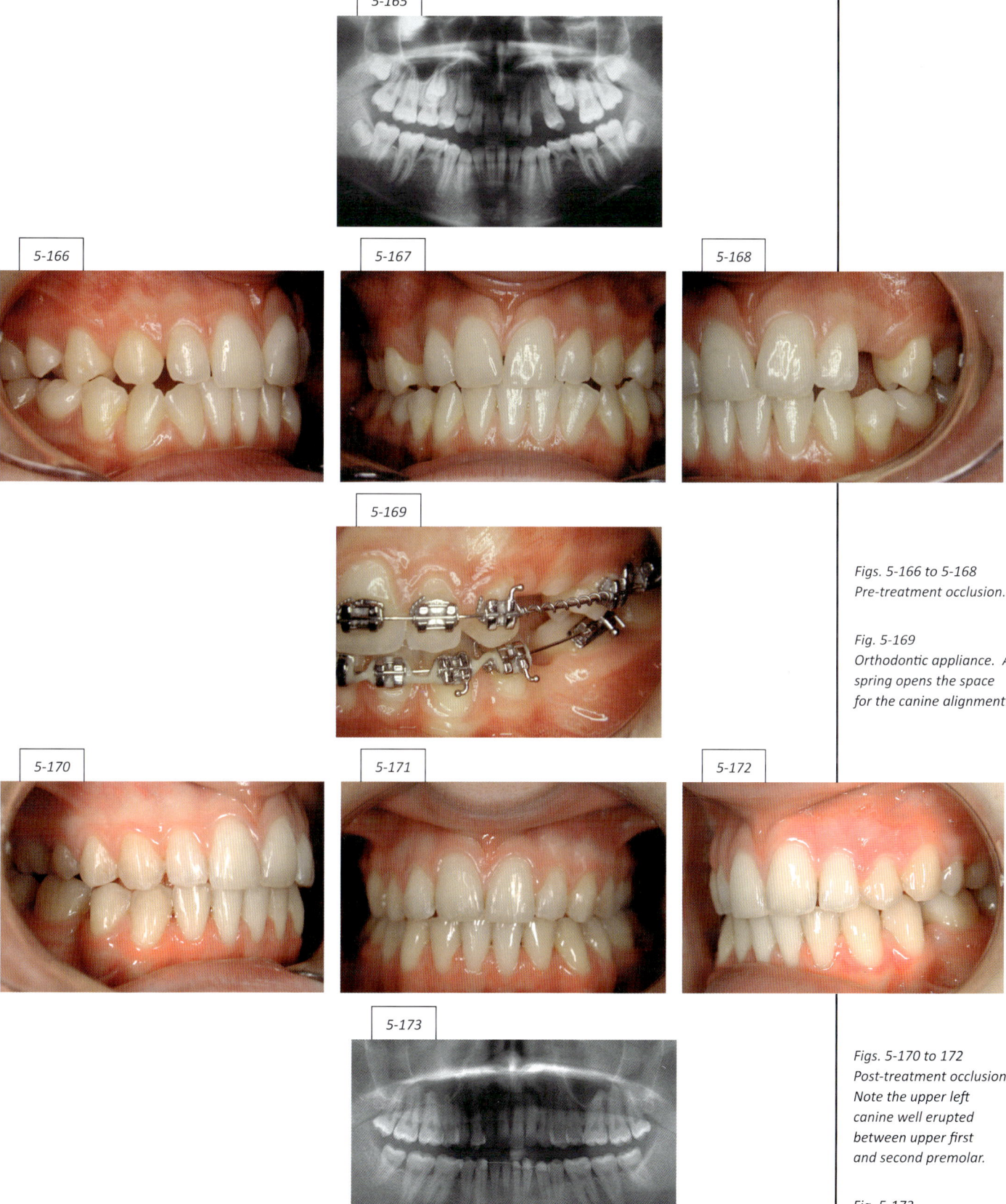

5-165

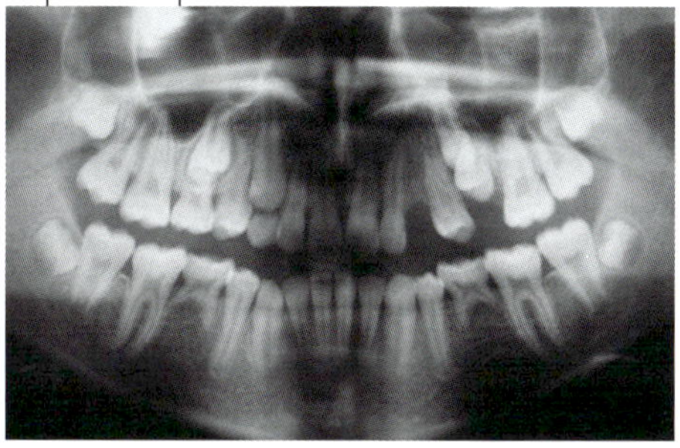

5-166

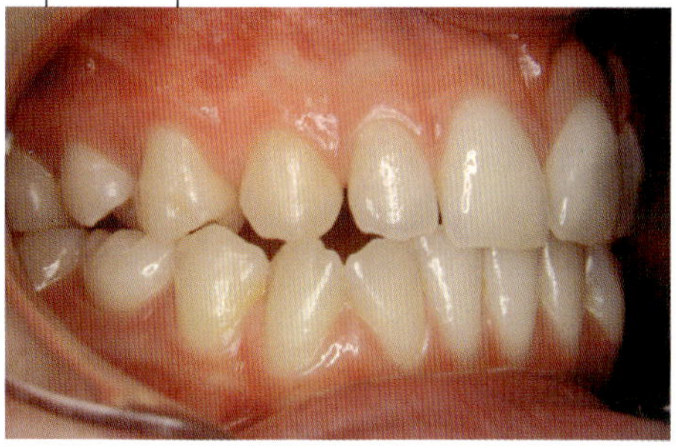

5-167

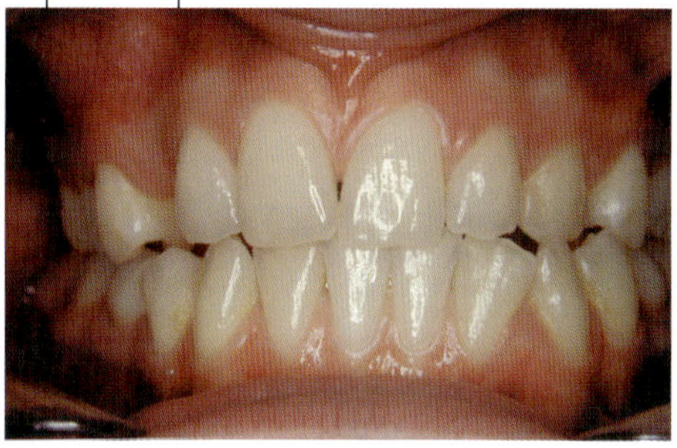

5-168

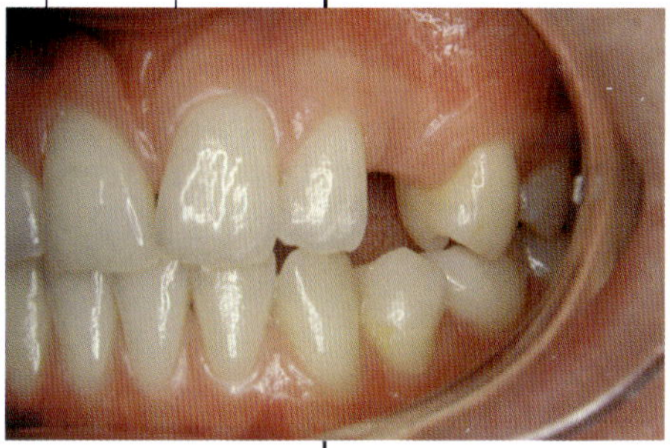

Figs. 5-166 to 5-168
Pre-treatment occlusion.

5-169

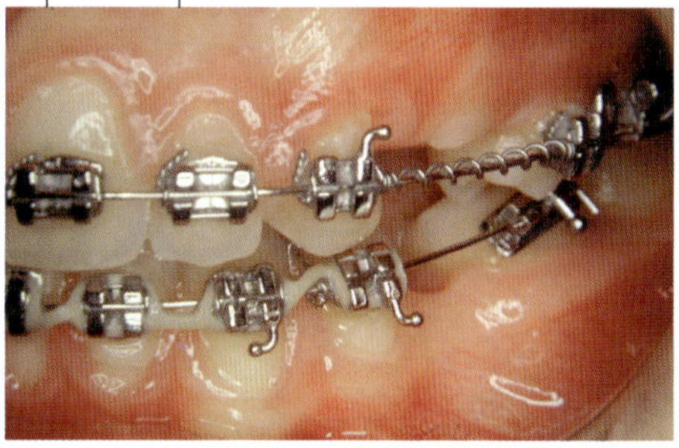

Fig. 5-169
Orthodontic appliance. A spring opens the space for the canine alignment.

5-170

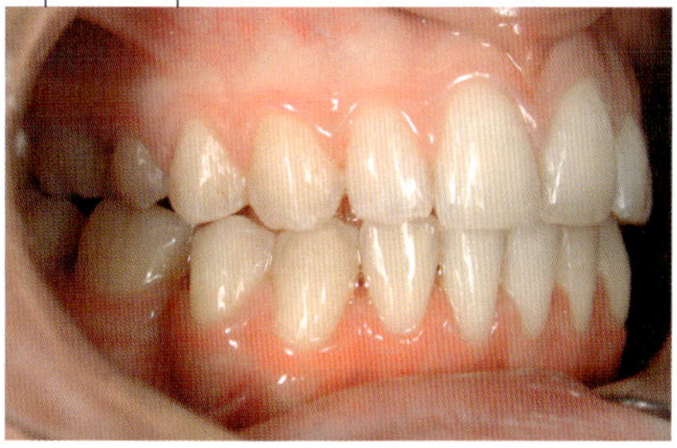

5-171

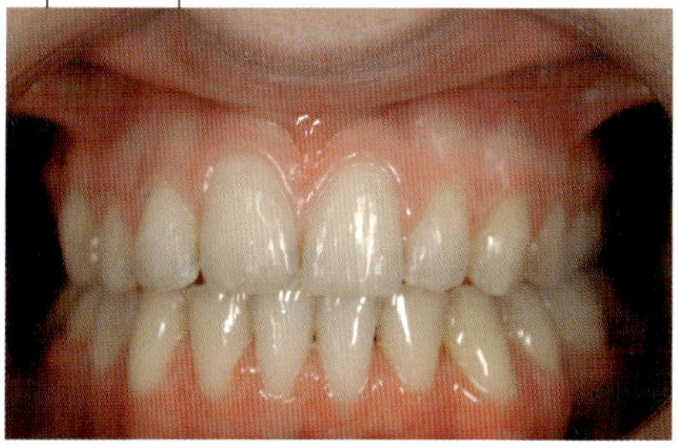

5-172

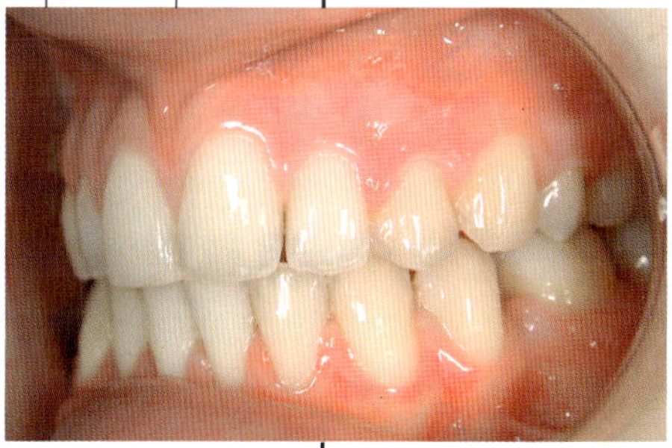

Figs. 5-170 to 172
Post-treatment occlusion. Note the upper left canine well erupted between upper first and second premolar.

5-173

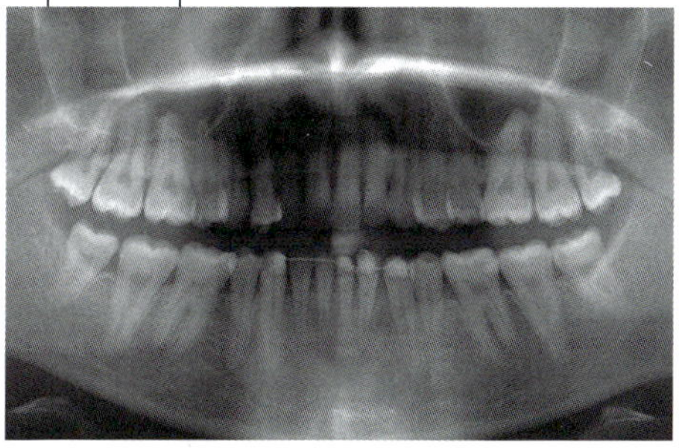

Fig. 5-173
Post-treatment panoramic occlusion.

CASE NUMBER 23

In this case the transposed upper right canine has been aligned in the correct position.

5-174

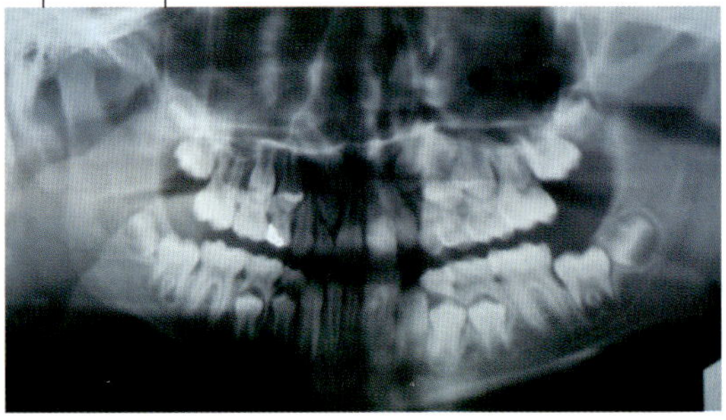

5-175

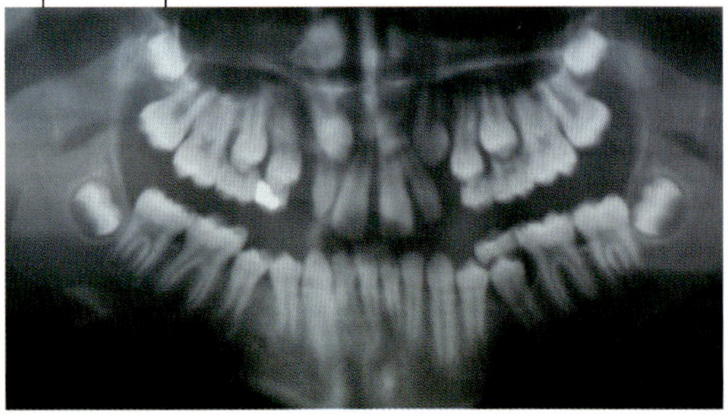

Fig. 5-175 Panoramic radiograph taken at different times, confirming the transposition of the upper right canine.

5-176

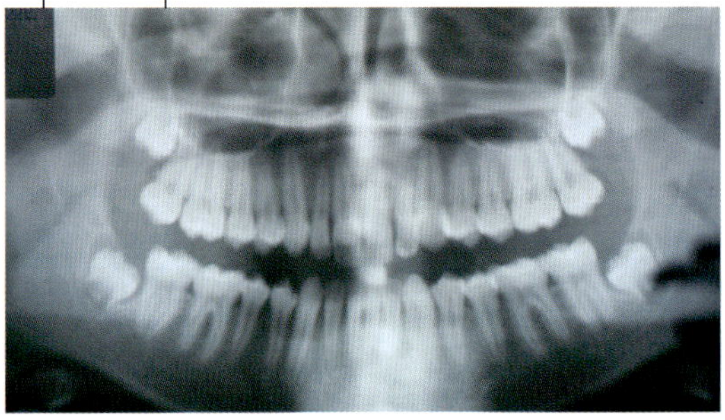

Fig. 5-176 Post-treatment panoramic radiograph.

5-177

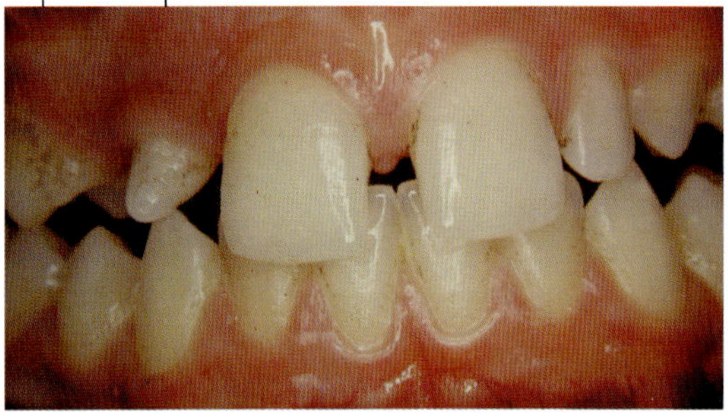

Fig. 5-177 Pre-treatment clinical view. A conoid upper right lateral incisor is present.

5-178

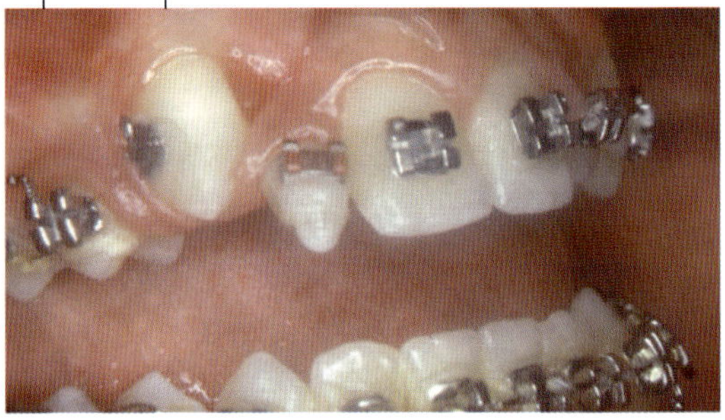

5-179

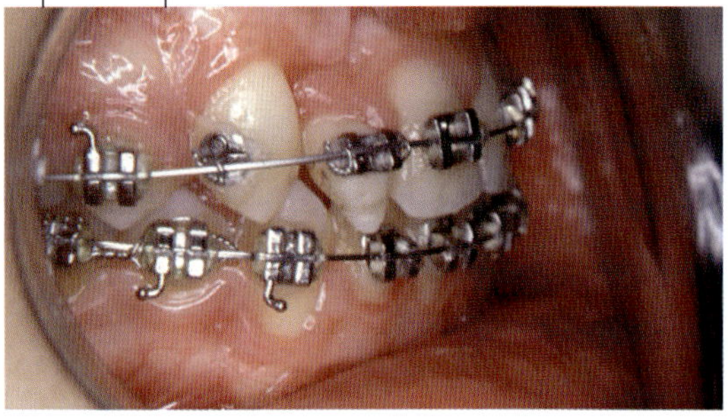

Figs.5-178 & 5-179 Phases of the orthodontic treatment.

5-180

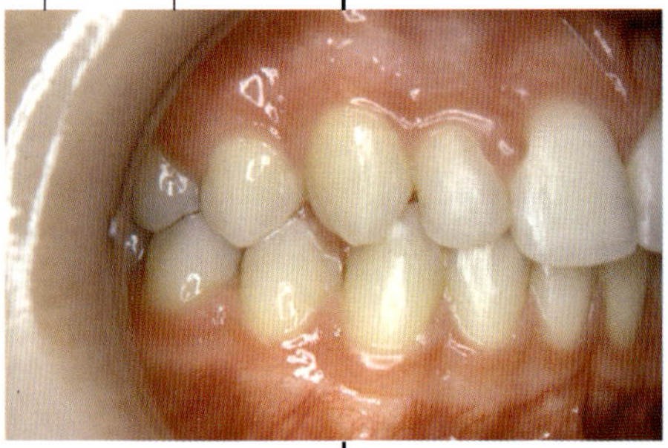

5-181

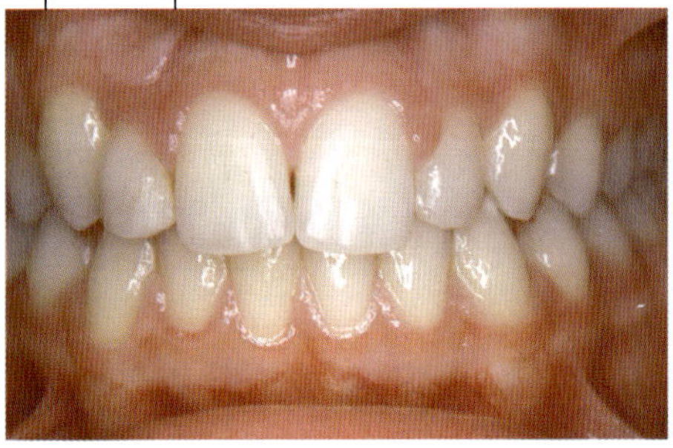

5-182

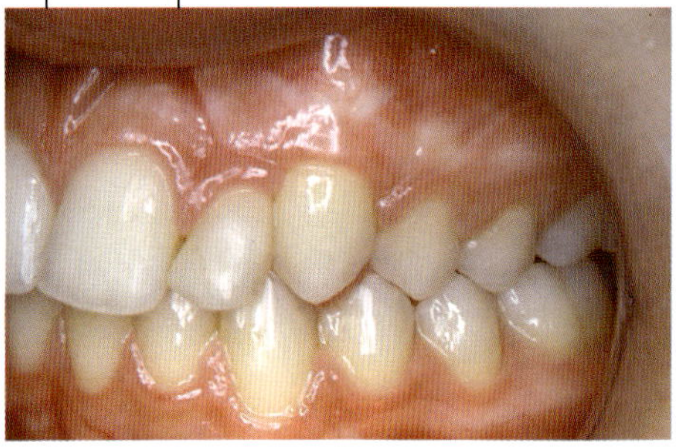

Fig. 5-180/181/182 Post-treatment occlusion. The conoid crown has been widened with the help of composite.

Orthodontics in Clinical Practice

Chapter VI:

Multidisciplinary Treatments: the Relationship between Orthodontics and Other Disciplines

ORTHODONTICS AND PERIODONTOLOGY

Every day we see patients affected by periodontal problems where teeth move in an unwanted way. For example, all dentists are aware of the negative consequences provoked by proclined incisors: they are one of the main causes of interdental spaces, functional and aesthetic issues.

I strongly believe that periodontal treatment limited to scaling, root planning and eventually followed by surgery, is unacceptable for a modern dentistry practice. In many cases orthodontic correction is necessary.

One problem is that usually periodontologists do not know much about orthodontics. Similarly, many orthodontists are not knowledgeable about periodontology. Another problem is that orthodontic treatment can be very dangerous for the periodontal status of many patients. Moreover, the periodontal patient is usually adult while orthodontists mainly treat young people.

However, when we see situations of extreme occlusal disorder such as in Figs. 6-1 to 6-6 an ortho-perio treatment is the best. What other possible solutions do we have? In situations like this, prosthetics give a bad aesthetic result. Also, many patients prefer to keep their natural teeth and accept the orthodontic treatment.

CASE NUMBER 1

6-1

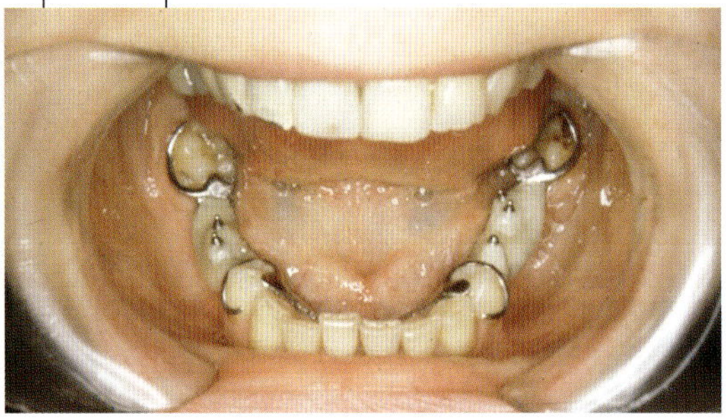

6-2

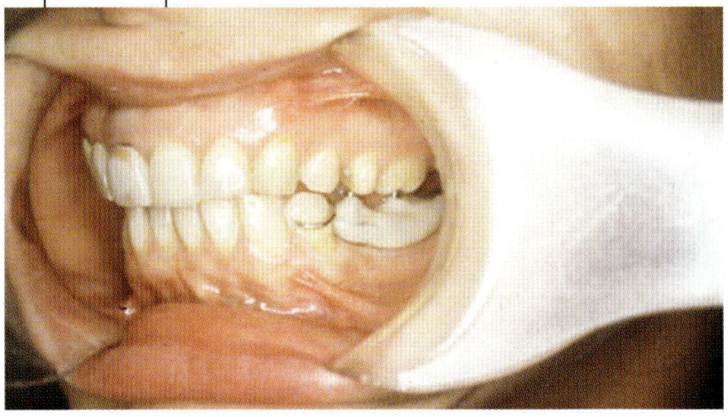

6-3

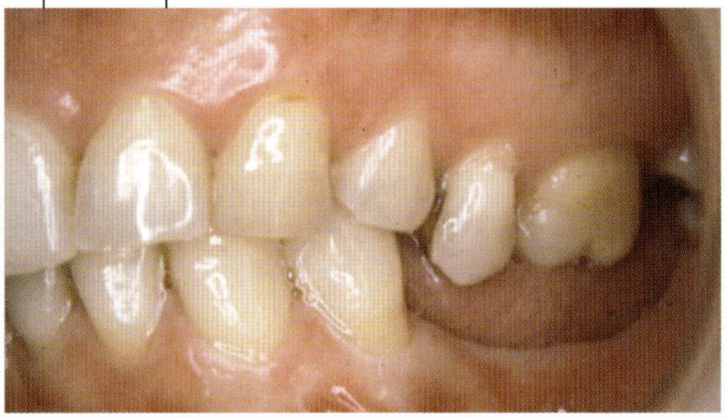

6-4

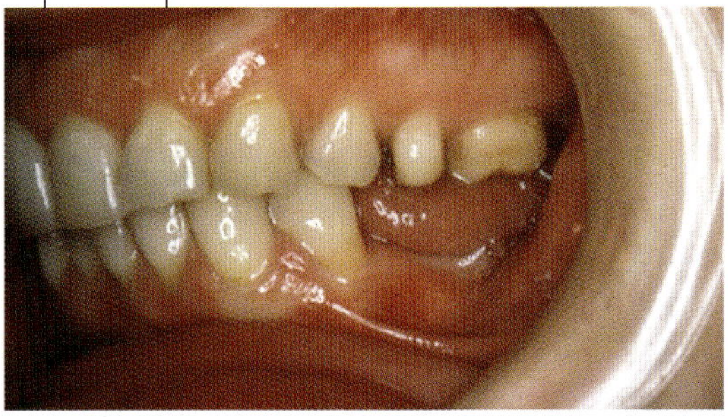

6-5

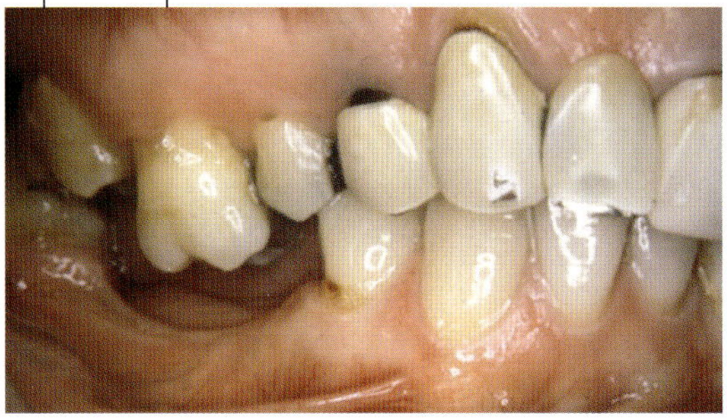

6-6

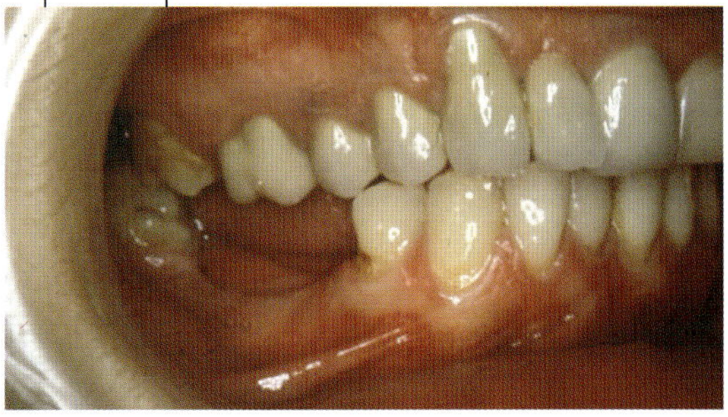

Fig. 6-1 intraoral view of the device with coil spring screws to intrude the extruded upper molars.

Fig. 6-2 4 months later. Note the change of the upper occlusal plane.

Fig. 6-3 intraoral view left. Note the upper margin of the dental filling on the second upper left premolar.

Fig. 6-4 4 months later, wearing the device for at least 20 hours a day. Note the upper margin of the dental filling on the upper left premolar. Compare it with fig. 3

Fig. 6-5, 6-6 On the right side a ceramic bridge has been applied.

6-7

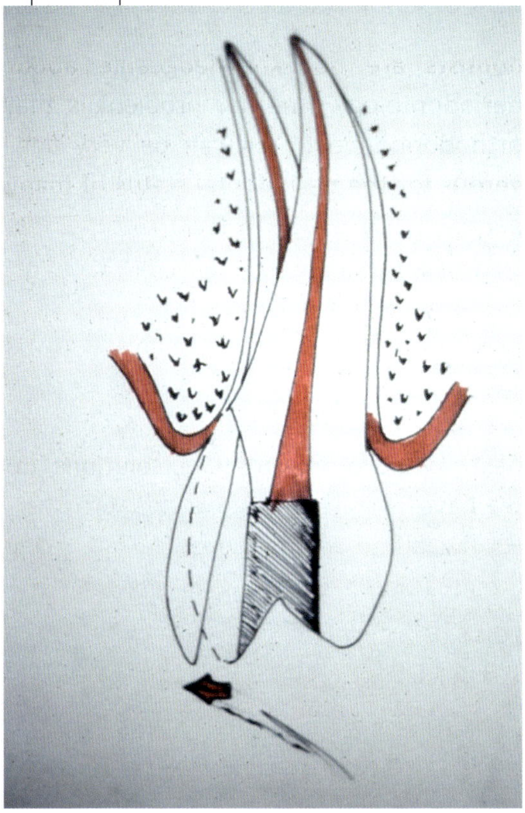

6-8

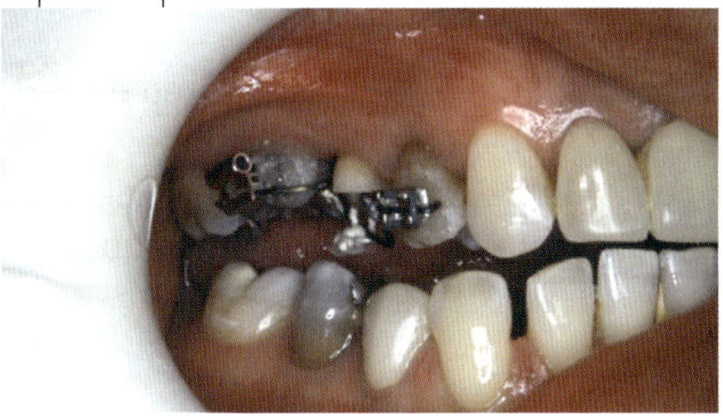

Fig. 6-7
Crown fracture under the gingival level. Extrusion is important in order to gain a correct biological width.

Fig. 6-8
Second upper premolar root where with traction between a pin in the root canal and a sectional fixed appliance it is possible to perform the tooth extrusion.

At that point, a more satisfactory prosthetic or cosmetic dentistry can follow.

HOW CAN TEETH WITH PERIODONTAL PROBLEMS BE MOVED?

Every author suggests the use of light force only. Hygienic dental plaque control is very important, to avoid decay but above all to prevent gingival inflammation, which can worsen the periodontal status. In fact, if the inflammation extends more deeply it can lead to periodontitis, which can cause alveolar bone resorption.
When compared to a traumatic occlusion, an orthodontic movement can worsen the situation. Even though some authors disagree, I personally suggest prudence and caution, so, in a case of periodontitis, start with a medical treatment and refrain from orthodontic movement.

INTRUSION

In order to intrude a tooth, very light forces (10–15g for one root) are necessary. The periodontal risk of infection derives from the change of bacterial dental plaque from Gram+ to Gram -. Melsen[168] explains clearly how many wonderful treatments are possible in adult patients with periodontal problems. Intrusion has an important part in all those cases.

EXTRUSION

Orthodontic dental extrusion is usually well accepted by periodontologists because it keeps dental plaque away from deeper structures and in this way there is less risk of infections.
There are two modalities of extrusion, slow or rapid. With a slow extrusion the root moves "with" the bone and can improve vertical infrabony pockets. A rapid extrusion is obtained with a weekly fiberotomy of superficial periodontal fibers around the root. This method allows the rescue of roots which move "through" the bone and gain a correct biological width in 1-2 months.

GINGIVAL RECESSIONS

Keratinized gingiva is very important for periodontal health. It is a barrier around the tooth that protects deeper structures from, for example, bacterial migration. Gingival recessions are mainly caused by the inflammatory action of dental plaque and by traumatic tooth brushing. Various studies have been carried out on the subject:-
Wennström et al.[1*1] found a relationship between the width of keratinized gingiva and the development of gingival recession during orthodontic dental movement in monkeys. In particular they stated that a

thin keratinized gingiva is the determinant factor of gingival recession.

Patterson et al.[1*2] found that in patients who received incorrect orthodontic treatment with excessive anterior dental proclination there was less keratinized gingiva.

Yared et al.[1*3] concluded that after orthodontic treatment, severe gingival recessions are more frequent when lower incisors have a thin attached gingiva and are more than 95° proclined.

Vanzin et al.[1*4] noted that with an excessive incisor proclination there are more risks of gingival recessions in an adult patient than in a youth.

Artun and Grobéty[1*5] found that the pronounced advancement of the mandibular incisors may be performed on adolescent patients with a dentoalveolar retrusion without increasing the risk of recession.

Allais and Melsen[1*6] concluded that pre-existing gingival retractions appeared or worsened in only a few orthodontic treatments performed on adults whom they examined.

Considering those contradictory results, how should a good orthodontist behave? Once again, I suggest prudence! It is especially important when treatments are planned for expanding dental arches with a minimal or thin keratinized gingiva. In those cases, does mucogingival surgery have to be performed before or after orthodontic treatment?

Before:

- when there is an absence or a minimal level of keratinized gingiva and the teeth need to be moved to a risky position (expansion).
- in doubtful cases.

After:

- when there is a traumatic occlusion (deep bite, cross bite)
- when the teeth need to be moved to a more favourable position (more centred in the alveolar bone).

The following cases can help us better understand the situation.

CASE NUMBER 2

In this case there was a gingival recession on the lower central incisor caused by dental plaque and by an anterior cross bite (traumatic occlusion). Orthodontic treatment with four first premolar extractions was planned. This way the lower incisors were moved to a more centred position in the alveolar bone without mucogingival surgery.

6-9

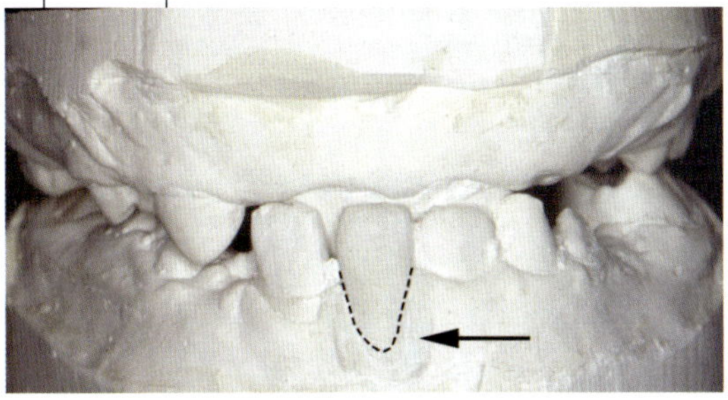

Fig. 6-9
Pre-treatment dental casts. Note the recession on the lower central incisor.

6-10

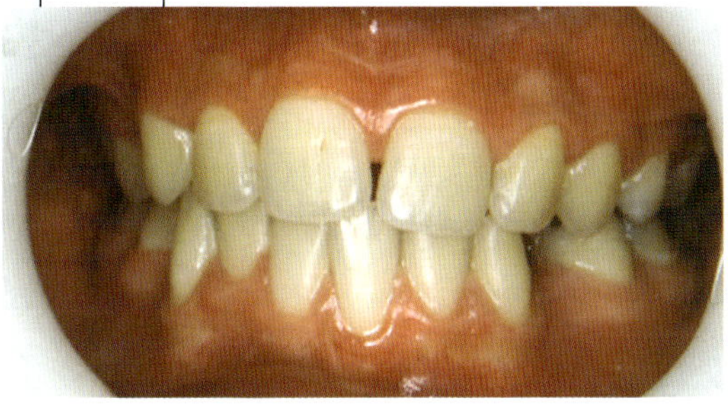

Fig. 6-10
Clinical view after extraction of the first four premolars and the cross bite correction.

6-11

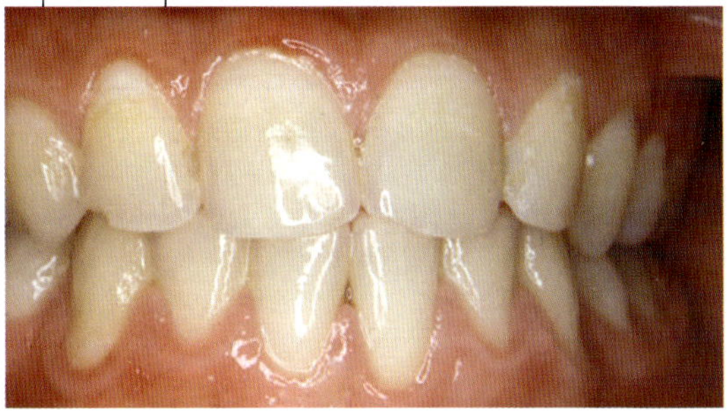

Fig. 6-11
Occlusion 10 years later. Note the good periodontal status without mucogingival surgery.

CASE NUMBER 3

In this case there is also a lower central incisor recession caused by dental plaque and an anterior cross bite. However, here an orthodontic treatment without extraction is planned.

An incisor proclination is expected, so mucogingival surgery precedes the orthodontic treatment.

6-12

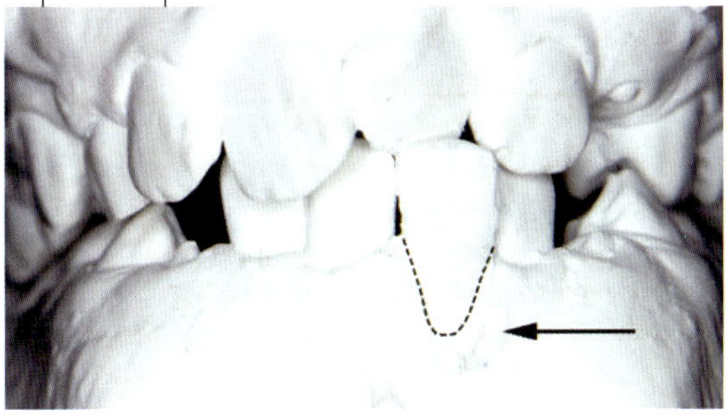

Fig. 6-12
Pre-treatment dental casts. Anterior cross bite and gingival recession on the lower central incisor.

6-13

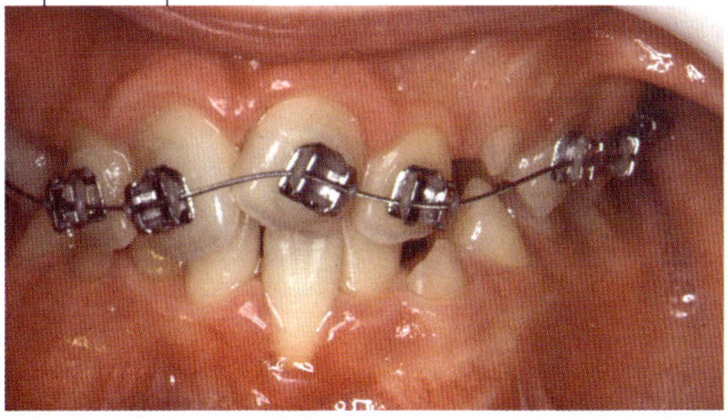

Fig. 6-13
After the cross bite correction, a mucogingival surgery (free gingival graft) is performed before the orthodontic treatment.

6-14

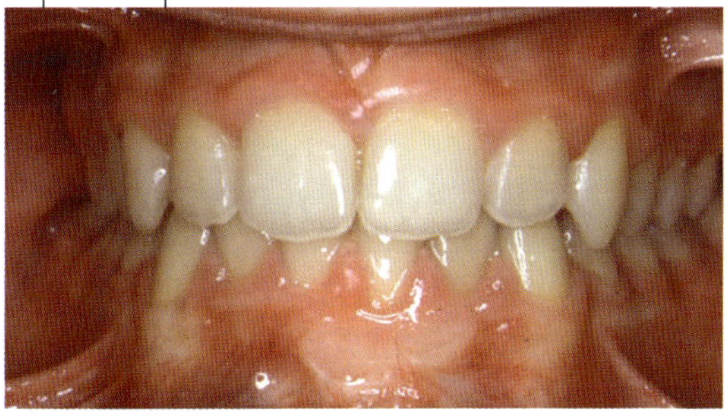

Fig. 6-14
Post-treatment occlusion. Notice the gingival graft which gives a good amount of keratinized gingiva.

CASE NUMBER 4

In this case there is advanced periodontal disease with deep pockets in the lower arch as well.
Would you accept the results of the conventional periodontal treatment shown?

6-15

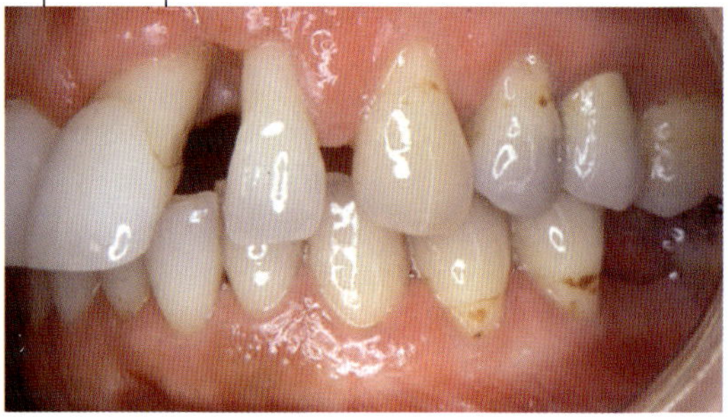

6-16

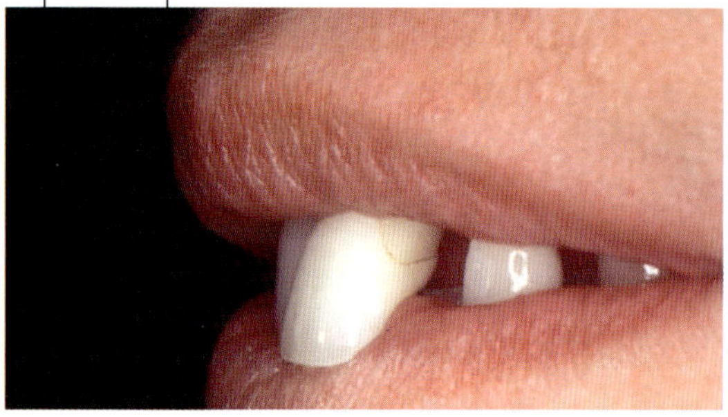

Figs. 6-15 & 6-16 Clinical view after questionable periodontal treatment on the upper arch..

While respecting the correct informed consent procedure I always explain to my patients the following different choices they have in order to improve a situation like this:

a) Dental crown enlargements with composite, prosthetic crowns. They lead to an unsatisfactory aesthetic result with wide interdental spaces.
b) Extractions followed by prosthetic bridges or implants. *Very often they lead to poor aesthetic results.*
c) More extractions followed by an over-denture on implants. *Good aesthetic result but irreversible mutilation.*
d) Ortho-perio treatment.

In my practice, 90% of my patients choose the ortho-perio treatment. To all of them I suggest that choice only if “they want to keep their teeth for as long as possible”. After the treatment they are very satisfied. The psychological aspect is extremely important because many patients identify the loss of teeth with an overall physical decay.

The treatment ends with a fixed teeth retainer (Figs. 6-17 & 6-18). The splint reduces teeth mobility and does not improve the periodontal situation but, by eliminating excessive movement, does provide good comfort to the patient.

6-17

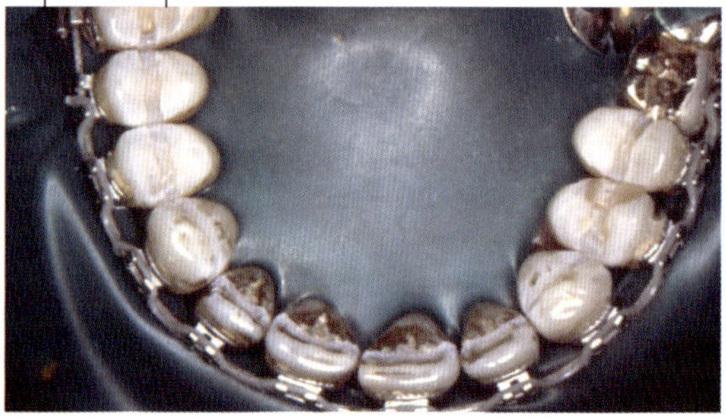

6-18

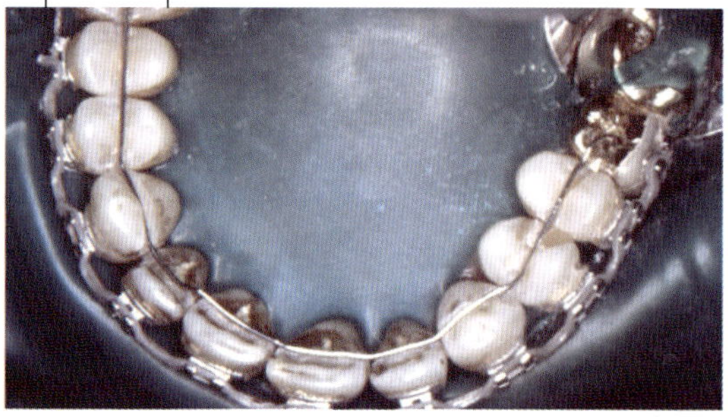

6-19

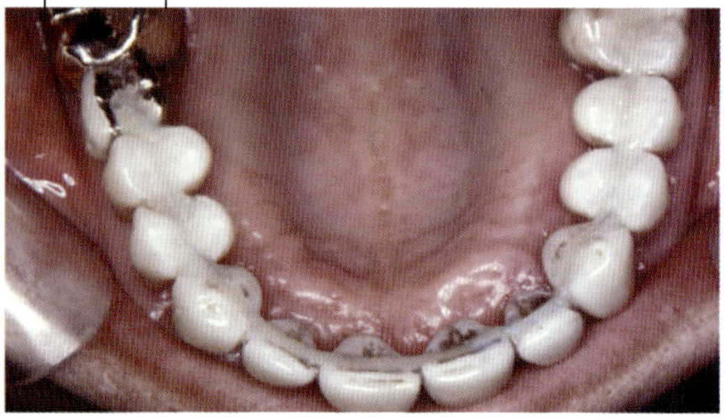

6-20

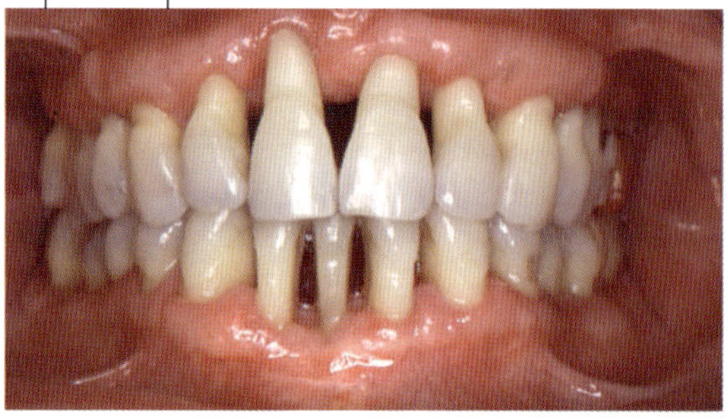

Fig. 6-17 The crowns are drilled to allow the insertion of the retainer.

Fig. 6-18 The stainless steel arch 0.18" retainer.

Fig. 6-19 Composite to cover the arch retainer.

Fig. 6-20 Post-treatment occlusion.

CASE NUMBER 5

The case involves a 21 year old female patient who has already had some unsuccessful periodontal treatment (Fig. 6-21). Evidently the lower left central incisor has been lost. What should we do? Prosthetic solutions are possible but would maintain the cross bite between the upper right lateral incisor and the lower right canine. Orthodontic space closure is in my opinion the best solution (Fig. 6-27), but what about the alveolar bone resorption? If we move the teeth are they going to end up in a "black hole"? No. With correct biomechanics, the use of light forces and good dental hygiene the teeth move "with" the bone and a new periodontal unit is created.

6-21

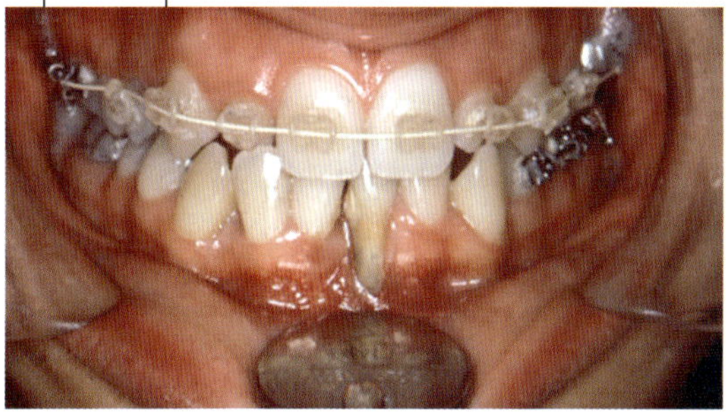

Fig. 6-21
First treatment phase. Clinical view.

6-22

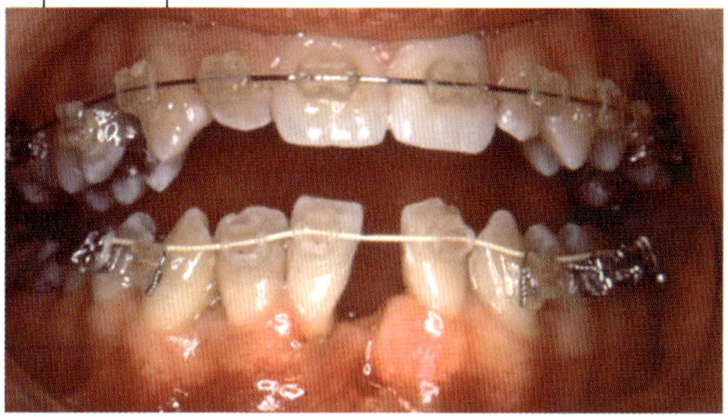

Fig. 6-22
Second treatment phase. Note the bone resorption where the lower central incisor has been lost.

6-23

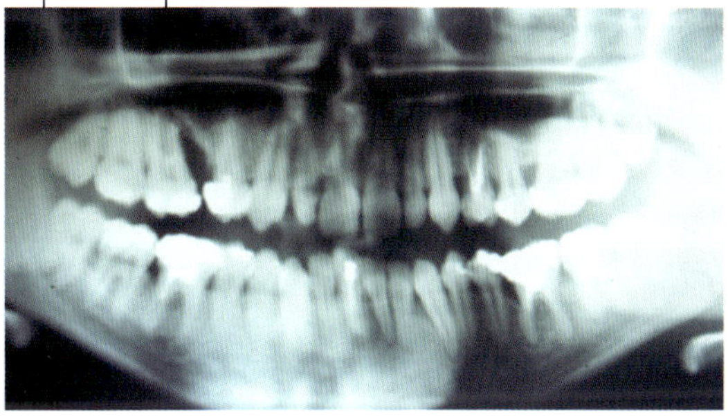

Fig. 6-23
Pre-treatment panoramic radiograph.

6-24

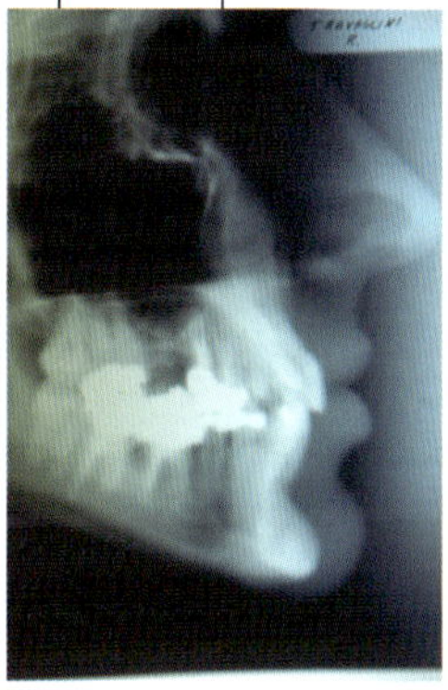

Fig. 6-24
Pre-treatment lateral cephalogram.

6-25

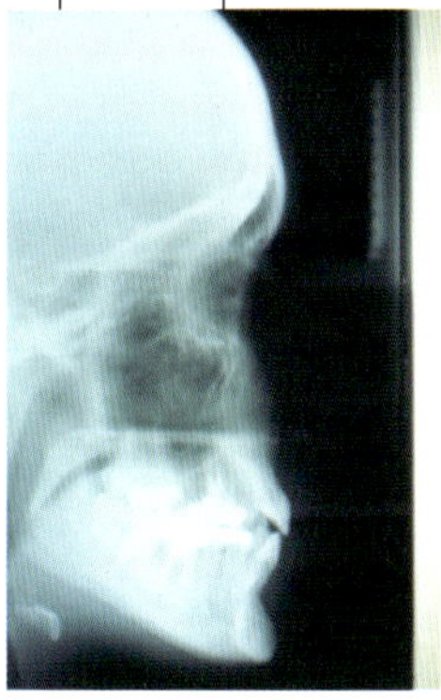

Fig. 6-25
Post-treatment lateral cephalogram.

6-26

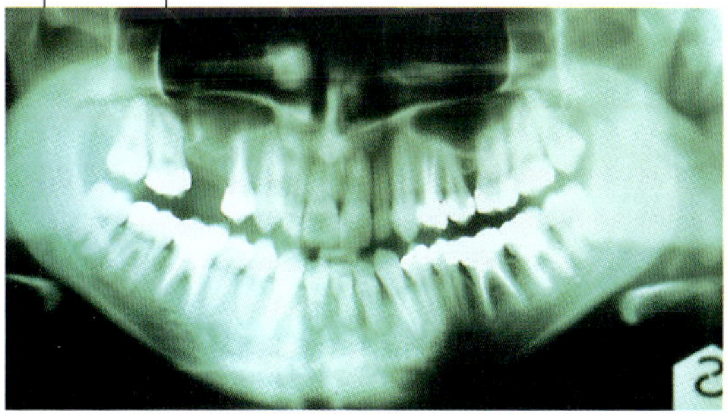

Fig. 6-26
Post-treatment panoramic radiograph

6-27

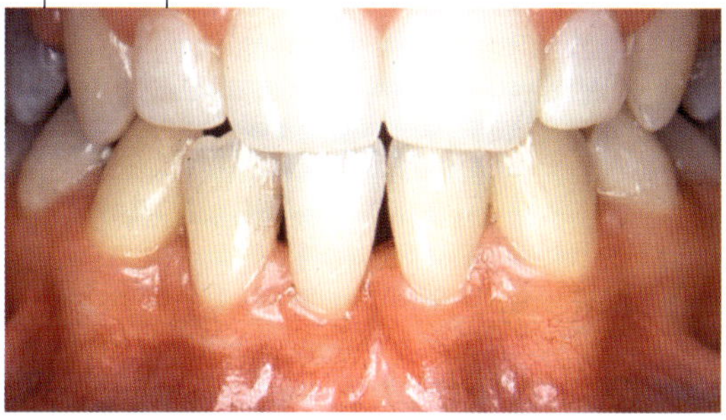

Fig. 6-27
Post-treatment occlusion.

CASE NUMBER 6

The case is a 24 year old female patient with advanced periodontal disease sustained by an evident large amount of calculus (Fig. 6-28). After scaling and root planning there is an improvement of the periodontal condition but the aesthetics are poor (Fig. 6-29). Orthodontic teeth alignment and intrusion of the upper incisors change the smile (Figs. 6-30 & 6-31).

6-28

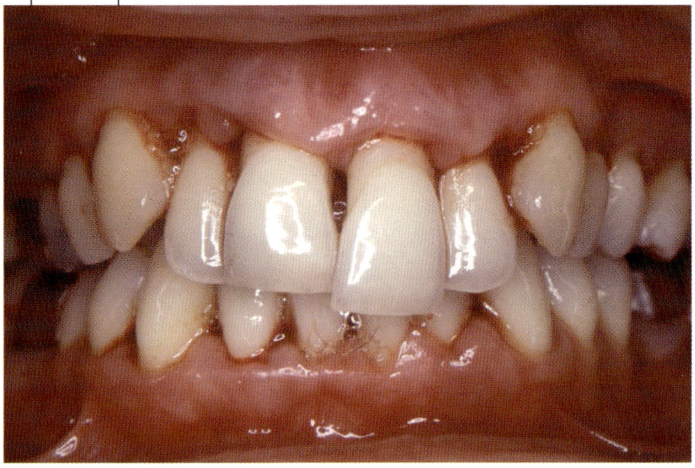

6-29

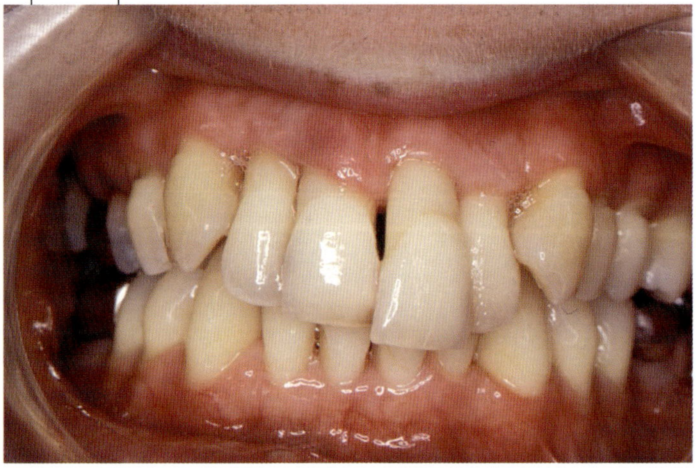

6-30

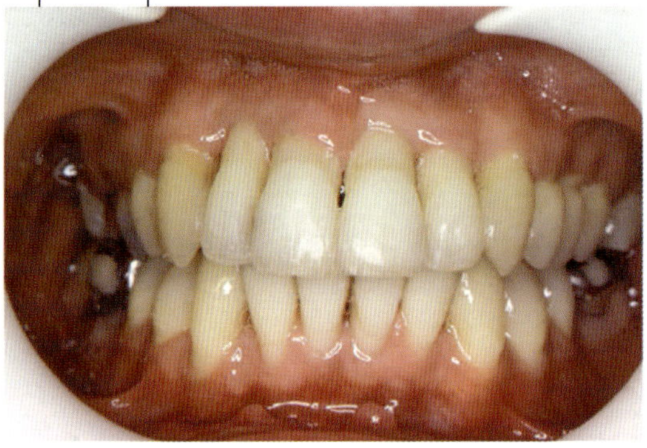

6-31

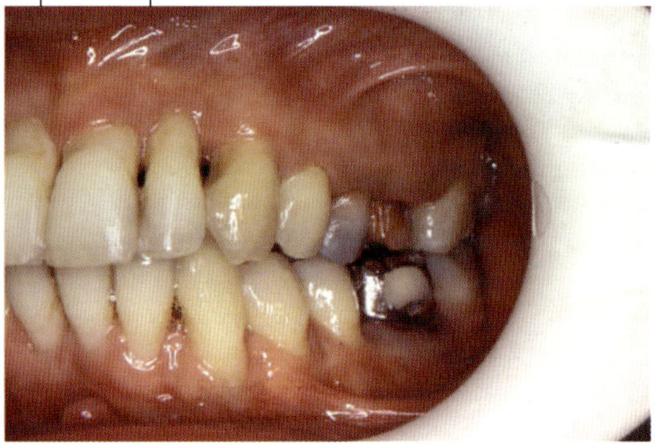

CASE NUMBER 7

Periodontal probing (Fig. 6-33) reveals deep infrabony pockets worsened by an anterior traumatic occlusion (cross bite). Without orthodontic treatment, is there an alternative prosthetic solution that can offer a good functional and aesthetic result? It would probably require extracting all the upper incisors.
In this case there is an excellent occlusion after the orthodontic treatment: notice in particular the correction with bone regeneration technique of the deep infrabony pocket between the first and second lower right premolars. How was it achieved? The treatment required upper teeth alignment with a straight wire technique using low forces. A temporary increase in the anterior vertical dimension with a lower bite guard was very helpful for correction of the anterior cross bite.

6-32

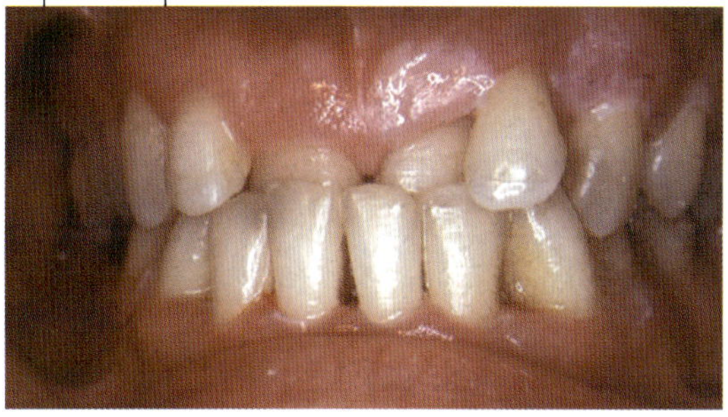

6-33

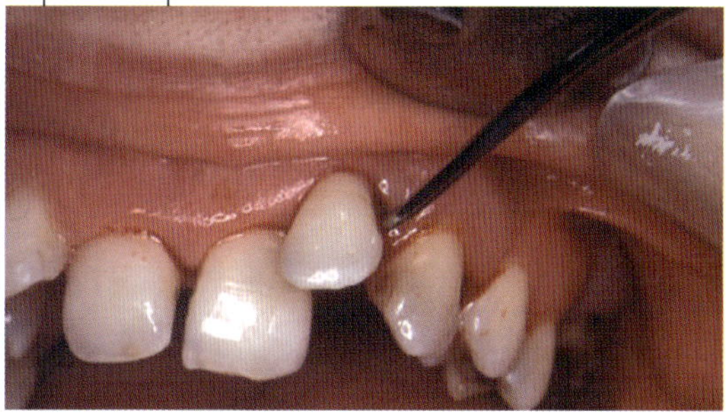

6-34

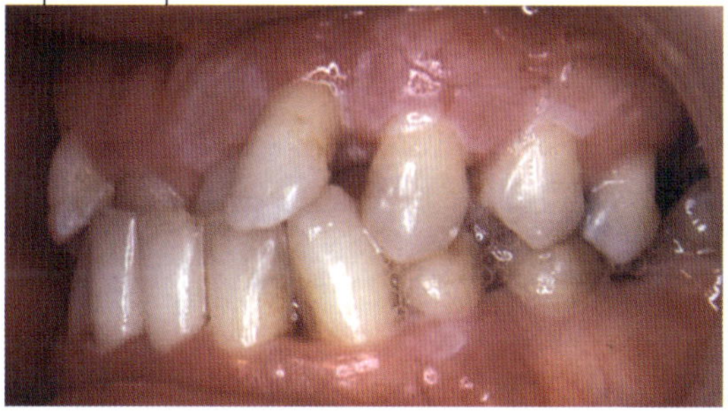

Figs. 6-32 to 6-34
Pre-treatment clinical situation.

6-35

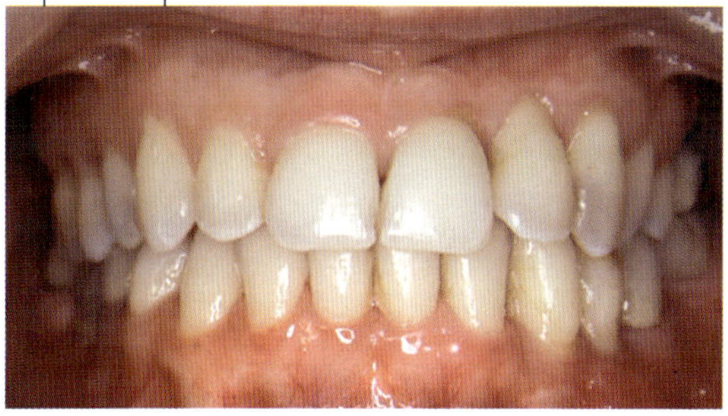

6-36

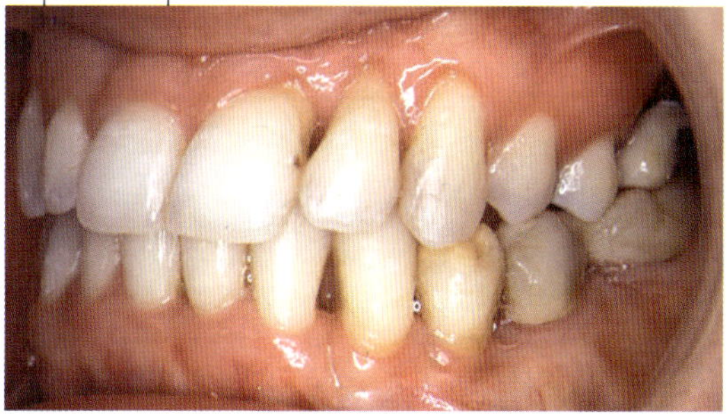

Figs. 6-35 & 6-36
Post-treatment occlusion.

6-37

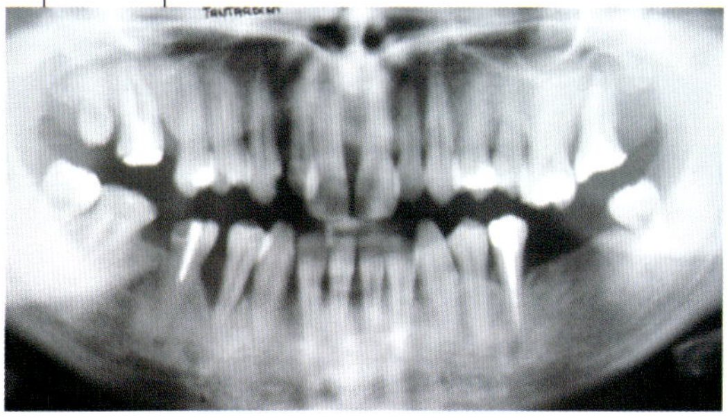

6-38

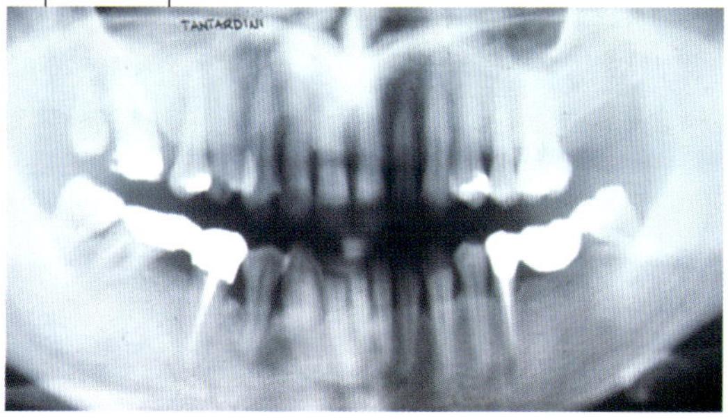

Fig. 6-37
Pre-treatment panoramic radiograph.

Fig. 6-38
Post-treatment panoramic radiograph.

CASE NUMBER 8

The case features a 16 year old girl with very serious periodontal disease. With conventional treatments many teeth would have been extracted. In light of her young age, the parents asked to go for the best that could be done in order to avoid the extractions. An ortho-perio treatment with bone regeneration techniques followed. Considering the initial seriousness of the case and the stability of the outcome 3 years later, we can be very satisfied with the way the job was performed.

6-39

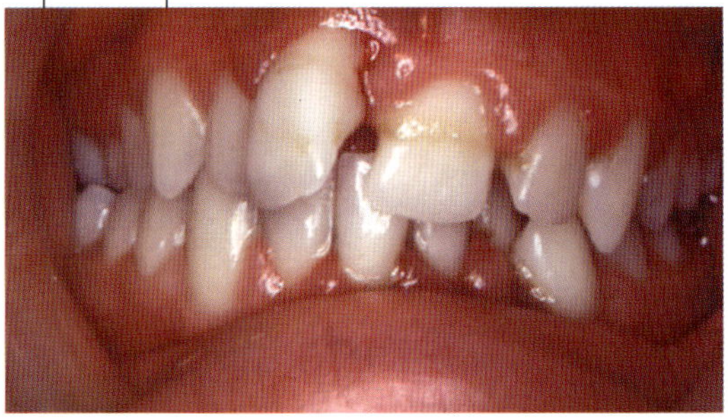

6-40

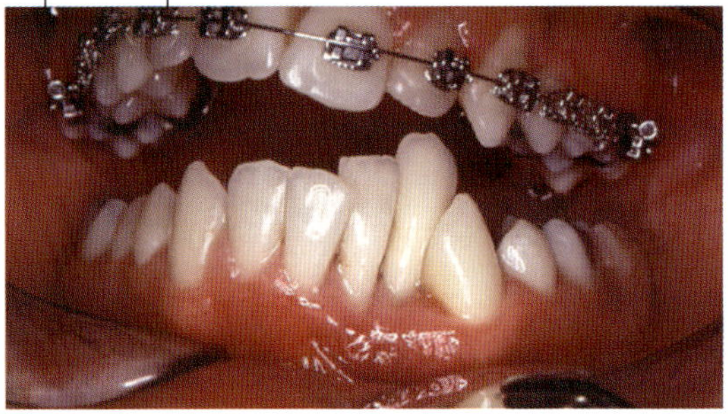

Fig. 6-39
Pre-treatment occlusion.

Fig. 6-40
First phase of orthodontic treatment with an edgewise appliance on the upper arch.

6-41

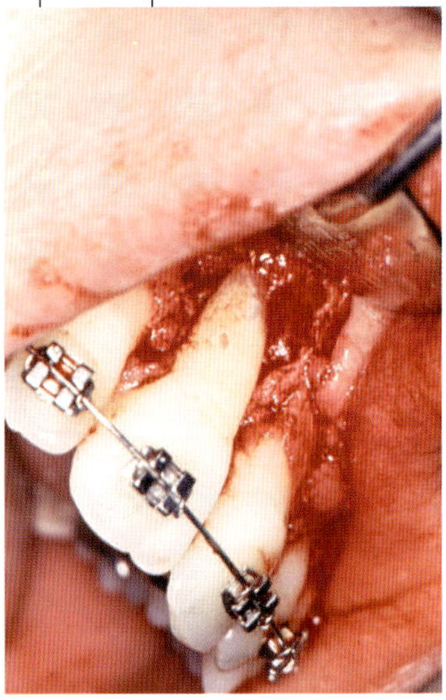

6-42

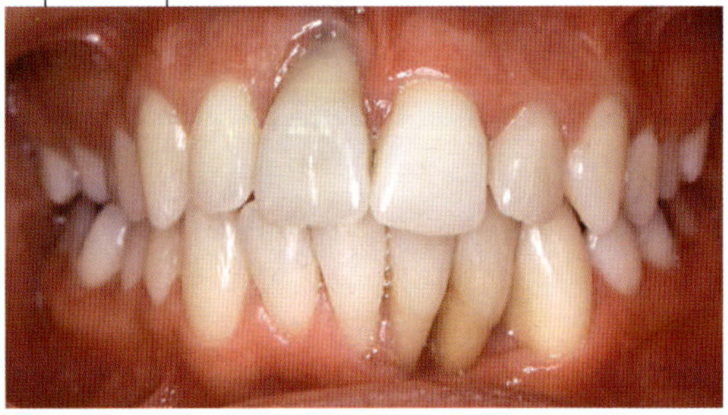

Fig. 6-41
A periodontal flap shows the amount of bone loss.

Fig. 6-42
Post-treatment occlusion.

6-43

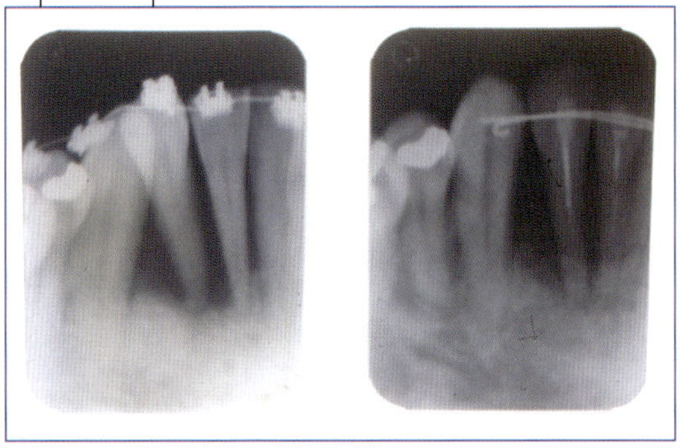

Fig. 6-43
Lower incisors X-ray. Left: the bone loss is evident. Right: a few days after the treatment and bone regeneration technique.

CASE NUMBER 9

The case featured a 45 year old female patient. The dentist suggested extracting the lower molars but the patient wanted to try to recover those molars. With an orthodontic treatment, a molar uprighting with closure of space was possible.

6-44

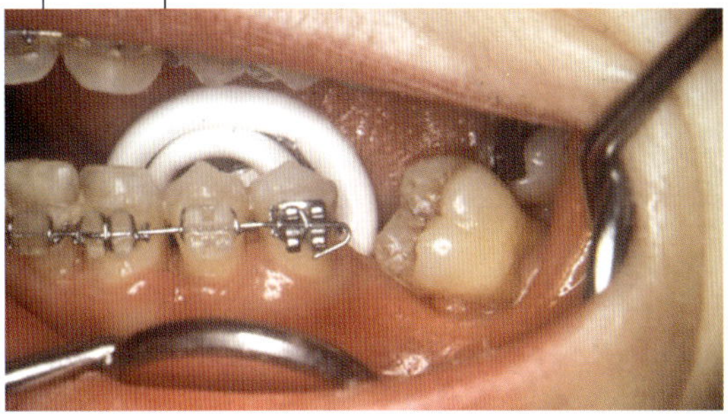

6-45

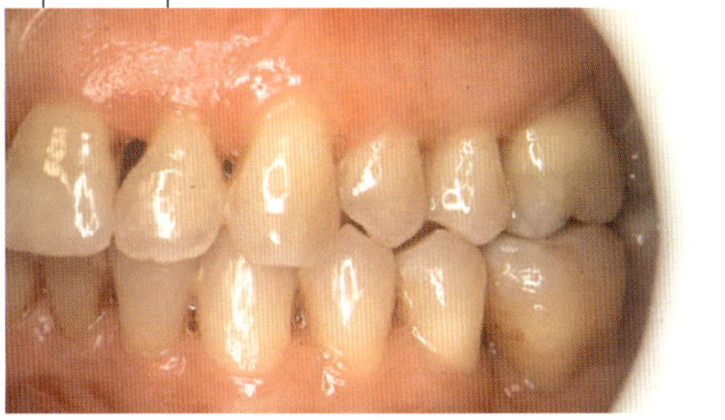

Fig. 6-44
Pre-treatment occlusion.

Fig. 6-45
Post-treatment occlusion.

6-46

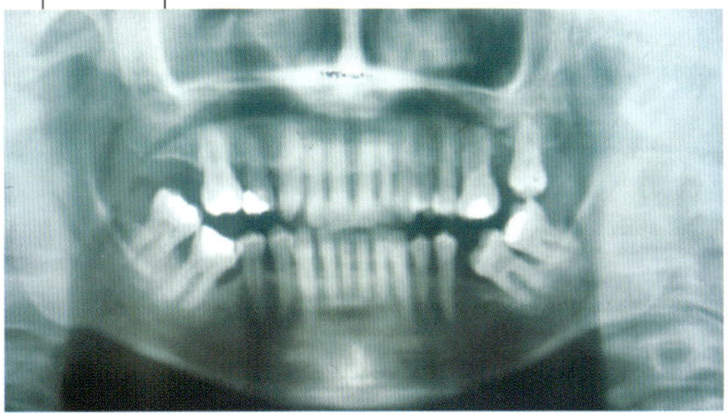

6-47

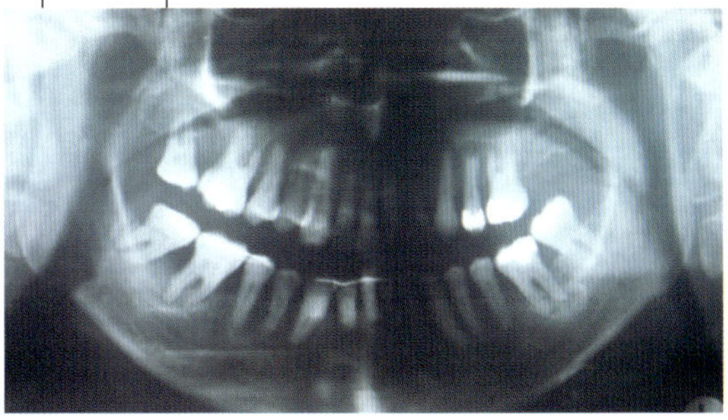

Fig. 6-46
Pre-treatment panoramic radiograph.

Fig. 6-47
Post-treatment panoramic radiograph.

CONCLUSIONS

Ortho-perio treatments can offer incredible and wonderful solutions. All my patients, including of course the cases above, have been very satisfied at the end of treatment. Many of them would have had this treatment before but they were not informed about the chances offered by orthodontics because many dentists and even orthodontists ignore the potential of ortho-perio treatments.

Once again let me stress the importance of correct informed consent regarding different solutions. Most people want to keep their teeth for as long as possible and I am one of them.

ORTHODONTICS AND PROSTHESIS

I like to say that between orthodontics and prosthesis there is a "love/hate" relationship; "love" when an orthodontic treatment moves the teeth allowing the realization of a better prosthesis, "hate" when an orthodontic treatment, by closing a space, prevents a prosthetic tooth replacement. "Love" refers to pre-prosthesis orthodontics, which allows the best functional and aesthetic solutions. Those are the goals of modern dentistry.

Many patients are adults and some dentists or even orthodontists believe that in these cases, moving teeth is more difficult because the bone is "hard". The truth is that in adults, with aging, movement can be slower due to a reduction in cellular activity.

Bone resorption increases while its formation decreases leading to possible bone porosity.

Vanarsdall and Musich[248] showed that it is possible to move teeth at all ages.

A tooth moves because an applied force activates a cellular reaction (osteoblasts and osteoclasts cf. http://www.youtube.com/watch?v=78RBpWSOI08), which is followed by bone remodelling. The use of light forces is important.

When it comes to choosing between a removable or fixed appliance, a removable one allows greater hygiene control but needs the patient's cooperation. It also has biomechanical limitations, and is recommended for minor movements. With fixed appliances teeth are better controlled, the action is more continuous and the results are more predictable.

In adult patients, of course, the orthodontist must be ready to use aesthetic and non-compliance braces. Can you imagine a businessman wearing a headgear?

Where it is possible I prefer to opt for the orthodontic replacement of missing teeth. I believe that progress in medicine is made whenever we are able to preserve natural body parts and to avoid prosthetics. I would do that on myself or on my relatives. However, make sure to be open-minded and avoid blinkered thinking because the consequences could be very negative. For example an orthodontist shouldn't try to resolve all cases with an orthodontic treatment. Likewise a dentist shouldn't try to solve them with a prosthetic one. As illustrated by the following case study number 11 (Cristiano)

INCISORS

In the case of missing incisors, if the anterior teeth are crowded or proclined, I would prefer an orthodontic space closure (see also Case Number 18 in Chapter II and Case Number 5 in Chapter VI). Otherwise, a prosthesis is indicated.

CASE NUMBER 10

As Zachrisson[259] showed, when the upper lateral incisors are congenitally missing in a Class II division 1 or in a Class I with proclination of the upper central incisors, one of the best solutions is an upper dental arch contraction with closure of spaces as explained in this case. This way you will not have a canine protection, while a group disclusion can be an acceptable alternative. With canine remodelling a good aesthetic result can be achieved.

For psychological reasons I would do anything possible in order to avoid a prosthesis. (That is exactly what I did to my daughter who, 25 years later, is extremely satisfied.) In a Class I without upper incisor proclination or in a Class III, a prosthesis is more commonly indicated.

In case 10 presented here the second lower premolars are congenitally missing as well, but there is a deep bite. Therefore, an orthodontic space closure is contraindicated: they will be replaced by a prosthesis.

6-48

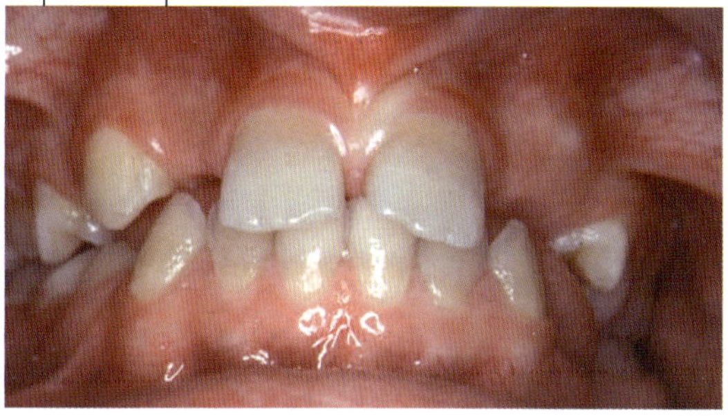

6-49

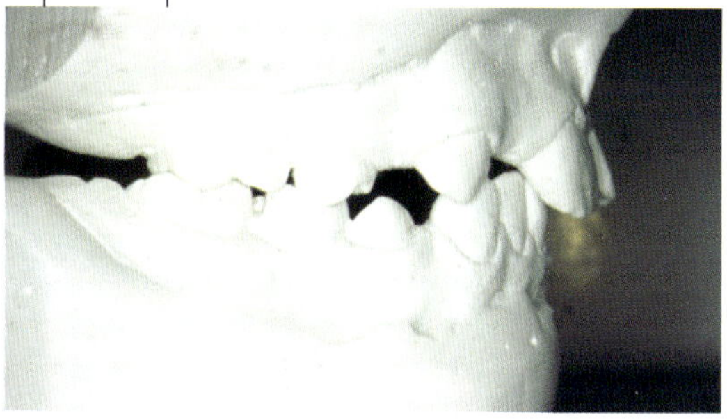

Fig. 6-48
Pre-treatment occlusion.

Fig. 6-49
Pre-treatment dental casts.

6-50

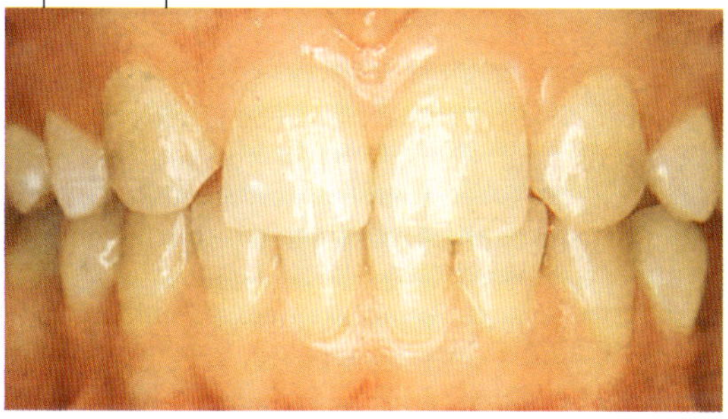

6-51

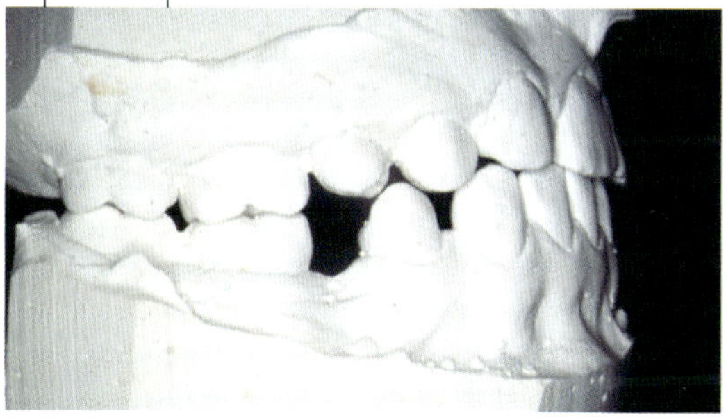

Fig. 6-50
Post-treatment occlusion.

Fig. 6-51
Post-treatment dental casts. The missing lower second premolars will be replaced by a prosthesis.

CASE NUMBER 11

THE CASES OF TWO BROTHERS

Cristiano is a Class I (ANB : +1.5°) with an edge-to-edge anterior occlusion. The right upper lateral incisor is congenitally missing and there is a left conoid lateral incisor. Many orthodontists would suggest the extraction of the left conoid and the orthodontic closure of spaces. The treatment with a fixed appliance seems to be good. Five years later the results speak for themselves (Fig. 6-58 & 6-59), disaster!

6-52

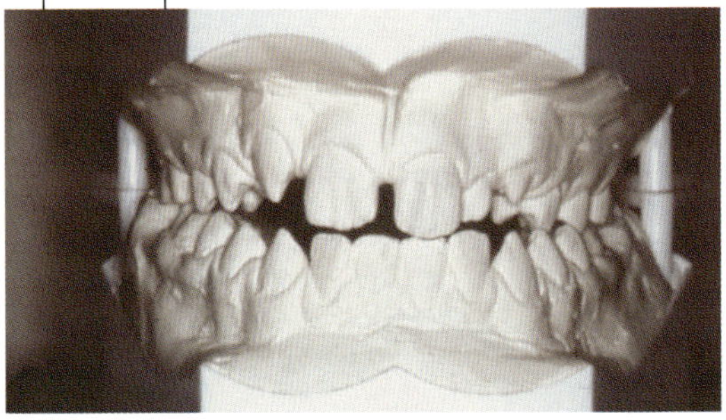

6-53

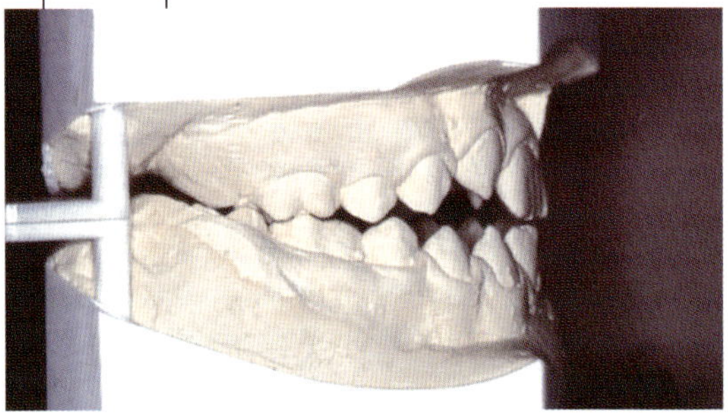

Figs. 6-52 & 6-53
Pre-treatment dental casts.

6-54

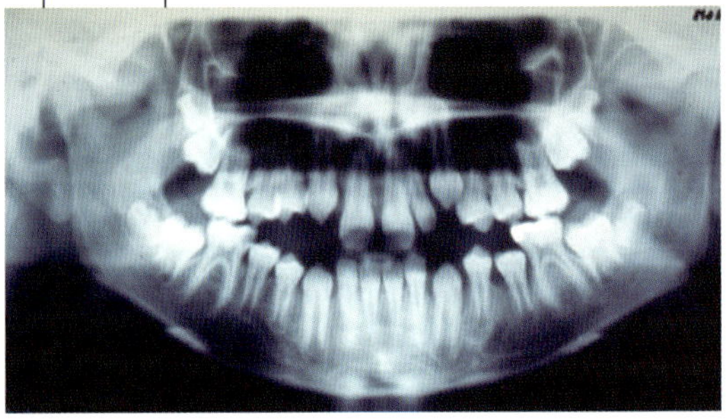

6-55

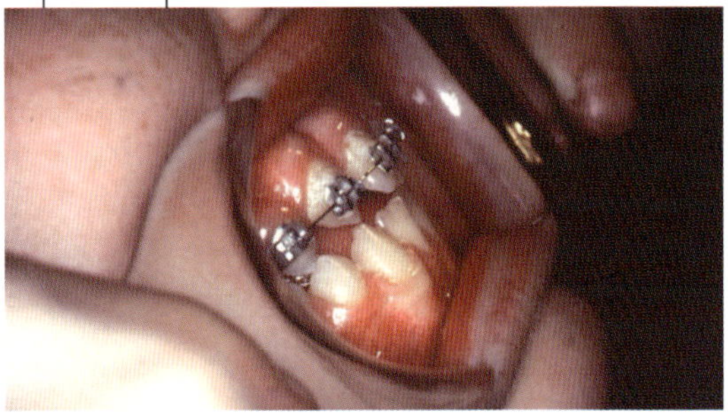

Fig. 6-54
Pre-treatment panoramic radiograph.

Fig. 6-55
Orthodontic treatment: initial phase.

6-56

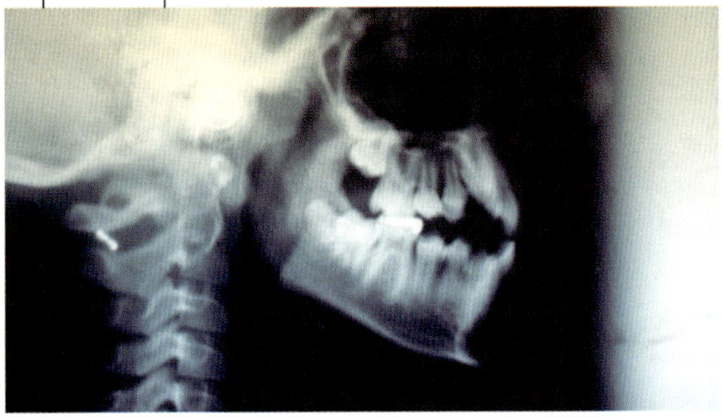

6-57

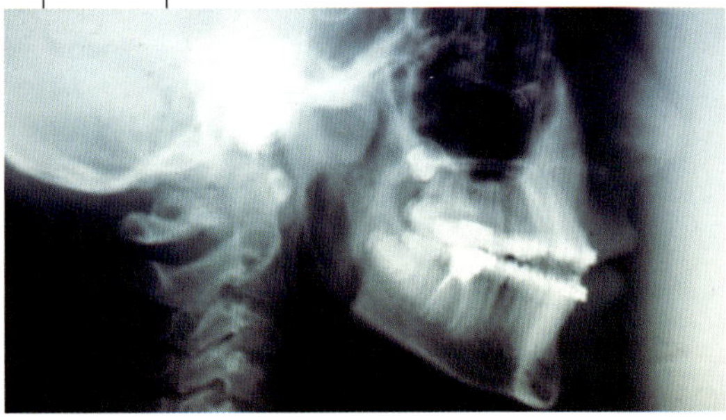

Fig. 6-56
Pre-treatment lateral cephalogram.

Fig. 6-57
Lateral cephalogram 12 months later.

6-58

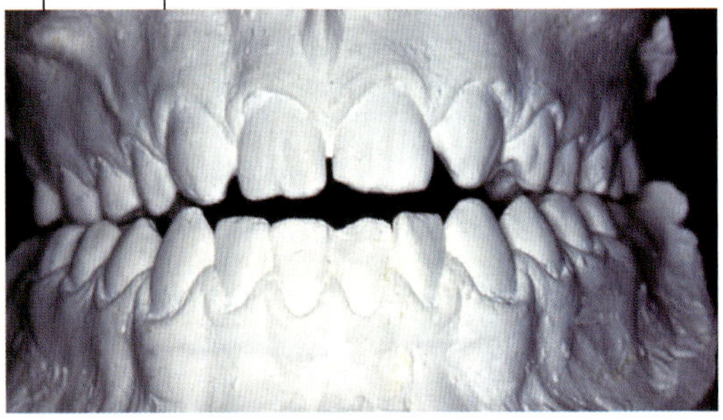

6-59

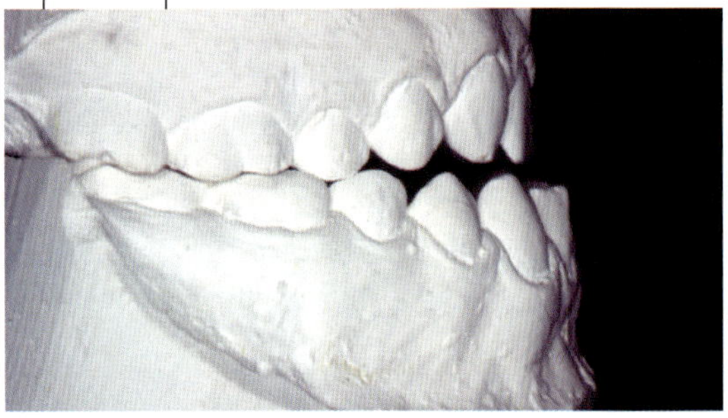

Figs. 6-58 & 6-59
Dental casts five years after the end of the treatment. The spaces are closed but the occlusion is a failure.

CASE NUMBER 12

6-60

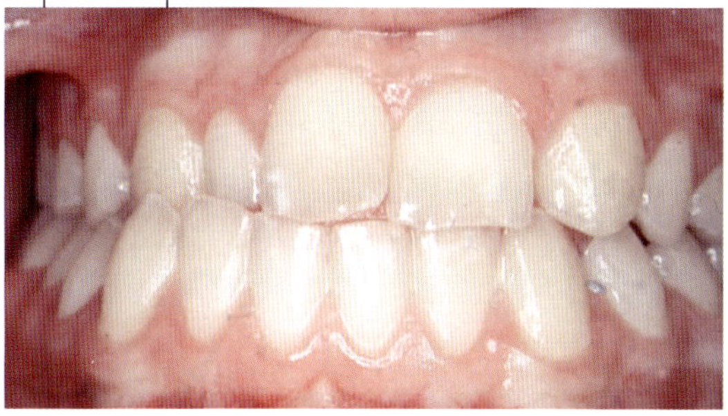

6-61

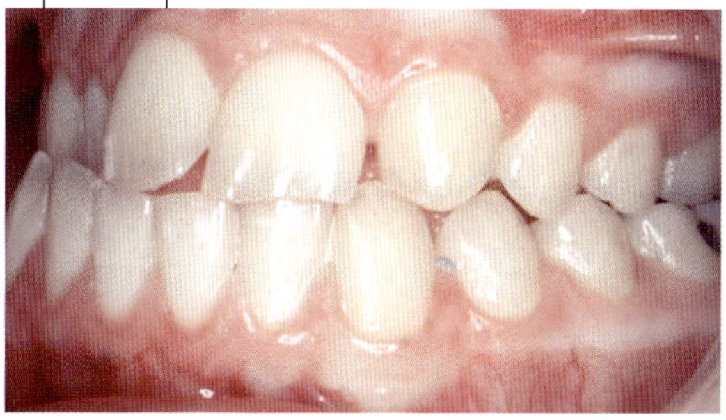

Figs. 6-60 & 6-61 Pre-treatment occlusion. Right: anterior cross bite. Left: missing upper lateral incisors.

6-62

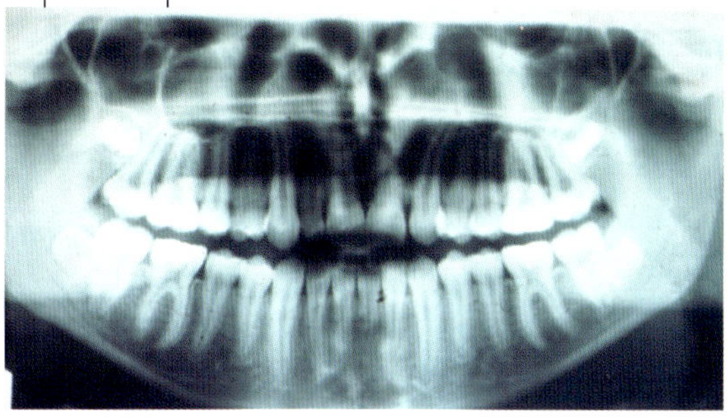

6-63

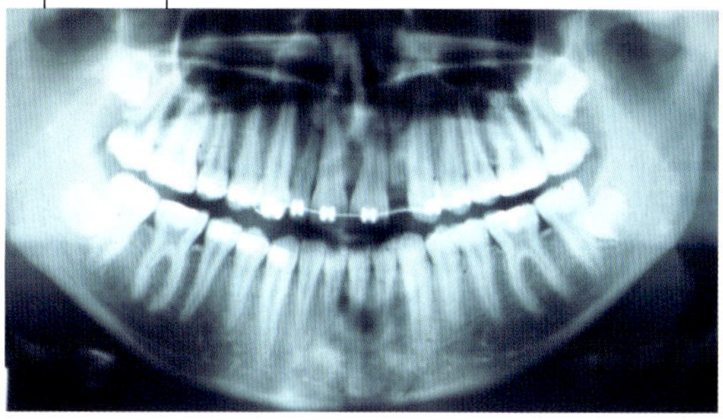

Fig. 6-62 Pre-treatment panoramic radiograph.

Fig. 6-63 Post-treatment panoramic radiograph.

6-64

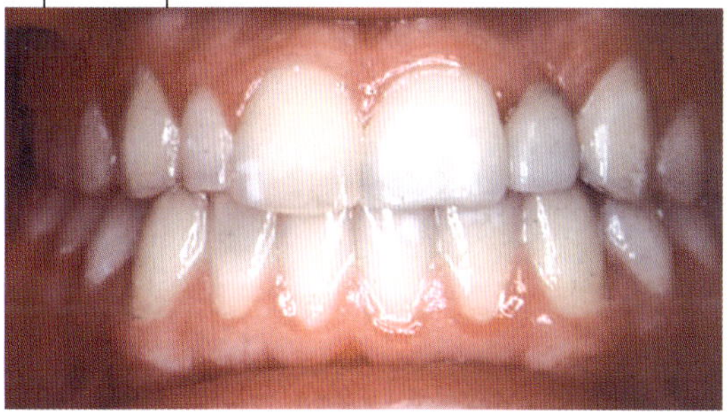

6-65

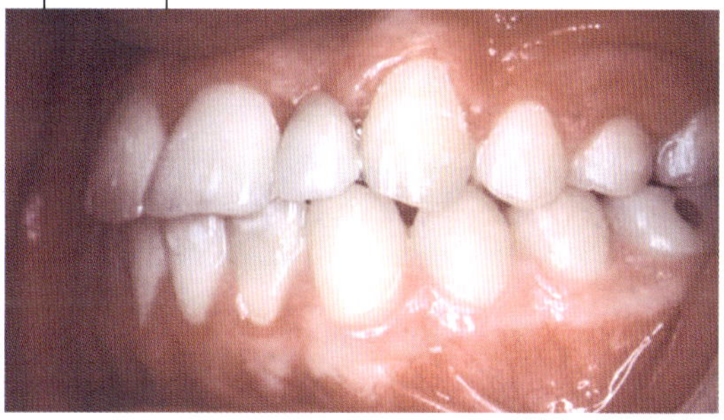

Figs. 6-64 & 6-65 Post-treatment occlusion.

6-66

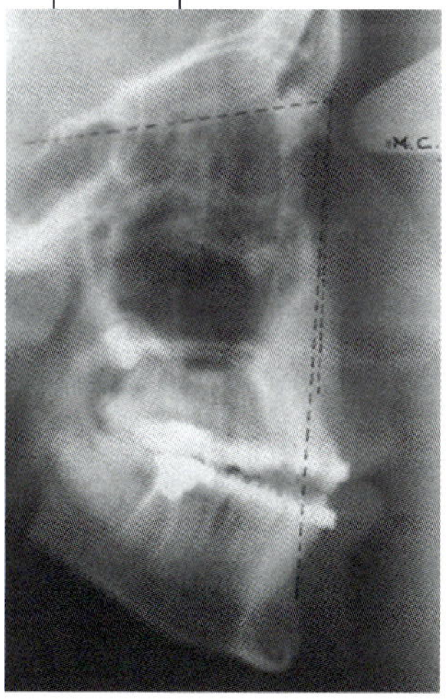

6-67

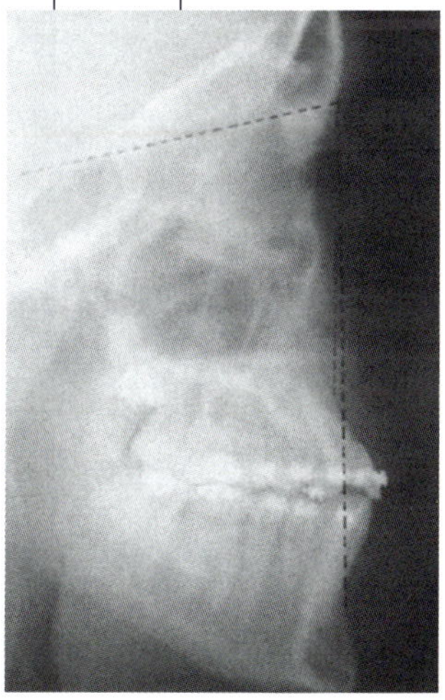

Figs. 6-66 & 6-67 Comparison between post-treatment lateral cephalogram. Left (66): Cristiano, who had a better skeletal situation (ANB: +1.5°), in the end had a worse result. Right (67): Federico, who had a worse skeletal situation (ANB: -1.5°), had a better result.

Cristiano's brother, Federico, is four years younger and has a skeletal Class III (ANB : -1.5°) with the upper left lateral incisor congenitally missing and an anterior right cross bite.

When remembering what happened to his brother, the right thing to do now is clear: open the space to replace the missing lateral incisor. Once the space has been opened with orthodontic treatment, a

Maryland bridge was applied. In the end, the patient who began the treatment in a better condition had a worse result and vice versa.

What happened to Cristiano? With the upper lateral incisors missing there was a constriction of the premaxillary area, which did not follow the mandible during his growth.

Thus his final outcome was a Class III relationship.

This case is useful because it shows the importance of growth. Do not forget that good orthodontics does not simply refer to only "teeth alignment".

CANINES

Canine agenesis is rare: there is a prevalence of maxillary inclusions. Very often there is a lack of space when it comes to alignment. When more space is needed and a solution could come from a first premolar extraction, the question is whether we are sure or not about canine recovery after that extraction. It would be very embarrassing to lose two teeth instead of one (see Chapter V).

In the following case, with orthodontic treatment there was an excellent recovery of the upper right canine. Alternatively, with the pre-treatment occlusion, it might have been sensible to open the space between the first premolar and the lateral incisor and to replace the canine with a prosthesis.

CASE NUMBER 13

6-68

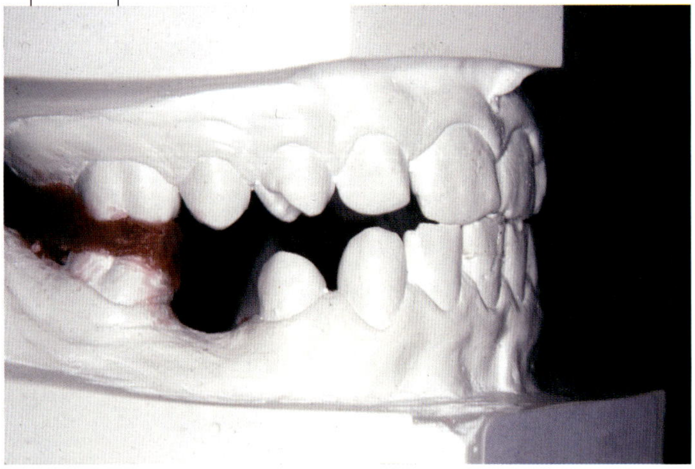

6-69

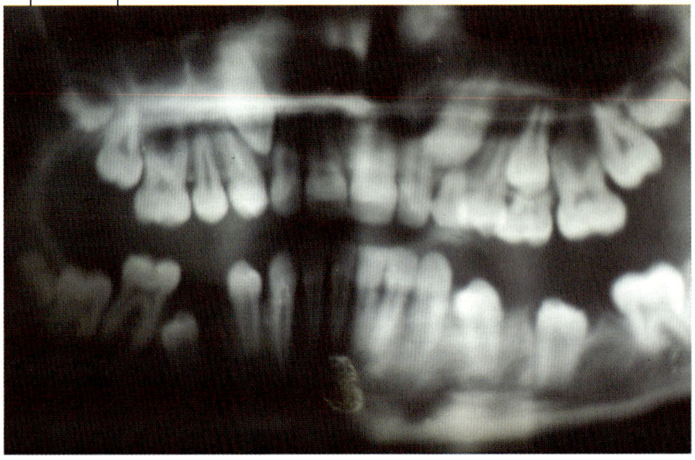

Figs. 6-68 & 6-69
Pre-treatment dental casts and panoramic radiograph. Skeletal Class I with an edge-to-edge anterior occlusion, dental posterior open bite and right maxillary canine included. The lack of space for the canine eruption is evident.

6-70

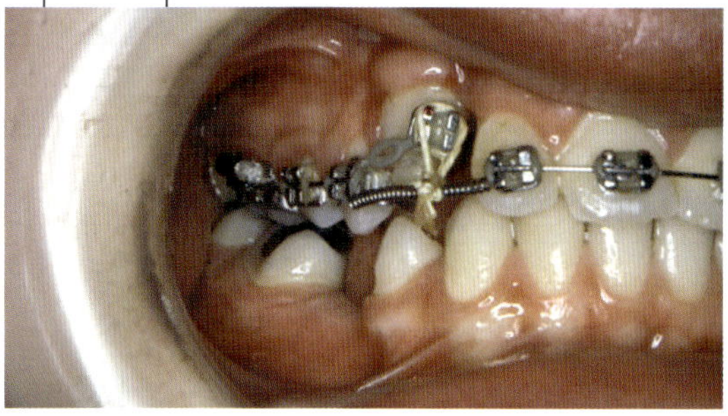

6-71

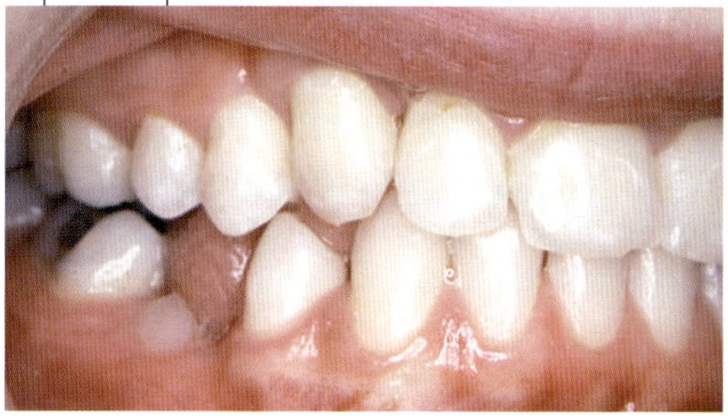

Fig. 6-70
Fixed appliance with a coil spring to open the space and align the canine.

Fig. 6-71
Post-treatment occlusion. The lower right space will be occupied by a prosthesis.

6-72

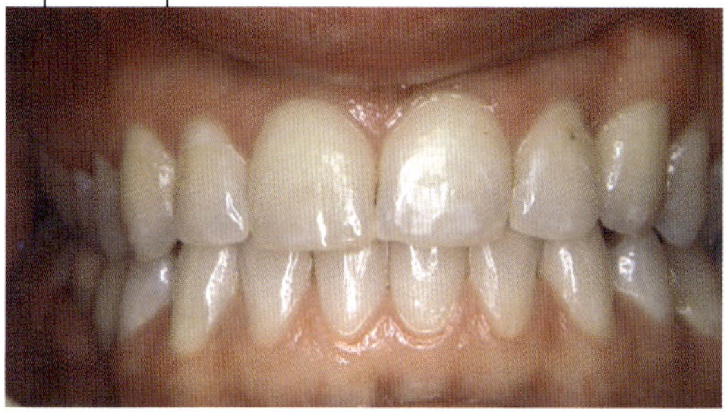

6-73

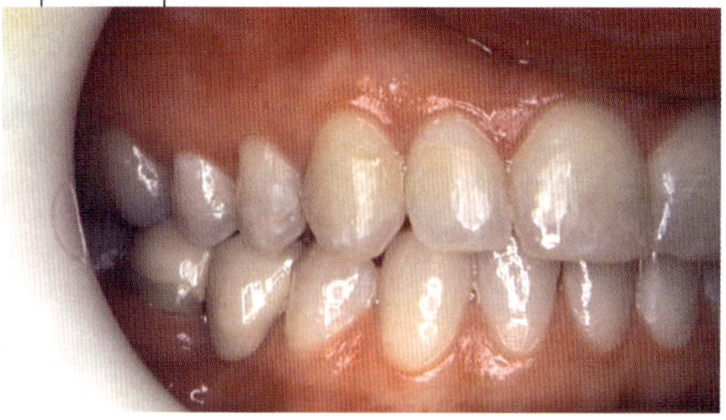

Figs. 6-72 & 6-73
Occlusion after the prosthesis application.

MOLARS AND PREMOLARS

Molars are fundamental for good mastication, a correct intermaxillary relationship and occlusion stability. When molars are missing it is usually necessary to replace them with a prosthesis. However, as an alternative, is it possible to perform an orthodontic treatment in order to close the extraction space? After the first lower molar extraction, is it possible to move mesially the second and third molars? The answer is yes! (See also Chapters II ,III ,V.)

In my opinion this is the best solution. It frequently allows for the recovery of a third molar in a bad distal periodontal condition.

However there are cases where the mesial displacement of molars is contraindicated because such a movement, by reducing the verticality, worsens deep bites, Class III, and can cause periodontal problems. We have already seen that by extracting premolars we can use the spaces to correct a Class II or a crowded arch.

CASE NUMBER 14

6-74

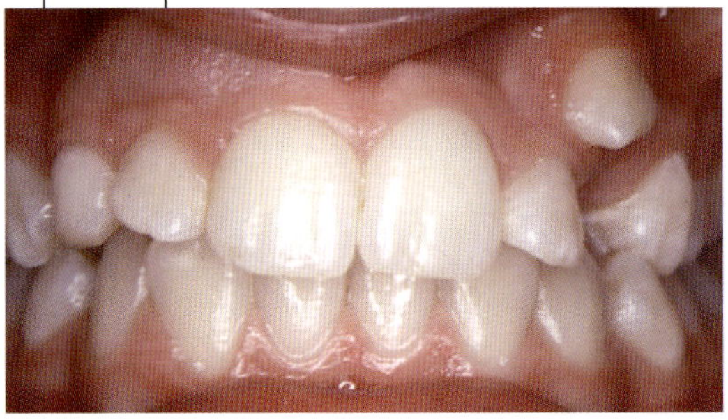

6-75

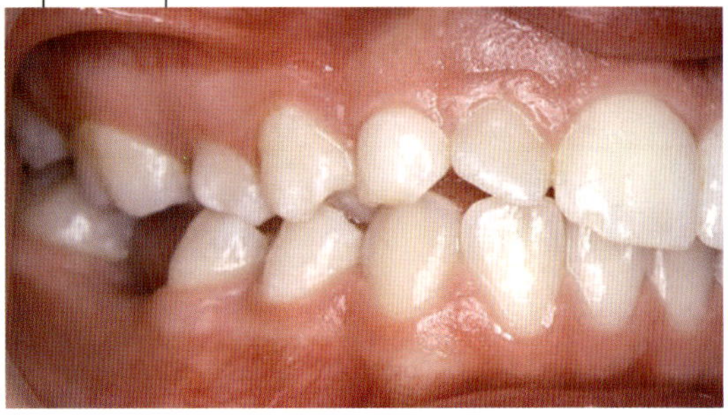

Figs. 6-74 & 6-75
Pre-treatment occlusion. The first right lower molar extraction space is evident while the upper right deciduous canine is still present because the permanent one is displaced.

6-76

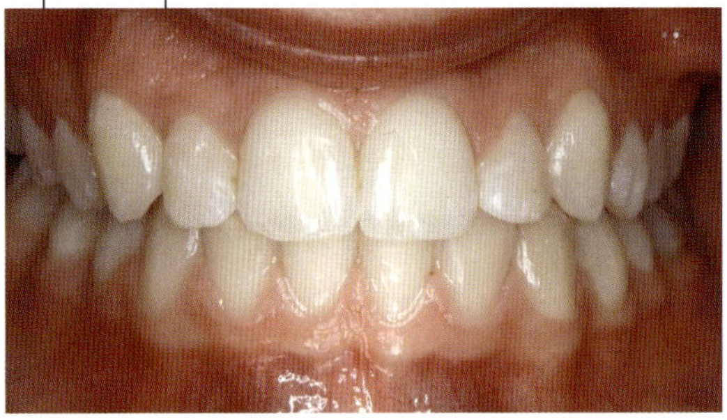

6-77

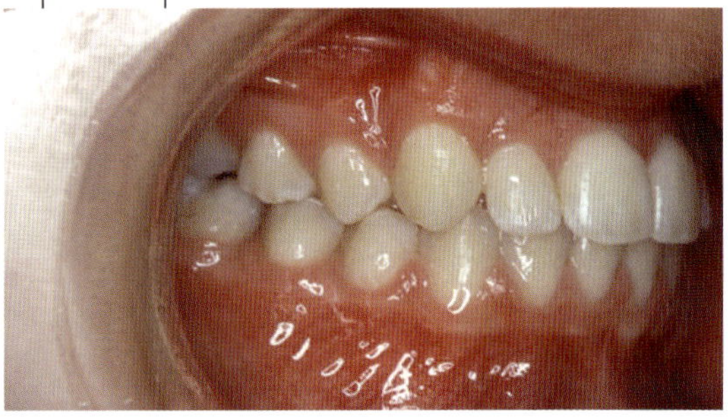

Figs. 6-76 & 6-77
Post-treatment occlusion. The second right lower molar has been mesially moved with a fixed appliance.

6-78

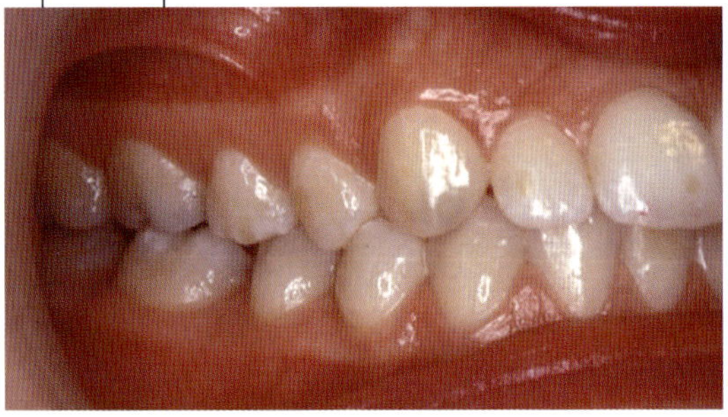

Fig. 6-78
Five years later. The third right lower molar is now well erupted in the previous second molar place. When a treatment like this is planned, it is important to control the eruption of the antagonistic tooth with a retainer in order to avoid undesired occlusal interferences.

6-79

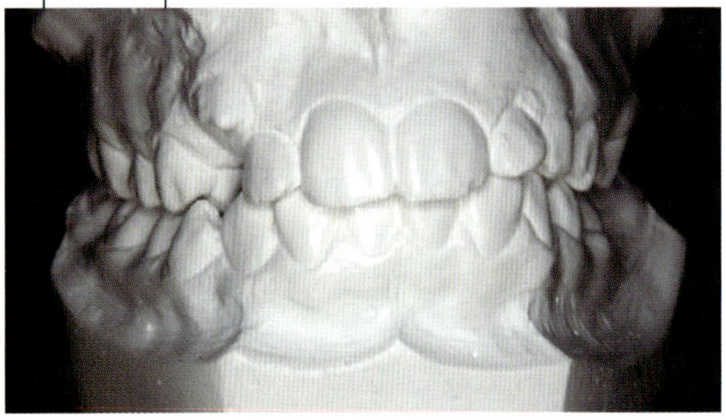

6-80

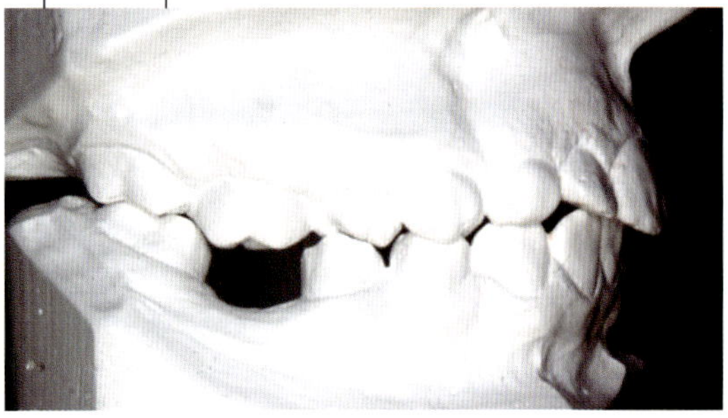

Figs. 6-79 & 6-80
Dental casts of the pre-treatment occlusion.

6-81

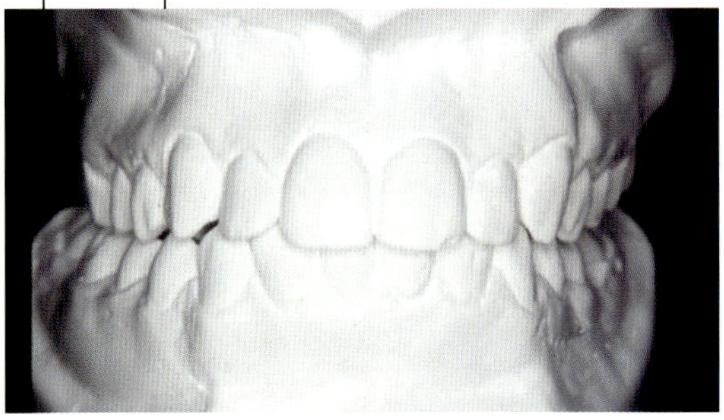

6-82

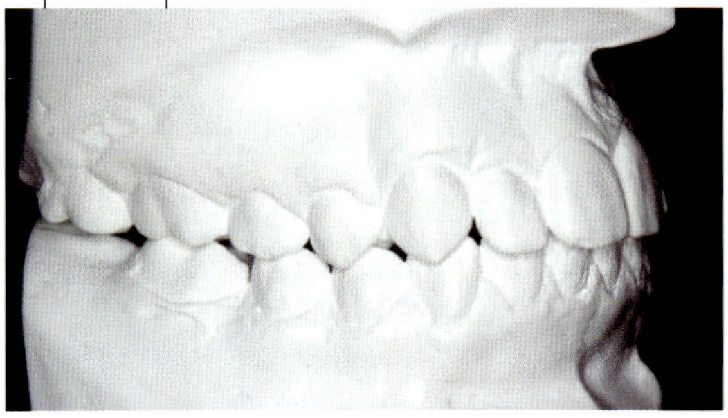

Figs. 6-81 & 6-82
Dental casts of the post-treatment occlusion. A following retainer on the upper arch is recommended in order to avoid upper second molar extrusion while waiting for the lower third molar eruption.

6-83

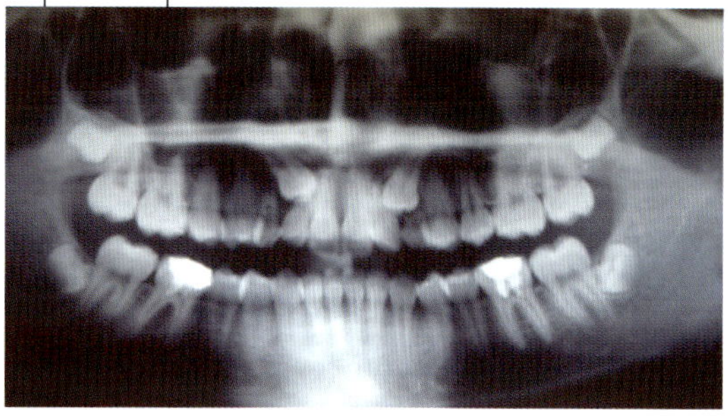

6-84

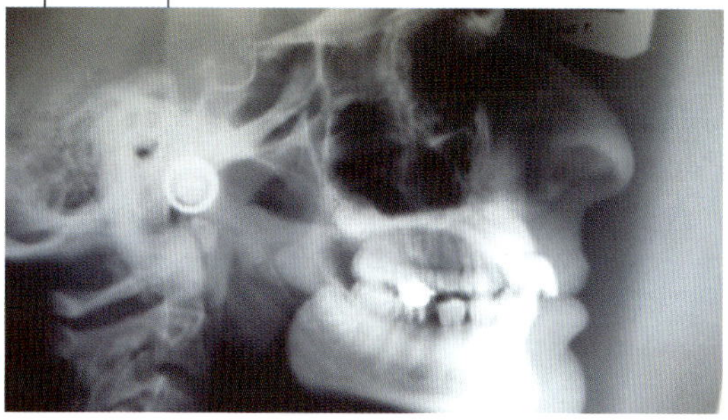

Figs. 6-83 & 6-84
Pre-treatment panoramic and cephalometric radiograph.

6-85

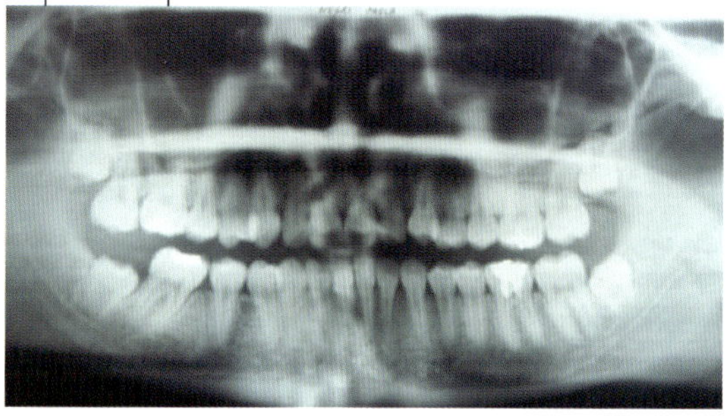

6-86

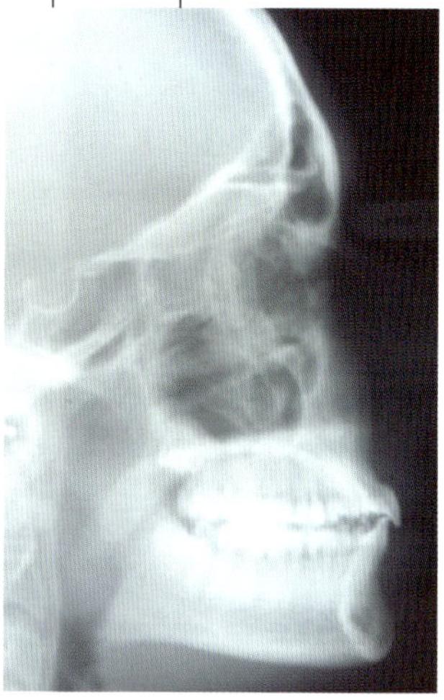

Figs. 6-85 & 6-86
Post-treatment panoramic and cephalometric radiograph.

MOLAR UPRIGHTING

It is very common to have situations with lower second molars that are mesially tipped after the extraction of the first molars. To prevent this tipping, the solution is the replacement of the missing teeth soon after extraction.

For orthodontic uprighting fixed appliances must be used. They are important for a prosthetic rehabilitation with a bridge because often we incur paralleling or space problems. For example, to obtain a parallelism between bridge abutments an endodontic treatment could be necessary. One controversial aspect is that a tipped molar causes mesial periodontal sufferance. This could continue despite 20 to 30 years of good periodontal health.

6-85

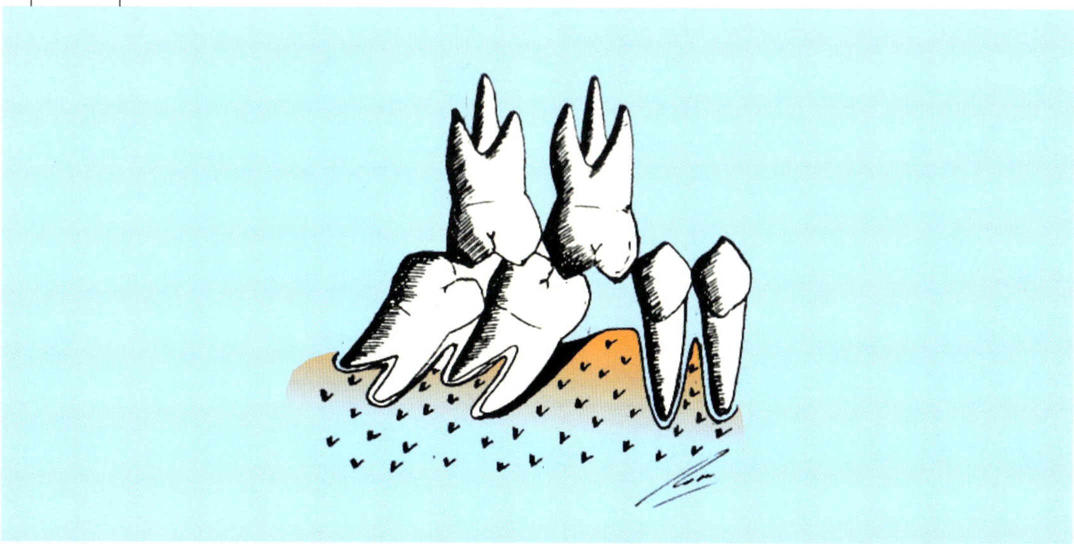

Fig. 6-87
Occlusal situation after the extraction of a lower first molar without the closure of the space with orthodontic treatment or a prosthesis. A mesial infrabony pocket is not always present.

6-88

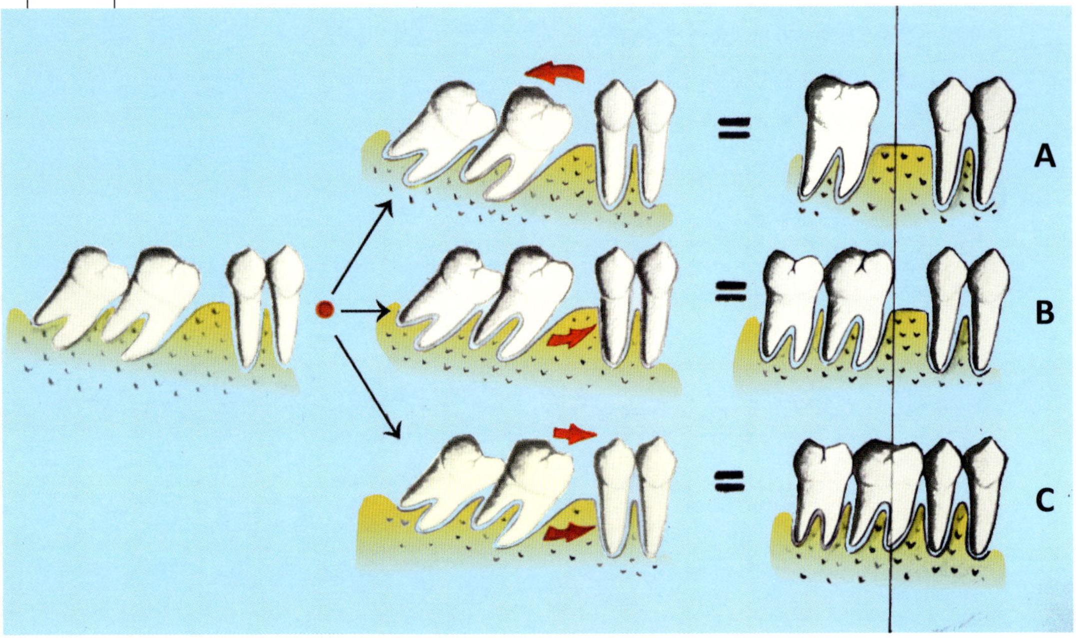

Fig. 6-88
There are three approaches in orthodontic uprighting:
A. Second molar uprighting and distal displacement after the third molar extraction
B. Second and third molar uprighting followed by their partial mesial displacement
C. Second and third molar uprighting followed by the extraction space closure.

Uprighting can be done in three ways (Fig. 6-88). In A, the uprighting follows third molar extraction and the second molar is displaced distally. Be careful because in this way the extrusion of the second molar often occurs, causing occlusal interferences which usually then need grinding. Sometimes the grinding leads to an endodontic treatment.

CASE NUMBER 15

A – B MODALITIES.

Uprighting of the lower second molars followed by two bridges. The uprighting has been achieved by using a fixed appliance in which the arch determined a rotary moment at molar level. The treatment time in this case was around 6 months.

Be careful because this procedure can lead to unwanted molar extrusion. Often in these cases there are prematurities that, if minimal, can be eliminated by grinding the tooth. If the premature condition is more serious then it's better to add an intrusive component using for example a double arch.

6-89

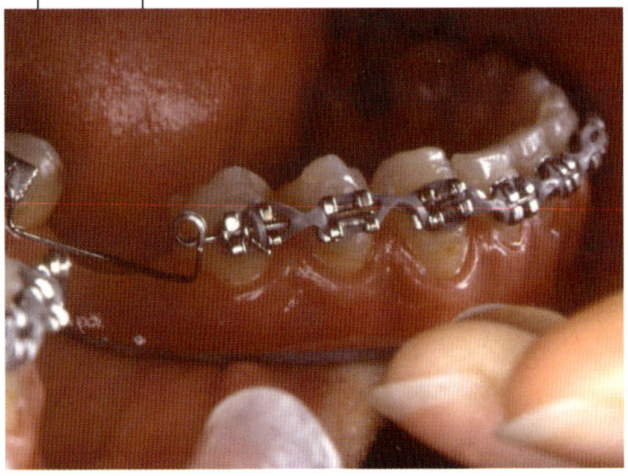

Fig. 6-89
Phase of orthodontic treatment.

6-90

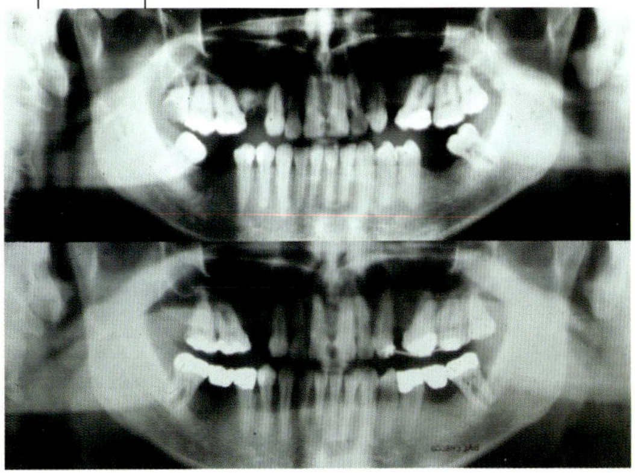

Fig. 6-90
Panoramic radiographs.
Pre-treatment: above.
Post-treatment: below.

CASE NUMBER 16

SECOND LOWER RIGHT MOLAR UPRIGHTING "C WAY" (MY FAVOURITE!).

This treatment was done on a female patient of 45 years old with active periodontal disease.

Note where we want to displace the second molars and how narrow the bucco-lingual dimension is. Do not move the teeth before their uprighting! In this case the treatment lasted 16 months.

6-91

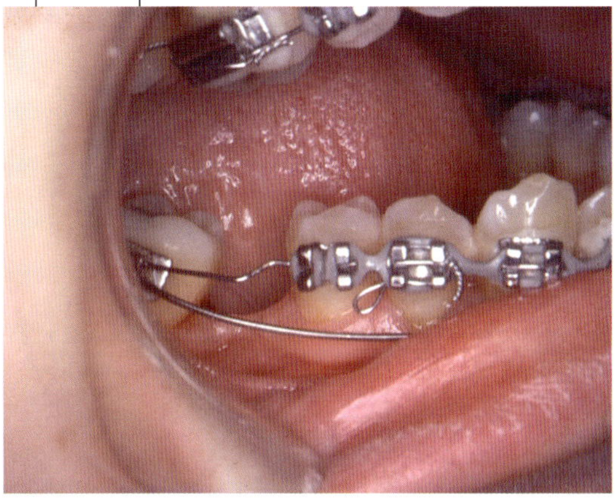

Fig. 6-91
Phase of the orthodontic treatment.

6-92

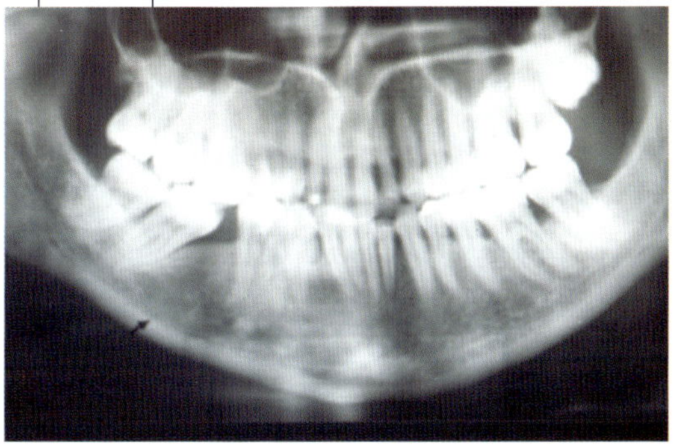

Fig. 6-92
Pre-treatment panoramic radiograph.

6-93

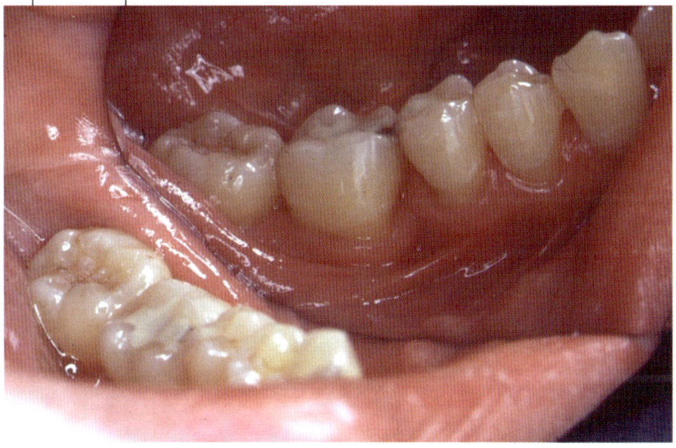

Fig. 6-93
Post-treatment occlusion. Note the uprighted lower second right molar and, together with the third lower right molar, the closure of the mesial space. The picture is taken using an intraoral mirror.

6-94

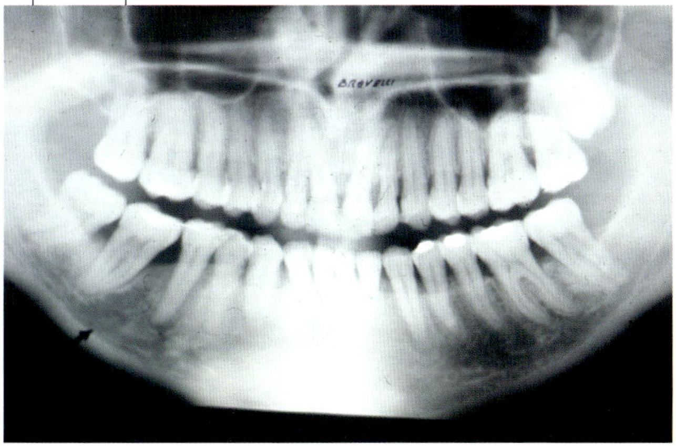

Fig. 6-94
Post-treatment panoramic radiograph.

MORE CASES TO ILLUSTRATE THE ORTHO-PROSTHESIS RELATIONSHIP

Since the goal of modern dentistry is to achieve optimal function and aesthetics, the best way to show the potential of orthodontic-prosthetic treatments is by presenting a gallery of case studies. In a few cases a prosthesis alone can give acceptable results (Figs. 6-95 to 6-98).

Otherwise, only multidisciplinary treatments can guarantee the best result.

6-95

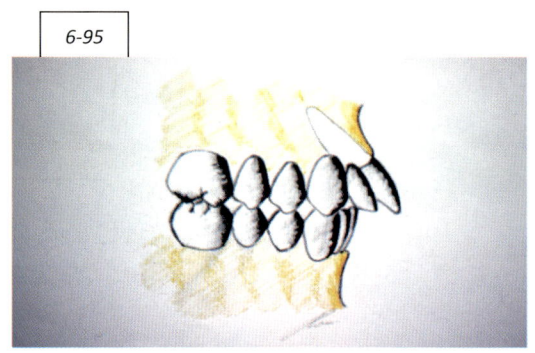

6-96

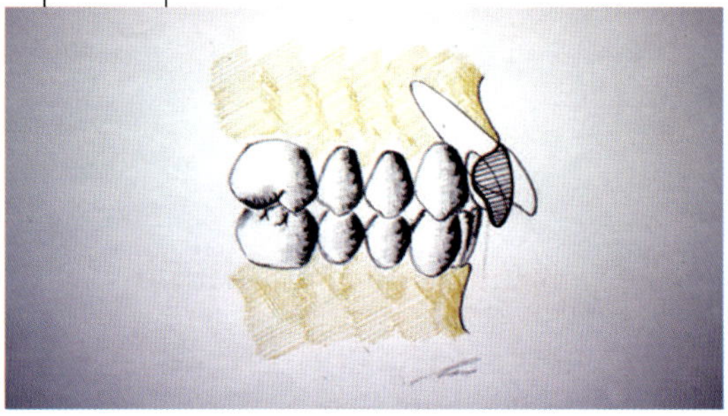

Figs. 6-95 & 6-96 Class II division 1 correction with a prosthesis.

6-97

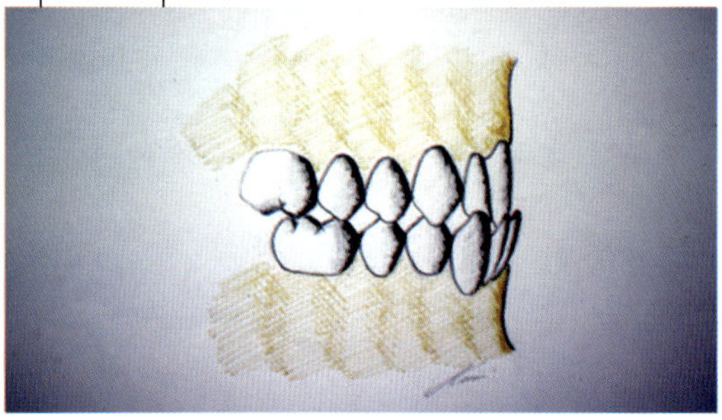

6-98

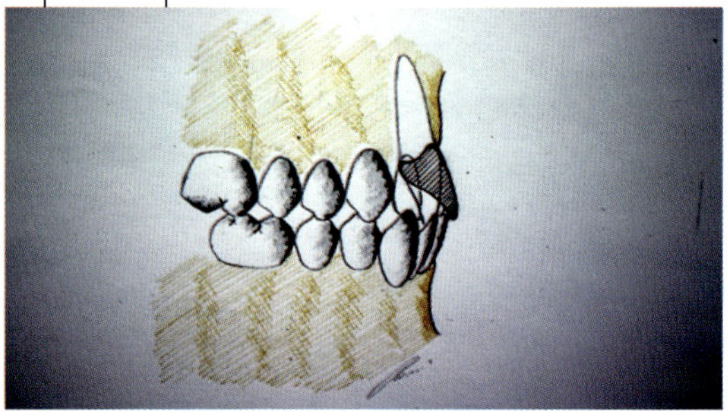

Figs. 6-97 & 6-98 Class III correction with a prosthesis.

CASE NUMBER 17

6-99

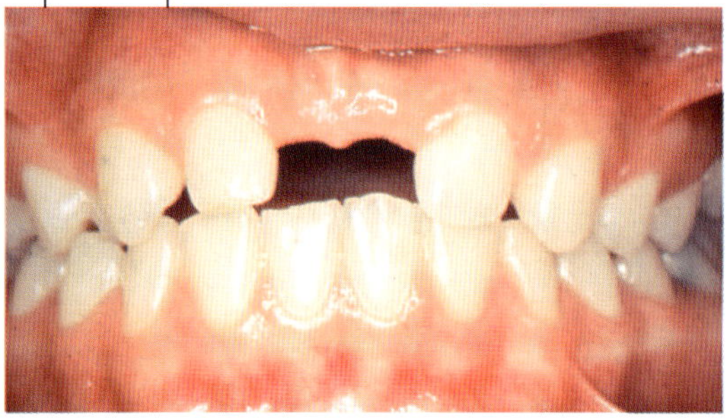

Fig. 6-99 Five years after the traumatic loss of maxillary central incisors: the mesial movement of other teeth reduced the space available for the incisor replacement. In this condition, an acceptable prosthesis cannot be realized.

6-100

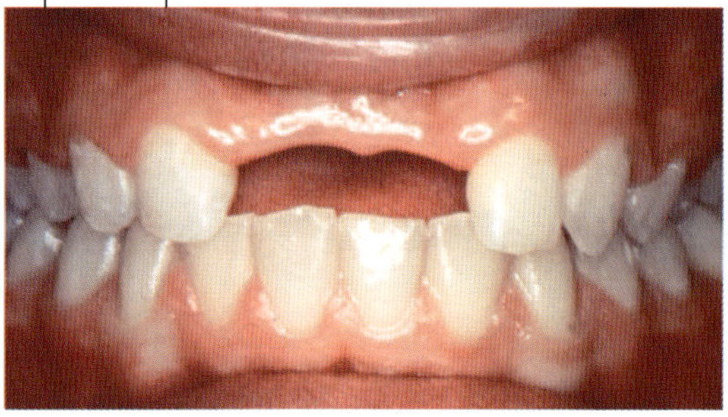

Fig. 6-100 With orthodontic treatment the correct space can be gained.

6-101

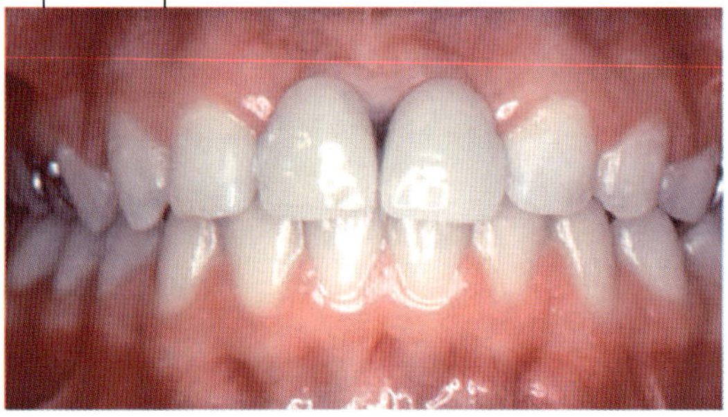

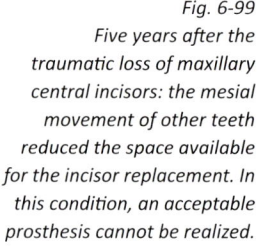

Fig. 6-101 After the orthodontic treatment a temporary removable prosthesis is applied.

CASE NUMBER 18

6-102

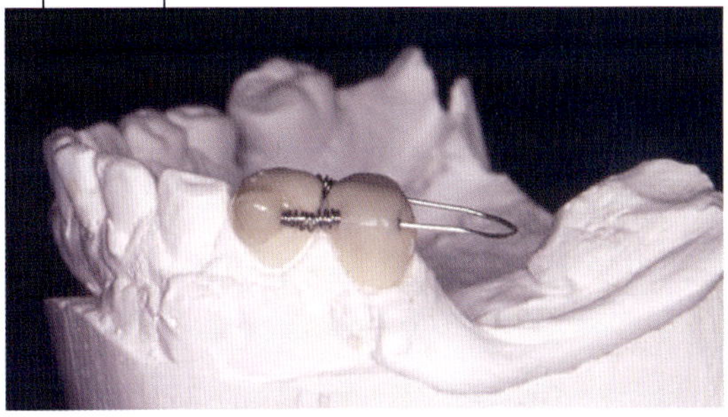

6-103

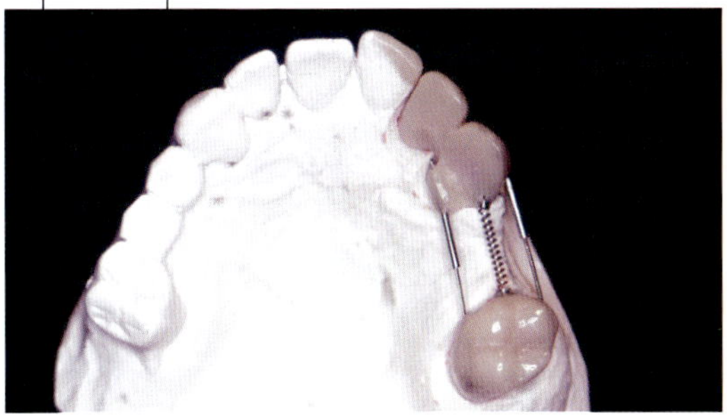

Fig. 6-102
Lower arch: ortho-prosthetic appliance for the distal displacement of the second premolar. On the premolars there are two acrylic crowns with one buccal and one lingual tube 0.20" where a stainless steel sectional 0.18" can slide, pushed by two open NiTi coil springs compressed between the teeth. The anterior teeth are lingually splinted.

Fig. 6-103
Upper arch: ortho-prosthetic appliance for the mesial displacement of the first molar. A closed NiTi coil spring pulls the molar mesially. The movement is guided by two 0.18" stainless steel sectionals sliding into two 0.20" tubes fixed on the canine.

6-104

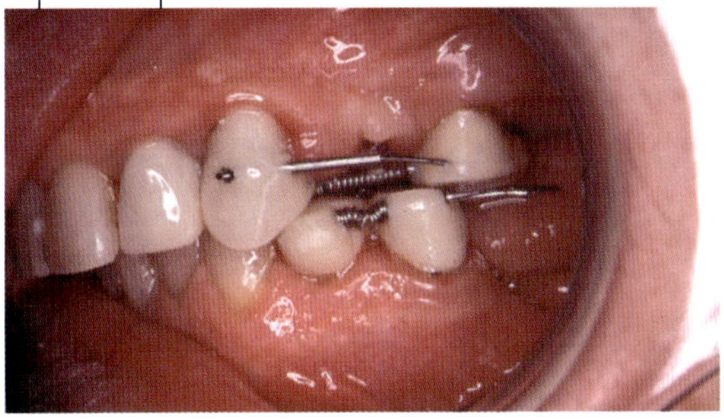

Fig. 6-104
The aim is to widen the masticatory surface in a 70 year old woman who refuses to opt for a removable prosthesis. The conditions for implants are not good. Thus the idea of two bridges after moving the upper molar mesially and the lower second premolar distally.

6-105

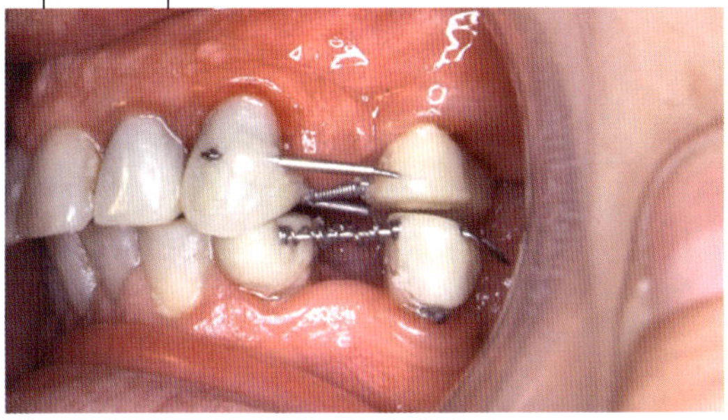

Fig. 6-105
Post-orthodontic phase of treatment. Two bridges will follow to end the treatment.

CASE NUMBER 19

6-106

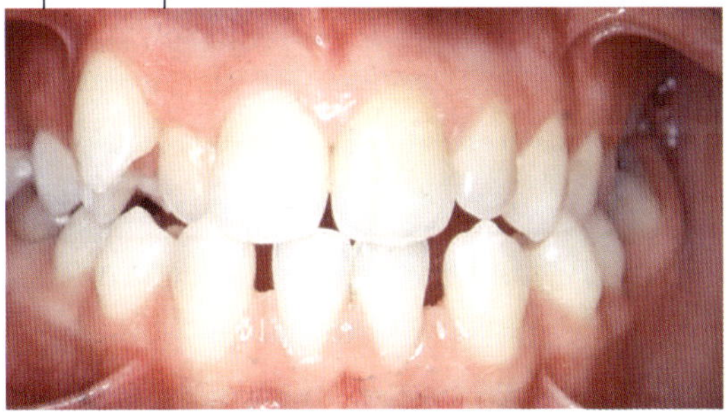

6-107

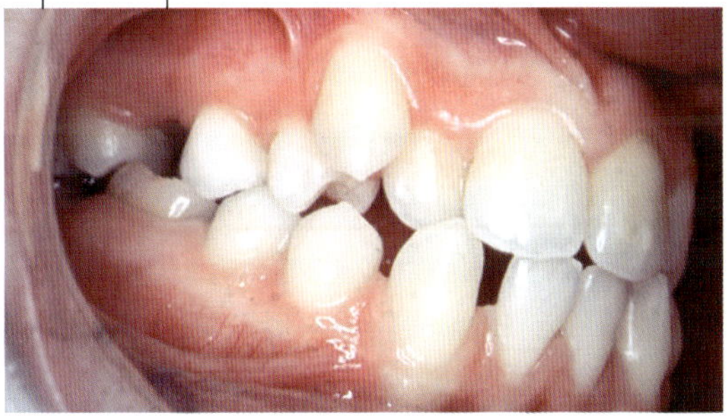

Figs. 6-106 & 6-107
Class I
Upper arch: space of extraction of first right molar, lack of space for right canine alignment, cross bite of right lateral incisor.
Lower arch: lateral incisors congenitally missing.
Treatment Plan
Upper arch: close orthodontically the molar extraction space while aligning the teeth.
Lower arch: open the space of the missing lateral incisors and replace them with a prosthesis.

6-108

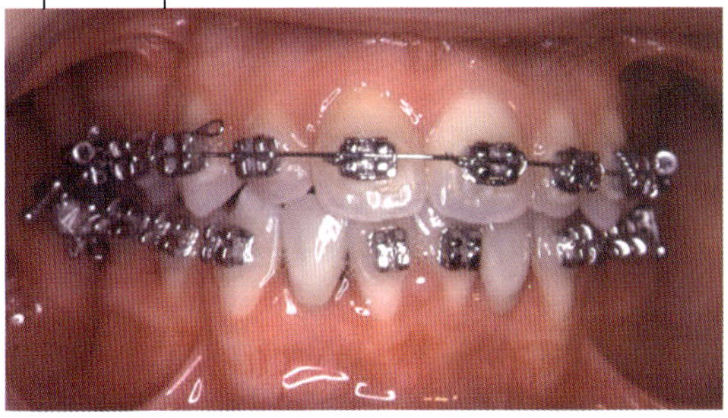

Fig. 6-108
At the end of the orthodontic treatment a Maryland bridge is applied. The alveolar bone was not thick enough for implants.

6-109

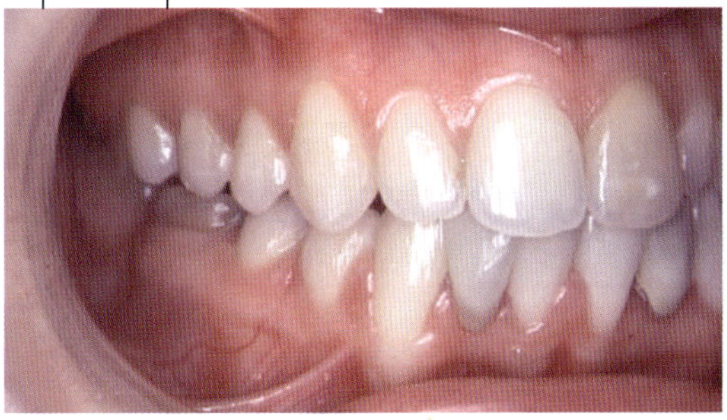

Fig. 6-109
Post-treatment occlusion.

CASE NUMBER 20

Fig. 6-110

Fig. 6-111
The case is a 45 year old patient.
Top: fixed prosthesis. Bottom: advanced periodontal disease with teeth migration. Which prosthesis should be considered under these circumstances?

6-110

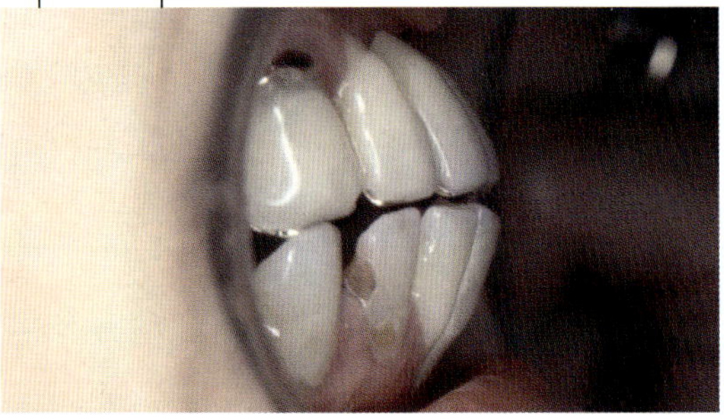

6-111

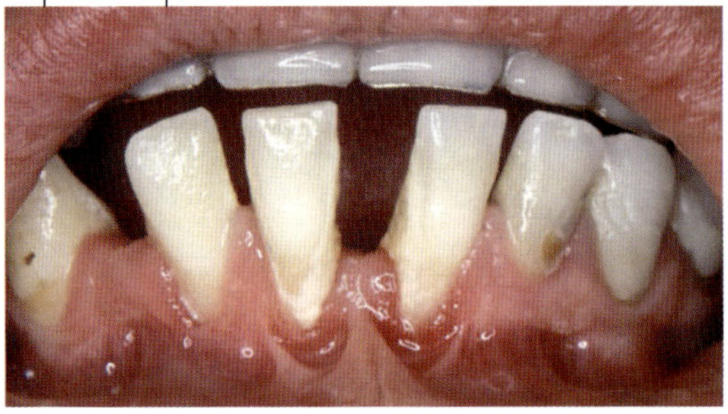

Figs. 6-112 & 6-113
Lower temporary prosthesis after a periodontal and orthodontic treatment. Notice the new lateral relationship between upper and lower dental arch.

6-112

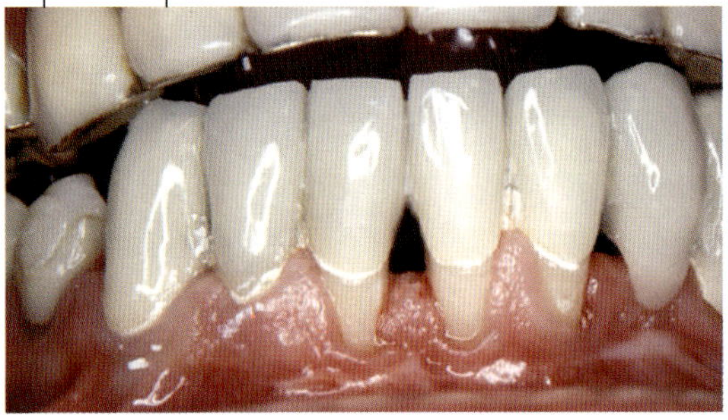

6-113

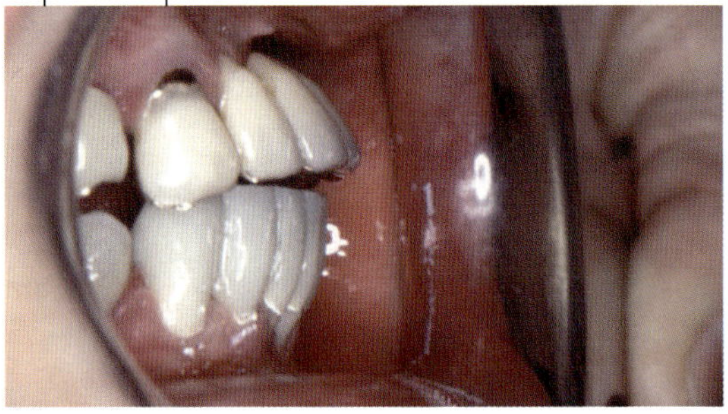

Fig. 6-114
Upper and lower new temporary prosthesis. There is a distal vertical space created to check whether the change in vertical dimension occurs without any consequences.

Fig. 6-115
Pre-treatment dental casts.

6-114

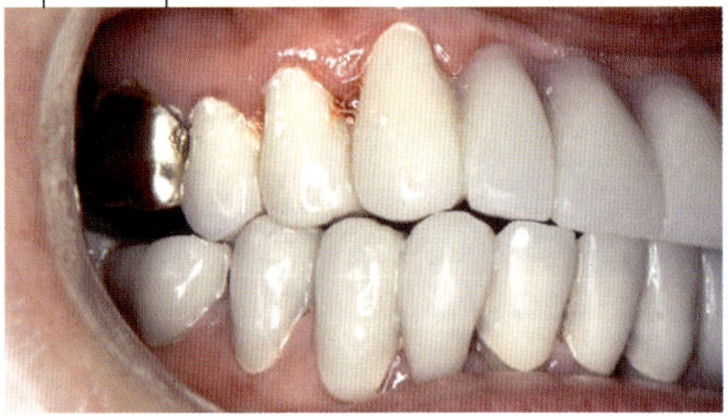

6-115

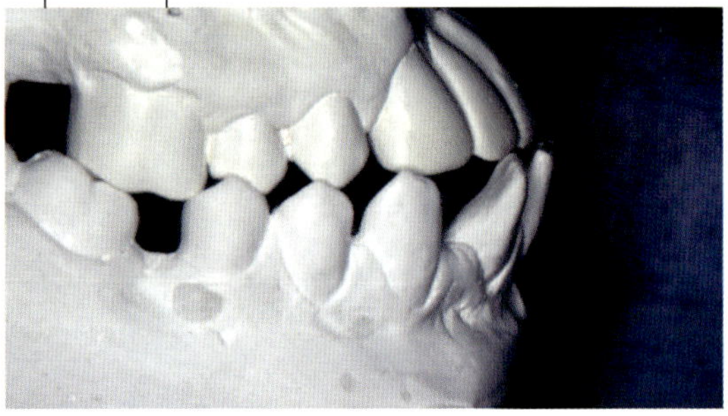

CASE NUMBER 21

6-116

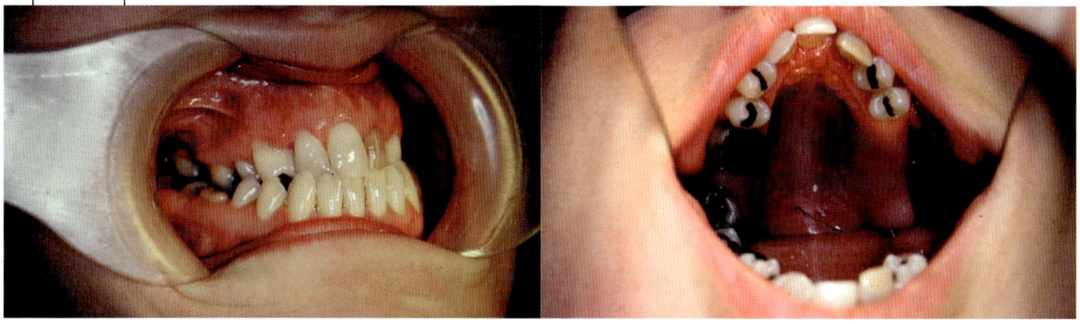

Fig. 6-116
Pre-treatment clinical situation in a 43 year old patient. There is an evident constriction of the upper dental arch as a consequence of many missing teeth.

6-117

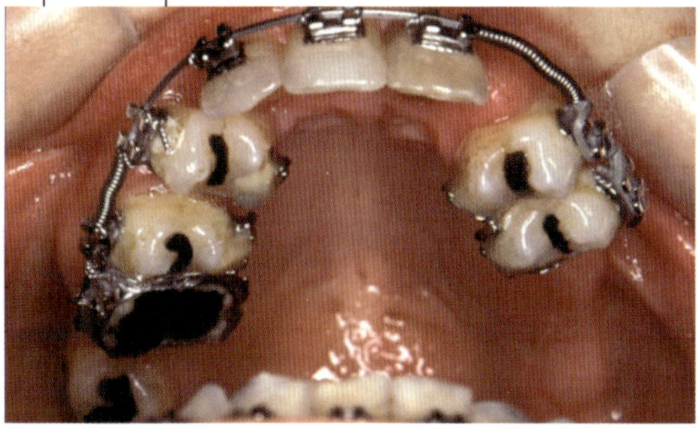

6-118

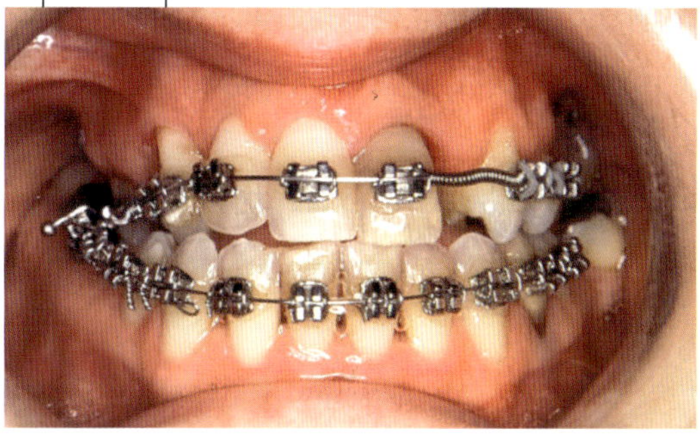

Figs. 6-117 & 6-118
The patient wants the best smile that can be obtained without surgery. By opening the spaces and changing the teeth torque, an orthodontic treatment is the premise for a satisfying fixed prosthesis.

6-119

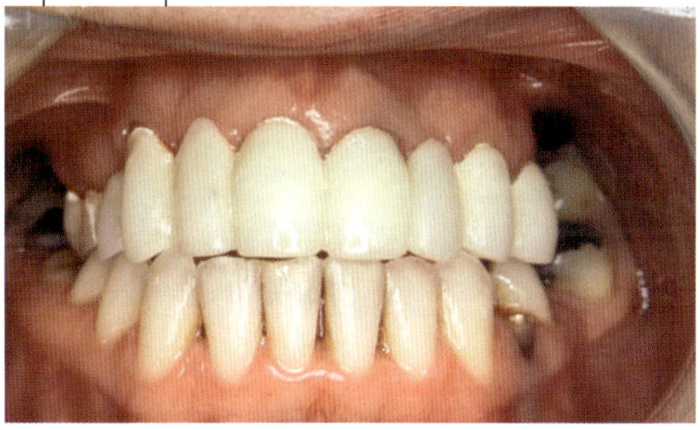

6-120

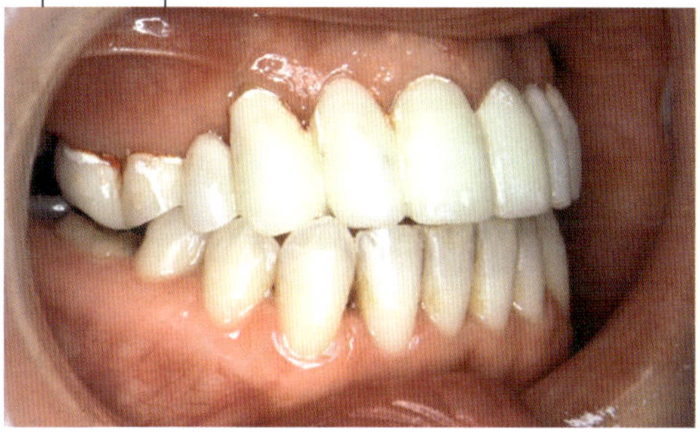

Figs. 6-119 & 6-120
Upper arch temporary prosthesis.

6-121

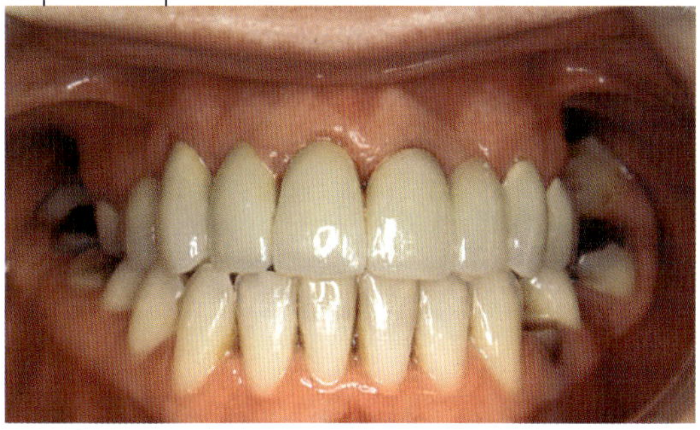

6-122

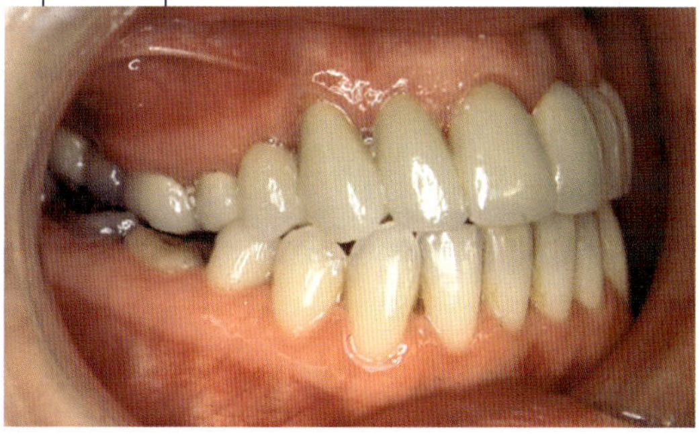

Figs. 6-121 & 6-122
Upper arch definitive prosthesis. Lower arch still under treatment.

ORTHODONTICS – IMPLANTOLOGY

Implantology is the basis of a prosthetic procedure. Consequently, many of the problems pointed out with ortho-prosthesis are the same as those with ortho-implants.

Once again, I would like to stress that it is better to place an implant in a mouth that has the best possible occlusion. There are cases where, in order to place an implant, more space between two teeth is needed and orthodontic treatment can be helpful. Do not forget that the space must be gained not only between the crowns but also between the roots. Above all, the implants must be placed at the end of growth in aesthetic areas, because where there is an implant the alveolar bone cannot grow and over the years an anti-aesthetic levelling of dental crowns can occur.

When a root has been lost in a growing patient because it has been fractured, before performing the extraction it is worth considering its orthodontic extrusion. That could be the best way to maintain a good bone level for an implant at the end of growth.

How do we know that growth has come to an end? A radiograph of the hand will allow us to evaluate the ossification stage of the carpus bones, the ulna – radius distal epiphysis.

Or, a lateral cephalogram can be repeated after one year. If there are no changes, growth has ended.

WHAT CAN IMPLANTOLOGY DO FOR ORTHODONTICS?

Implants, just like ankylosed teeth, do not move when a force is applied because there is no periodontal ligament (Figs. 6-123 & 6-124). Therefore, an implant provides ideal orthodontic maximum anchorage.

Once we thought that only osteointegrated implants (fixed to stay beyond the orthodontic treatment) could work. However, we now know that mini implants (which will be removed at the end of the orthodontic treatment) can also work in the same way. With the help of implants we can move teeth in all directions without undesired effects.

6-123

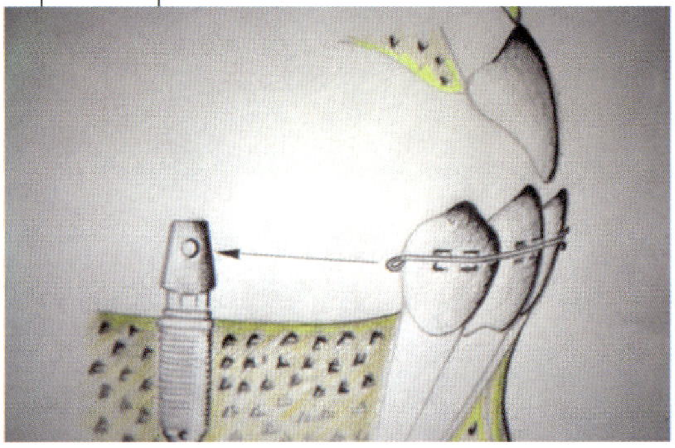

6-124

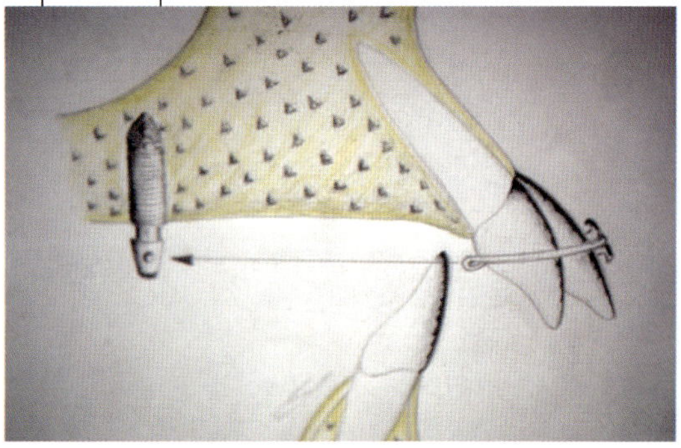

CASE NUMBER 22

This case underlines the importance of orthodontic treatment followed by implantology for the correction of a serious situation. The 21 year old female has a skeletal and dental open bite. After extraction of the roots, a fixed orthodontic appliance allows an excellent correction. All the roots appearing on the pretreatment panoramic radiograph were extracted. Then a fixed straight wire appliance was used to align the teeth and close the anterior open bite
Top: complete closure of the extraction spaces. Bottom: partial closure of the extraction spaces and implants.

6-127

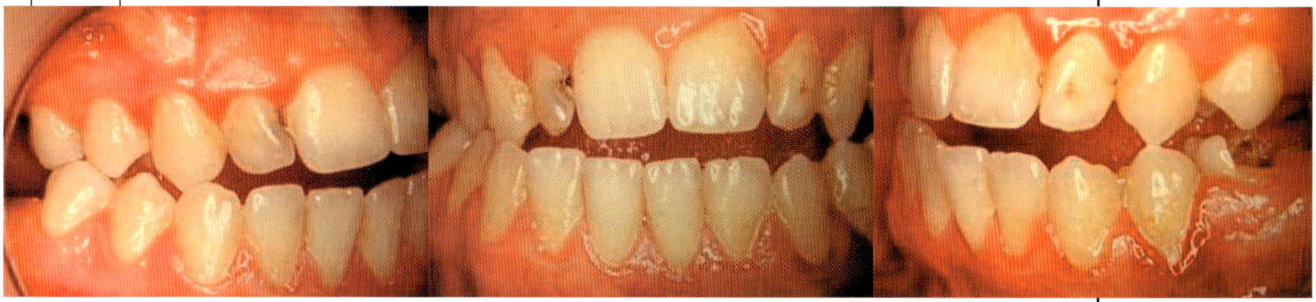

Fig. 6-127
Pre-treatment occlusion.

6-128

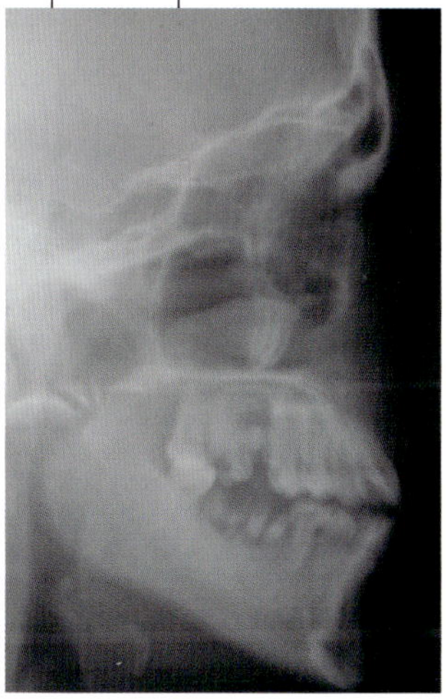

Fig. 6-128
Pre-treatment lateral cephalogram.

6-129

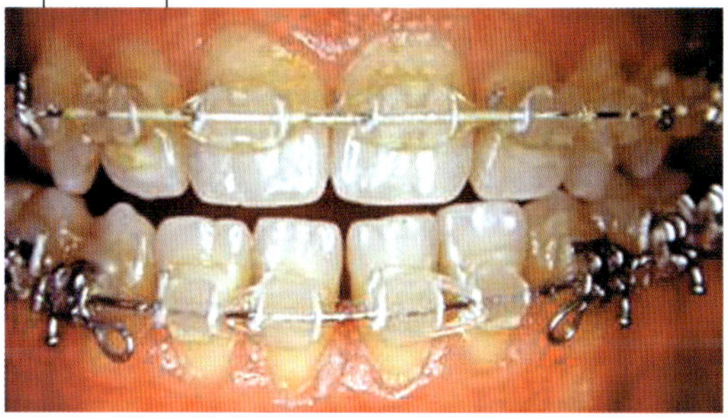

Fig. 6-129
Phase of orthodontic treatment.

6-130

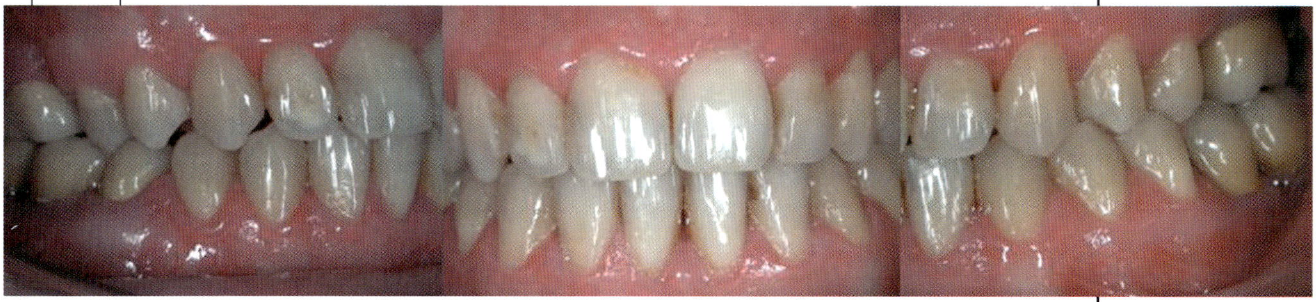

Fig. 6-130
Post-treatment occlusion.

6-131

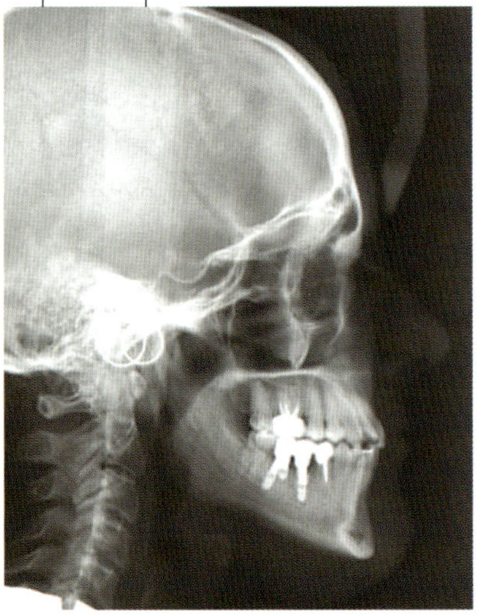

6-132

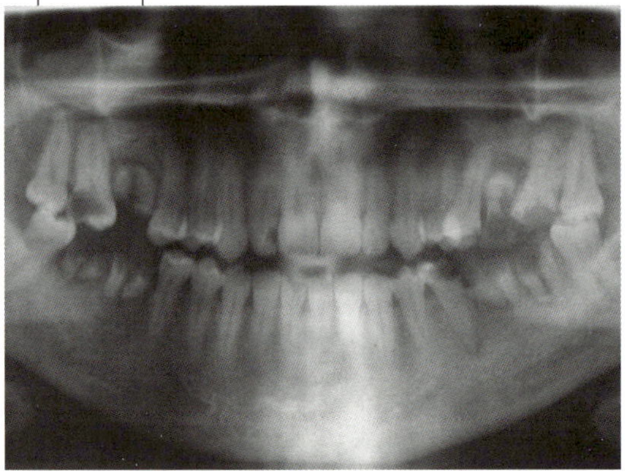

Fig. 6-131
Post-treatment lateral cephalogram.

Fig. 6-132
Pre-treatment panoramic radiograph.

6-133

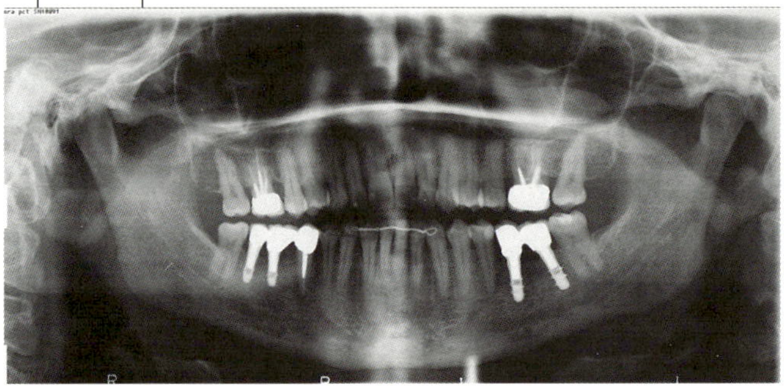

Fig. 6-133
Post-treatment panoramic radiograph.

CASE NUMBER 23

The case features missing lower left molars and consequent extrusion of the upper molars. With a simple NiTi sectional, intrusion of the first upper molar is possible. The second molar intrusion follows.

6-134

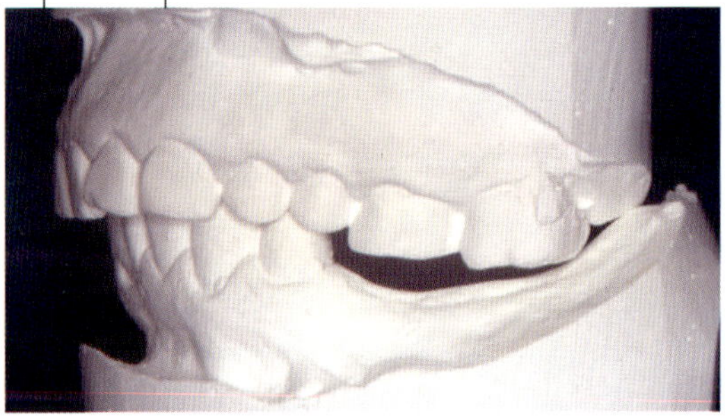

6-135

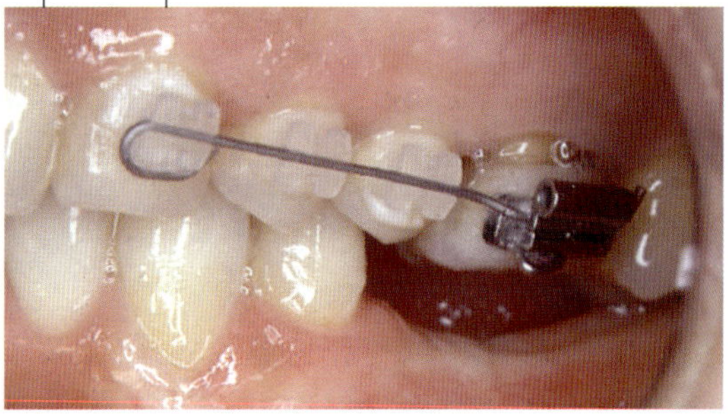

Fig. 6-134
Pre-treatment dental casts.

Fig. 6-135
NiTi sectional.

6-136

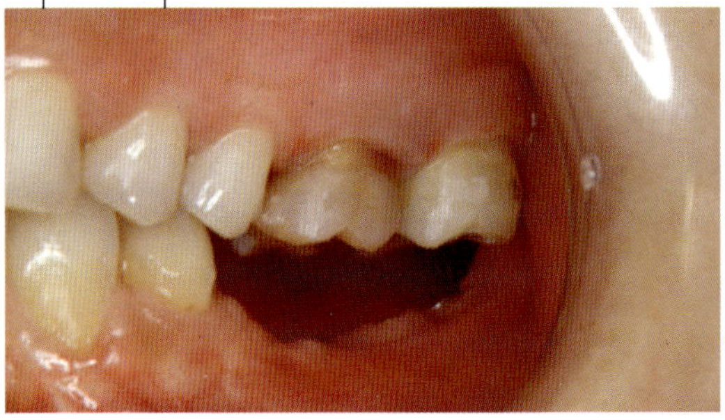

6-137

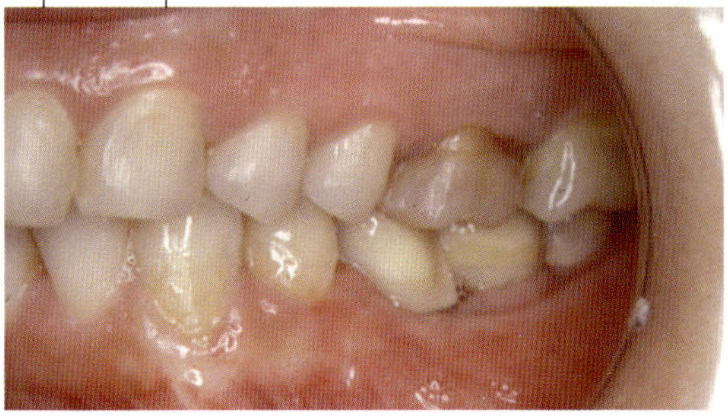

Fig. 6-136
After the intrusion and a gentle grinding of first molar.

Fig. 6-137
Temporary prosthesis on lower implants.

CASE NUMBER 24

WHAT IMPLANTOLOGY CAN DO FOR ORTHODONTICS.

The 27 year old patient has the lower left second premolar congenitally missing, the first molar with serious lesions, and the third molar partially erupted. She works at a dentist's office. Knowing the alternatives, she asks for an extraction of the first molar and of the deciduous tooth. She also wants to place an implant as anchorage in order to move the second and third molar mesially. She agreed to an experimentally short implant. The aim was to test the validity of the anchorage for an important movement (13 mm). Seven years later, the implant is still in a good condition.

6-138

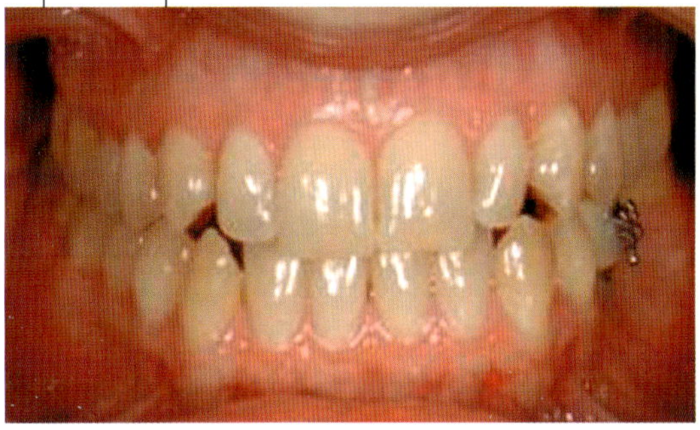

6-139

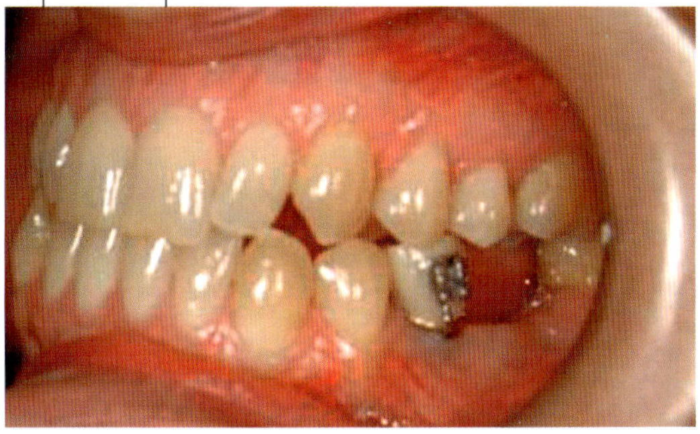

Figs. 6-138 & 6-139 Occlusion after placement of the implant. Crown on the implant. The crown has a bracket for the mesial traction of second molar.

6-140

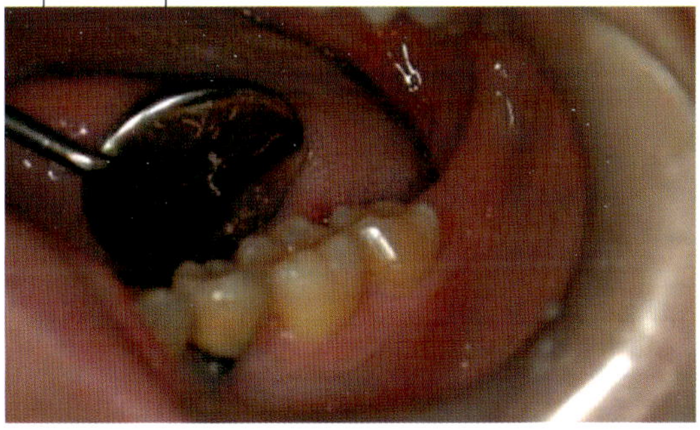

6-141

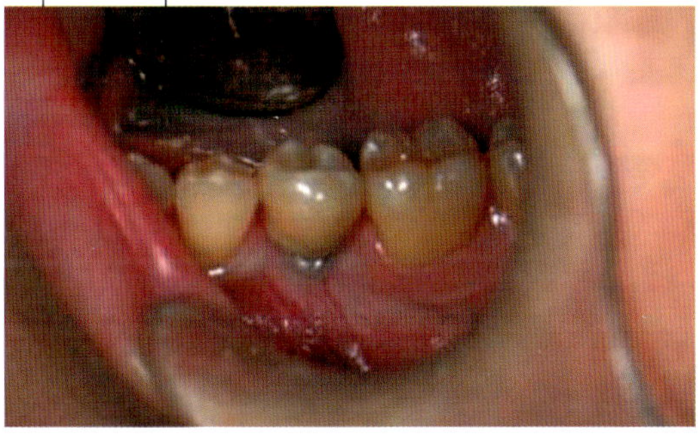

Figs. 6-140 & 6-141 Post-treatment situation.

6-142

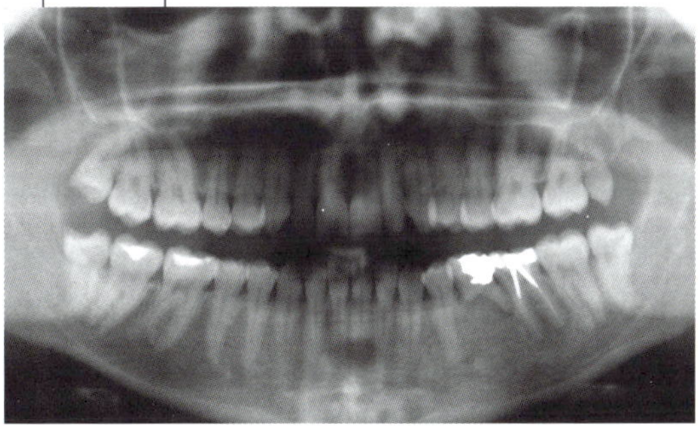

6-143

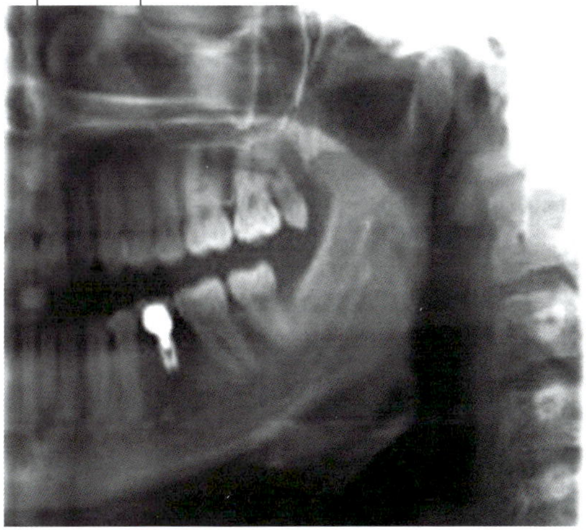

Fig. 6-142 Pre-treatment panoramic radiograph.

Fig. 6-143 Post-treatment panoramic radiograph.

SPECIAL THANKS TO THE AUTHORS OF THE FOLLOWING SECTION.

SURGICAL MANAGEMENT OF MINISCREW INSERTION AND REMOVAL: A STEP-BY-STEP APPROACH*

AUTHORS: DR. REINHART MEURSINGE REYNDERS AND DR. LAURA RONCHI

INTRODUCTION

Osteointegrated dental implants have been reliable sources of anchorage in orthodontics. The large size of these devices has limited their usage and smaller implants have therefore been developed. Currently, research on orthodontic mini-implants (OMIs) is still in its infancy.[1]

Success rates of OMIs range from 0% to 100%, but most clinical studies report success rates greater than 80% if mobile and displaced implants are included.[1] Little information about the adverse effects of OMI insertion (e.g. biological damage, inflammation, pain and discomfort) is available in dental literature. The orthodontic profession should therefore demand more scientific evidence for the application of these devices and companies that market OMIs should be involved in financing randomized clinical trials.[2] The current advice for using these devices is therefore "Doctor be prudent".

Prior to starting the insertion of OMIs we recommend:

1) evaluating the orthodontic devices necessary for the treatment
2) evaluating alternative devices for the treatment
3) carefully studying the dentofacial anatomy
4) studying the literature on mini-implant insertion
5) considering the risk of possible biological damage
6) considering the risk of mobility and displacement of OMIs
7) enrolling on several courses teaching the use of different implant systems, preferably practising on cadavers.

As a result of the vast amount of information on mini-implants and the limited space available in just one chapter we will focus exclusively on two procedures: the surgical management of the insertion of OMIs and their removal. Two types of OMIs are available: self-drilling and pre-drilling. The self-drilling type is currently the most frequently used and our insertion and removal protocols will only describe the procedures for this type of screw. These protocols should be used as general step-by-step guidelines and do not pretend to cover all aspects of the surgical management of the insertion and removal of OMIs. Furthermore, these protocols describe exclusively the process of interradicular insertion and have to be modified according to the location.

** Special note: This protocol is based on the clinical experience of the authors. Most additional information was retrieved from references 3, 10, 12, 15, and 16*

A PROTOCOL FOR SURGICAL MANAGEMENT OF THE INSERTION OF MINI-IMPLANTS

SURGICAL PHASES:

I) PREPARATION PHASE
II) SOFT TISSUE PHASE
III) CORTICAL BONE PHASE
IV) TRABECULAR BONE PHASE
V) FINAL POSITIONING PHASE

I) PREPARATION PHASE (STEPS 1-6)

RECORD TAKING (STEP 1)

Take new records at least 1 week prior to mini-implant insertion:
a) models of the dental arches
b) panoramic radiographs and or periapical radiographs and in complicated cases 3D images
c) extra and intra oral photographs.

INSERTION SITE SELECTION (STEP 2)

A) Clinical Intraoral Analysis:

Analyze the following clinical parameters, at least 1 week prior to mini-implant insertion:

1) Locate the mucogingival junction.
2) Analyze the soft tissue thickness.
3) Check the alveolar height.
4) Analyze potential intraoral barriers by pulling lips and cheeks, and possible frenum involvement.
5) Palpate the root prominence of neighbouring teeth.
6) Analyze the risk of soft tissue impingement by proposed orthodontic treatment devices.

B) Photographic Analysis:

1) Prepare a set of photographs with drawings of the mucogingival junction and the tooth axes of the neighbouring teeth using root prominence as a reference.
2) Prepare a set of photographs with drawings of the intended orthodontic treatment devices.

C) Radiographic Analysis:

1) Analyze the angulation of the roots.
2) Measure the interradicular space.

D) Model Analysis:

1) Design the mucogingival junction on the model.
2) Design the tooth axes of the neighbouring teeth using the root prominence as a reference.
3) Measure bone depth.
4) Analyze the alveolar curvature.
5) Analyze the risk of soft tissue impingement by the proposed treatment devices on the model.

Finally, select the insertion site based on the clinical, photographic, radiographic and model analyses and mark this site on the model and the photograph.

SELECTION OF MINISCREW (STEP 3)

Select the proper mini-implant (diameter, length, neck, and head) based on the analyses described under Step 2. The length of the neck has to be verified when the soft tissue thickness is measured (see Step 14).

CLINICAL VERIFICATION OF INSERTION SITE (STEP 4)

Thirty minutes prior to surgery: Check if the insertion site selected with the records can be confirmed clinically. Although this step seems redundant it is better to establish a possible error in insertion site selection prior than during surgery.

ORTHODONTIC PREPARATION (STEP 5)

1) **Thirty minutes prior to surgery**: Position surgical reference wire (.021 x .028 wires in a .022 slot) in the bracket of a neighbouring tooth (Fig. 1). It has also been recommended to bend a rectangular wire with an occlusal arm over the interproximal contact area.[3] This wire can be used to orient the X-ray beam and later the screwdriver during the insertion phase (see Step 13).
2) **Take a periapical radiograph.** A panoramic radiograph is not sufficiently reliable because of magnification and distortion of the image.[4-7] Vertical magnification in panoramic radiographs has been reported to be approximately 18-21%, whereas horizontal magnification is more unreliable.[6] Schnelle et al found the highest horizontal magnification (22%) in the mandibular molar area.[5] Further, there is a clinically significant variation between the radiographic and true root angulations.[4] Mckee et al found exaggerated root divergence in maxilla between the canine and first bicuspid, and in the mandible an exaggerated root convergence between canines and lateral incisors.[7]

SURGICAL PREPARATION (STEP 6)

Factors to consider with regard to surgical preparation:

1) Bring all records to the surgical area.
2) Aim to use pre-sterilized miniscrews. Touch only the head of miniscrew with the screwdriver. Never touch the screw part with any instrument or gloves! The label on the box of the pre-sterilized miniscrew should be attached to the patient's chart at the end of the insertion procedure!
3) Experience counts so aim for the same surgeon.[8,9]
4) Prepare the surgical set-up. Following is a basic checklist of instruments that are necessary for mini-implant insertion:
   a) Dental instruments and anaesthetics: dental probe, periodontal probe, mirror, tweezers, surgical scalpel, suction tip, cheek retractors, local extraoral topical anaesthetic and gauzes with chlorhexidine 0.12%.
   b) Mini-implant instrumentarium (Fig. 2): soft tissue punch, round burr and mini-implant burrs, hand drill for cortical bone penetration, surgical handpiece with NaCl solution, short and long screwdrivers and accessories, and a torque ratchet.
5) The doctor should wear a face mask and a surgical cap and after a surgical handwash, a pair of sterile gloves.

1

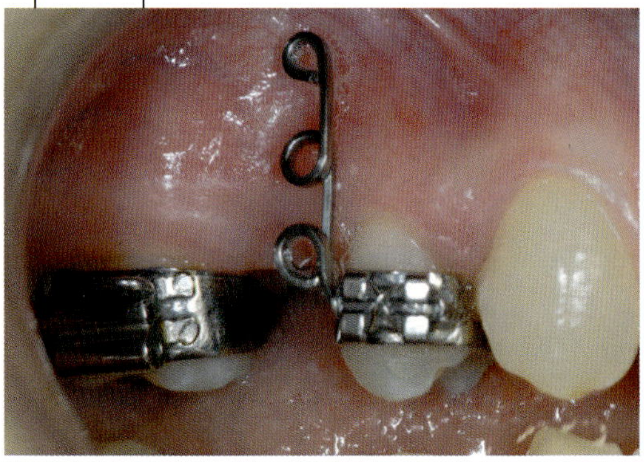

2

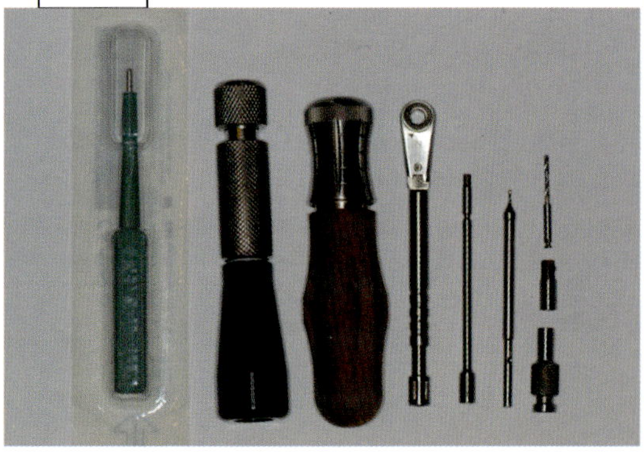

II) SOFT TISSUE PHASE (STEPS 7-15)

CLEANING WITH CHLORHEXIDINE (STEP 7)

Clean with chlorhexidine 0.12% (Fig. 3).

3

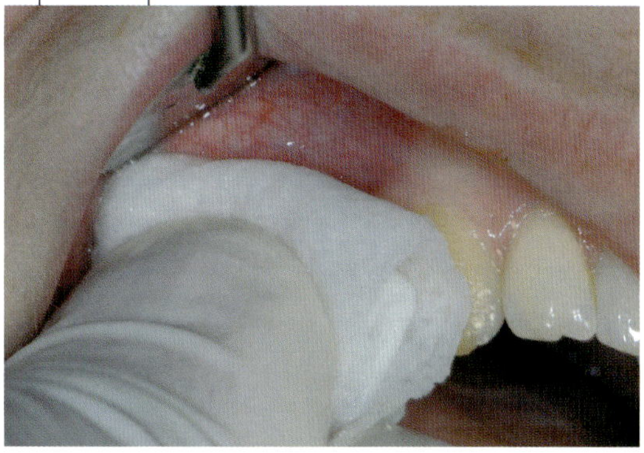

ANAESTHETIC PHASE (STEP 8)

The clinician should not try to achieve profound anaesthesia of the teeth, but only of the soft tissue. Therefore the patient can assess pain and react to warn the operator if the drill or the implant goes in too far. TADs placed on the buccal do not require anaesthetic on the lingual surfaces. One fourth of a lidocaine ampule is administered per insertion site.[10]
The epinephrine content is determined based on the patient's general condition. The injection point should be adjacent to the estimated insertion site and not in the depth of the vestibule because "block" anaesthesia is generally not necessary. An apical and distal injection is ideal considering the trajectory of the neurovascular bundle.[10]

REVIEW RECORDS AND CLINICAL ANALYSIS (STEP 9)

Prior to establishing the insertion site it is recommended to review all factors described under steps 1-3. It is particularly important to evaluate the direction of the orthodontic forces because a potential displacement of the screw could lead to biological damage.

VERTICAL POSITION OF THE INSERTION SITE (STEP 10)

1) Put a cheek retractor into place. This device greatly improves viewing during the entire process of mini-implant insertion. The patient should be instructed not to open the mouth too wide so that the lips are relaxed and retraction is readily possible.[3]
2) Check the periapical radiograph with the orthodontic reference wires.
3) Analyze the amount of bone in the coronal and apical areas. Take into consideration the conical shape of the roots.
4) Locate the mucogingival junction (Fig. 4). Don't make the insertion closer to the apex than the mucogingival junction if possible because this might lead to soft tissue irritation and inflammation (Fig. 5). If it is not possible to place the implant coronally to the mucogingival junction, it will be necessary to attach an extension wire

4

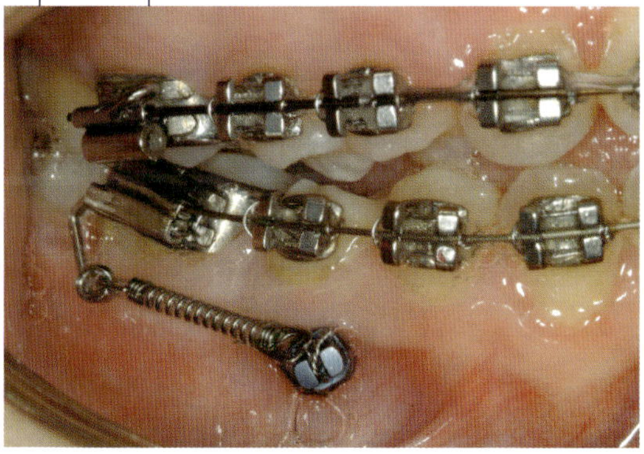

5

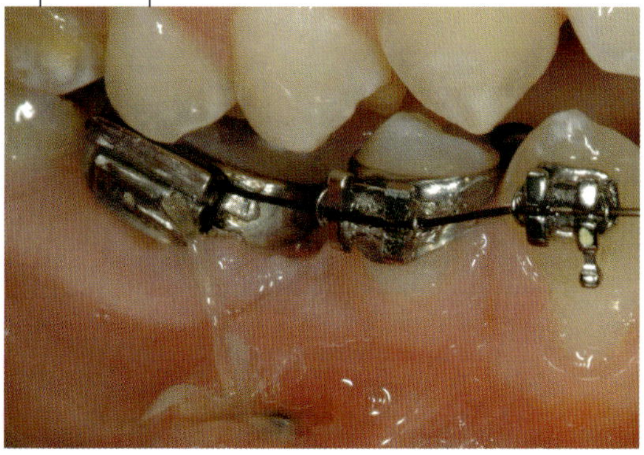

to the implant during the insertion phase. If the implant gets embedded in the soft tissues, it will still be usable by attaching orthodontic forces to the extension wire.

6

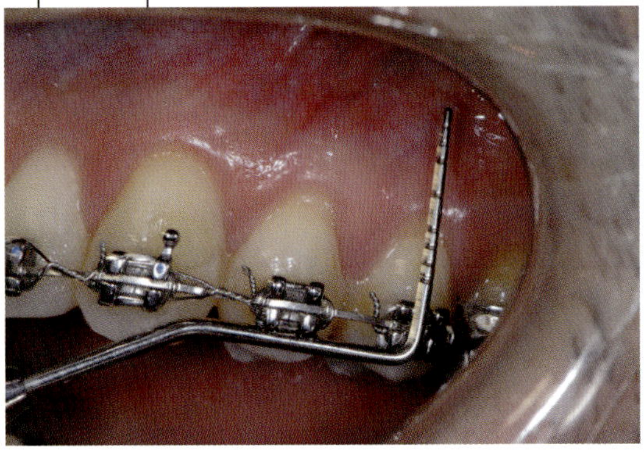

HORIZONTAL POSITION OF THE INSERTION SITE (STEP 11)

1) Check the root proximity on the periapical radiograph with the orthodontic reference wires.
2) Establish the angulation of the neighbouring teeth clinically and radiographically.
3) Feel the root contour with your fingers.
4) Mark with a perio probe an indentation in the soft tissue over the roots of the teeth neighbouring the insertion sites. This procedure can be helpful with horizontal orientation (Fig. 6).
5) Check the insertion site from the lateral view first and then from the occlusal view.
6) Check the orientation and location of the miniscrew also with the mouth mirror. Using a mirror from the occlusal side helps to confirm the miniscrew location.[3]
7) Check the rotation of the teeth.
8) To create an interdental reference line, mark with a perio probe the depression in the alveolar bone between the roots.

THE VERTICAL DIRECTION OF INSERTION (STEP 12)

1) Review all factors described under steps 1, 2, 3 and 9-11.
2) Prior to establishing the vertical direction of insertion the following factors should be considered:
   a) Vertical angulation may prevent root contact or other surgical damage.[8]
   b) Vertical angulation may increase cortical bone contact.[8]
   c) A vertical angulation of 45 degrees to the occlusal plane is generally acceptable.
   d) Excessive vertical angulation could:
      a) weaken the cortical bone[10]
      b) lead to slippage of the miniscrew
      c) decrease the contact between platform and cortical bone
      d) leave part of the threaded portion exposed.[10]

THE HORIZONTAL DIRECTION OF INSERTION (STEP 13)

1) Review all factors described under steps 1, 2, 3 and 9-11.
2) Check the site from the lateral view first and then from the occlusal view.
3) The proximal contact area is a good reference for determination of the proper insertion path because the interradicular space reflects the direction of the contact surface viewed from the occlusal surface (Fig. 7).[10] Rectangular orthodontic wire with an occlusal arm over the inter-

7

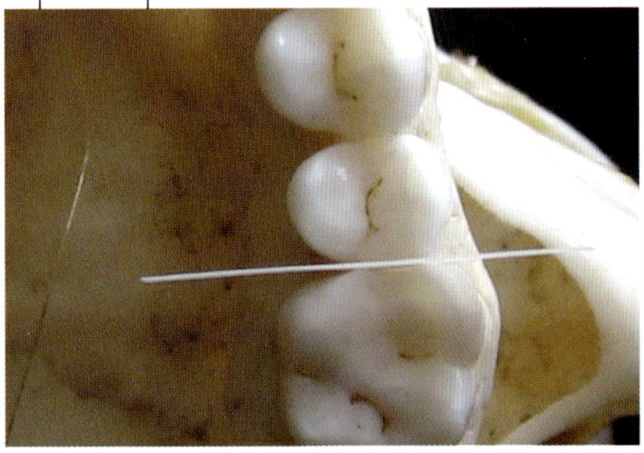

proximal contact area can facilitate finding the proper direction[3] (see Step 5). It is important to note that the maxillary labial cortical bone is not exactly perpendicular to the interproximal contact, especially in the buccal segment.[10]

4) Check the rotation of teeth from the occlusal surface (Fig. 8) and possible anomalies of root formation (Fig. 9).
5) Bear in mind that close root proximity can lead to miniscrew failure.[11]

8

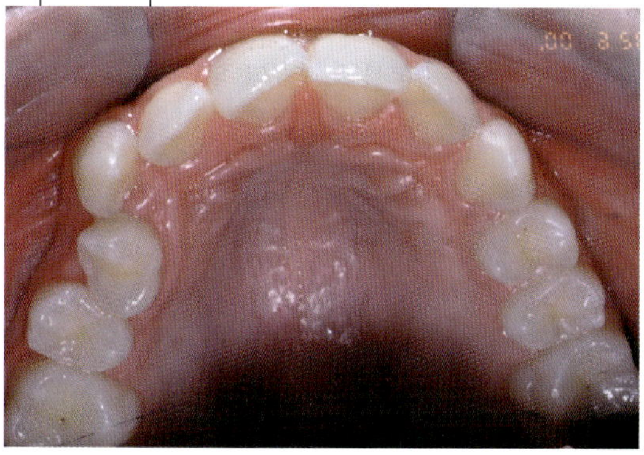

9

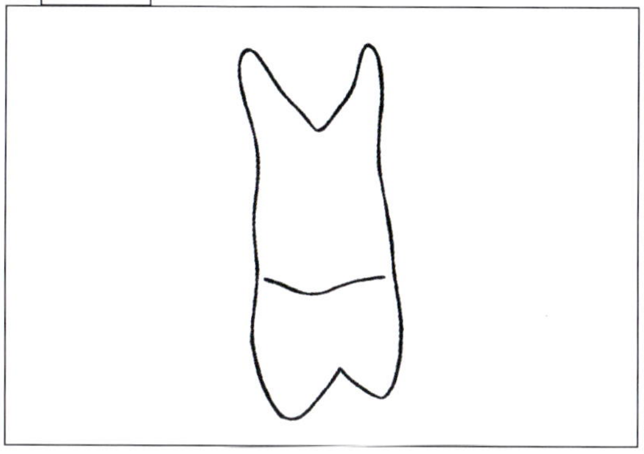

MARKING THE INSERTION SITE AND MEASURING THE GINGIVAL THICKNESS (STEP 14)

1) After careful evaluation of the vertical and horizontal positioning and direction, the insertion site can be marked with the point of an explorer or a perio probe.
2) With a periodontal probe the thickness of the gingiva can be measured and an implant with the proper neck length can be selected. Gingival thickness is generally 1-2 mm in the buccal premolar and molar area in both maxilla and mandible.
3) At this point the orthodontic vertical reference wire is removed.

SOFT TISSUE PENETRATION (STEP 15)

Three modes of soft tissue penetration:

1) Direct soft tissue penetration without a soft tissue punch. This procedure is indicated in areas with thin soft tissues and when pilot hole drilling in the cortical bone is not indicated. The soft tissue is directly penetrated by the screw at the insertion site. Penetration should be performed by pressing the self drilling screw through the gingiva without turning the screw because this might lead to tissue injuries.[12]

10

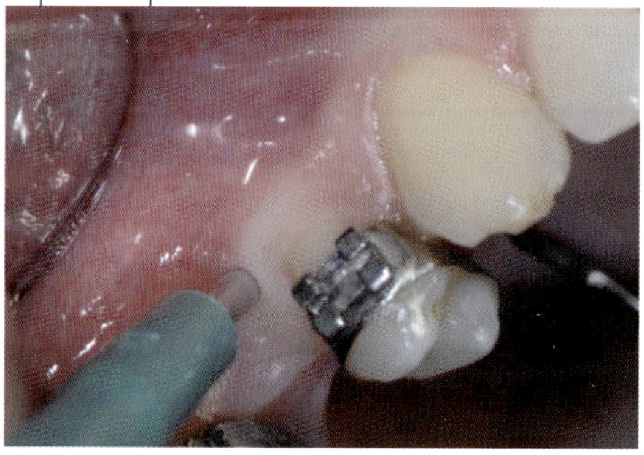

2) Soft tissue penetration with a tissue punch (mini flap) (Fig. 10). This procedure can be helpful in areas with thicker soft tissues. Tearing of this tissue should be avoided because this may lead to infection or inflammation. To avoid tissue tear, always use a new tissue punch for each insertion site. Use the same size diameter punch as the diameter of the screw, a 1.5 mm diameter punch for a 1.5 mm screw. The tissue excised by the tissue puncher needs to be removed with tweezers or a sharp surgical scalpel.

3) Soft tissue penetration with a flap. The size of a soft tissue flap is generally between 2-5 mm. Advantages of this procedure are:
   a) Direct viewing of the bone which is particularly indicated in areas with movable mucosa or areas that are technically challenging.
   b) Less risk of soft tissue spinning around the burr.
   c) Less risk of soft tissue getting embedded into the hole.[13]

Flap procedures generally lead to greater discomfort.[1]

III) CORTICAL BONE PHASE (STEP 16)

CORTICAL BONE PENETRATION WITHOUT A STARTER PILOT HOLE (STEP 16A)

A) Indications for cortical bone penetration without a starter pilot hole

1) In cases of thin cortical bone (pilot holes are rarely indicated in the maxilla).
2) When access is relatively easy.
3) When no excessive angulation is necessary (no risk of slippage).

B) Technique

1) Insertion direction

A short screwdriver can be used initially to get a feel for the bone density. Longer screwdrivers with large handles allow for easier insertion but at the same time increase the risk of breakage.[15] The screw is placed in the screwdriver and is positioned at the insertion site. Always start with a perpendicular approach to the bone at the beginning. First penetrate the bone perpendicularly and then angulate. This approach avoids the risk of slipping (Fig. 11). If a risk of slipping exists, prepare a starter pilot hole in the bone first (see Step 16b).

2) Insertion path

The insertion path is generally established during the trabecular phase (see Step 17). However, in cases of very thick cortical bone, the insertion path is already defined in the cortical bone insertion phase.

3) Insertion pressure and movement

The first turns (2-4) require firm pressure to efficiently penetrate the cortical bone. Apply a constant force of 4-10 Ncm.[12] Turning should be done by twisting the thumb and forefinger and should not be done with the wrist.[12] The penetration of the cortical bone should be performed by virtue of the function of the screw, with rotational motion rather than with vertical force.[16] If the cortical bone is too hard, prepare a pilot hole with a hand piece (see Step 16b). Avoid wiggling movements because this can negatively affect the primary stability.

4) Insertion speed

Insert slowly, not faster than 30 rpm, which is almost impossible to achieve with rotations by hand.[10] Saline irrigation is not needed if the insertion speed does not exceed this recommended value.[3]

11

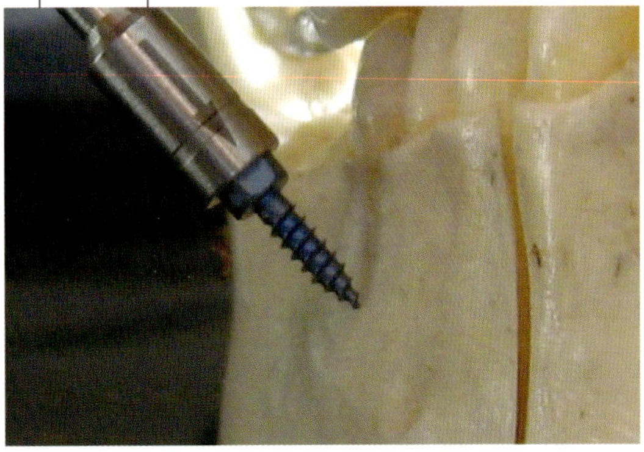

CORTICAL BONE PENETRATION WITH A STARTER PILOT HOLE (STEP 16B)

A) Indications for cortical bone penetration with a starter pilot hole

1) In cases of thick cortical bone (mid palatal suture, and buccal alveolus in the mandible).
2) In areas that are difficult to access.
3) When an excessive angulation is necessary. A pilot hole then helps to avoid slippage of the miniscrew.[12]

B) Techniques

Technique of starter pilot hole drilling of the cortical bone with hand drill

1) Just an indentation mark in the cortical bone is usually sufficient.
2) Avoid excessive pressure, especially in thicker cortical bone
3) Insertion speed should be slow, not faster than 30 rpm, which as mentioned is almost impossible to achieve with rotations by hand.

Technique of starter pilot hole drilling of the cortical bone with hand piece

1) Avoid wiggling of the shaft.[9] Inaccuracy of the shaft can cause wiggling and therefore loosening. The drill should be checked before surgery to make sure it has no bends that might cause it to wobble and inadvertently enlarge the opening.
2) Usually cortical bone penetration can be performed directly with a pilot hole drill. However, in areas with dense bone or areas that are hard to access or when the implant needs to be inserted at an excessive angulation it is recommended to prepare a small initial indentation in the bone. Use a small round drill (1 mm rose drill) for this procedure.
3) Use pilot hole drills with a smaller diameter than the diameter of the screws. The diameter of the drill should be 70-85% of the external diameter of the screw.[17] Therefore use 1 mm drills for 1.5 mm diameter miniscrews and 1.5 mm drills for 2 mm miniscrews.
4) Use sharp and new drills.[8] Frequently replace screws because drills age with use and sterilization procedures.
5) Change pilot hole burrs for each implant site (avoids risk of contamination).[18]
6) To keep the insertion site clean and cool, spray cooled (5°C) physiological saline solution into the surgical site using a sterile syringe (Fig. 12).
7) Monitor carefully the drill speed (500 to 800 rpm) and the temperature.[8]
8) Avoid excessive pressure.
9) Pay attention to avoid soft tissue impaction into the surgical site.

12

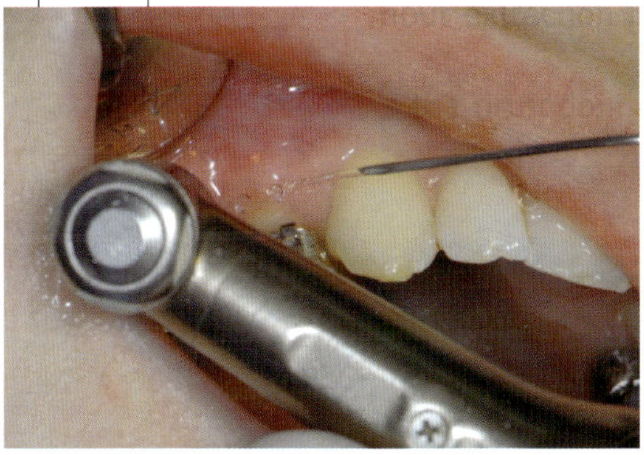

IV) TRABECULAR BONE INSERTION PHASE (STEP 17)

1) Insertion Path

The proximal contact points should be used as a reference line for the insertion path (Fig. 7). Keep watching this line during the entire trabecular bone insertion phase. During this phase the neighbouring roots should be checked for possible mobility caused by a contact between the miniscrew and the root. Be aware of rotated teeth (palatal root involvement). In case of insecurity about the correct direction of the insertion path, a periapical radiograph can be taken to control progress after half of the miniscrew length has penetrated the bone.[3] Changing the direction of insertion can be done in the early phases of insertion but should be carried out with great caution because it could widen the implant shaft which could negatively influence the initial stability and result in implant failure. Furthermore, a late change in the direction of insertion could lead to the fracture of the screw.

2) Insertion Speed

Insertion speed should be slow, not faster than 30 rpm, (Fig. 13). Also, in cases that require predrilling, the speed of the hand piece should be adjusted to 25 rpm.[15]

3) Insertion Pressure and movement

Maintain a steady torque (4-10 Ncm).[12] Avoid wiggling, because this type of movement can negatively affect primary stability and increases the risk of fracture. Therefore firmly fix the handle of the driver in the palm of the hand. Delicate movements of the thumb and the index and middle finger are indicated and wrist movements should be avoided. A short screwdriver can be used initially to get a feel for the bone density. Longer screwdrivers with large handles allow for easier insertion, but at the same time increase the risk of breakage and damage to the bone.[15] As described under the penetration of the cortical bone, the trabecular bone should also be penetrated by virtue of the function of the screw, a rotational motion rather than vertical force.[16]

Remember that excessively compressed bone is more subject to local necrosis and in cases of extremely hard bone it is recommended to predrill. A torque ratchet (Fig. 14) with torque control is helpful to avoid excessive force levels, but manipulation of this instrument is difficult and could transmit undesirable lateral forces.

13

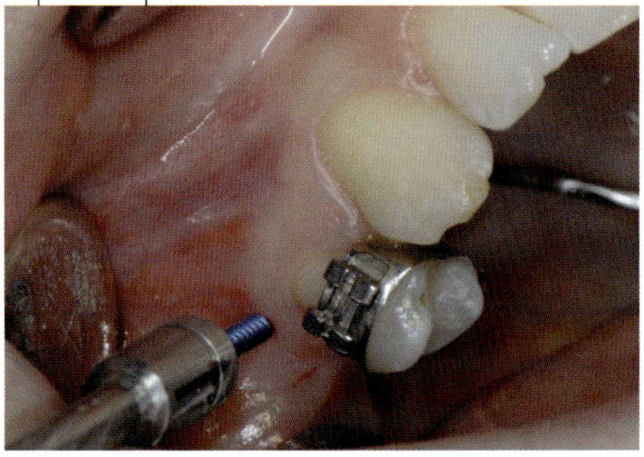

14

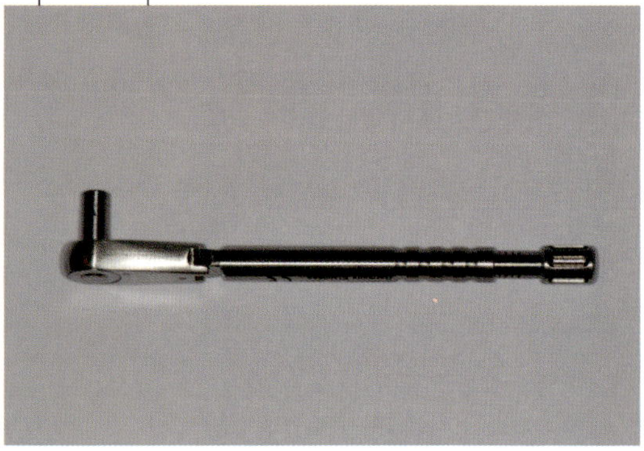

Tips to avoid root damage include:

1) Careful preoperative planning.
2) Preoperative radiography.
3) Use of reference wires.
4) Create spacing between roots during pre-surgical orthodontic phase.
5) Angulation of the screw to avoid root contact. With an oblique insertion, slippage is likely to occur instead of penetration of the root.[16]
6) Infiltrative anesthesia (small amount).
7) Patient response.
8) Tactile sense (direct from hands or indirect from adjacent tooth movement).
9) Periapical radiograph after initial penetration of the trabecular bone to check correct insertion path. Be attentive to the differences in hardness between the cementum and bone during the insertion procedure.

10) Post-operative X-ray to see how accurate predictions were and to help improve the learning curve.

Tips on how to avoid miniscrew fracture

1) Pilot drilling in cases of thick cortical bone.
2) Consistent insertion path.
3) Appropriate diameter.
4) Adequate vertical torque.
5) Avoid lateral movements.

V) FINAL POSITIONING PHASE (STEPS 18-24)

INSERTION TORQUE (STEP 18)

After approximately two thirds of the full length of the screw is inserted and its bone engagement is secured, implant placement should be finished with only a rotational movement.[16] The screw should be rotated carefully without vertical or lateral movements.

Excessive torque can damage the bone. Torque values for 1.6 mm screws of 5-10 Ncm have been recommended.[19,20] The torque ratchet can be used to set these torque values, but lateral movements are difficult to control with this instrument.

INSERTION DEPTH (STEP 19)

Opinions differ with regard to the insertion depth. Kuroda et al[11] recommend an insertion depth of at least 5-6 mm and Poggio et al[21] 6-8 mm.

REMOVAL OF SCREWDRIVER OR TORQUE RATCHET (STEP 20)

Detach the driver from the screw by removing the screwdriver in an exact line with the axis of the implant. Removal of the screwdriver or torque ratchet should be done with great care because lateral movements can traumatize the bone and therefore negatively affect primary stability.

CHECK PRIMARY STABILITY (STEP 21)

Primary stability should be checked with an explorer (Fig. 15). The stability of the mini-implant usually does not rely on osteointegration, but mostly on mechanical retention. Loosening of a mini-implant is probably related to a lack of initial stability.[13,20] Therefore, in cases of insufficient primary stability, a larger diameter screw should be used or a new insertion site should be chosen.

15

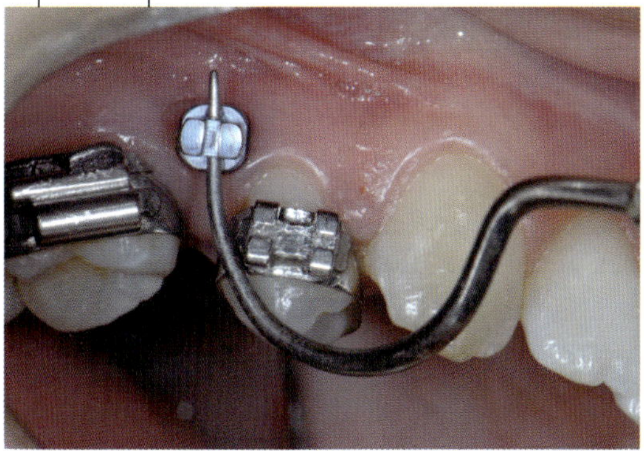

SOFT TISSUE CONTROL (STEP 22)

At the completion of the miniscrew insertion the soft tissues directly surrounding the miniscrews should be analyzed. Soft tissue release incisions are at times indicated. A tissue punch could also release circular tension of the soft tissues around the miniscrew head.

RADIOGRAPHIC CONTROL (STEP 23)

It is necessary to take a periapical radiograph after the insertion of the implant. One image with the tip of the miniscrew located between the roots is enough to verify safe placement, but if the miniscrew seems to overlap the root, a second radiograph at another angle needs to be taken.[3]

STABILIZING OF THE MINI-IMPLANT (STEP 24)

When implants are immediately loaded only light forces should be applied (less than 50 grams) (Fig. 16).[18,22]

16

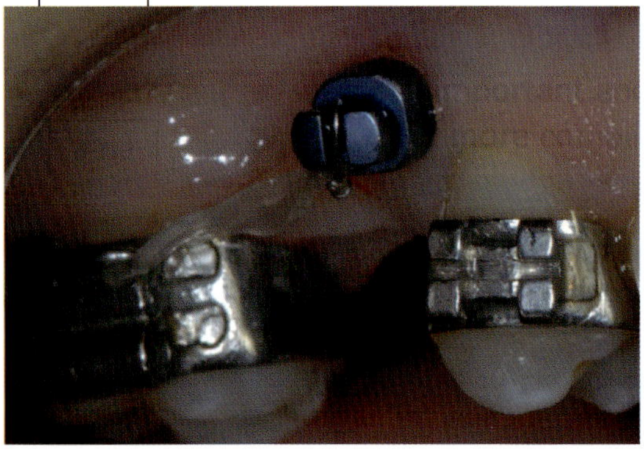

SURGICAL MANAGEMENT FOR THE REMOVAL OF MINI-IMPLANTS

Although the removal of OMI is generally easy, this procedure should be performed with great care.[23-25] The highest torsion forces are applied to the miniscrews during the removal process and special prudence is recommended when osseointegration has occurred. The miniscrew head could fracture from the neck of the shaft and a minimum diameter of 1.6 mm for self-drilling miniscrews of 8 mm or longer has therefore been recommended.[23] One study showed that 50% of 2 mm diameter implants required removal torque values greater than 8.7 Ncm and removal torque values were higher for the longer screws and in the mandible.[24] Kim et al[25] showed that the removal torque is proportional to the square of the radius of the screw. We advise checking the safe removal torque values with the implant company for each specific screw.

If the miniscrew fractures a small surgical procedure will be necessary. In the case that this procedure risks damage to neighbouring structures, the broken screw is either left in position or an orthodontic treatment can be performed to increase the area of access for a later surgical procedure to remove the broken fragment. Our protocol for the removal of OMIs is described under here.

PROTOCOL FOR THE REMOVAL OF MINI-IMPLANTS

LOCAL ANESTHESIA (STEP 1)

Generally, local anaesthesia is not necessary for the removal of mini-implants that are placed between dental roots.

USE OF REMOVAL DEVICES (STEP 2)

Set the torque ratchet at the proper safe removal torque value (as supplied by the implant company) and rotate the screw in a counterclockwise direction. The screwdriver that was used for the miniscrew insertion can also be used to remove the initial torque, but forces are more difficult to control. Howe pliers have been suggested[26] but turning is more complicated and these pliers also lack control over the torquing forces.

USE OF DENTAL FLOSS (STEP 3)

When the implant has been loosened to about a quarter way out of the bone, it is recommended to tie dental floss to it to prevent the implant from falling into the patient's oral cavity once fully extracted.

TIPS IN CASE OF DIFFICULTY WITH THE REMOVAL OF MINI-IMPLANTS (STEP 4)

When an implant cannot be removed with the appropriate screwdriver or torque ratchet, gentle touching of the screw head with a slow rotating round carbide burr can be a helpful clinical trick to facilitate loosening. This method is particularly useful when removing an implant in the posterior part of the dentition.[26]

REPEAT STEP 4 (STEP 5)

If no mobility is obtained, it is recommended to wait 3-7 days and then retry the same procedure. It has been suggested that microfractures or bone remodelling caused by the initial attempt will loosen the implant and facilitate removal during the second attempt.[27]

INSTRUCTIONS ON WOUND HEALING (STEP 6)

Wound healing is mostly fast and uneventful (Fig. 17). Patients should avoid eating hot and salty foods for 2 to 3 days to prevent pain or aggravation of the wound.[16]

17

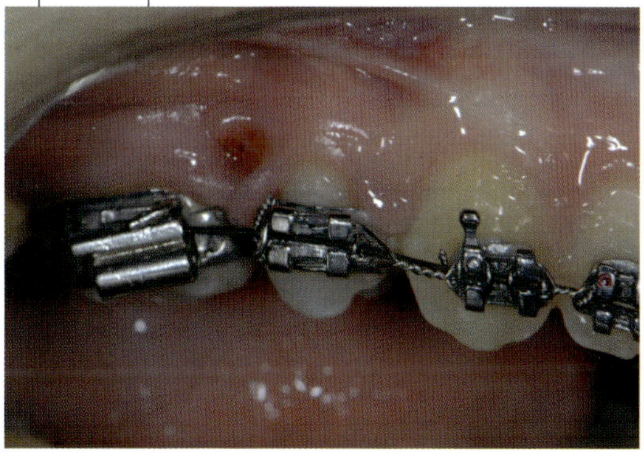

REFERENCES

1. Reynders R, Ronchi L, Bipat S. Mini-implants in orthodontics: a systematic review of the literature. *Am J Orthod Dentofacial Orthop* 2009;135:564.e1-564.e19.
2. Skeggs RM, Benson PE, Dyer F. Reinforcement of anchorage during orthodontic brace treatment with implants or other surgical methods. *Cochrane Database Syst Rev* 2007 Jul 18;(3):CD005098.
3. Paik CH, Park IK, Woo Y, Kim TW. *Orthodontic Miniscrew Implants: Clinical Applications*. 2009 Mosby Elsevier. Chapter 5 pp 33-57.
4. Owens AM, Johal A. Near-end of treatment panoramic radiograph in the assessment of mesiodistal root angulation. *Angle Orthod* 2008;78:475-481.
5. Schnelle MA, Beck FM, Jaynes RM, Huja SS. A radiographic evaluation of the availability of bone for placement of miniscrews. *Angle Orthod* 2004;74:832-837.
6. Larheim TA, Svanaes DB. Reproducibility of rotational panoramic radiography: mandibular linear dimensions and angles. *Am J Orthod Dentofacial Orthop* 1986;90:45-51.
7. Mckee IW, Williamson PC, Lam EW, Heo G, Glover KE, Major PW. The accuracy of 4 panoramic units in the projection of mesiodistal tooth angulation. *Am J Orthod Dentofacial Orthop* 2002;121:166-175.
8. Park HS, Jeong SH, Kwon OW. Factors affecting the clinical success of screw implants used as orthodontic anchorage. *Am J Orthod Dentofacial Orthop* 2006;130:18-25.
9. Luzi C, Verna C, Melsen B. A prospective clinical investigation of the failure rate of immediately loaded mini-implants used for orthodontic anchorage. *Prog Orthod* 2007;8:192-201.

10. Park YC, Lee KJ. Biomechanical principles in miniscrew-driven orthodontics. In Nanda R, Uribe FA, editors: *Temporary Anchorage Devices in Orthodontics*. 2009 Mosby Elsevier pp 93-144.
11. Kuroda S, Yamada K, Deguchi T, Hashimoto T, Kyung HM, Takano-Yamamoto T. Root proximity is a major factor for screw failure in orthodontic anchorage. *Am J Orthod Dentofacial Orthop* 2007;131:00.
12. Ludwig B, Glasl B, Landes C, Lietz T, Bowman SJ. Insertion of miniscrews. In Ludwig B, Baumgaertel S, Bowman SJ, editors: *Mini-implants in orthodontics*. 2007. Quintessence Books. pp 73-90.
13. Herman RJ, Currier F, Miyake A. Mini-implant anchorage for maxillary canine retraction: a pilot study. *Am J Orthod Dentofacial Orthop* 2006;130:228-35.
14. Kuroda S, Sugawara Y, Deguchi T, Kyung HM, Takano-Yamamoto T. Clinical use of miniscrew implants as orthodontic anchorage: success rates and postoperative discomfort. *Am J Orthod Dentofacial Orthop* 2007;131:9-15.
15. Lietz T, Baumgaertel S, Bowman SJ. Miniscrew-aspects of assessment and selection among different systems. In Ludwig B, Baumgaertel S, Bowman SJ, editors: *Mini-Implants in Orthodontics*. 2007 Quintessence Books. pp 11-73.
16. Lee JS. Kim JK, Park YC, Vanarsdall RL. *Applications of Orthodontic Mini-Implants*. 2007 Quintessence Publishing Co. Chapter 5 pp.87-110.
17. Gantous A, Phillips JH. The effects of varying pilot hole size on the holding power of miniscrews and microscrews. *Plast Reconstr Surg* 1995;95(7):1165-1169.
18. Melsen B, Mini-Implants: Where are we? *J Clin Orthod* 2005;39:539-47.
19. Motoyoshi M, Matsuoka M, Shimizu N. Application of orthodontic mini-implants in adolescents. *Int. J. Oral Maxillofac. Surg*. 2007;36:659-699.
20. Motoyoshi M, Hirabayashi M, Uemura M, Shimizu N. Recommended placement torque when tightening an orthodontic mini-implant. *Clin Oral Implants Res* 2006;17:109-114.
21. Poggio PM, Incorvati C, Velo S, Carano A. "Safe Zones": a guide for miniscrew positioning in the maxilla and mandibular arch. *Angle Orthodontist* 2006;76:191-197.
22. Dalstra M, Cattaneo PM, Melsen B. Load transfer of miniscrews for orthodontic anchorage. *Orthod* 2004;1:53-62.
23. Kravitz ND, Kusnoto B. Risks and complications of orthodontic miniscrews. *Am J Orthod Dentofacial Orthop* 2007;131:S43-S51.
24. Chen YJ, Chen YH, Lin LD, Yao CC. Removal torque of miniscrews used for orthodontic anchorage-a preliminary report. *Int J Oral Maxillofac Implants* 2006;21:283-9.
25. Kim JW, Ahn SJ, Chang YI. Histomorphometric and mechanical analyses of the drill-free screw as orthodontic anchorage. *Am J Orthod Dentofacial Orthop* 2005;128:190-194.
26. Kim H, Kim TK, Lee SJ. Convenient removal of orthodontic mini-implants. *Am J Orthod Dentofacial Orthop* 2006;101:S90-S91.
27. Melsen B, Verna C. Miniscrew implants: the Aarhus anchorage system. *Semin Orthod* 2005;11:24-31.

EXAMPLE OF MINISCREW APPLICATION

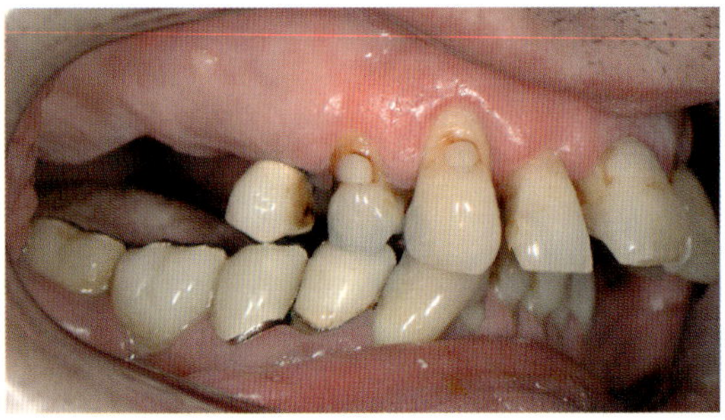

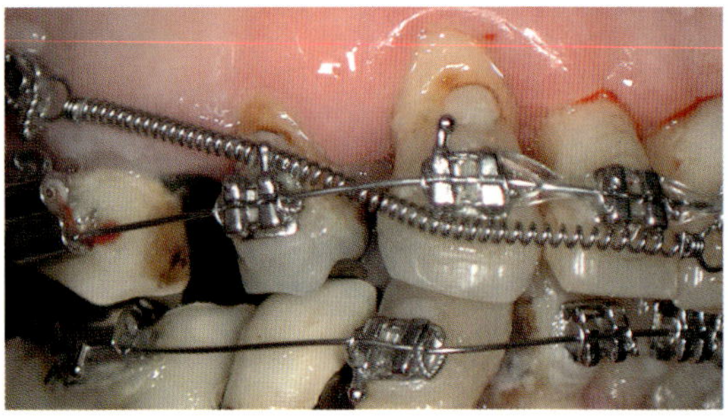

Miniscrews are used as maximum anchorage to move the anterior teeth distally in the absence of dental anchorage.

CASE NUMBER 25

The case features a 25 year old patient.

6-144

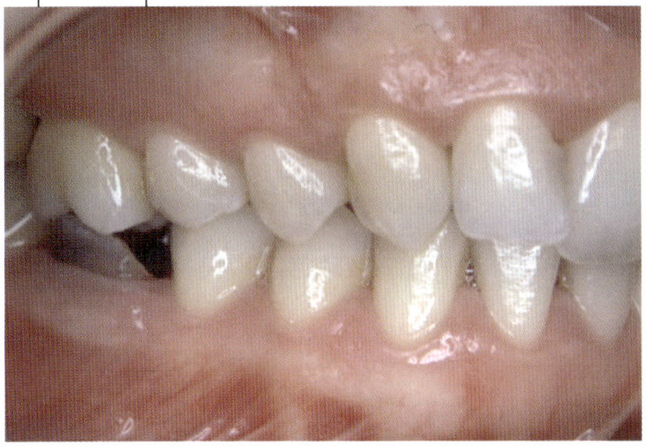

6-145

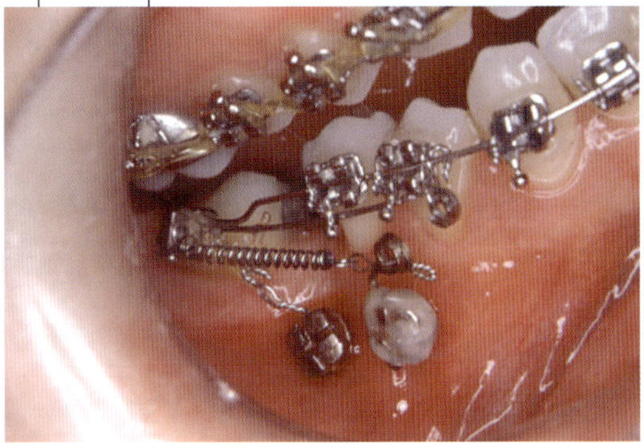

Fig. 6-144
Pre-treatment occlusion. Note the condition of the first lower right molar. Its extraction follows.

Fig. 6-145
During the orthodontic treatment, two titanium miniscrews are used to mesially displace the second lower right molar. One of the screws is lost after a few days while the other allows for complete space closure in 12 months of treatment.

6-146

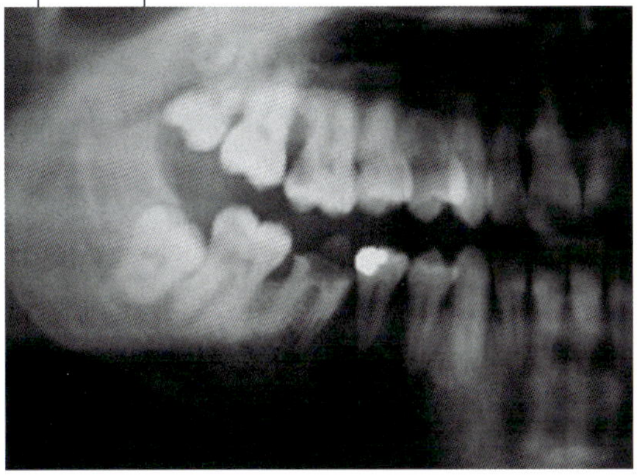

6-147

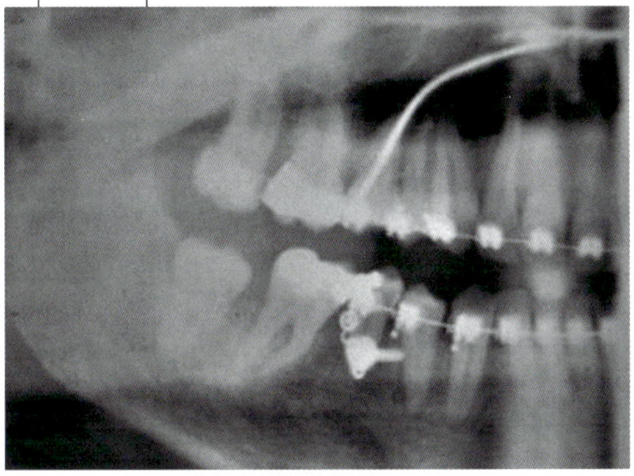

Fig. 6-146
Pre-treatment panoramic radiograph.

Fig. 6-147
Post-treatment panoramic radiograph.

6-148

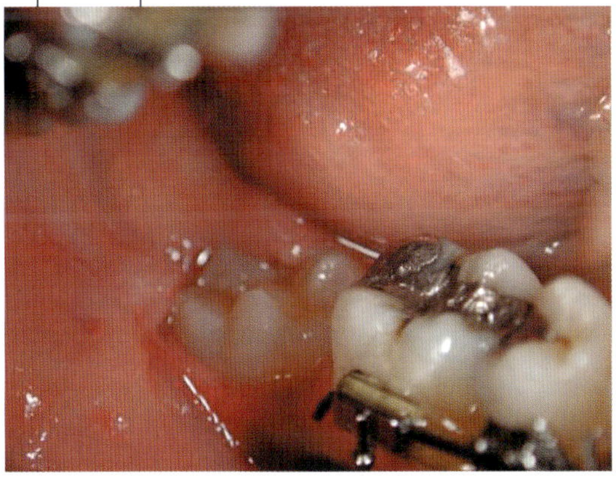

6-149

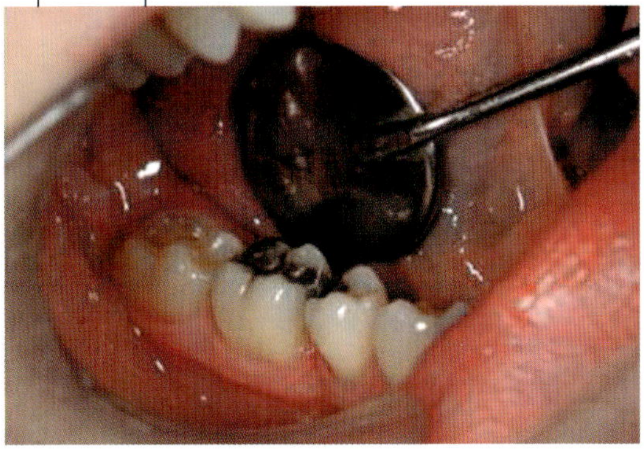

6-150

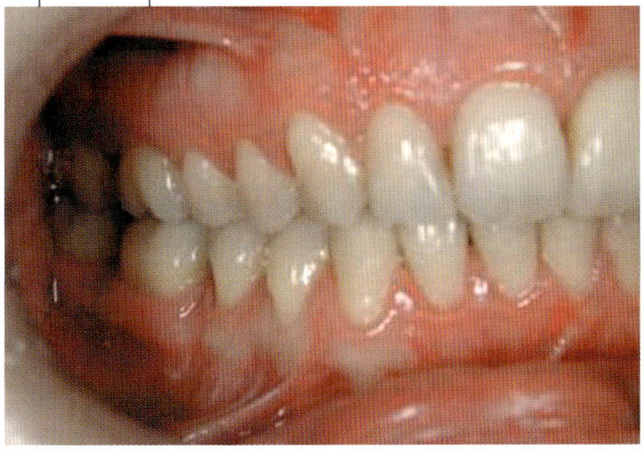

Figs. 6-148 to 6-150
Three different clinical moments after the second molar displacement. Note the spontaneous third molar eruption! A satisfactory final occlusion.

ORTHODONTICS AND THE TEMPOROMANDIBULAR JOINT (TMJ)

THE RELATIONSHIP BETWEEN ORTHODONTICS AND GNATHOLOGY

Anatomy and Function

The TMJ is the articulation between the condyle of the mandible and the articular fossa of the temporal bone. A fibrous meniscus also known as the articular disc divides the condyle and the fossa and is contiguous with the posterior bilaminar zone, which is a vascular, innervated structure. The anterior border of the disc is attached to the lateral pterygoid muscle. The meniscus supports the bones in the joint, preventing them from rubbing together and allowing the joint to move smoothly. When opening the mouth, the condyle first rotates and then translates with the meniscus. Together they move forward beneath the articular eminence. No clicks are present (Figs. 6-151: 1 & 2).

TEMPOROMANDIBULAR JOINT DISORDERS

Signs and Symptoms

If the meniscus is anteriorly displaced in front of the condyle, coordinated movement is not present and the posterior bilaminar zone is stretched. When the condyle moves forward at a certain point, it does so beneath the meniscus and the bilaminar zone returns to its normal position. In these cases we speak of anterior displacement with reduction - opening the mouth the disc returns to its correct position between the condyle and the articular fossa. As the mouth opens or closes there are characteristic popping or clicking sounds known as internal derangement (Fig. 6-151: 3 & 4).

In cases of anterior displacement without reduction, the disc is permanently displaced and the jaw's range of motion is limited. The mouth opening (which is normally 44–48 mm) is now 25–30 mm. This condition may be acute or, after repeated episodes, become chronic. When chronic, no sounds are present. There are several causes, for example bruxism, trauma and some misalignments of the teeth.

A common symptom is pain, not only in the joint but also elsewhere in the skull, face or jaw.

Muscle hyperactivity is often involved and can also cause internal derangement. Think about the anatomic relationship of the lateral pterygoid muscle, articular disc and condyle (Fig. 6-152).

6-151

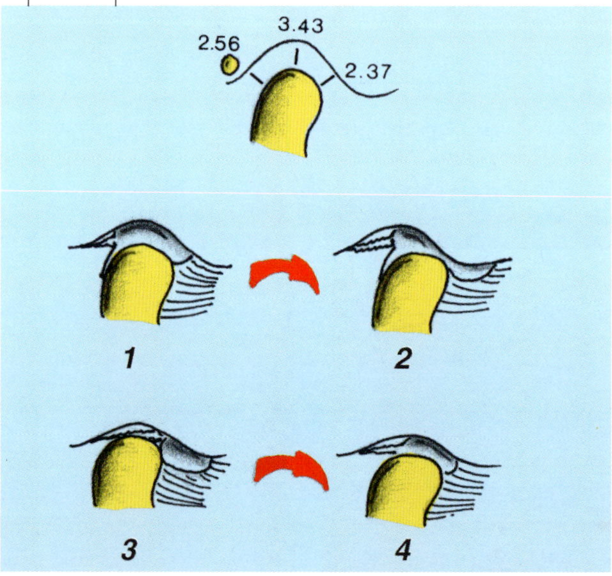

Fig. 6-151 Condyle well positioned in the articular fossa. Distance in mm between the two structures (Ricketts – Dumas 1984). 1-2 good relationship condyle-disc. They move together without making sounds. 3-4 condyle distally displaced. The disc is forward. During movement there are sounds (clicks).

6-152

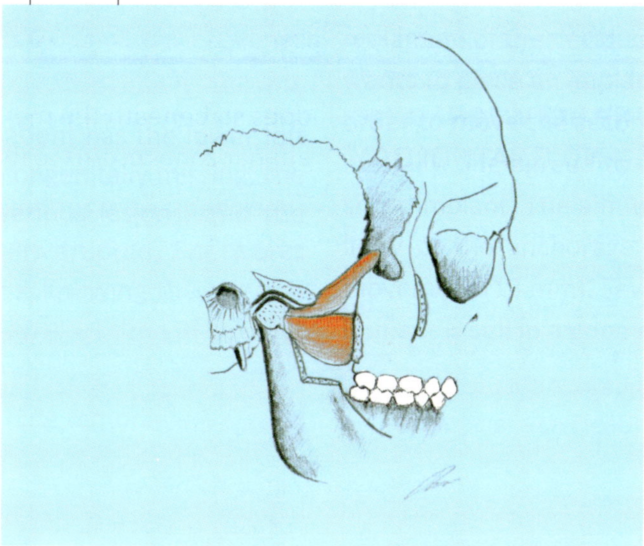

Fig. 6-152
Relationship between the lateral pterygoid muscle, articular disc, condyle.

An important role is played by stress or anxiety: they can trigger bruxism or muscle hyperactivity. TMJ disorders most commonly occur in women between the ages of 30 and 50, but can also be present in children.

Why should an orthodontist be interested in TMJ disorders? The reason is because there are gnathologists who suggest TMJ disorders are caused by:

a) dental occlusions
b) malocclusions
c) orthodontic treatments.

To which we ask: What type of occlusion/ malocclusion/orthodontic treatment?

Let us take a look at the answers below.

THE RELATIONSHIP BETWEEN THE TMJ AND ORTHODONTICS

Sagittal Evaluation

Can there be TMJ disorders in every dental occlusion? Yes, temporomandibular disorders are possible with every dental occlusion.

Among malocclusions, which ones are most common? Considering that disorders are present above all with the condyle distally displaced in the fossa, Class III and Class II division 2 are suspected the most.

For many gnathologists, in a Class III when an overjet-overbite tries to be achieved, the mandible can be pushed distally causing an internal derangement (Case Number 26).

In a Class II division 2, it is hyperactive labial musculature that pushes the mandible distally (Case Number 27).

In some Class II division 2 cases, by moving the upper incisors labially there is mandibular advancement, which would suggest distal mandibular entrapment with temporomandibular disorders. However, it is unpredictable. Moreover, in other Class II division 2 cases, as Langlade [150] said, the mandible does not move forward.

CASE NUMBER 26

6-153

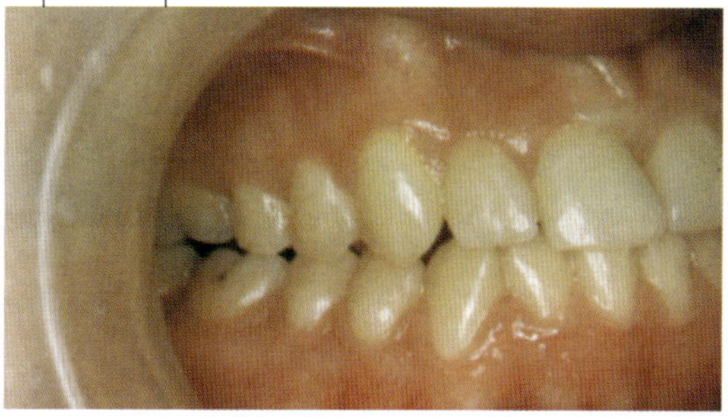

6-154

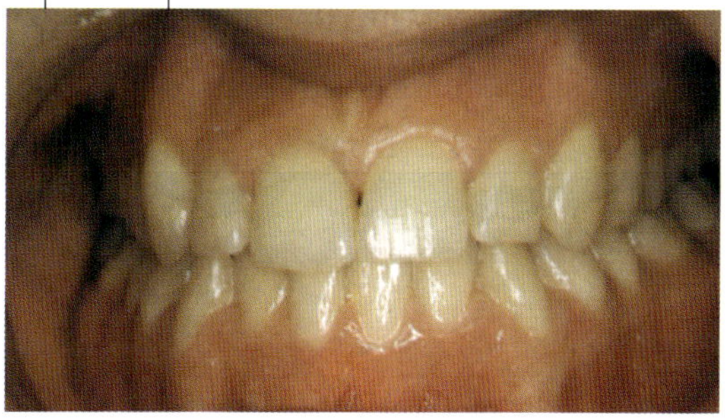

Figs. 6-153 & 6-154
Skeletal Class III with teeth compensation: upper incisors are proclined while lower incisors are lingually positioned.

CASE NUMBER 27

6-155

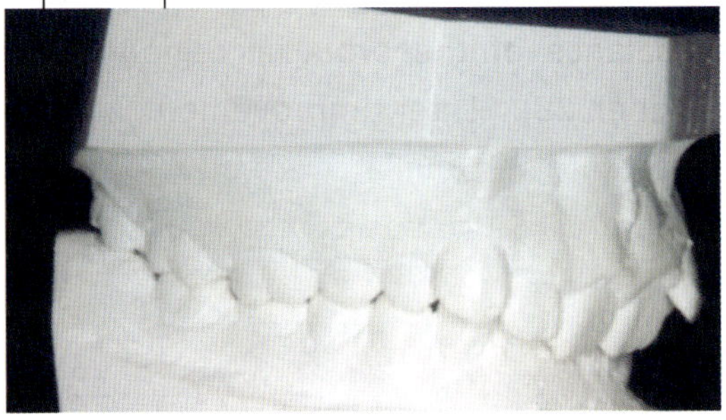

6-156

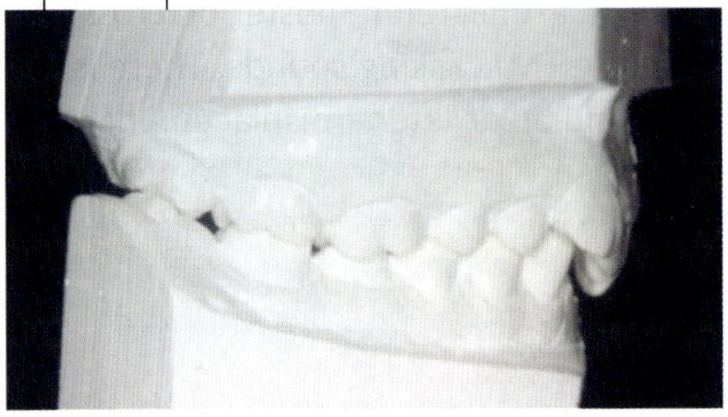

6-157

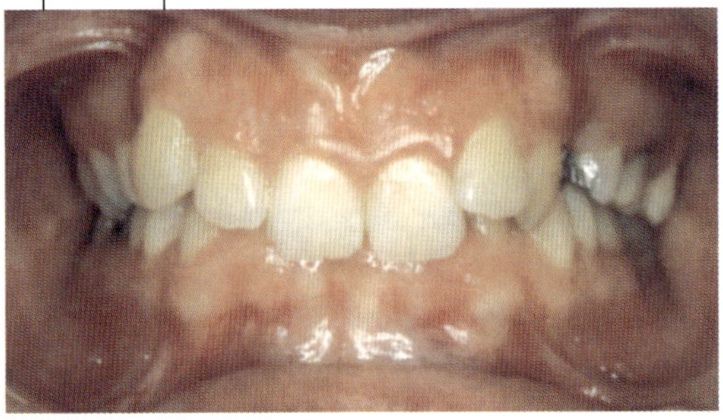

6-158

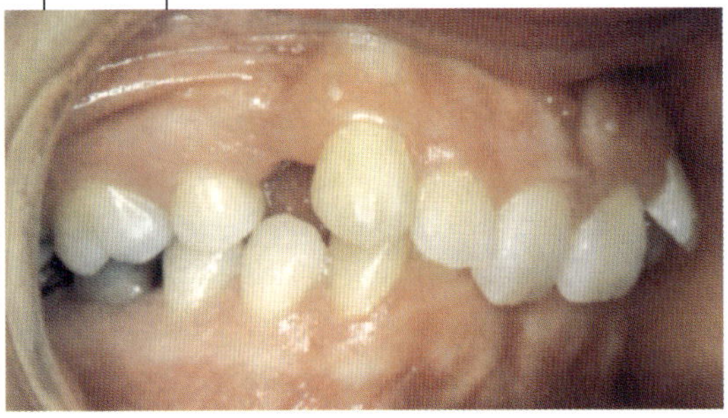

6-159

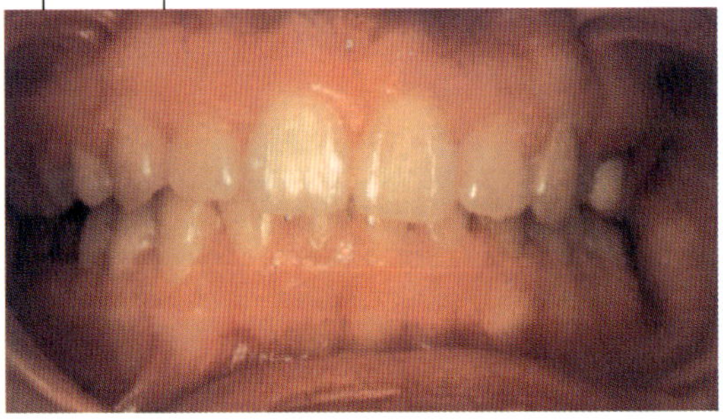

6-160

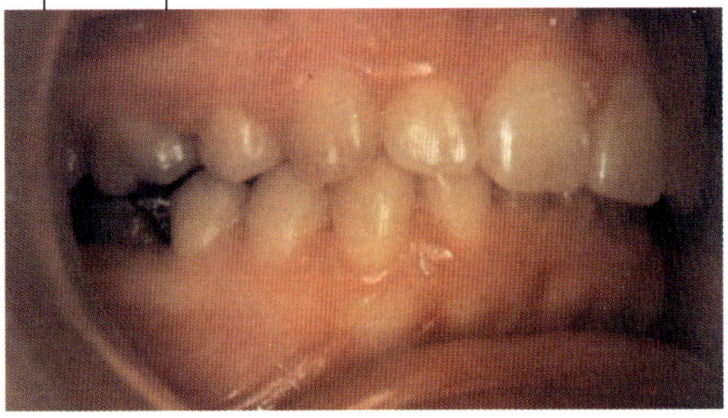

6-161

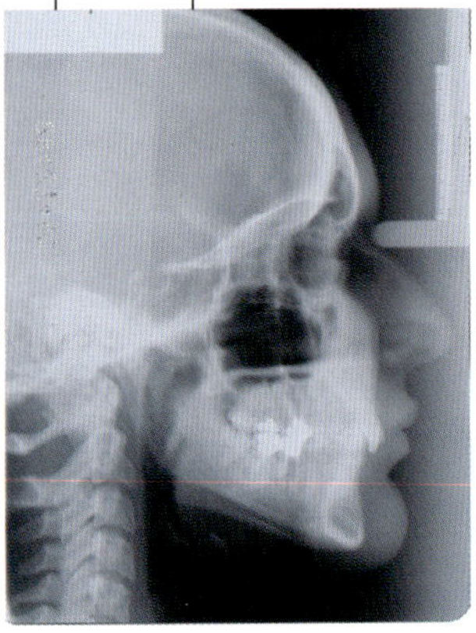

6-162

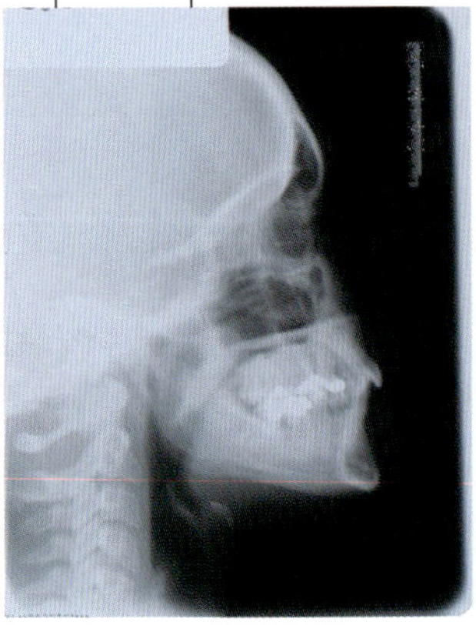

Figs.6-155 & 6-156 Class II division 2 in a 25 year old patient. Pre-treatment dental casts.

Figs. 6-157 & 6-158 Pre-treatment occlusion. For orthodontic correction at the end of growth, the two first upper premolars are extracted. It is usually recommended to avoid extractions in deep bites. However, every rule has its own exception and this is one of them. No signs and symptoms of temporomandibular disorders are present.

Figs. 6-159 & 6-160 Post-treatment occlusion. Note the deep bite correction with intrusion of the upper incisors. No signs and symptoms of temporomandibular disorders are present.

Fig. 6-161 Pre-treatment lateral cephalogram

Fig. 6-162 Post-treatment lateral cephalogram.

At this time there is no evidence that malocclusions per se are predisposing factors for the development of TMJ disorders.

TRANSVERSE EVALUATION

Clinically, in many cases (including children) of a unilateral posterior crossbite there are TMJ clicking sounds. There is often mandibular lateral displacement with condylar rotation, deviation of the chin, facial asymmetry and dental midline discrepancy. An early treatment, usually with an upper arch expansion, is necessary to re-establish the structural and functional balance of the orofacial region (case number 28). Later, improvement is possible (case 29) but at the end of growth surgery must be considered.

CASE NUMBER 28

The patient shows unilateral crossbite due to maxillary constriction which caused mandibular lateral displacement. If not treated before the end of growth, from "positional" it could become "structural" (see also Case Number 6, Chapter IV). At that time only surgery could give the best results.

6-163

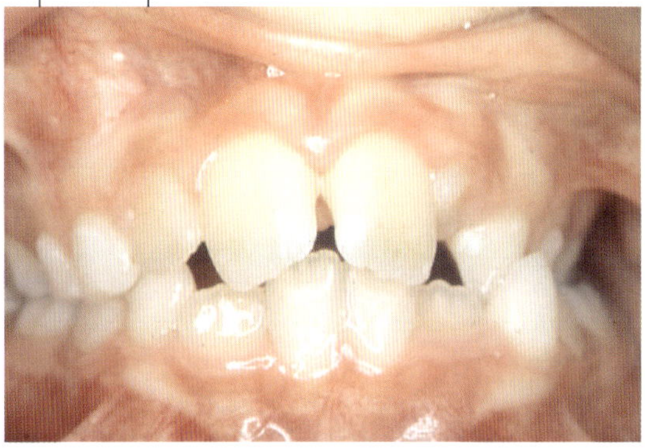

6-164

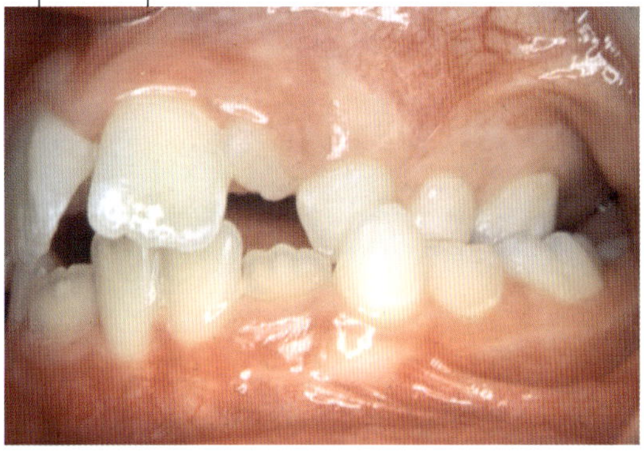

Figs. 6-163 & 6-164
Pre-treatment occlusion.
Left crossbite.

6-165

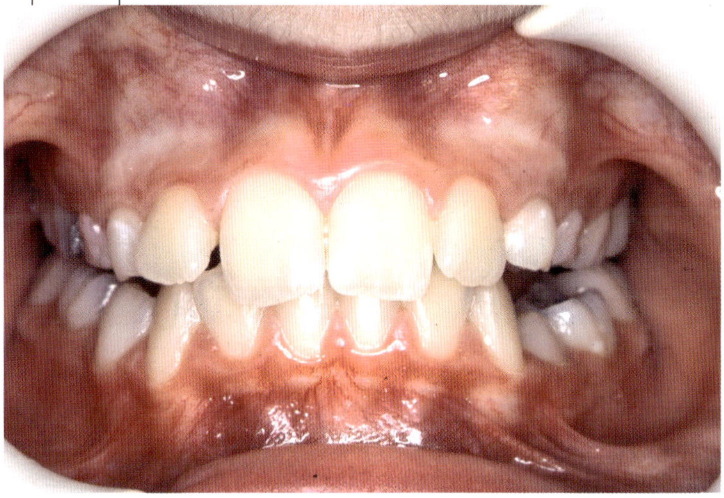

Fig. 6-165
Post-treatment occlusion
after cross-bite correction.

CASE NUMBER 29

6-166

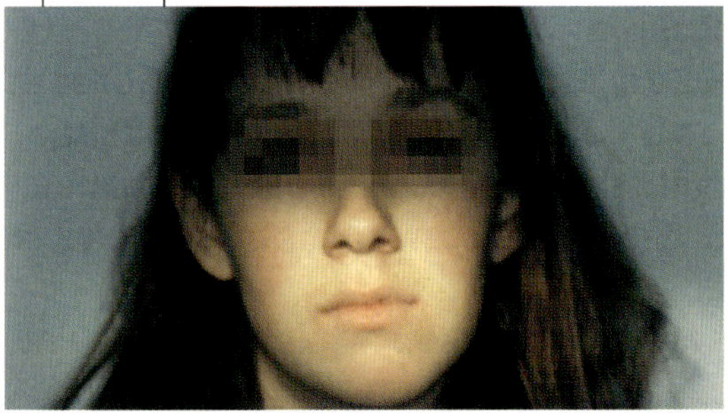

Fig. 6-166
Facial asymmetry in a female patient close to the end of her growth.

6-167

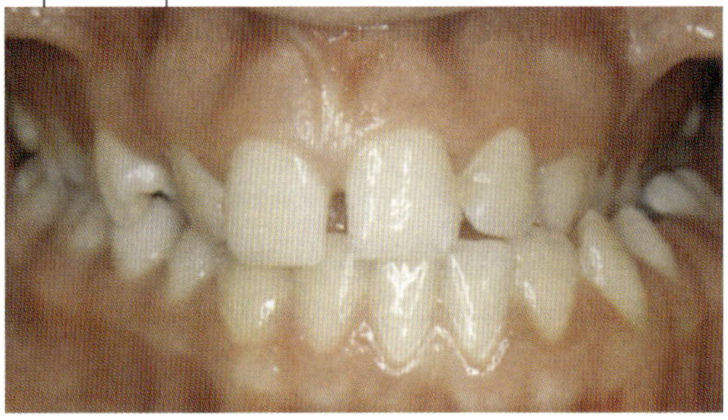

6-168

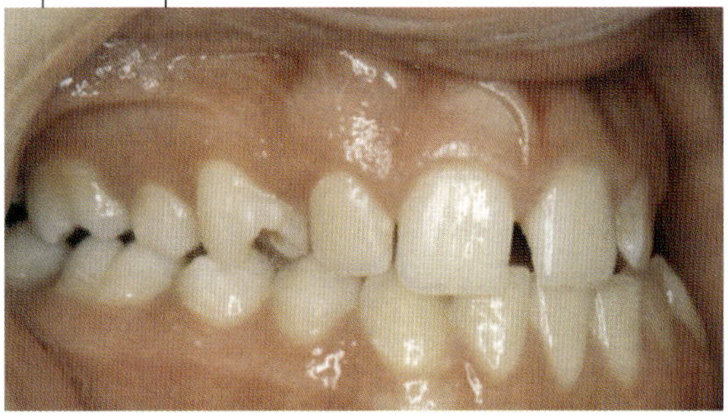

Figs. 6-167 & 6-168
Left crossbite with evident mandibular lateral displacement. There is an ectopic eruption of the upper right canine. Articular sounds are present.

6-169

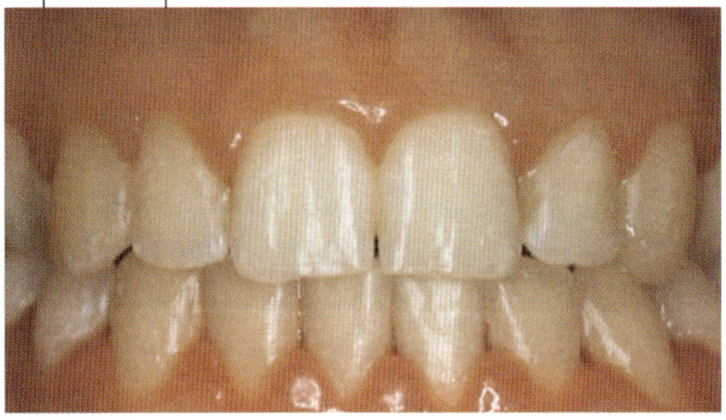

6-170

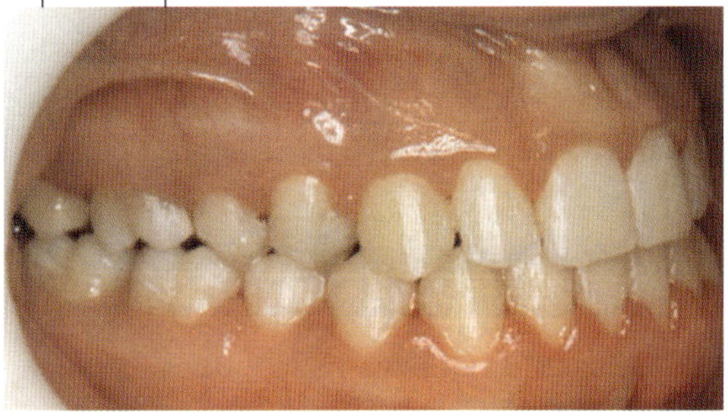

6-171

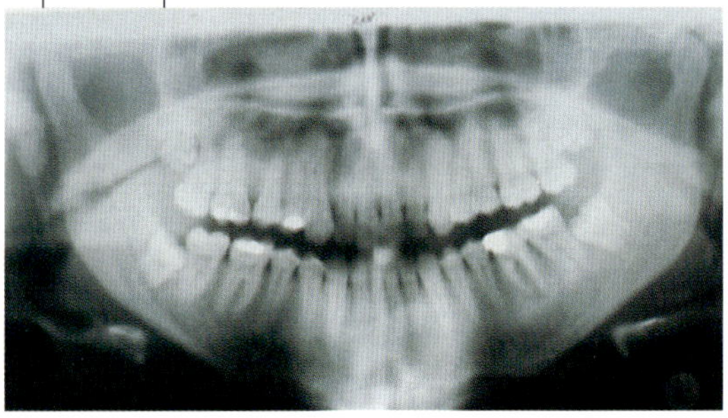

Figs. 6-169 to 6-171
Post-treatment occlusion and panoramic radiograph. Articular sounds have decreased but have not completely disappeared.

VERTICAL EVALUATION

Many gnathologists believe that a possible cause of TMJ disorders is a vertical dimension reduction, which is often associated with tooth extractions. It can occur when many molars are removed and therefore the condyle is not sustained by an adequate occlusal plane.

The mandible, like a boat, can "pitch" or "roll" with TMJ consequences (Case Number 32).

According to Ricketts, [209] sometimes a reduction of vertical height is possible (particularly when in a patient with bruxism or clenching) as there is a combination of great dental crown abrasion and molar intrusion (Case Number 30).

CASE NUMBER 30

Serious deepbite in a 60 year old female. The patient complains about articular pain and chronic headache.

6-172

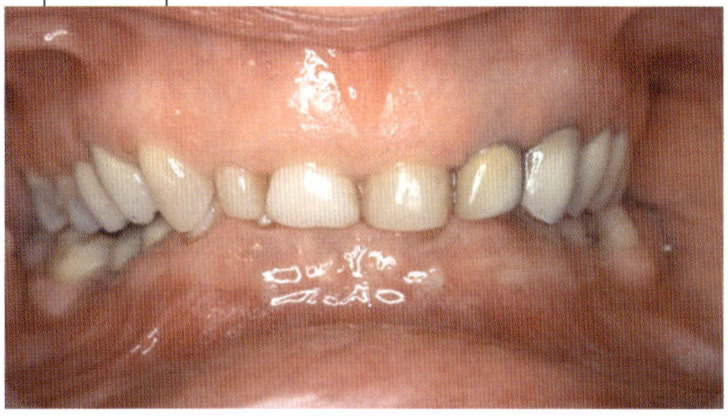

6-173

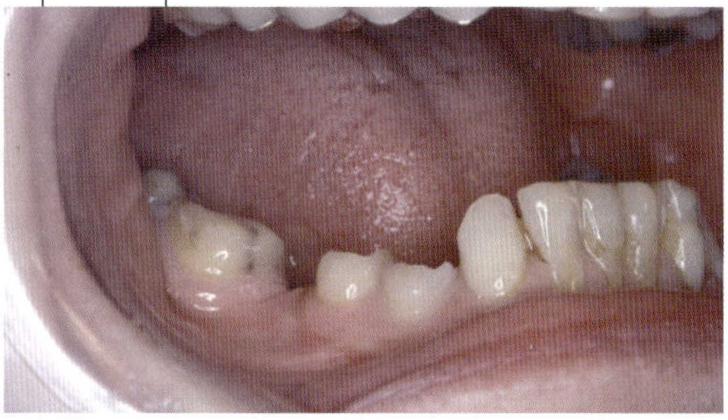

Fig. 6-172
Pre-treatment deepbite.

Fig. 6-173
Lower dental situation. Notice the abrasion and intrusion of the molars and premolars.

6-174

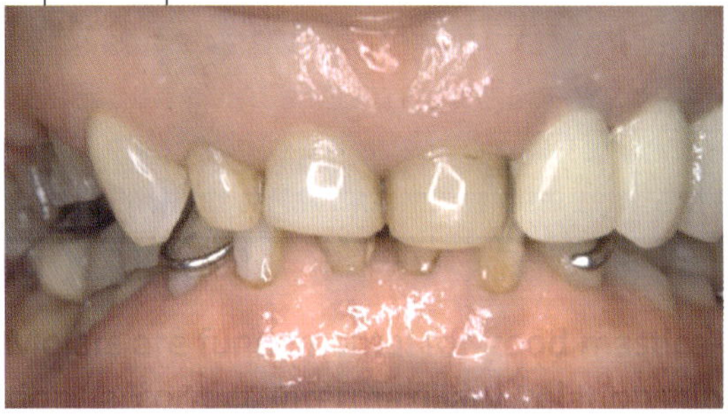

6-175

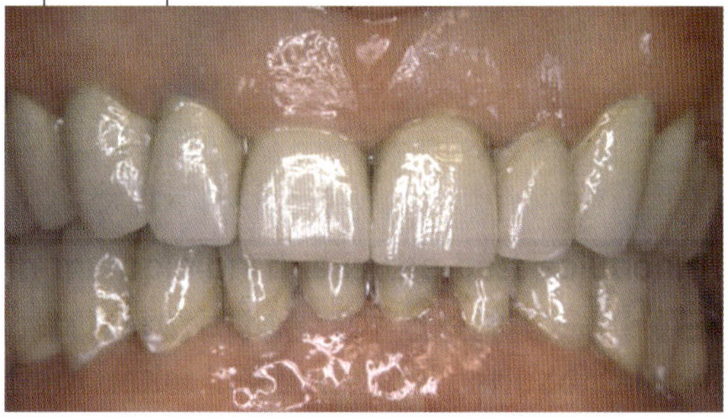

Fig. 6-174
On the lower arch a removable overdenture is applied to test a new vertical height.

Fig. 6-175
The patient feels so good that 12 months later, a lower and upper fixed prosthesis follow.

TMJ disorders can be present, not only in those with a reduced verticality, but also in openbite cases like the one below.

CASE NUMBER 31

In a 23 year old woman there is a mandibular right lateral displacement. With a fixed orthodontic appliance (straight wire) it was possible to coordinate the upper and lower dental arches, thus improving the occlusion.

6-176

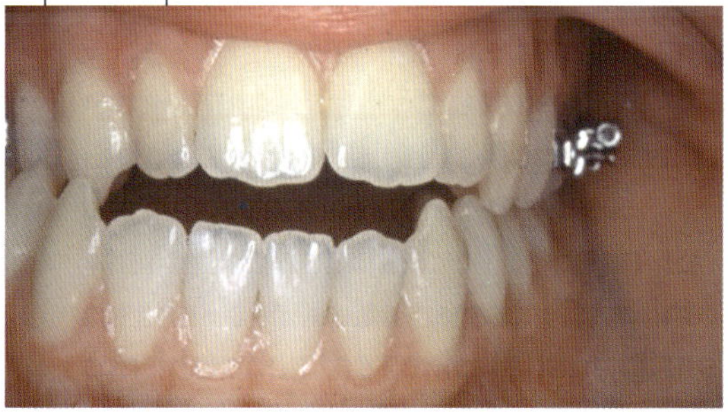

6-177

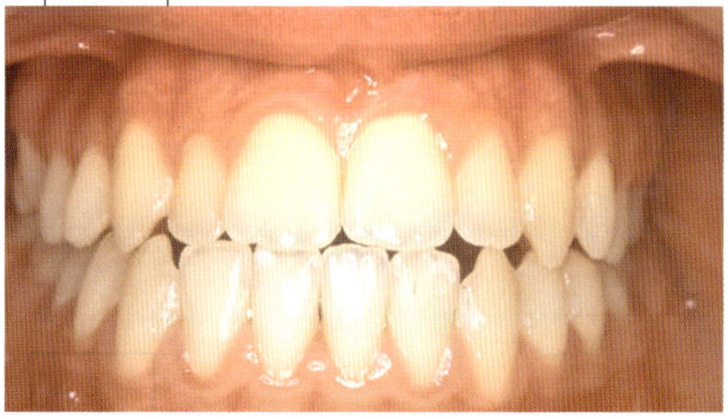

Fig. 6-176
Pre-treatment occlusion. Openbite with mandibular right lateral displacement. Articular sounds are present.

Fig. 6-177
Post-treatment occlusion. Articular sounds are reduced in intensity but have not completely disappeared.

6-178

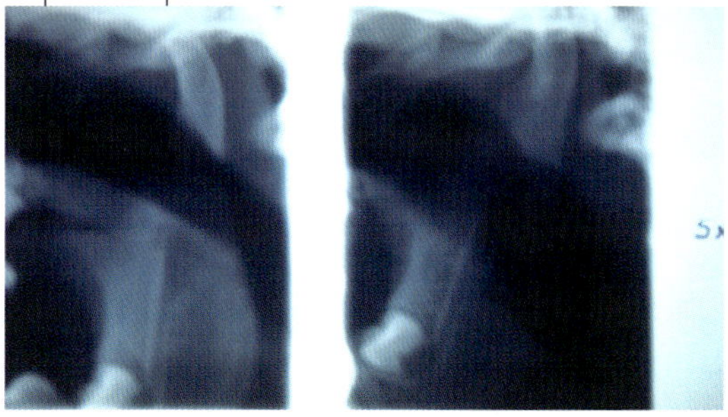

6-179

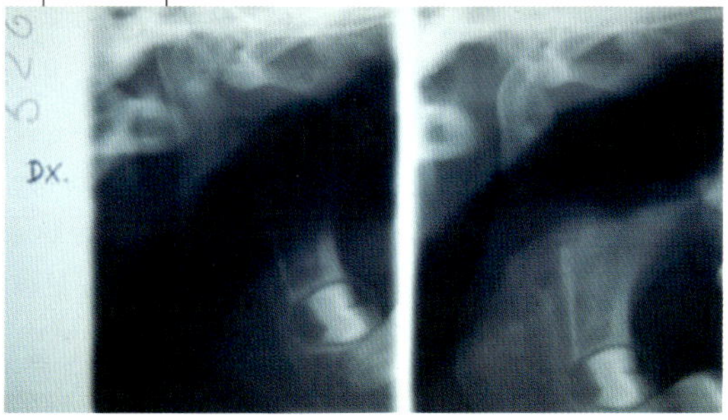

Fig. 6-178
Left condyle X-ray.

Fig. 6-179
Right condyle X-ray. Notice the calcified hypertrophy which interferes with the condylar movements.

CASE NUMBER 32

Very "bad bite" with lateral left crossbite in a 27 year old patient. Articular sounds are present. They disappear after treatment. The mandibular lateral displacement was corrected with a straight wire fixed appliance which aligned the teeth and coordinated upper and lower dental arches.

6-180

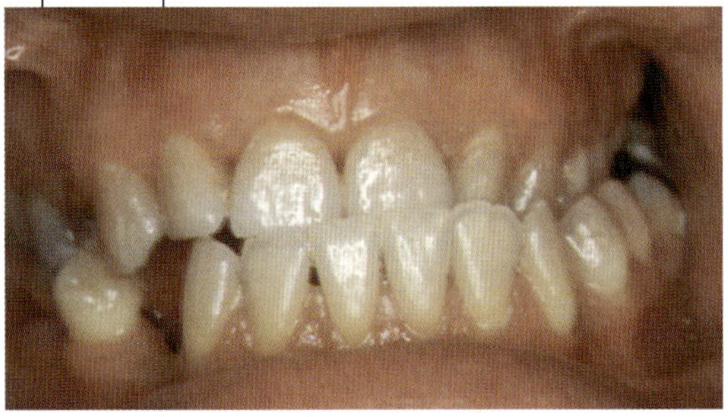

6-181

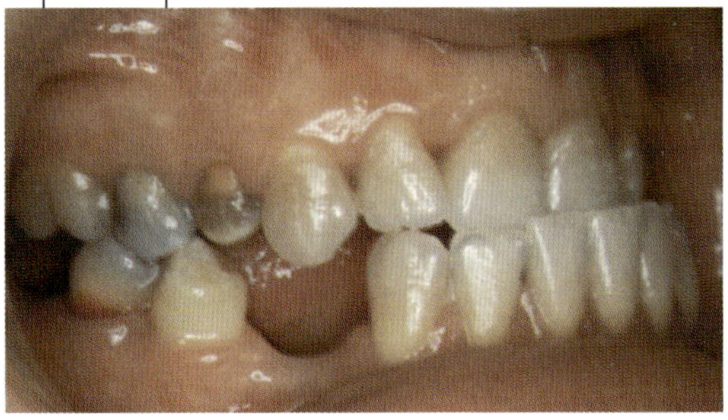

6-182

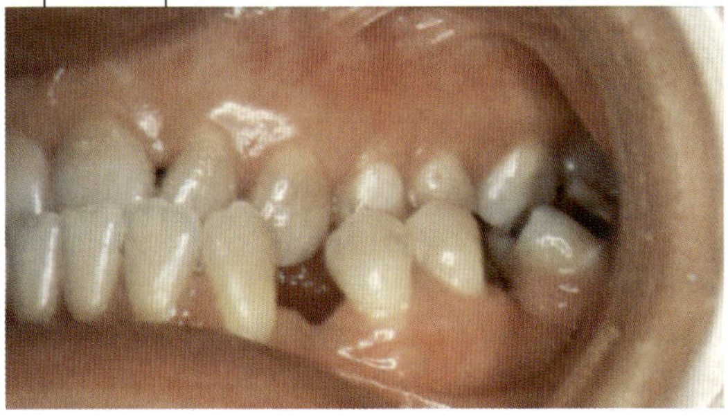

Figs. 6-180 to 6-182 Left lateral crossbite with mandibular "roll" on the same side.

6-183

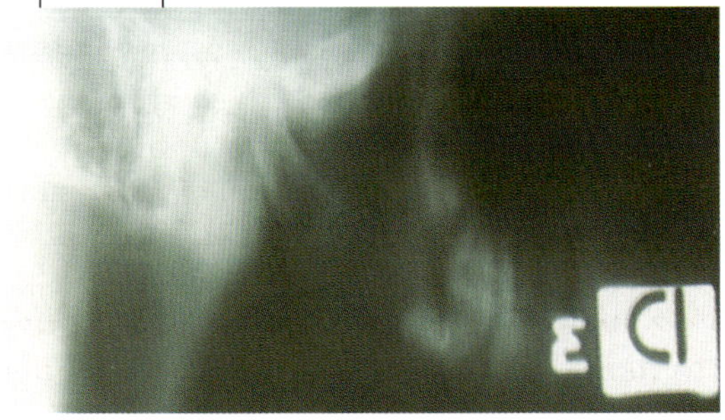

6-184

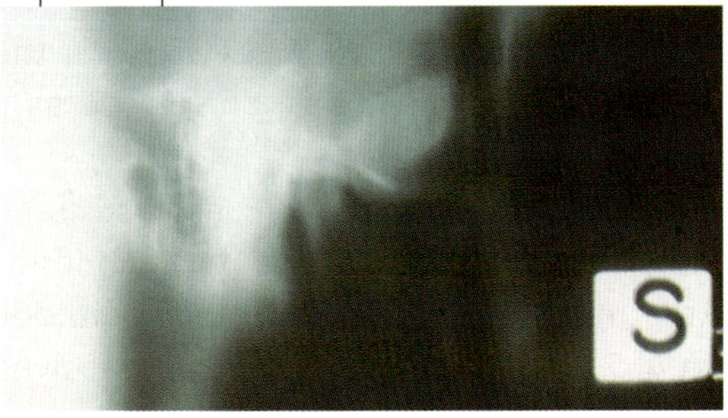

Fig. 6-183 Right TMJ radiograph.

Fig. 6-184 Left TMJ radiograph. The upper articular space is reduced compared to the right one.

6-185

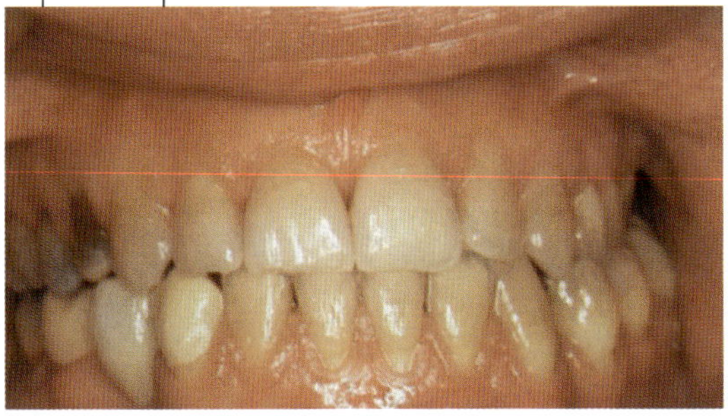

Fig. 6-185 Post ortho-prosthesis treatment. No surgery.

Now, what should we say to those who claim that orthodontic treatments cause TMJ disorders? Before evaluating clinical and personal matters, it is useful to consider what has been reported in the most qualified literature.

Reynders[7*1] pointed out that many personal opinions and case reports of poor scientific value with often contradictory results have been published. His paper concludes that "the most important studies suggest that orthodontic treatment does not increase the risk of developing TMJ". With that premise in mind it is interesting to remember that when Farrar and McCarty[87] state that premolar extractions can cause a mandible distal dislocation followed by TMJ disorders *they are just expressing an opinion.*

Dibbets and van der Weele[73] wrote in 1991 "from a comparison of treatments without extractions, with extractions of four premolars and with extractions of other teeth, the TMJ disorders eventually present are more probably caused by the pattern of growth instead of by the extractions".

Gianelly et al.[8*1] looked at the condylar position of those treated orthodontically with the extraction of maxillary first premolars compared with the condylar position of non-treated persons. They discovered no differences.

Luecke and Johnston[160] found that in their study of the effects on mandibular position of the extraction of upper first premolars and the retraction of upper incisors, the mandible was not distally displaced as a result.

Egermark and Thilander[1**1] analysed craniomandibular disorders and orthodontic treatment from childhood to adulthood in 402 subjects. Those who had received orthodontic treatment in the past showed fewer TMJ disorders than those who had never been treated.

Kremenak et al.[2**1] found that that 90% of their patients treated orthodontically showed an improvement of TMJ disorders.

Artun et al.[3**1] studied the relationship between orthodontic treatment, the condylar position and internal derangement in the TMJ. Their results did not "suggest increased prevalence of posteriorly-located condyles in patients treated with extractions of maxillary first premolars only".

Staggers[4**1] looked at vertical changes following first premolar extractions and concluded that "the results of this work showed that the vertical changes occurring after the extractions of first premolars were no different than those occurring in the non-extraction cases. This study doesn't support the theory that first premolar extractions reduce the vertical dimension of occlusion, and thus predispose extraction patients to TMJ disorders."

Katzberg et al.[5**1] concluded that their study of orthodontics and TMJ disorders suggested orthodontic treatments do not increase the risk of developing TMJ dysfunctions. Kim et al[6**1] support this view.

Rinchuse and McMinn[9**1] concluded that "traditional orthodontic treatment does not increase the prevalence of TMJ disorders. The occlusion, once considered the primary and sole cause of TMJ disorders, now has at best a secondary role in the cause of articular disorders. Occlusal adjustment is not recommended for the treatment or prevention of TMJ disorders. The use of occlusal splints might be beneficial in the treatment of TMJ disorders."

Current diagnosis and treatment of TMJ disorders is based on a patient's history and clinical examination, sometimes supported by TM joint imaging. Yet for some authors this is not enough and they feel that the use of electronic devices is necessary.

Interestingly, on this subject Mohl[7**1] wrote in 1993 "many electronic devices are suggested in the diagnosis of temporomandibular joint disorders: mandibular kinesiography, surface electromyography, silent period durations, sonography, thermography, TENS (transcutaneous electrical nerve stimulation)... The scientific criteria for the evaluation of diagnostic modalities are: Reliability, Validity, Sensitivity, Specificity."

Several reviews of the scientific literature have concluded that the proposed reliability, validity, sensitivity and specificity of electronic devices in the diagnosis of TMJ disorders have not been established.

In addition, an occlusal "analysis" with or without the use of articulated study casts is in most cases not diagnostic of a temporomandibular disorder per se. TMJ imaging can be useful in the detection of pathology within the joint, however, the assessment of the condylar position as a diagnostic criterion for temporomandibular disorders has very poor reliability and validity.

Fifteen years later those conclusions were generally reconfirmed by Gonzales et al.[8**1]

TREATMENT

It must be considered that the aetiology of TMJ disorders is multifactorial and the subject excites many contradictory opinions. According to the recommendations of the National Institute of Dental and Craniofacial Research (USA), treatments for TMJ disorders should not alter the jaw or teeth and need to be reversible.

Among the most common interventions are:

- stretching or relaxation exercises for the jaw
- stabilization splint (biteplate, night-guard)
- pain relief medications.

CONCLUSIONS

I think that on the basis of what has been discussed, an orthodontist can be proud of his job.

We have seen that TMJ disorders are a multifactorial disease. Dental occlusion is now less important than in the past. If an occlusion must be changed, it is possible to do so only with an orthodontic treatment, in a comprehensive, reliable and reversible manner. With a prosthesis or by grinding the teeth, the changes are minor and irreversible.

Personally, I suggest prudence in the orthodontic treatment of a Class III at the end of growth.

We have looked at results from highly qualified literature. There is no evidence to indicate orthodontics as a cause of TMJ disorders. On the contrary, we know that early treatment can prevent or improve TMJ disorders – for instance consider mandibular lateral displacement.

Even adult patients who have a very "bad bite" often feel better after orthodontic treatment.

When pain is present it can disappear. Articular sounds may decrease but usually do not go away. One of the problems is that good results are unpredictable.

INTERDISCIPLINARY CASES

In clinical practice it is common to encounter cases where only an interdisciplinary approach can assure a good functional and aesthetic result. I personally like to describe the orthodontist as an architect: he realizes a project and uses the other disciplines to accomplish it.

In an interdisciplinary treatment, the first step is to assure good periodontal health with hygienic procedures (scaling, root planning etc.). Then it is the turn of orthodontic treatment.

Prosthesis, when needed, follows at the end of the treatment. Sometimes periodontal surgery and implants precede the orthodontic treatment.

CASE NUMBER 33

The case is a Class II division 1 in a 40 year old patient. Many teeth are missing and they have a bad periodontal status. Clicks are present in both TM joints. Could you imagine good functional and aesthetic improvement without orthodontic treatment? Close cooperation between orthodontics, periodontology, prosthetics and gnathology is necessary. It is impossible to achieve a good result in this case without dental plaque hygiene control as a basis for gingival health. And gingival health allows a good orthodontic treatment to be followed by a good prosthesis with the optimal gnathologic condition. The final result is evident. It is only possible to obtain it with a multidisciplinary approach, even in adult patients with a very serious initial situation as here.

6-186

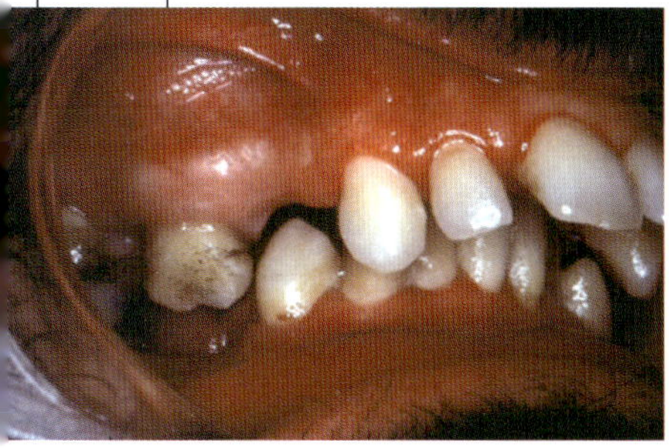

6-187

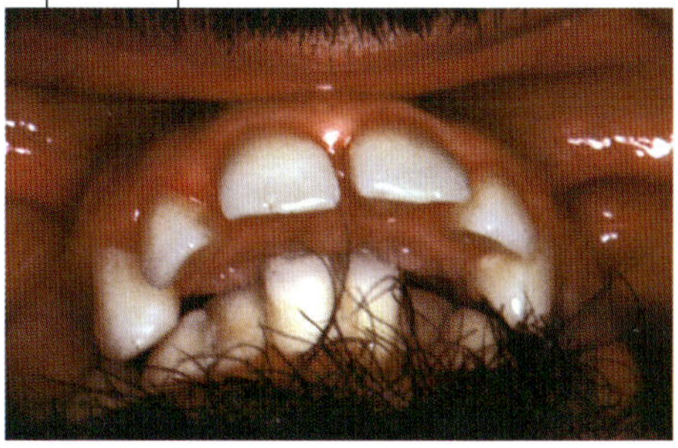

6-188

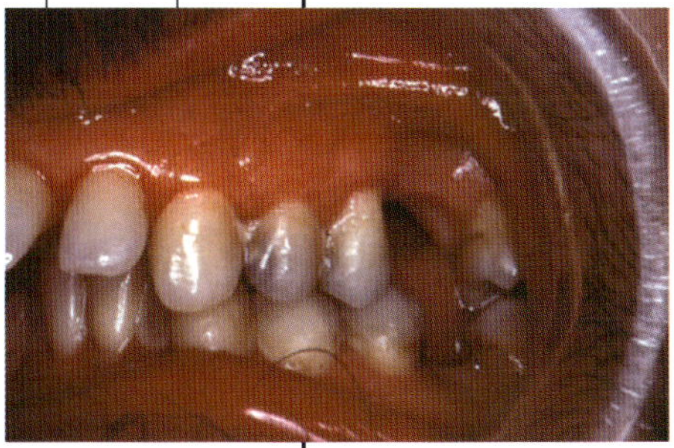

6-189

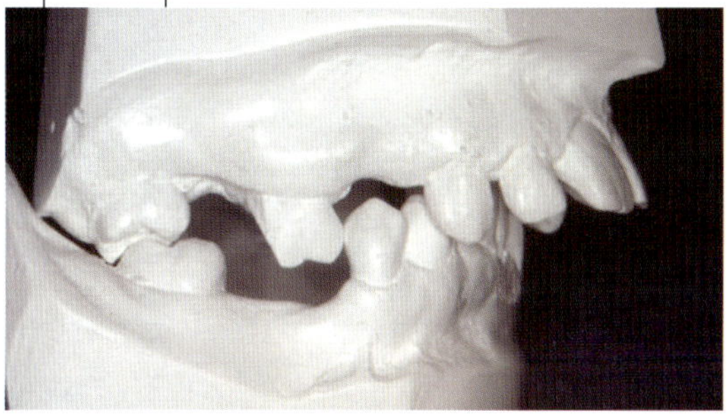

6-190

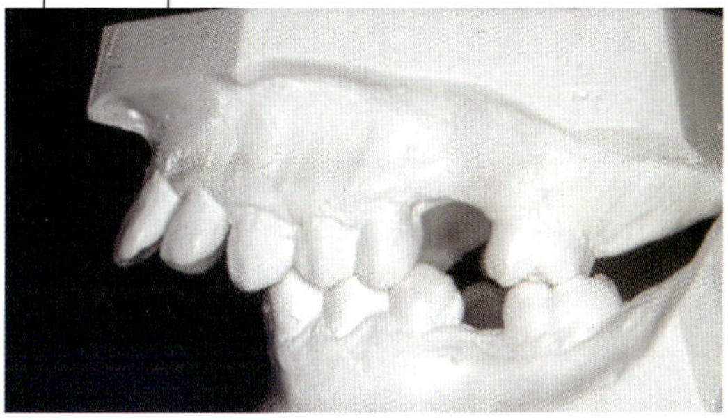

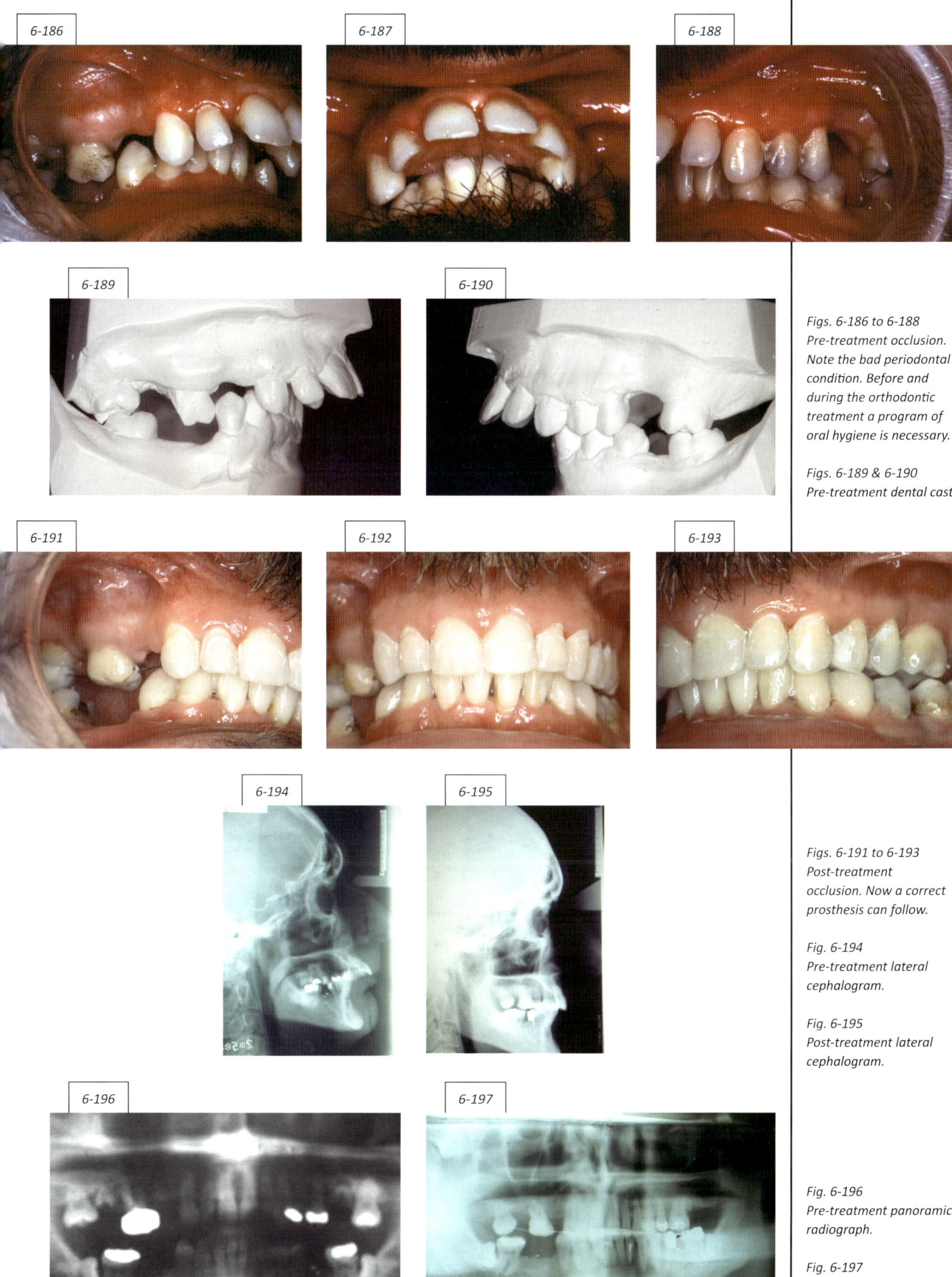

Figs. 6-186 to 6-188 Pre-treatment occlusion. Note the bad periodontal condition. Before and during the orthodontic treatment a program of oral hygiene is necessary.

Figs. 6-189 & 6-190 Pre-treatment dental casts.

6-191

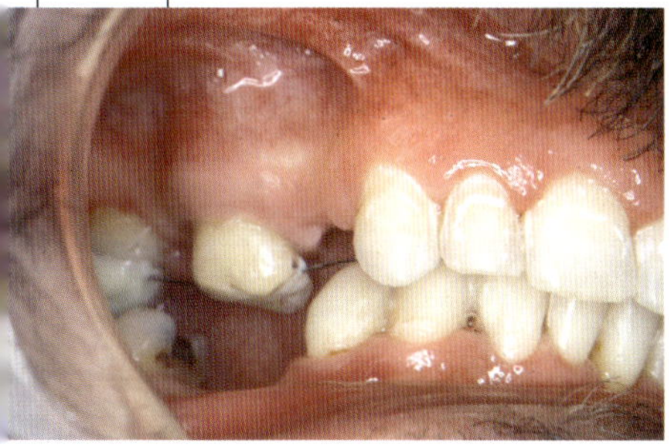

6-192

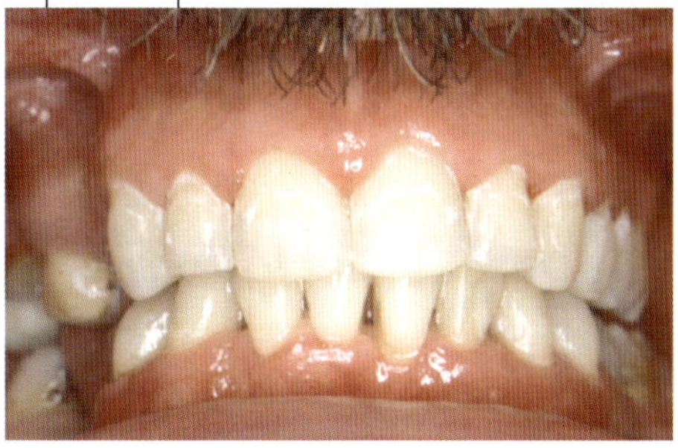

6-193

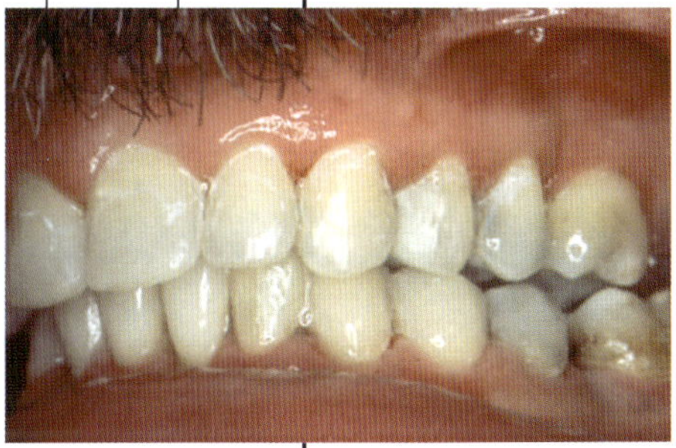

6-194

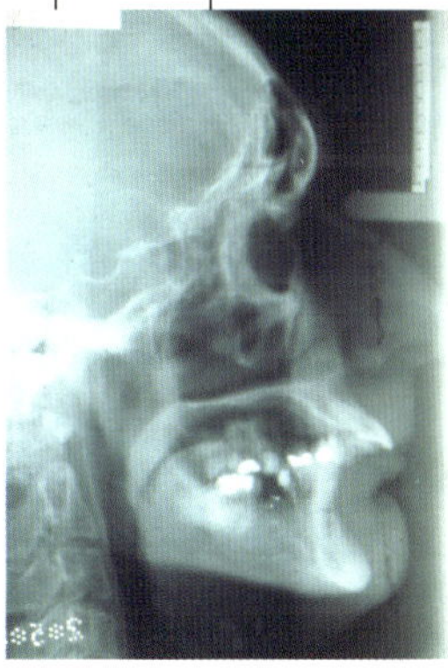

6-195

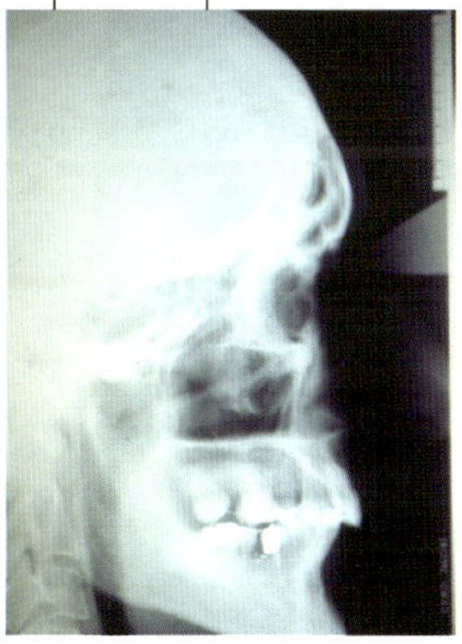

Figs. 6-191 to 6-193 Post-treatment occlusion. Now a correct prosthesis can follow.

Fig. 6-194 Pre-treatment lateral cephalogram.

Fig. 6-195 Post-treatment lateral cephalogram.

6-196

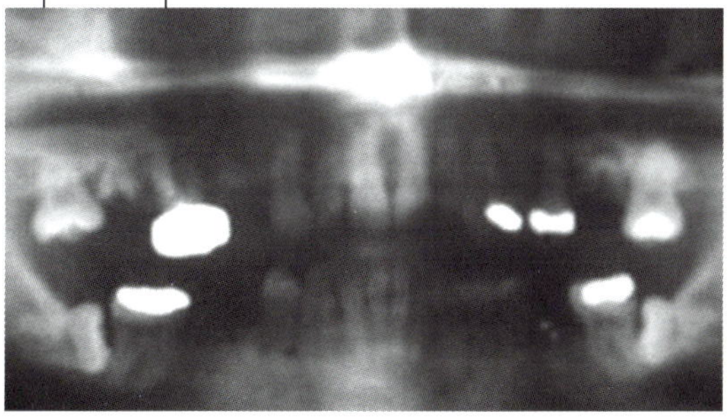

6-197

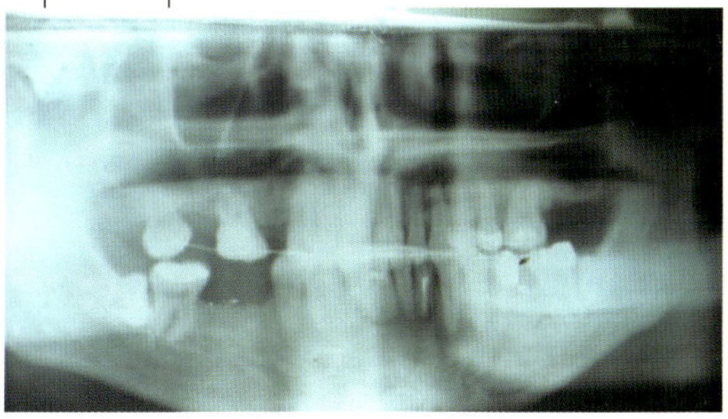

Fig. 6-196 Pre-treatment panoramic radiograph.

Fig. 6-197 Post-treatment panoramic radiograph.

CASE NUMBER 34

The case is a 45 year old female patient with a Class II division 2 and a deepbite. She wants to change the prosthesis and replace the missing teeth but her dentist does not know what to do under those circumstances. Orthodontic treatment can be precious and extremely helpful.

6-198

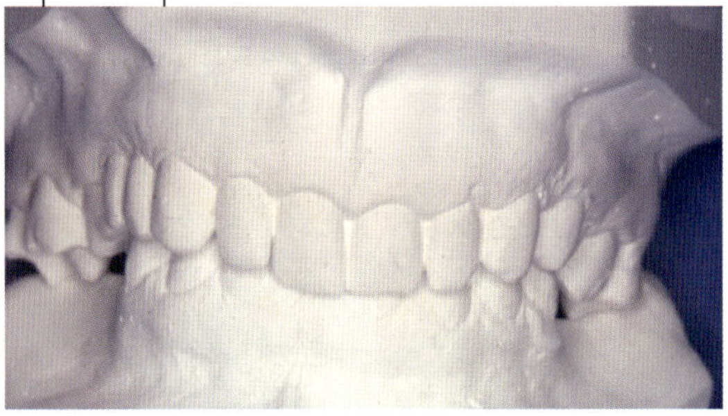

6-199

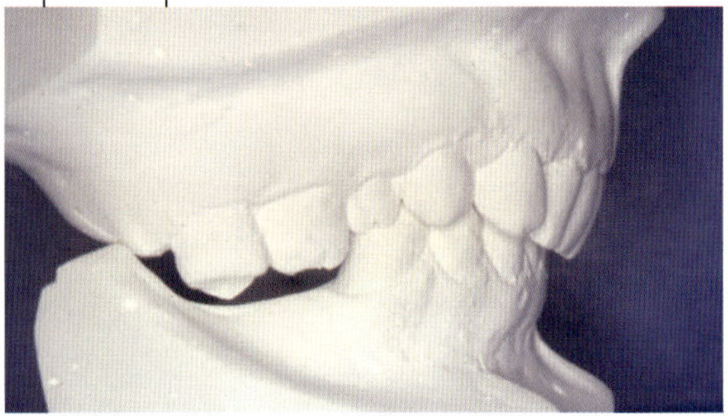

6-200

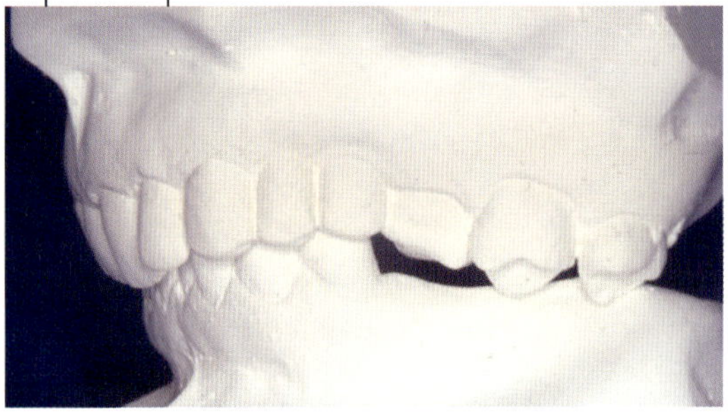

Figs. 6-198 to 6-200
Pre-treatment dental casts.

6-201

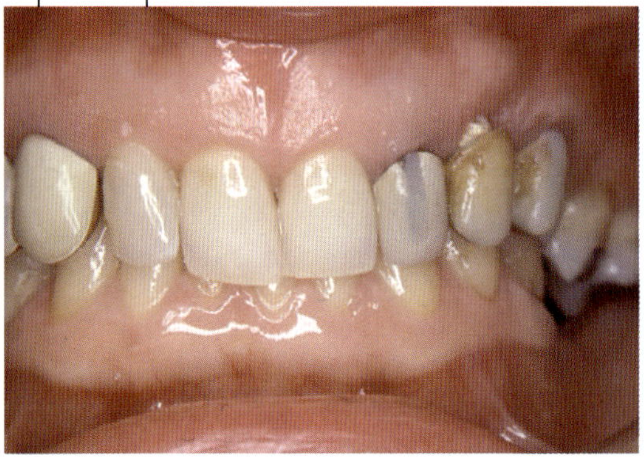

6-202

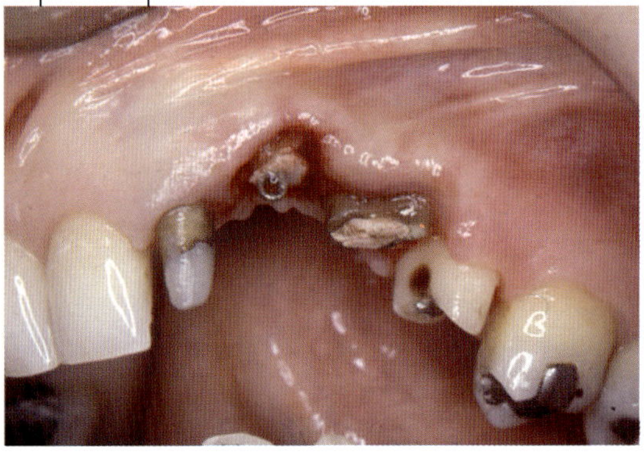

Fig. 6-201
Pre-treatment occlusion.

Fig. 6-202
After removal of the crowns.

6-203

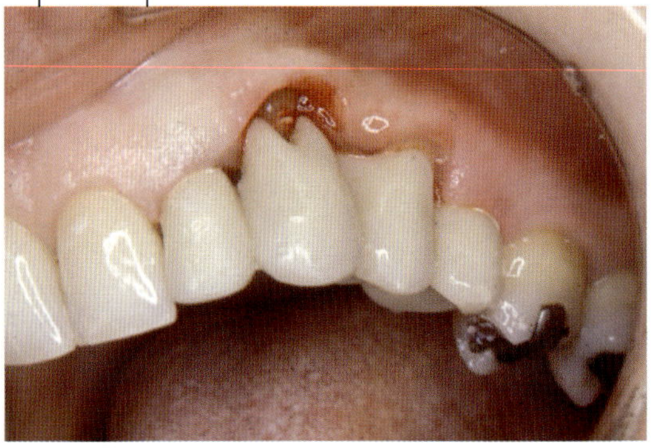

Fig. 6-203
Temporary crowns are applied.

6-204

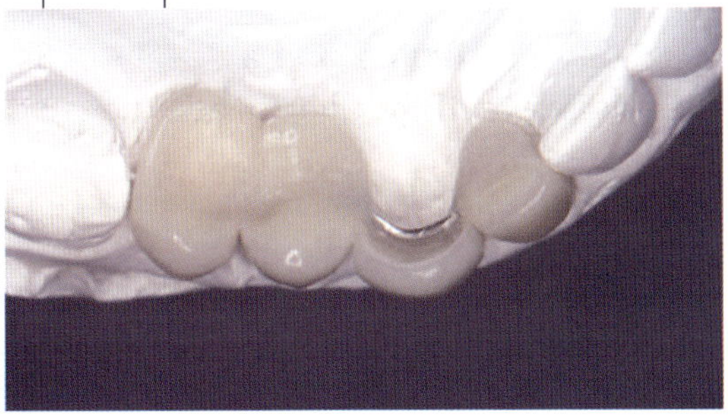

6-205

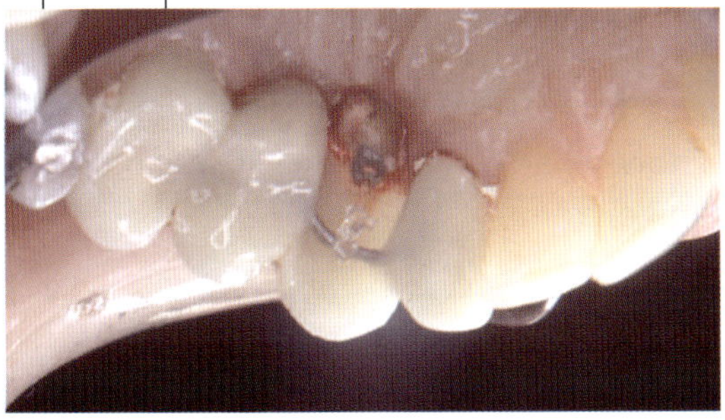

Figs. 6-204 & 6-205
Temporary crowns: palatal view. Note the small bar to which an elastic traction can be applied for the left canine root extrusion.

6-206

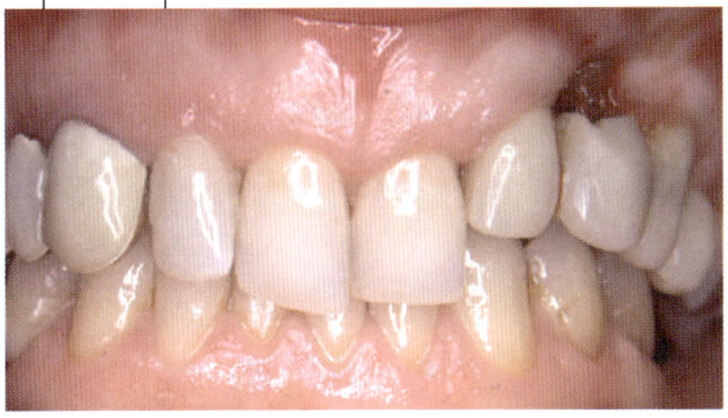

6-207

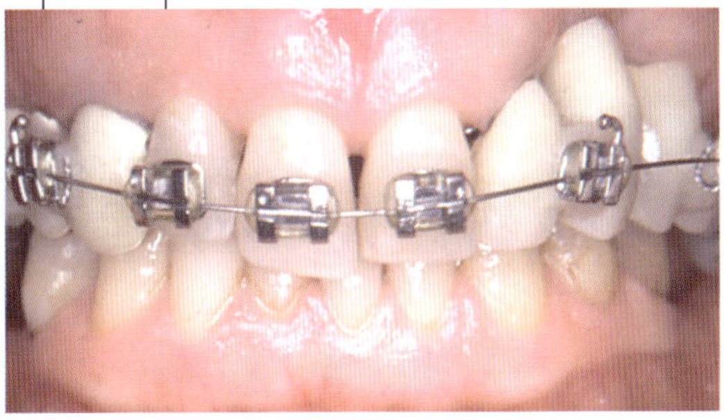

Fig. 6-206
A rapid extrusion was attempted but instead of the root extrusion there was an intrusion of other teeth. Ankylosis of the canine root was assumed.

Fig. 6-207
This unexpected intrusion permitted, with the help of a fixed appliance, the intrusion of the upper incisors and the correction of the dental deepbite. Now, an acceptable prosthesis can follow. In this case a removable prosthesis was applied.

6-208

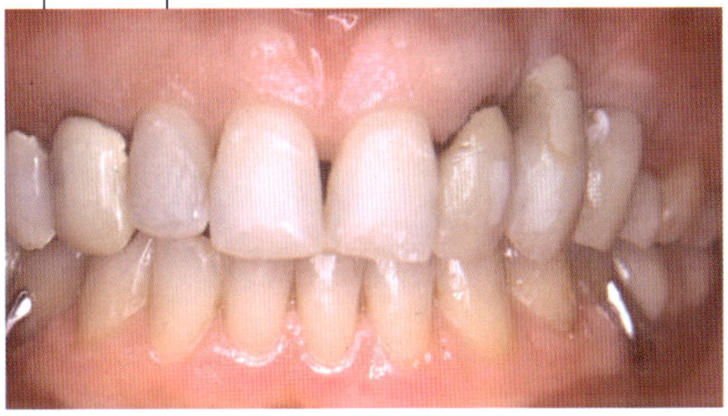

6-209

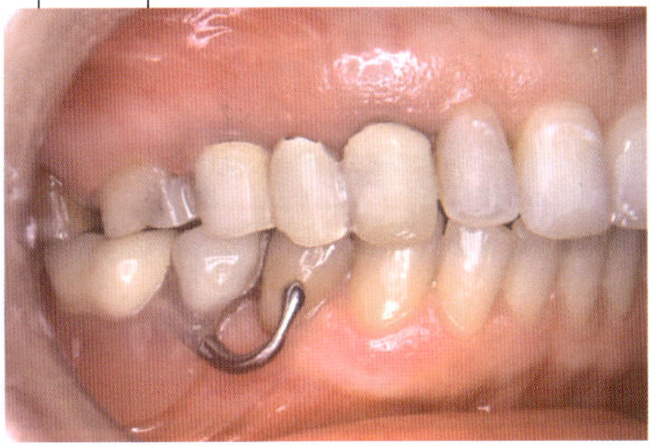

6-210

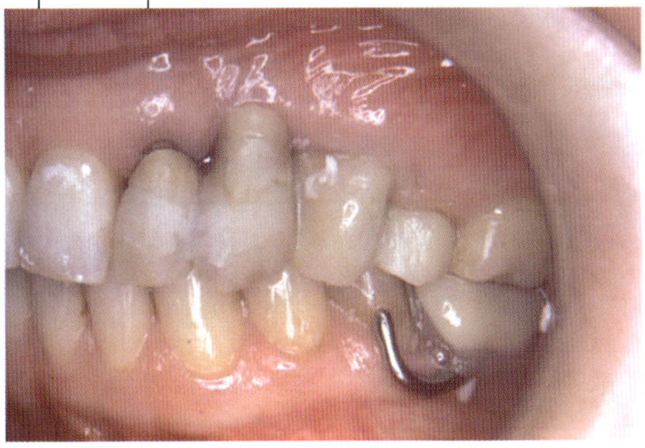

Figs. 6-208 to 6-210
Post-treatment occlusion. Temporary prostheses are still applied.

CASE NUMBER 35

The case is a Class II division 1 with upper crowding and a skeletal openbite. For many orthodontists its correction would be surgical. The lower second molars are mesially tipped and the lower third molars are distally displaced.

6-211

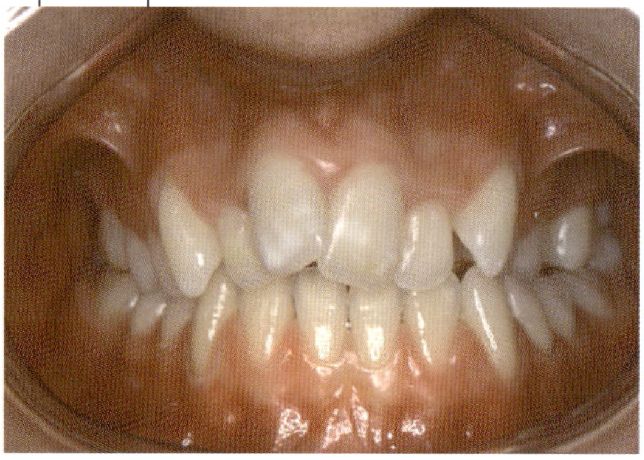

6-212

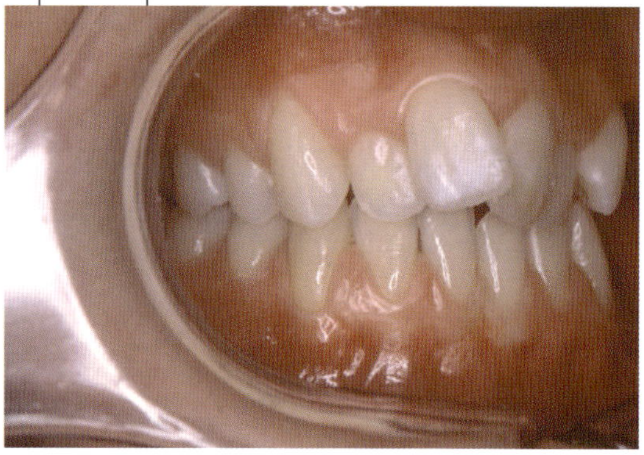

Figs. 6-211 & 2-212 Pre-treatment occlusion.

6-213

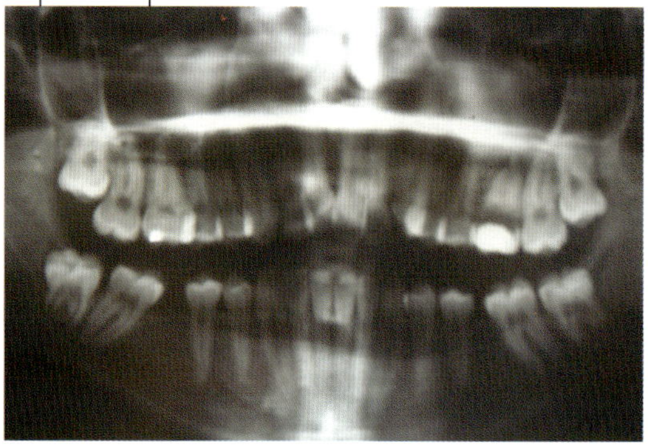

6-214

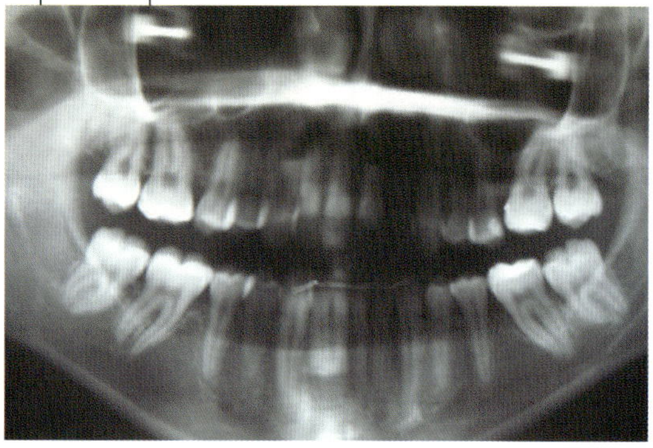

Fig. 6-213 Pre-treatment panoramic radiograph. Note the conditions of the first upper molars and the lower molars.

Fig. 6-214 Post-treatment panoramic radiograph. Notice the space closure of the first molars.

6-215

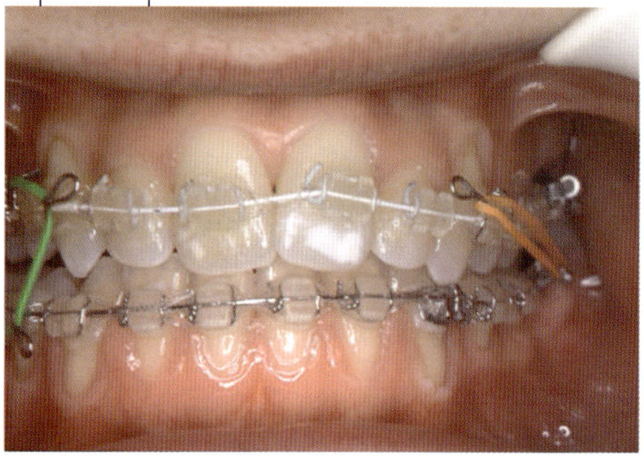

6-216

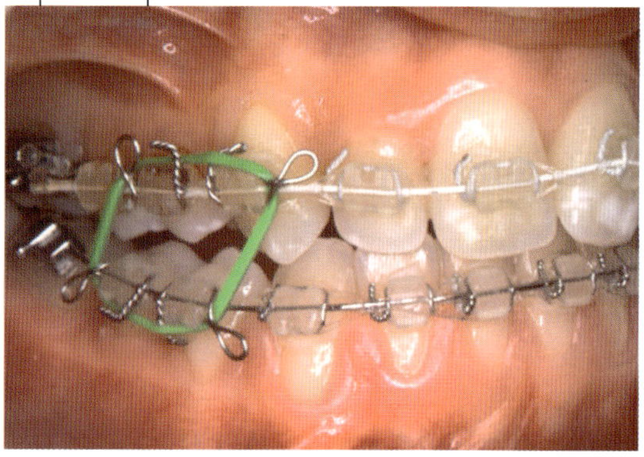

Figs. 6-215 & 6-216 After extraction of the upper first molars, a fixed appliance is placed.

6-217

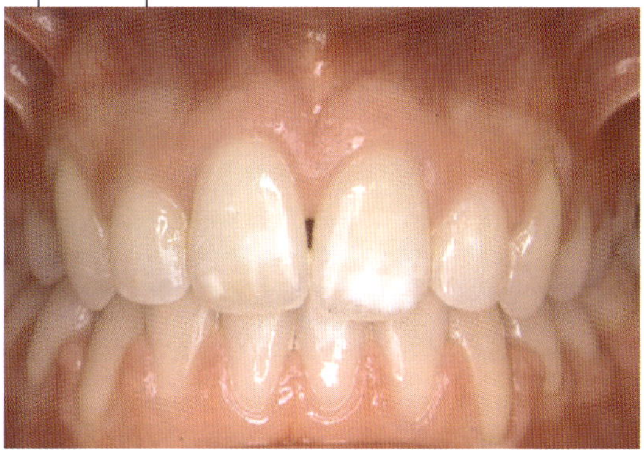

6-219

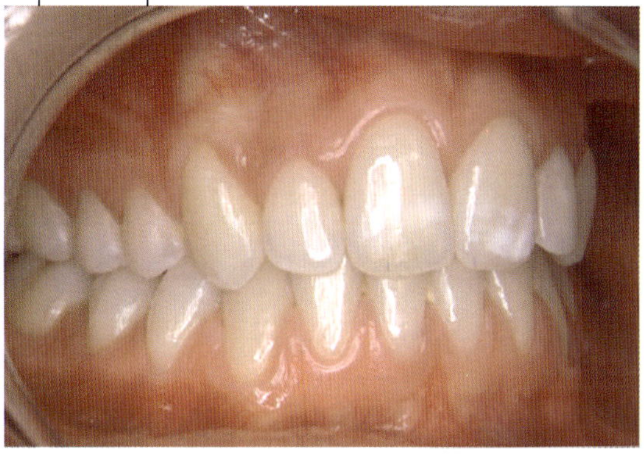

6-218

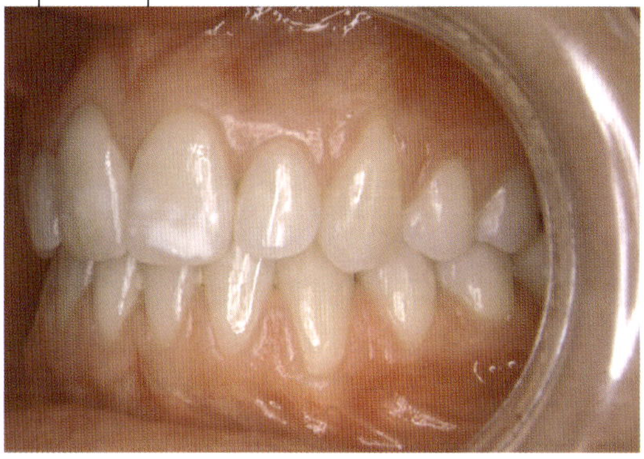

Fig. 6-217 to 6-219
Post-treatment occlusion after 18 months of treatment.

6-220

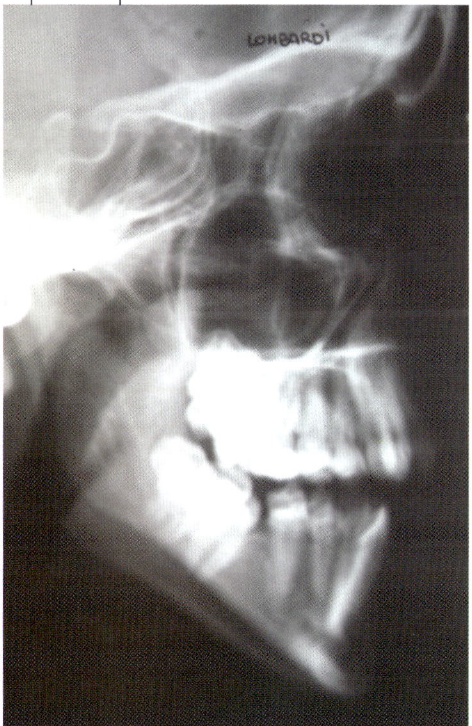

6-221

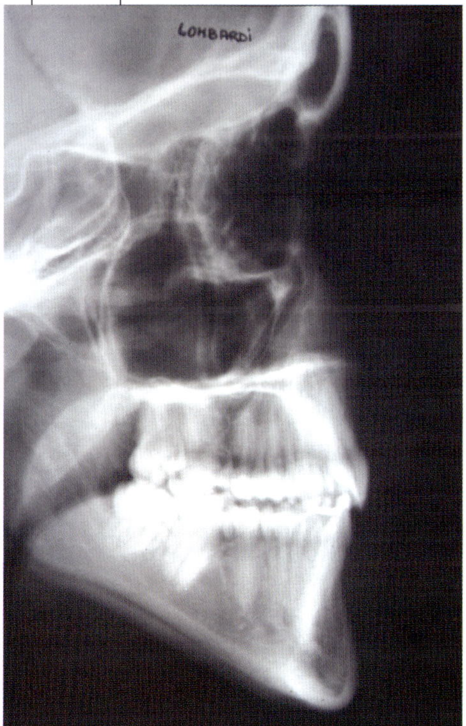

Fig. 6-220
Pre-treatment lateral cephalogram. The skeletal openbite is evident.

Fig. 6-221
Post-treatment lateral cephalogram. No surgery was performed.

Orthodontics in Clinical Practice

Chapter VII:
Orthognathic Surgery

ORTHOGNATHIC SURGERY

At the end of a patient's growth, a malocclusion with mild skeletal discrepancy can be partially corrected by orthodontic treatment. It is possible to achieve dentoalveolar compensation. In a Class III for example, the lower incisors are lingually inclined while the upper incisors are proclined. But if the aim of modern orthodontic treatment is the improvement of dental occlusion and facial aesthetics, then in the presence of severe skeletal discrepancies dentoalveolar compensation is unacceptable.

A modern orthodontist cannot ignore the treatment opportunities offered by surgery. Orthognathic surgery is performed to correct malocclusions characterized by severe jaw discrepancies. In these cases orthodontic treatment cannot offer a satisfactory functional and aesthetic facial and dental result.

With osteotomies (cuts in the bones), the jaws are moved to the desired alignment in all three planes. The cuts are made intra-oral thus offering a pleasing aesthetic outcome.

After surgical movement, the parts of jaws can be held in place with either titanium plates or screws. The surgery is usually performed under general anaesthesia with nasal intubation.

The main surgical treatments are: maxillary Le Fort I osteotomy (Fig.7-1) and mandibular bilateral sagittal split osteotomy (Fig. 7-3). With them, in a skeletal Class III, the following are possible: isolated mandibular set-back, isolated maxillary advancement (Fig.7-5) and simultaneous maxillary advancement and mandibular set-back procedures (Fig. 7-2).

When it comes to the mandible some surgeons prefer a vertical split of the ramus (Fig. 7-4).

In a Class I or II open bite, the maxilla can be repositioned superiorly and the sagittal discrepancy corrected by a mandibular counterclockwise rotation.

In a non-open bite Class II a bilateral sagittal split osteotomy followed by a mandibular advancement can be performed. Deep bite cases are best treated with ramus and subapical surgery.

Transverse problems of the upper jaw can be corrected cutting the maxilla in 2–3 pieces. The maxilla can be expanded laterally or constricted with reasonable stability. To

7-1

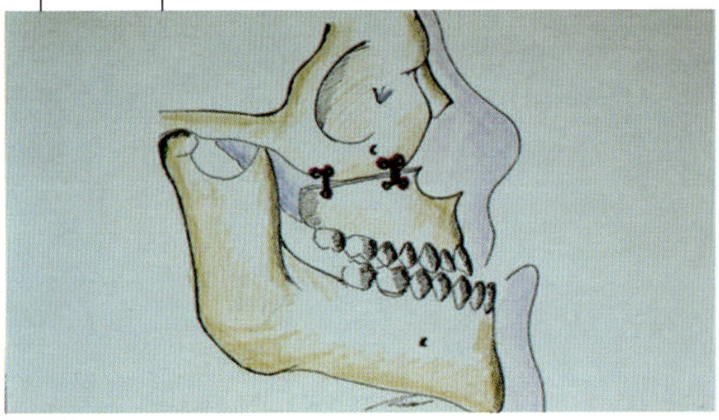

7-2

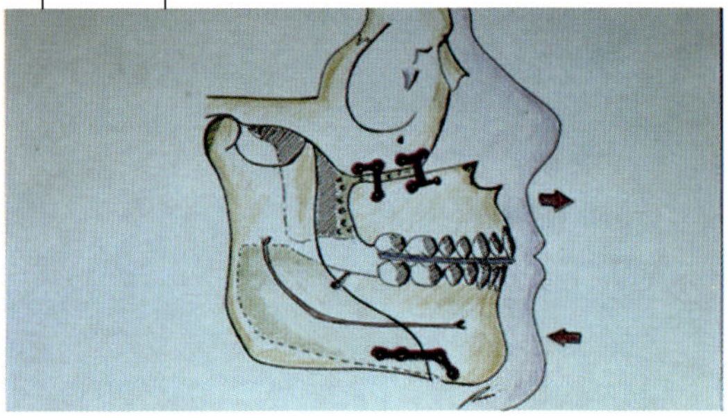

7-3

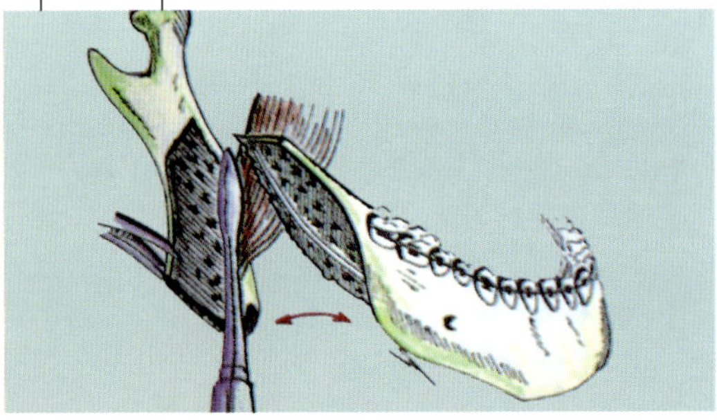

7-4

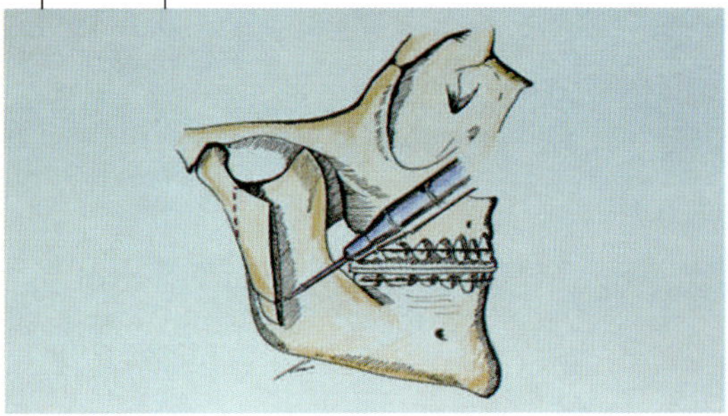

Figs. 7-1 to 7-4
The main treatments of orthognathic surgery.

Fig. 7-1
Le Fort I

Fig. 7-2
Maxillary advancement - mandibular set-back

Fig. 7-3
Mandibular sagittal split osteotomy

Fig. 7-4
Ramus vertical osteotomy (Epker modification)

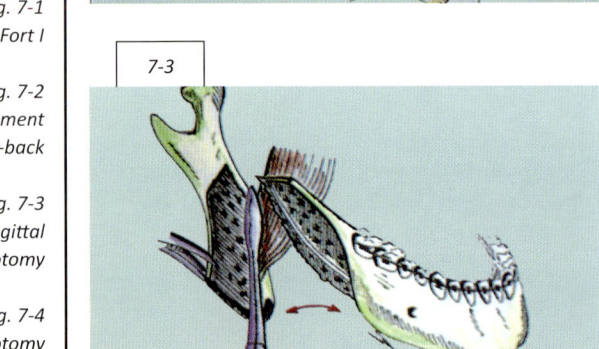

7-5

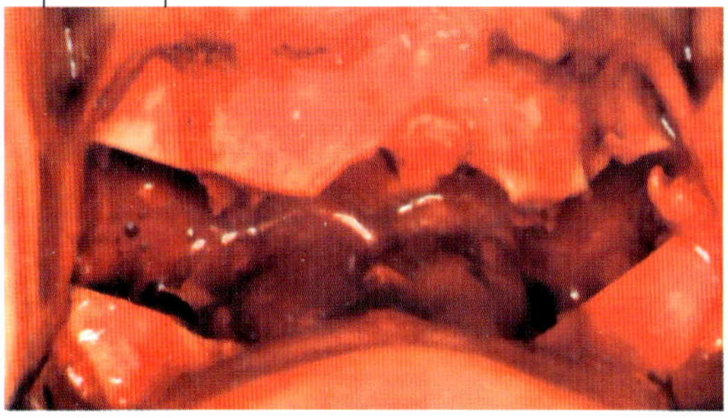

7-6

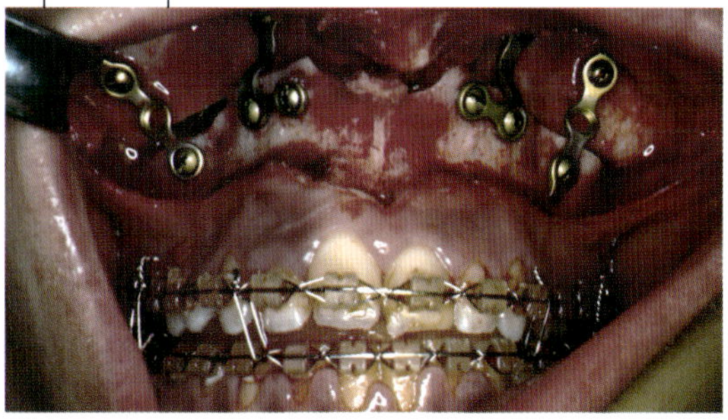

Fig. 7-5
Le Fort I. Maxillary detachment phase.

Fig. 7-6
The maxilla is advanced and held in place with titanium plates.

improve the aesthetic outcome, a surgical chin correction (genioplasty) is often performed.

Before surgery, it is very important to remove, by orthodontic treatment, the dentoalveolar compensation of the skeletal discrepancy, which often worsens the occlusion.

However, with well-aligned teeth and coordinated dental arches it is possible, by moving the bones, to achieve a good and stable result. A post-surgical orthodontic phase is then required.

In 4-6 months the final detailing of the occlusion is evident.

CASE NUMBER 1

Treated by Drs. Massimo Pricca, Luca Maria Banfi, Fabio Mazzoleni.

The case is a Class III in a 25 year old patient. It is clearly a surgical one. With combined ortho-surgical treatment, not only does the occlusion change, but also the look of her face.

7-7

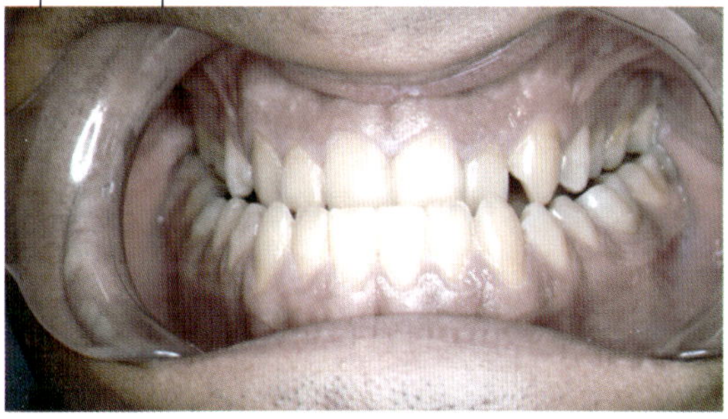

7-8

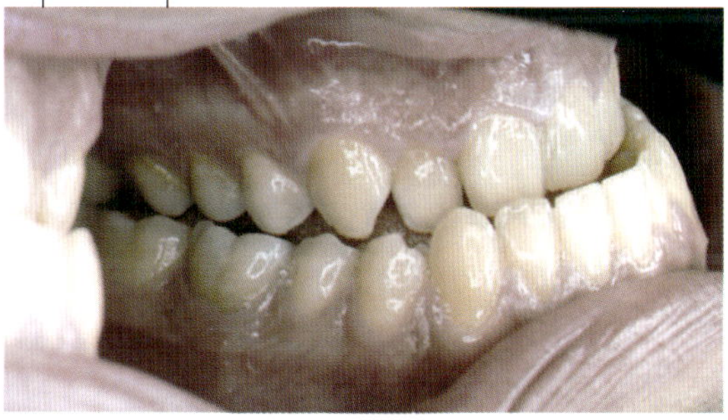

Figs. 7-7 & 7-8
Pre-treatment occlusion.

7-9

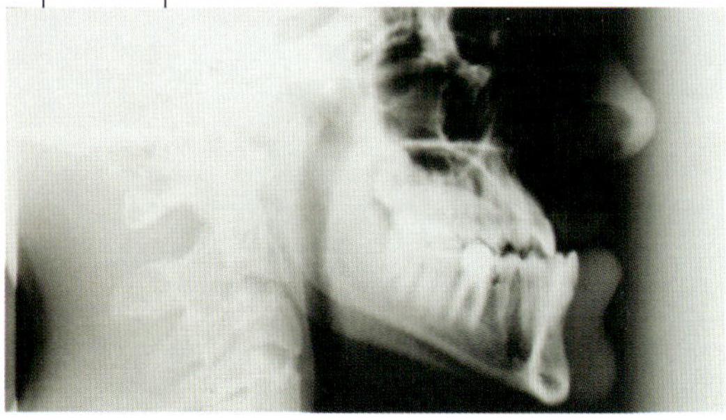

7-10

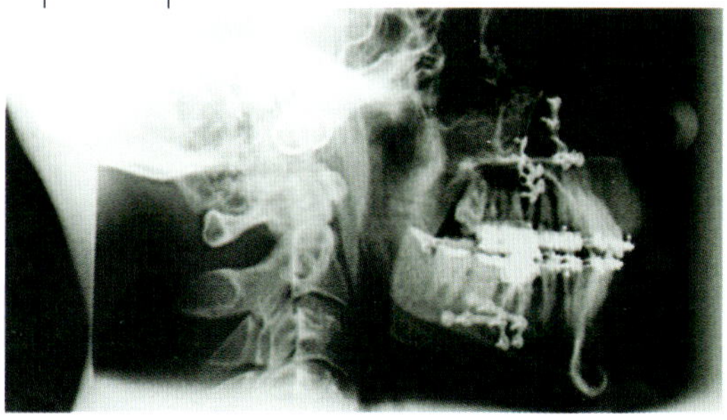

Fig. 7-9
Pre-treatment lateral cephalogram.

Fig. 7-10
Post-treatment lateral cephalogram.

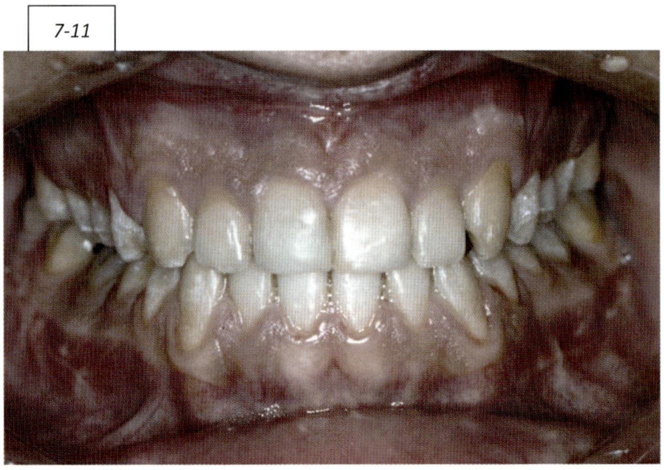

Fig. 7-11
Occlusion 3 months after surgery.

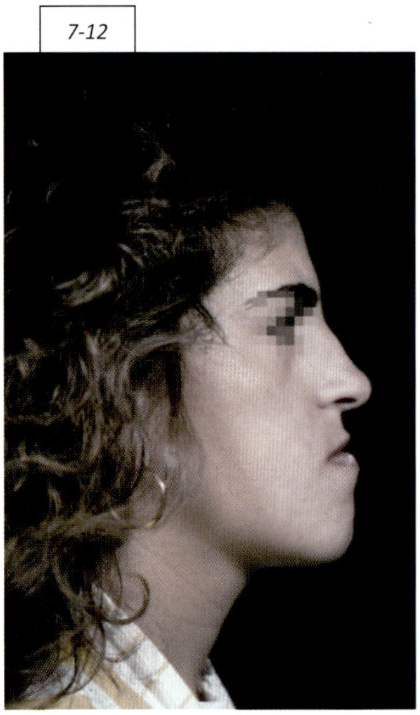

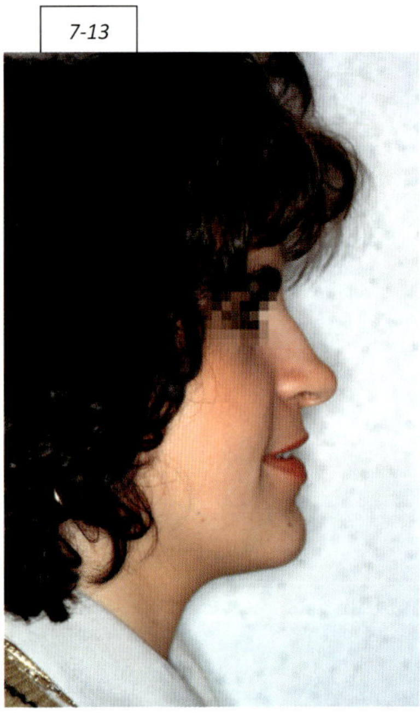

Fig. 7-12
Pre-treatment profile.

Fig. 7-13
Post-treatment profile.

Special thanks to Prof. Aldo Bruno Giannì and Dr. Alessandro Baj of the Department of Maxillo-Facial Surgery, University of Milan, who performed the surgical treatment of the following cases, which demonstrate the results of collaboration in clinical practice between orthodontist, maxillofacial surgeon and implantologist.

CASE NUMBER 2

The patient in this case has long face syndrome, a Class II with open bite. There is transverse maxillary deficiency. One of the main goals of treatment is not only a better occlusion but also a better maxilla/mandible relationship with evident aesthetic improvement.

7-14

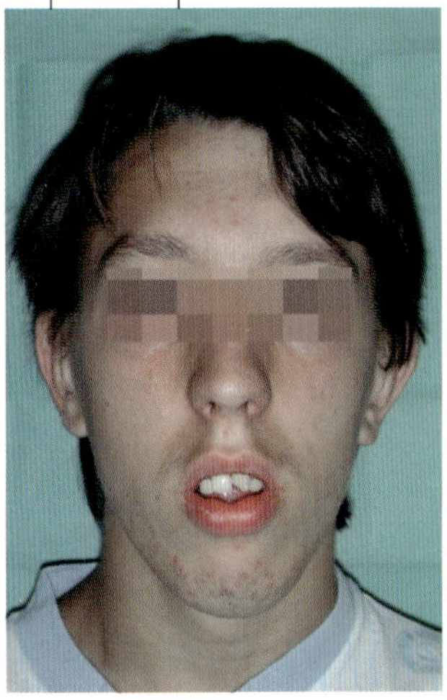

7-15

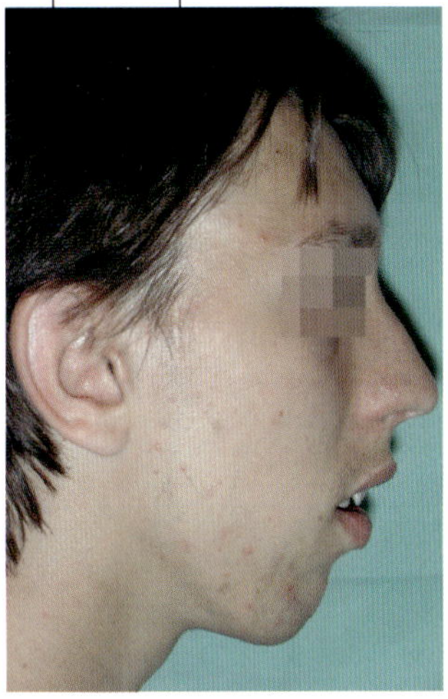

7-16

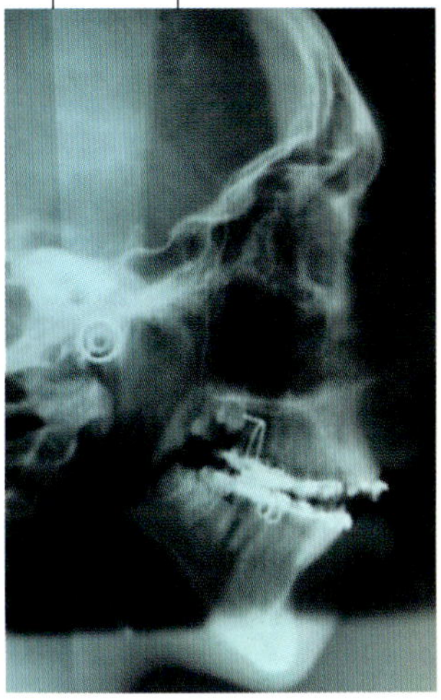

7-17

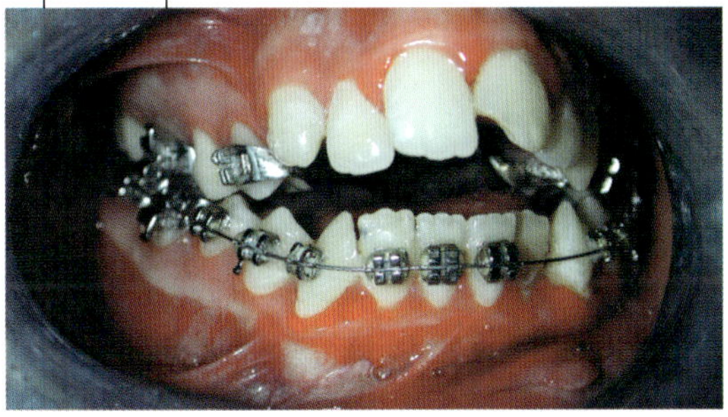

Figs. 7-14 to 7-17
Orthodontic/surgical expansion where the upper jaw defect is larger than 7mm. The expansion is necessary to carry out the correct presurgical dental realignment. Then follows osteotomy of the upper jaw in 2 or more fragments.

TREATMENT:

Phase I: surgically assisted rapid palatal expansion. Orthodontic treatment (Figs 7-18 to 7-22).

7-18

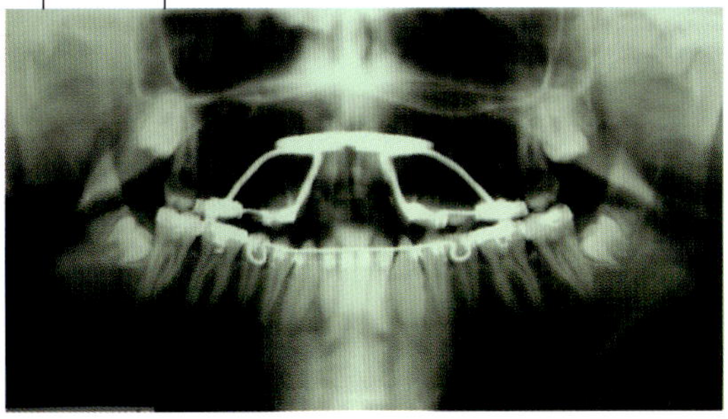

7-19

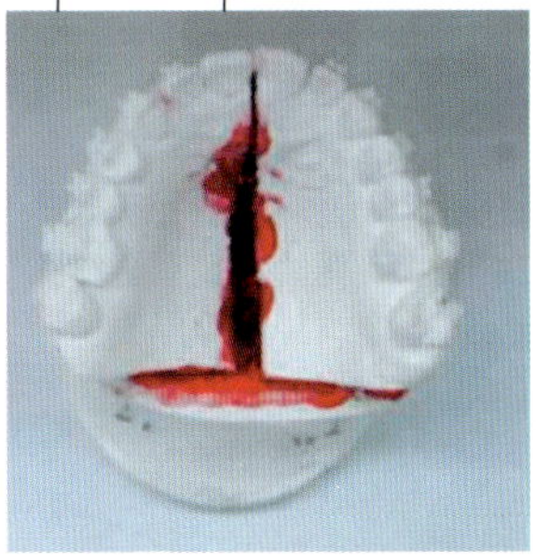

Fig. 7-18
Rapid parietal expander shown in X ray.

Fig 7-19
Cast to simulate the expansion pre-surgery.

7-20

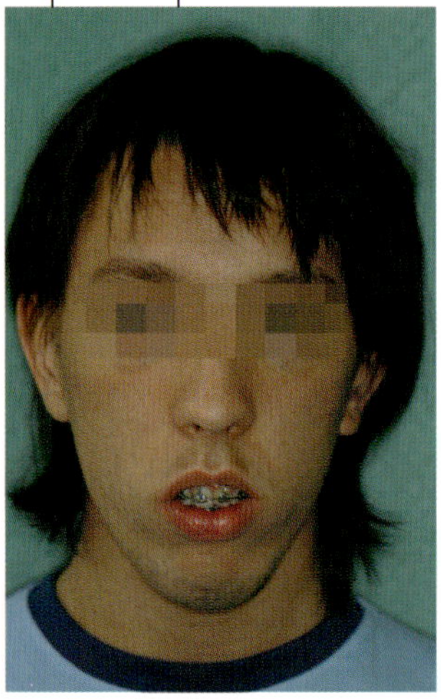

7-21

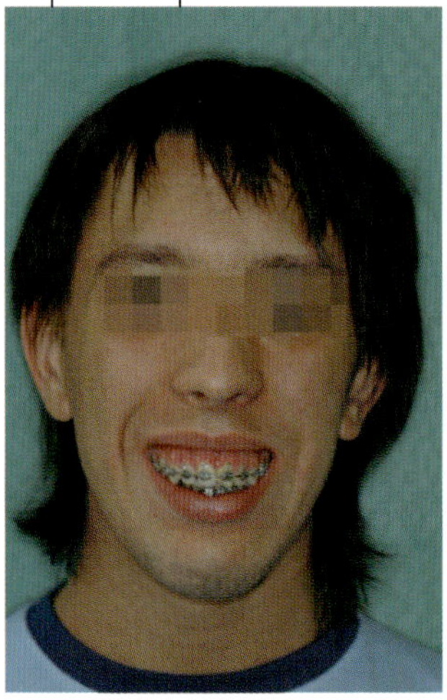

7-22

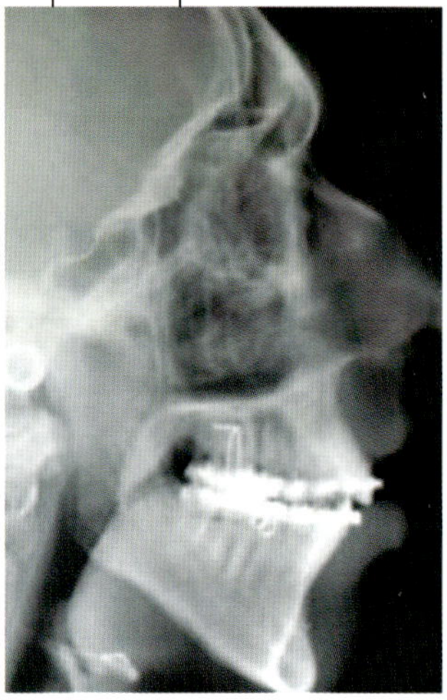

Phase II: bimaxillary surgery. Anterior verticality reduction. Genioplasty. Bone fixture using titanium screws and plates (Figs. 7-23 to 7-25).

7-23

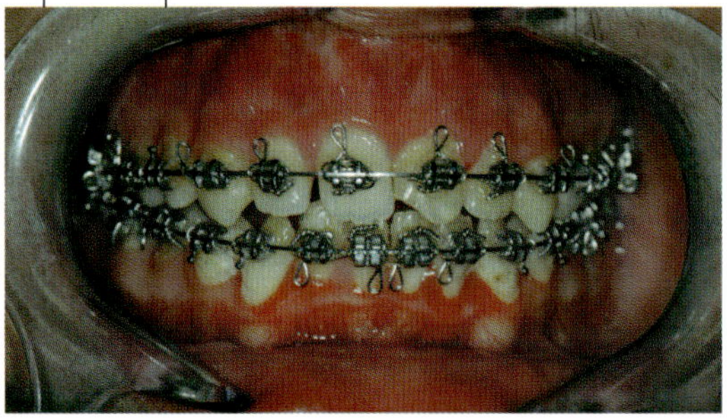

7-24

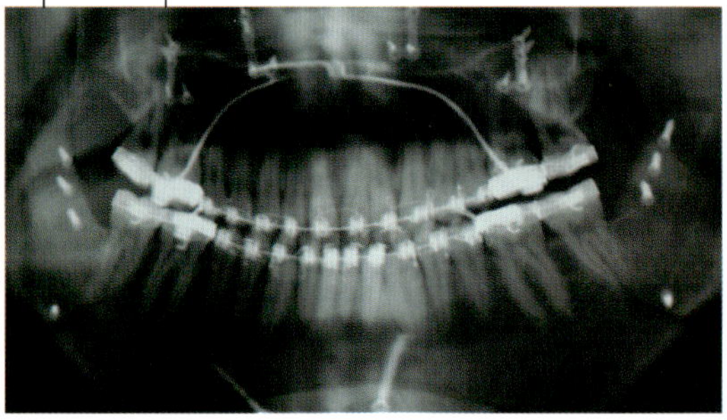

7-25

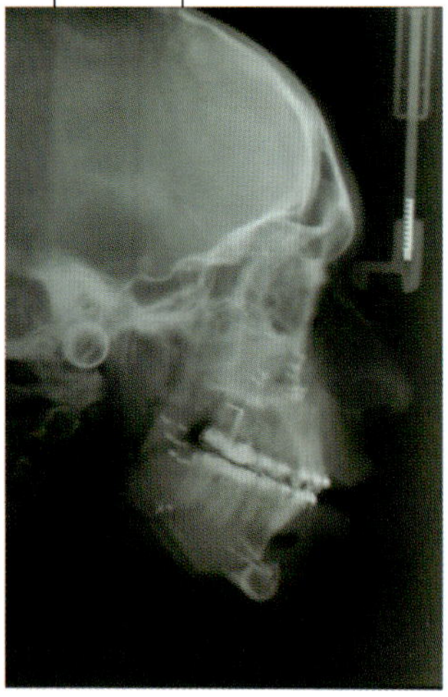

7-26

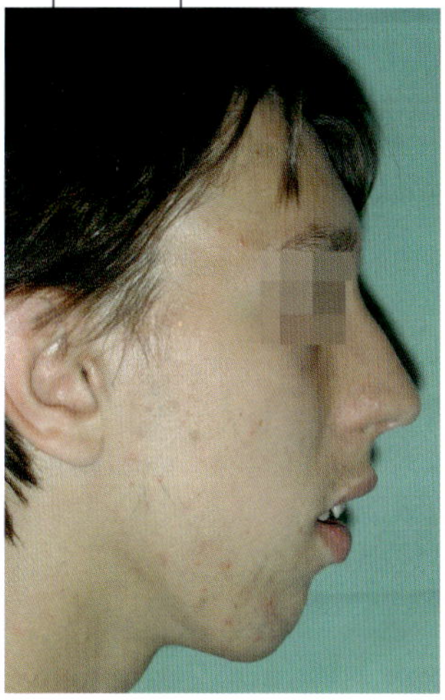

7-27

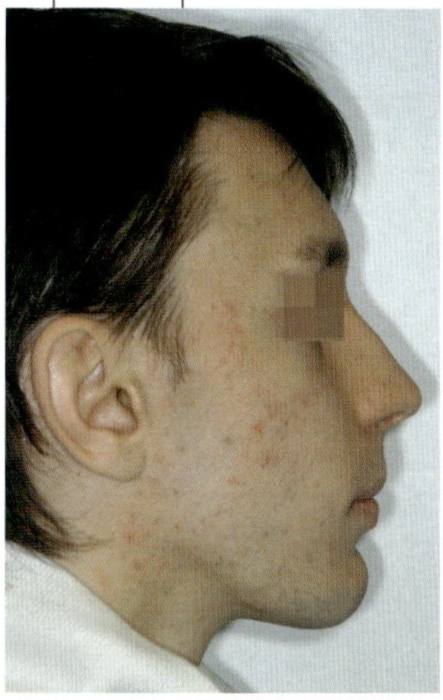

Fig. 7-26
Pre-treatment profile.

Fig. 7-27
Post-treatment profile.

7-28

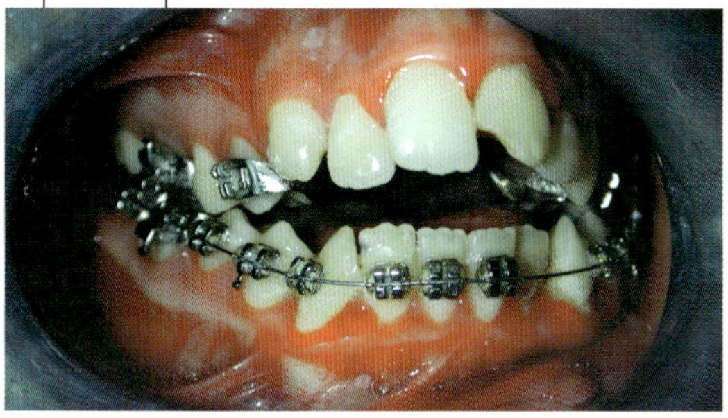

7-29

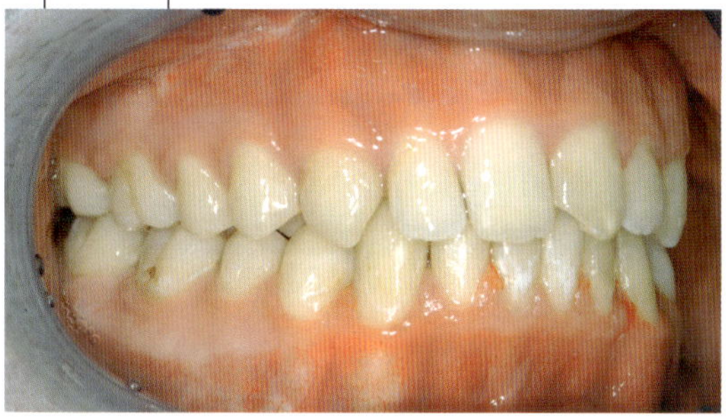

Fig. 7-28
Pre-treatment occlusion.

Fig. 7-29
Post-treatment occlusion.

7-30

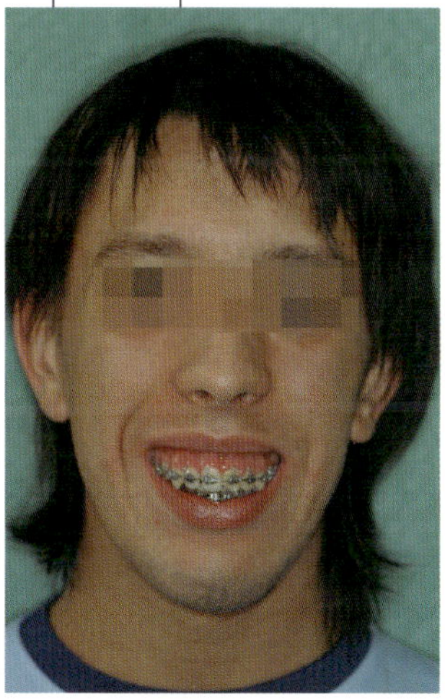

7-31

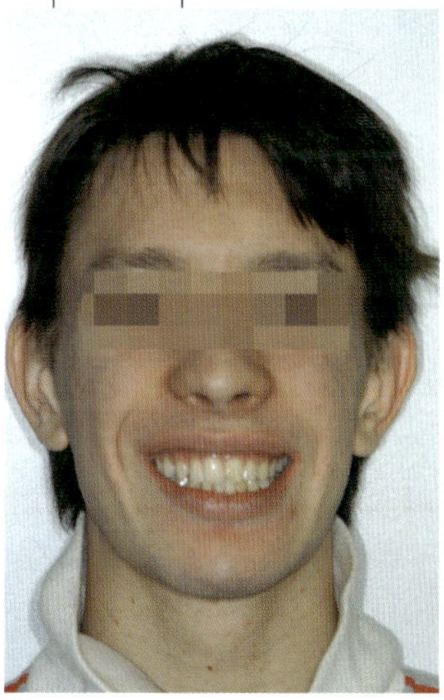

Fig. 7-30
Smile during the treatment.

Fig. 7-31
Smile after the treatment.

Orthodontic treatment performed by Dr. G. Perrotti.

CASE NUMBER 3

The patient has a short face, a Class II with deep bite (Figs. 7-32 & 7-33)

7-32

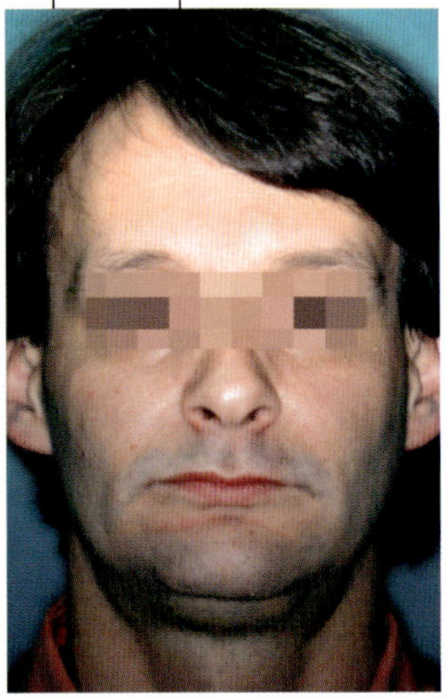

7-33

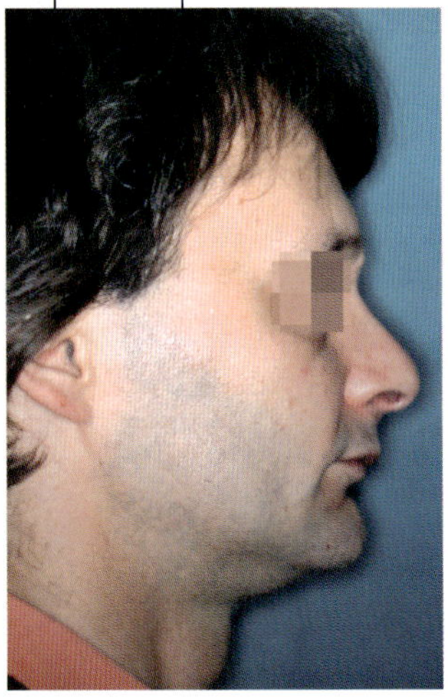

7-34

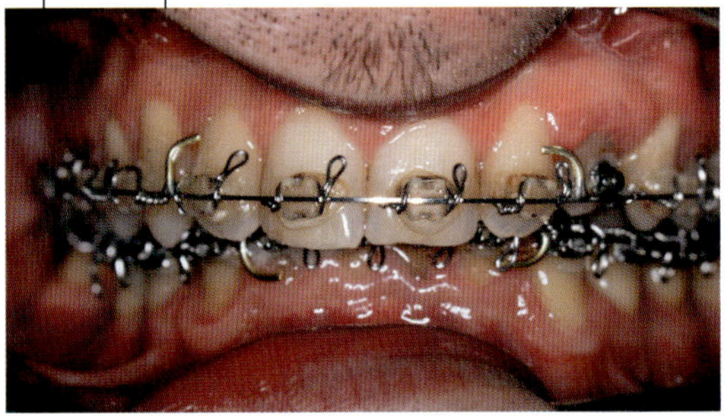

7-35

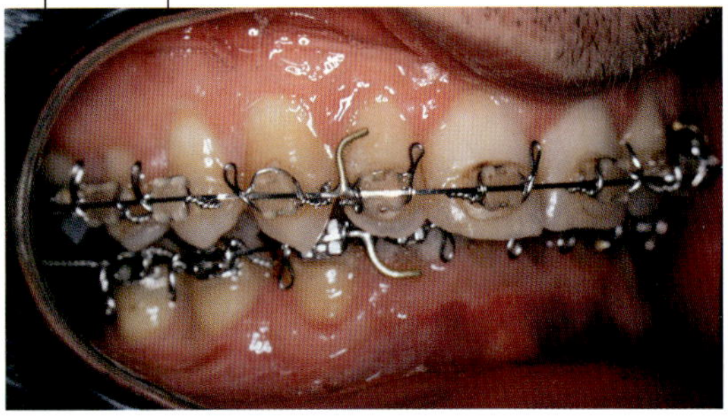

Figs. 7-34 & 7-35 Pre-surgical orthodontic treatment.

7-36

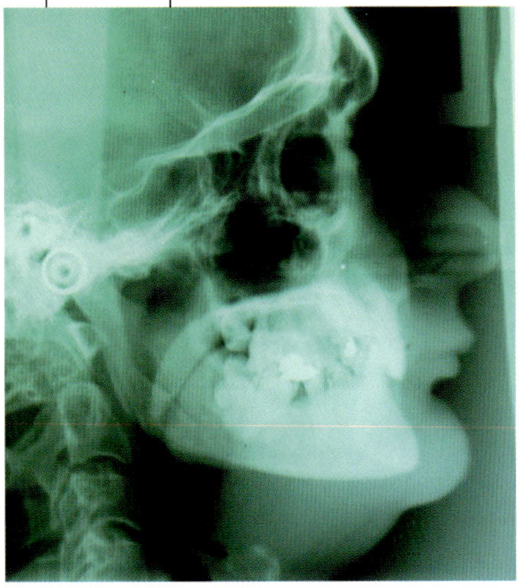

7-37

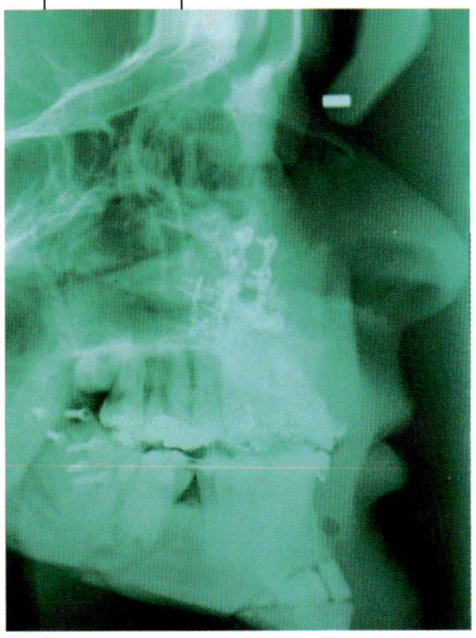

Figs. 7-36 & 7-37 Bimaxillary osteotomies with genioplasty, giving vertical increase. Bone fixture with titanium screws and plates.

7-38

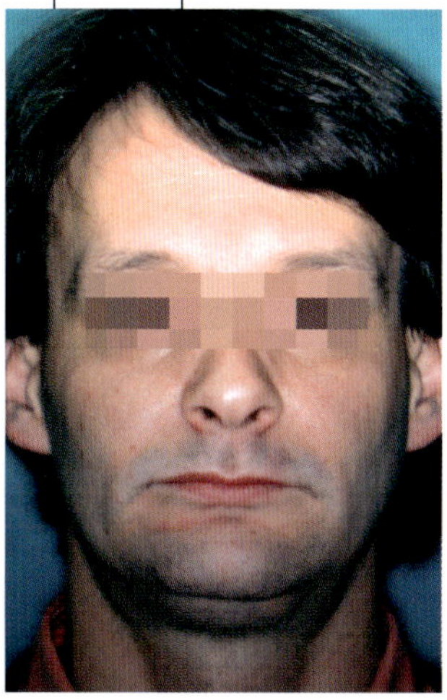

7-39

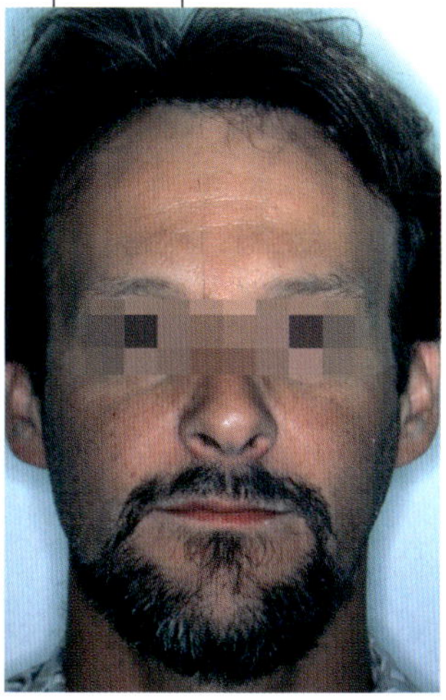

Fig. 7-38
Face before treatment.

Fig. 7-39
Face after treatment.

7-40

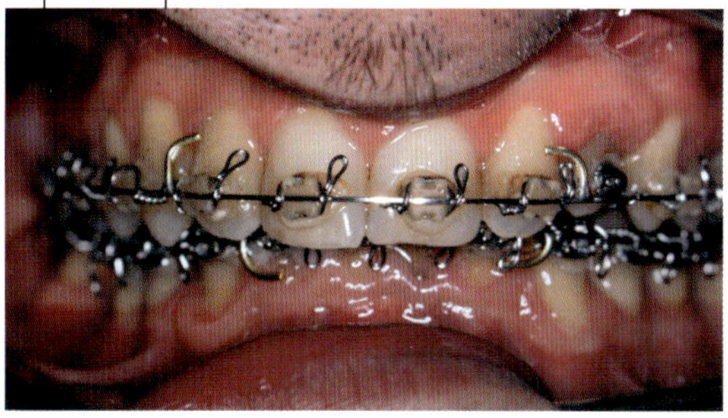

7-41

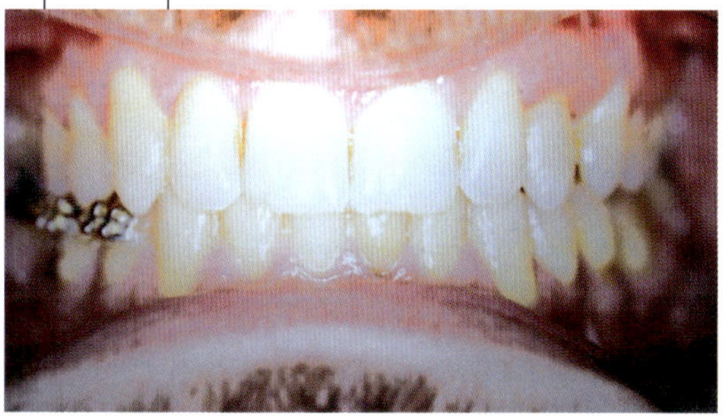

Fig. 7-40
Occlusion during treatment.

Fig. 7-41
Occlusion after treatment.

Orthodontic treatment performed by Dr. C. de Colle.

CASE NUMBER 4

The patient has a long face, a Class II and a gummy smile. Orthodontic treatment was followed by bimaxillary surgery.

7-42

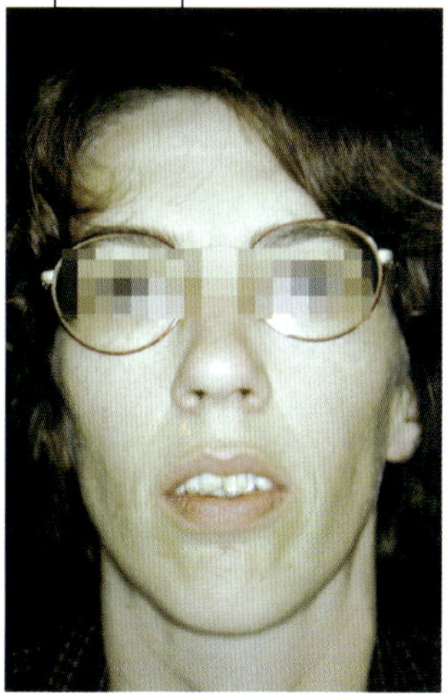

7-43

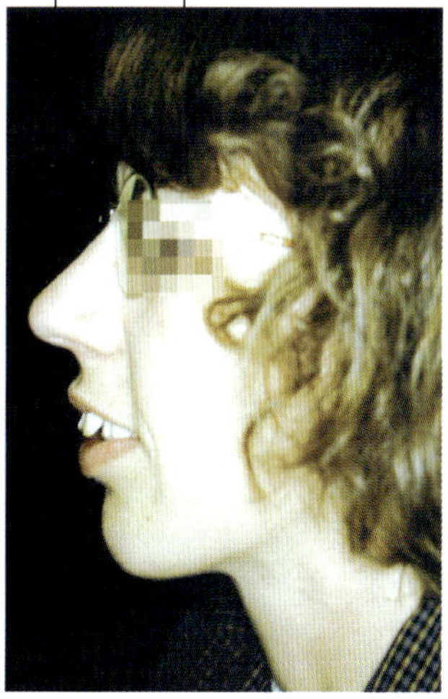

Figs. 7-42 & 7-43
Pre-treatment face and occlusion.

7-44

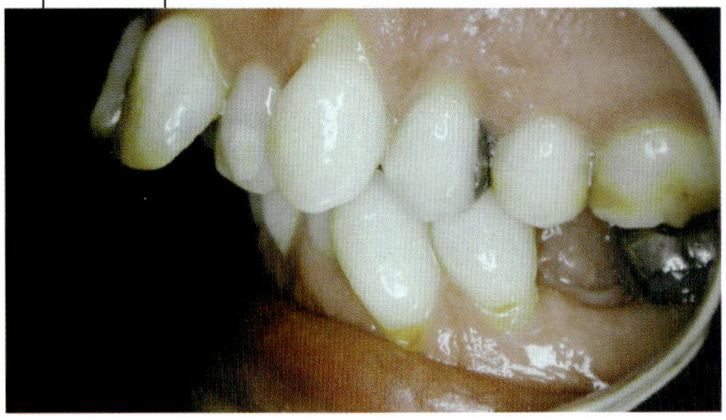

Fig. 7-44
Pre-treatment occlusion.

7-45

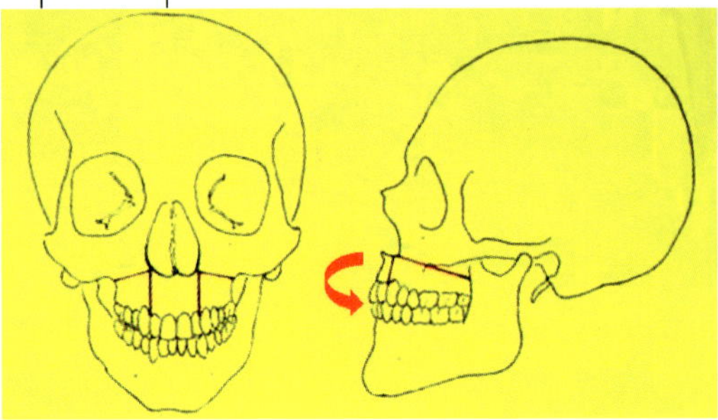

Fig. 7-45
Schematic representation of maxillary surgery.

7-46

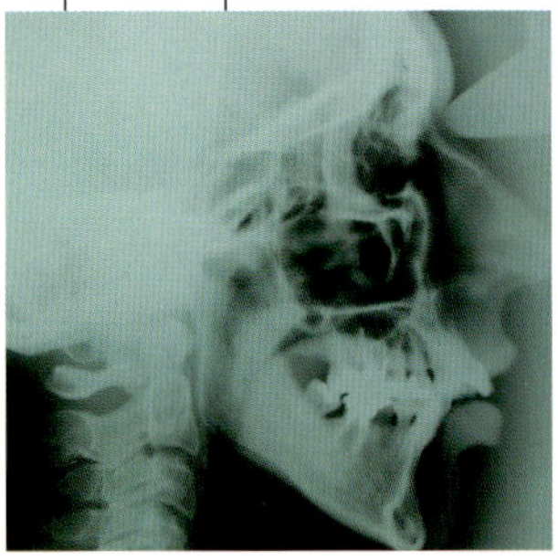

Fig. 7-46
Pre-treatment lateral cephalogram.

7-47

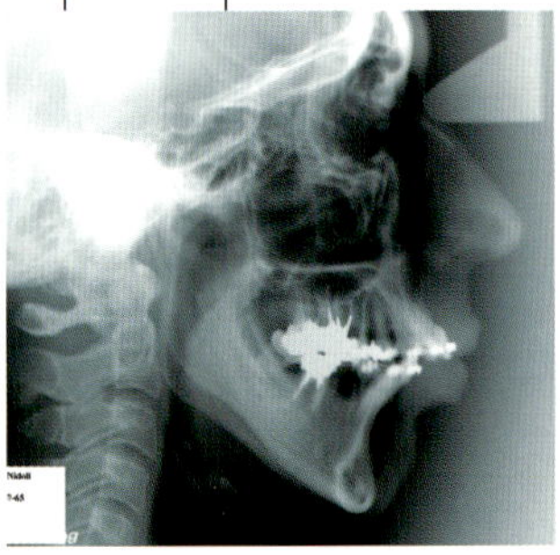

Fig. 7-47
Lateral cephalogram after the orthodontic treatment.

7-48

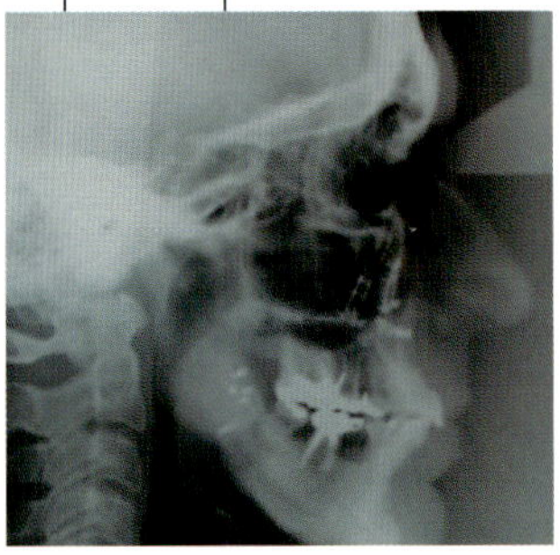

Fig. 7-48
Post-treatment lateral cephalogram.

7-49

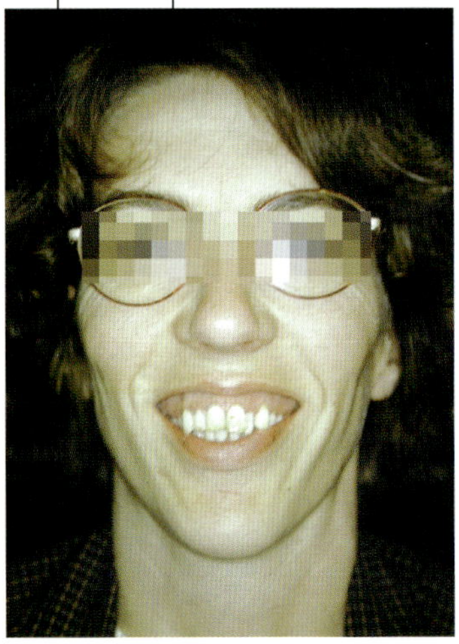

7-50

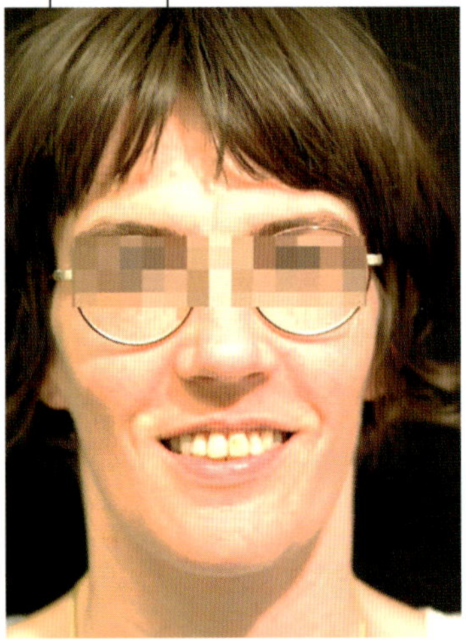

7-51

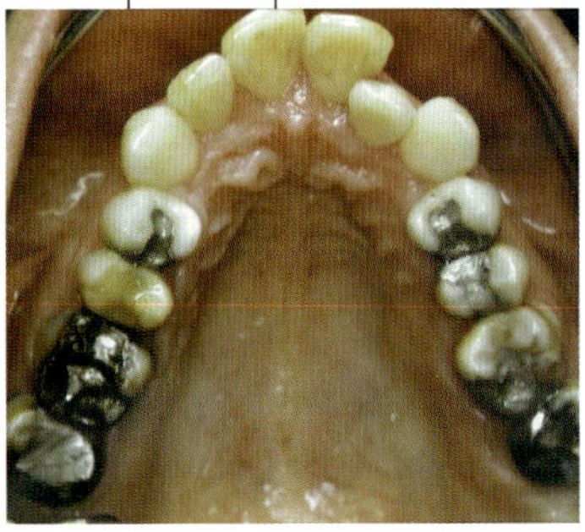

7-52

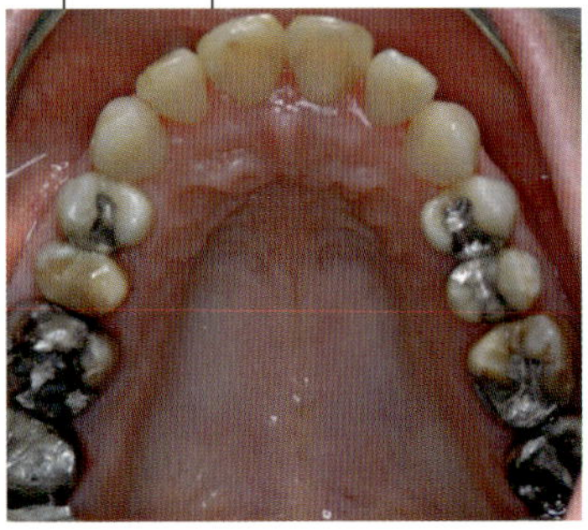

Figs. 7-49 & 7-51
Pre-treatment.

Figs. 7-50 & 7-52
Post-treatment.

7-53

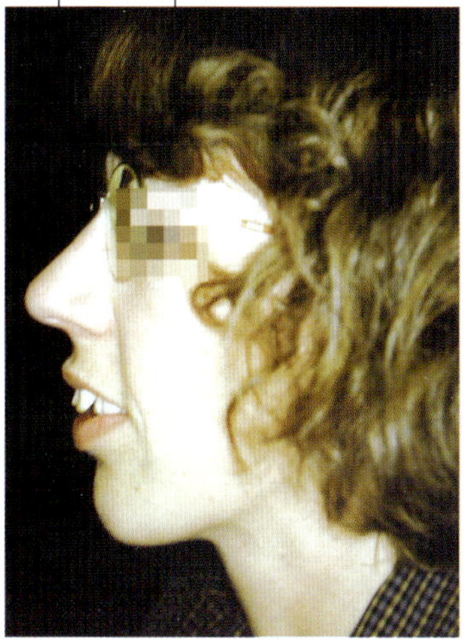

7-54

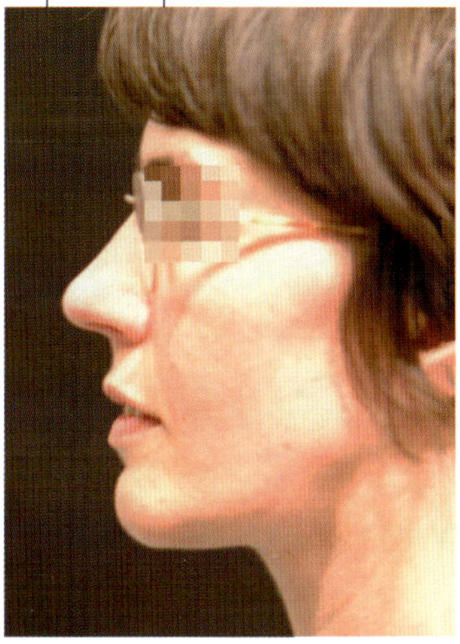

7-55

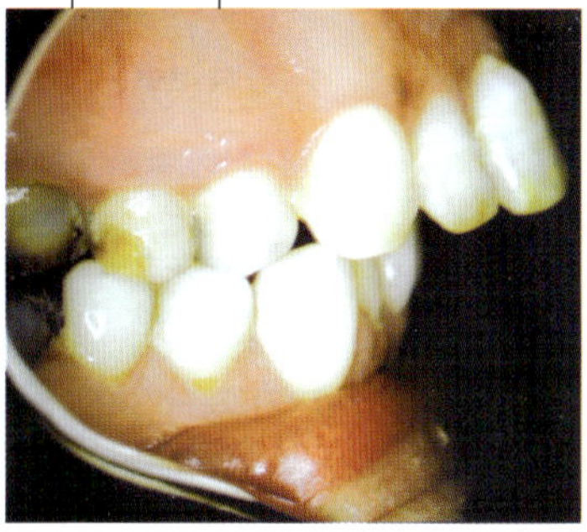

7-56

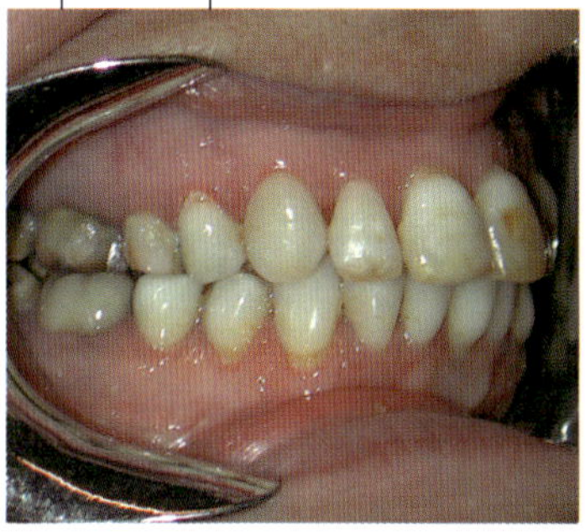

Figs. 7-53 & 7-55
Pre-treatment.

Figs. 7-54 & 7-56
Post-treatment.

Orthodontic treatment performed by Dr. A. Macchi.

CASE NUMBER 5

The patient has a Class II, a mandibular retrusion and a convex profile.

TREATMENT:

1.Sagittal split osteotomy to advance the mandible.
2.Genioplasty.
3.Bone fixture with titanium screws.

7-57

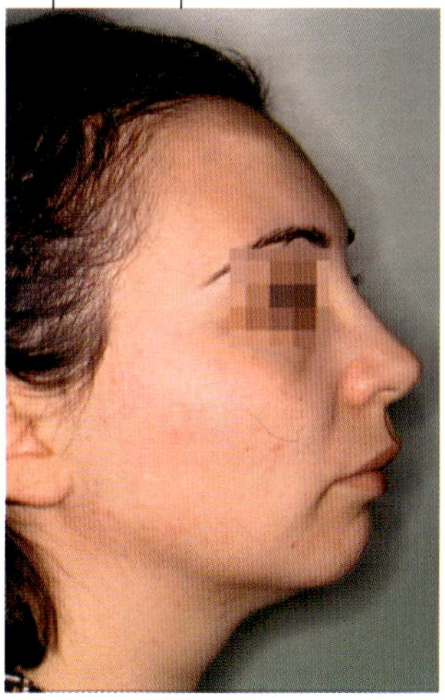

7-58

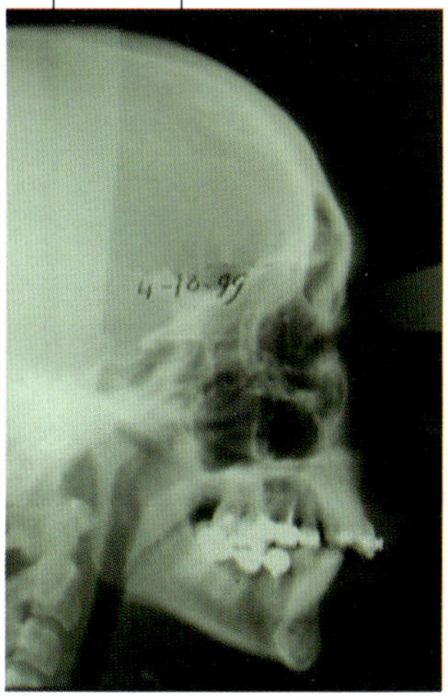

7-59

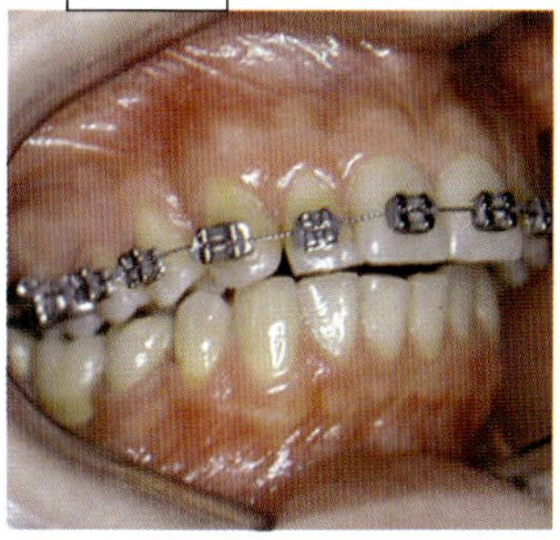

Figs. 7-57 to 7-59
Pre-treatment.

7-60

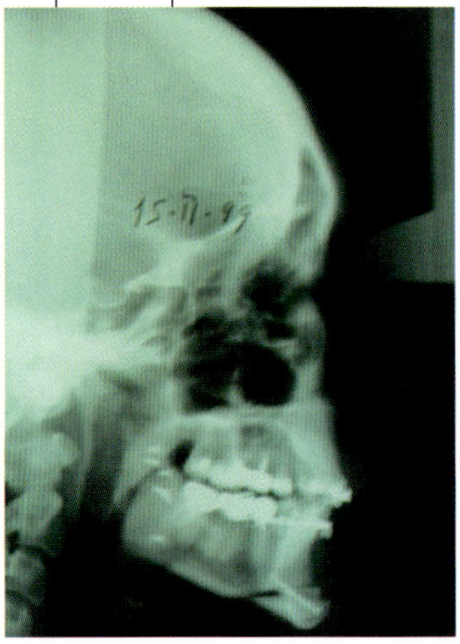

7-61

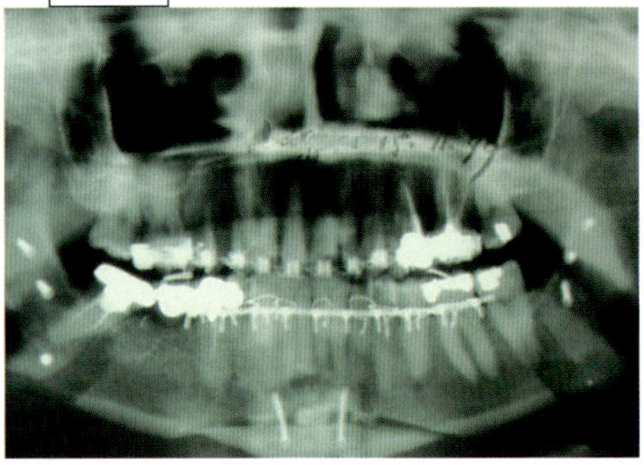

Figs. 7-60 & 7-61
Post-treatment X-rays.

7-62

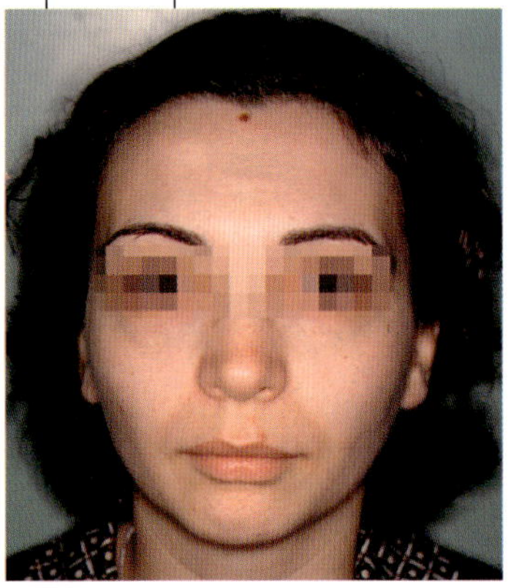

7-63

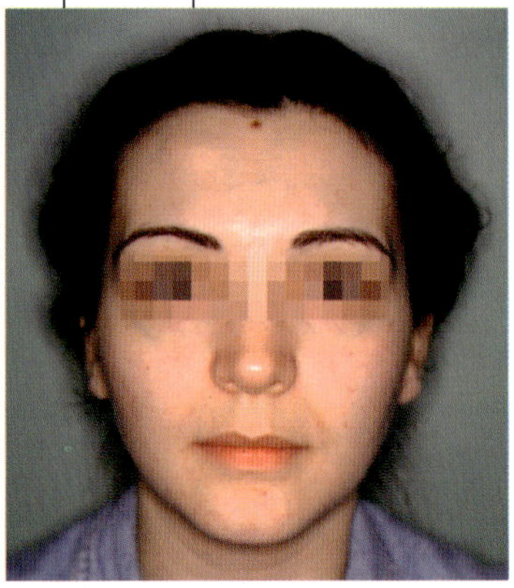

7-64

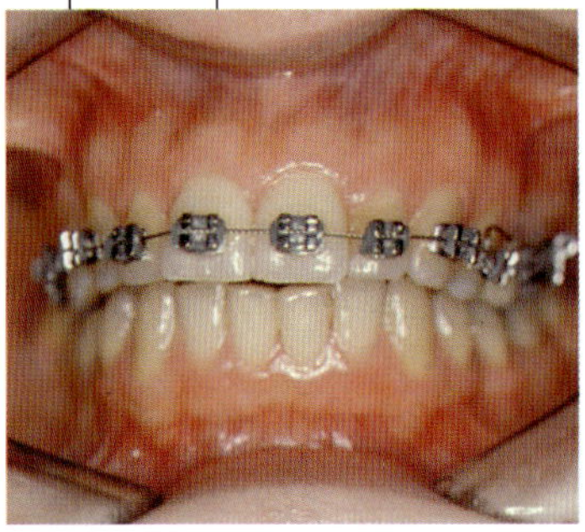

7-65

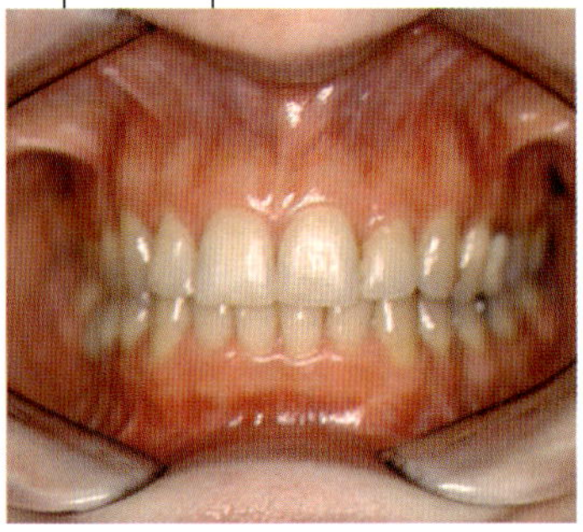

7-66

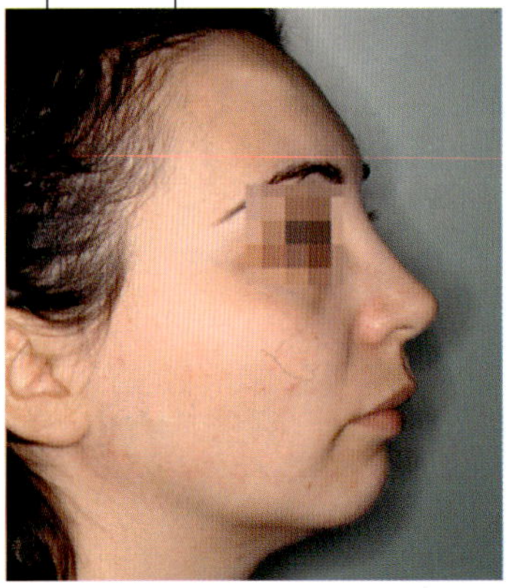

7-67

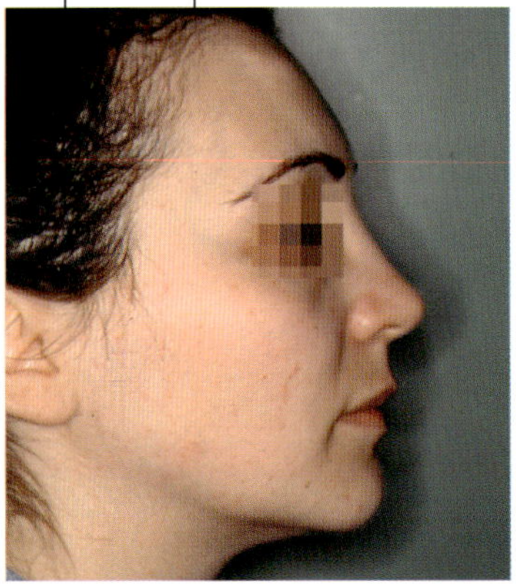

Figs. 7-62, 7-64, 7-66
Pre-surgical treatment.

Figs. 7-63, 7-65, 7-67
Post-surgical treatment.

7-68

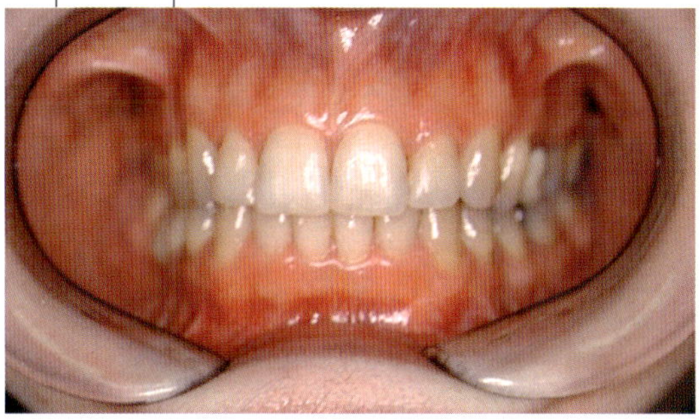

7-69

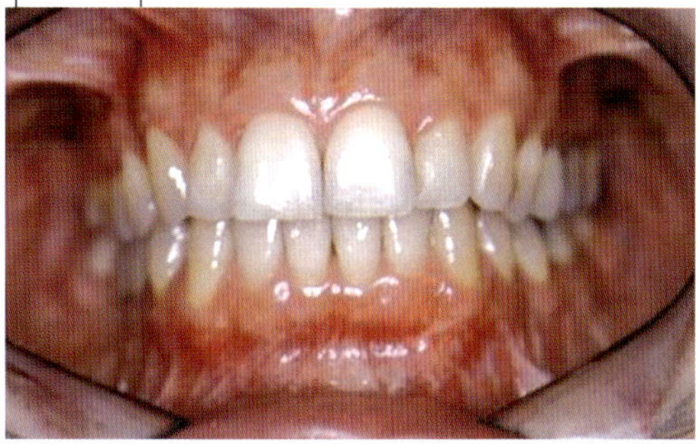

Fig. 7-68
Occlusion 3 months after treatment.

Fig. 7-69
Occlusion 28 months after treatment.

7-70

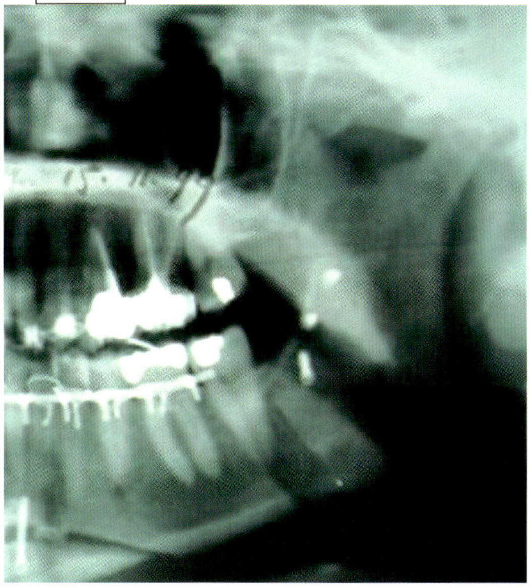

7-71

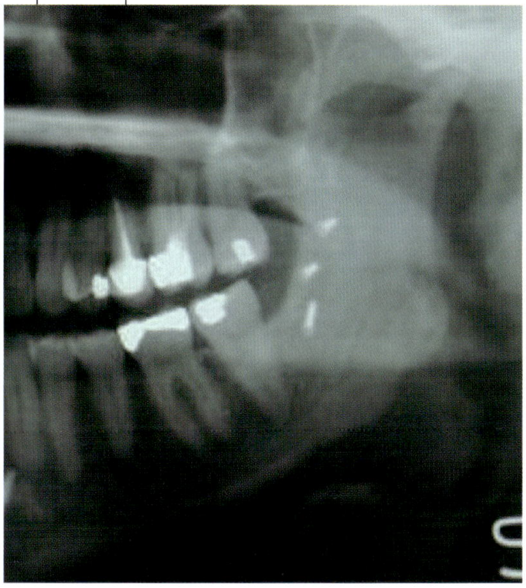

Fig. 7-70
Radiograph 1 month after surgery.

Fig. 7-71
Radiograph 28 months after surgery.

General Bibliography

Please note that this english language edition of *Orthodontics in Clinical Practice* has been updated and enlarged since the publication of the original italian edition. Consequently there are many new references, as a result of which different numbering referral systems have been used within the text.

1. Accivile E et al. Valutazione statistica sulla posizione del canino mascellare incluso. *Mondo Ort.* 1995, 5: 453-9.
2. Adkins MD, Nanda RS & Currier GF. Arch perimeter changes on rapid palatal expansion. *Am J Orthod Dentofacial Orthop.* 1990, 97(3): 194-9.
3. Alexander RG. *The Alexander Discipline*. Lerici: Biaggini ORMCO Italia, 1993.

1*6 Allais D & Melsen B. Does labial movement of lower incisors influence the level of the gingival margin? A case-control study of adult orthodontic patients. *Eur J Orthod.* 2003, 25(4): 343–52.

4. Andlaw RJ & Rock WP. *A Manual of Pedodontics.* Churchill Livingstone: Edinburgh, 1982.
5. Andreasen GF & Bishara S. Comparison of alastik chains with elastics involved with intra-arch molar-to-molar forces. *Angle Orthod.* 1970, 40(3): 151-8.
6. Andreasen JO. *Traumatic Injuries of the Teeth.* Copenhaghen: Munksgaard. 2th edn, 1981.
7. Andresen V. The Norwegian system of functional gnatho-orthopedics. *Acta Gnathol.* l936, l: 5-36.
8. Andrews LF. *Straight Wire: the concept and appliance*. San Diego: LA Wells, 1989.

6** Angelieri F et al. Dentoalveolar and skeletal changes associated with pendulum appliances followed by fixed orthontic treatment. *Am J Orthod Dentofacial Orthop.* 2006, 129 (4): 520 -7.

1*5 Artun J & Grobéty D. Peridontal status of mandibular incisors after pronounced orthodontic advancement during adolescence: a follow-up evaluation. *Am J Orthod Dentofacial Orthop.* 2001, 119(1): 2-10.

9. Artun J, Hollender LG & Truelove EL. Relationship between orthodontic treatment, condylar position, and internal derangement in the temporomandibular joint. *Am J Orthod Dentofacial Orthop.* 1992, 101(1): 48-53
10. Balters W. *Representation Figurative du Principe du Bionator, Son Action lors du Redressement Fonctionnel de l'espace Buccal*. RFOS. Fevrier, 1964.
11. Bass NM. Bass orthopedic appliance system. *J Clin Orthod.* 1987, Part 1: 21(4): 254-65, Part 2: 21(5): 312-20, Part 3: 21(6): 384-94.
12. Bass NM. The aesthetic analysis of the face. *Eur J Orthod.* 1991, 13(5): 343-50.
13. Bassigny F. Les traitements avec extraction; des premières molaires. *Orthod Fran.* 1979, 50: 131-272.

14. Bassigny F. Riassorbimenti radicolari di origine ortodontica. Analisi di una ricerca clinica. *Dental Cadmos.* 1992, 2049-57.
15. Betteridge MA. The effects of interdental stripping on the labial segments evaluated one year out of retention. *Br J Orthod.* 1981, 8(4): 193-7.
16. Baumrind S et al. Quantitative analysis of orthodontic and orthopedic effects of maxillary traction. *Am J Orthod.* 1983, 84(5): 384-98.
17. Baumrind S, Kom EL & West EE. Prediction of mandibular rotation: an empirical test of clinician performance. *Am J Orthod.* 1984, 86(5): 371-85.
18. Bishara SE et al. Management of impacted canines. *Am J Orthod.* 1976, 69(4): 371-87.
19. Becker A. Periodontal splinting with multistrand wire following orthodontic realignment of migrated teeth: report of 38 cases. *Int J Adult Orthodon Orthognath Surg.* 1987, 2(2): 99-109.
20. Begg PR & Kesling PC. *Begg Orthodontic Theory and Technique*. The University of Michigan: 3rd edn, 1977.
21. Bennett JC & McLaughlin RP. Controlled space closure with a preadjusted appliance system. *J Clin Orthod.* 1990, 24(4): 251-60.
22. Berard R. *Pèdodontie.* Paris: Julien Prélat Ed, 1980.
23. Bery A. Gli inddenti causati dalle forze extraorali. *Ortognatodonzia Italiana.* 1993, 2(3): 508-11.
24. Bimler HP. Dynamic functional therapy. The Bimler appliance. *Trans Eur Orthod Soc.* 1973: 451-6.
25. Bjerregaard J, Bundgaard AM & Melsen B. The effect of the mandibular lip bumper and maxillary bite plate on tooth movement, occlusion and space conditions in the lower dental arch. *Eur J Orthod.* 1980, 2(4): 257-65.
26. Björk A. The use of metallic implants in the study of facial growth in children: method and application. *Am J Phys Anthropol.* 1968, 29(2): 243-54.
27. Björk A. Prediction of the mandibular growth rotation. *Am J Orthod.* 1969, 55(6): 585-99.
28. Björk A & Skieller V. Normal and abnormal growth of the mandible. A synthesis longitudinal cephalometric implant studies over a period of 25 years. *Eur J Orthod.* 1983, 5(1): 1-46.
29. Björk A & Skieller V. Postnatal growth and development of the maxillary complex. In: *Factors Affecting Growth in the Midface.* Namara JA, editor. Ann Arbor, University of Michigan Centre for Human Growth and Development, 1976.
30. Boese LR. Fiberotomy and reproximation without lower retention, nine years in retrospect. *Angle Orthod.* 1980, Parts I: 50(2): 88-97, Part II: 50(3): 169-78.
31. Bolton WA. The clinical application of a tooth-size analysis. *Am J Orthod.* 1962, 48(7): 504-29.
9** Bonetti G A et al. Preventive treatment of ectopically erupting maxillary permanent canines by extraction of deciduous canines and first molars: a randomized clinical trial. *Am J Orthod Dentofacial Orthop*. 2011, 139(3): 316-23.
***** Boyd RL. Esthetic orthodontic treatment using the invisalign appliance for moderate to complex malocclusions. *J Dental Educ.* 2008, 72(8): 948-67.
32. Bradlaw R. An inheritance of dwarfed or absent maxillary lateral incisors in three generations. *Inter J Orthod & Dent Child.* 1935, 21(5): 439-44.
33. Brusotti C & Collesano V. [Etiology and pathogensis of impacted teeth.] *Dental Cadmos.* 1980, 48(7): 21-5.
34. Brudevold F, Tehrani A & Bakhos Y. Intraoral mineralization of abraded dental enamel. *J Dent Res.* 1982, 61(3): 456-9.

35. Buisson C. Examen radiographique des canines incluses et indications thérapéutiques. *Anneles Odt Stomatologiques.* 1957, 6: 293-310.
36. Burstone CJ & Koenig HA. Forces systems from an ideal arch. *Am J Ort* .1974, 65(3): 270-89.
37. Burstone CJ. Variable-modulus orthodontics. *Am J Orthod.* 1981, 80(1): 1-16.
38. Burstone CJ & Goldberg AJ. Beta titanium: a new orthodontic alloy. *Am J Orthod.* 1980, 77(2): 121-32.
39. Burstone CJ, Qin B & Morton JY. Chinese NiTi wire – a new orthodontic alloy. *Am J Orthod.* 1985, 87(6): 445-52.
40. Burstone CJ & Koenig HA. Creative wire bending – the force system from step and V bends. *Am J Orthod Dentofacial Orthop.* 1988, 93(1): 59-67.
41. Burstone CJ. The segmented arch approach to space closure. *Am J Orthod.* 1982, 82(5): 361-78.
42. Burstone CJ & Koenig HA. Precision adjustment of the transpalatal lingual arch: computer arch form predetermination. *Am J Orthod.* 1981, 79(2): 115-33.
43. Burstone CJ & Pryputniewicz, RJ. Holographic determination of centres of rotation produced by orthodontic forces. *Am J Ort.* 1980, 77: 396-409.
44. Byloff-Clar, H. Argumentaciòn al tema [Extraction of first molar.] *Trans Eur Orthod Soc.* 1970, 46° Congress, 426.
45. Canut JA. Clinical management of the mandibular molars. *Am J Orthod.* 1975, 68(3): 277-89.
46. Case CS. The question of extraction in orthodontia. Reprint. *Am J Orthod.* 1964, 50(9): 660-91.
47. Cervera JA. *Syllabo de Ortodontia*. CEOA, 1973.
48. Cetlin NM & Ten Hoeve A. Nonextraction treatment. *J Clin Orthod.* 1983, 17(6): 396-413.
49. Chateau P, Heskia JE & Chassignol J. Contribution à l'etude des relations entre le voies respiratoires et l'ortopedie dento-faciale. *Orthod FR.* 1959, 30: 5-120.
50. Chimenti C, Colangelo P & Accivile E. Classificazioni ed eziopatogenesi dell'inclusione del canino superiore. *Min Stom.* 1990, 8(1): 59-69.
51. Christensen J & Fields HW. Space maintenance in the primary dentition. In: Pinkham JR et al, editors. *Pediatric Dentistry*. Philadelphia: WB Saunders, 1988.
52. Clark CA. Method of ascertaining the relative position of unerupted teeth by means of film radiographs. *Proc Ray Soc Med.* 1910, 3: 87-90.
53. Conforth G. A computerized study of the behavior of the axis during treatment and posttreatment MS Thesis, Lorna Linda University, 1976.
54. Cox NH & van der Linden FP. Facial harmony. *Am J Orthod.* 1971, 60(2): 175-83.
55. Crain G & Sheridan JJ. Susceptibility to caries and periodontal disease after posterior air-rotor stripping. *J Clin Orthod*, 1990, 24(2): 84-5.
56. Creekmore TD & Radney LJ. Fränkel appliance therapy: orthopedic or orthodontic? *Am J Orthod.* 1983, 83(2): 89-108.
57. Creekmore TD. The importance of interbracket width in orthodontic tooth movement. *J Clin Orthod*. 1976, 10(7): 530-4.
58. Cryer BS. Third molar eruption and the effect of extraction of adjacent teeth. *Dent Practit.* 1967, 17: 405-18.
59. Dake ML & Sinclair PM. A comparison of the Ricketts and Tweed-type arch levelling techniques. *Am J Orthod Dentofacial Orthop*. 1989, 95(1): 72-8.
60. Dale JG. Guidance of occlusion: serial extraction. In: Graber TM, Swain BF, editors. *Orthodontics: current principles and techniques*. St Louis: Mosby, Year Book, 1985.

61. Damon OH. Clinical study of extraoral high-pull tradition to the maxilla utilizing a heavy force: a cephalometric analysis of dentofacial changes. MSD Thesis, University of Washington, 1970.
62. Darque-Boileau MJ. Influence des forces extra-orale sur l'ange ANB. *J Edg.* 1986, 13: 58-78.
63. Daugaard-Jensen I. Extraction of the first molars in discrepancy cases. *Am J Orthod.* 1973, 64(2): 115-36.
64. David JA. Functional appliance does job of oral surgeon. *Funct Ort.* 1988, 5(1): 29-33.
65. Dawson PE et al. *Les problèmes de l'occlusion: évaluation, diagnostic et traitement.* Paris: J Prélat, 1977, Chap 20: 243.
66. Delaire J. Considérations sur la croissance faciale (en particulier du maxillaire supérieur). (Deductions thérapeutiques). *Rev Stom.* 1971, 72: 57-76.
67. Delaire J. Considérations sur l'accroissement du prémaxillaire chez l'homme. *Rev Stom.* 1974, 75: 951-70.
68. Delaire J. Le syndrome prognathique mandibulaire. *Orthod Fr.* 1976, 1: 203-19.
69. Delaire J et al. Quelques resultats des tractions extra-orales à appui fronto-mentonnier dans le traitement des malformations maxillo-mandibulaires de classe III et des sequelles osseuses des fentes labio-maxillaires. *Rev Storm.* 1972, 73: 633-42.
70. Demange C & François B. Measuring and charting interproximal enamel removal. *J Clin Orthod.* 1990, 24(7): 408-12.
71. Dermaut LR, De Munck A. Apical root resorption of upper incisors caused by intrusive movement: a radiographic study. *Am J Orthod Dentofacial Orthop.* 1986, 90(4): 321-6.
72. Dewel BF. A critical analysis of serial extraction in orthodontic treatment. *Am J Orthod.* 1959, 45: 424-55.
73. Dibbets JMH & van der Weele LT. Extraction, orthodontic treatment, and craniomandibular dysfunction. *Am J Orthod Dentofacial Orthop.* 1991, 99(3): 210-9.
74. Di Malta E. *Le Terze Classi.* Milano: Masson, 1989.
75. Drescher D, Bourauel C & Schumacher HA. Frictional forces between bracket and arch wire. *Am J Orthod Dentofacial Orthop.* 1989, 96(5): 397-404.
76. Drobocky OB & Smith RJ. Changes in facial profile during orthodontic treatment with extraction of four first premolars. *Am J Orthod Dentofacial Orthop.* 1989, 95(3): 220-30.
77. Ducheyne P & Hastings GW. *Metal and Ceramic Biomaterials. Vol II. Strength and Surface.* Boca Raton, Fla: CRC Press, 1984.
78. Edwards J. The diastema, the frenum and the frenectomy: a clinical study. *Am J Orthod.* 1977, 71(5): 489-508.
79. Egermark-Eriksson I, Carlsson CE & Ingervall B. Prevalence of mandibular dysfunction and orofacial parafunction in 7-, 11- and 15-year-old Swedish children. *Eur J Ort.* 1981, 3(3): 163-72.
1**1 Egermark I &Thilander B. Craniomandibular disorders and orthodontic treatment: an evaluation from childhood to adulthood. *Am J Orthod Dentofacial Orthop.* 1992, 101(1): 28-34.
161. El-Mangoury NH et al. In-vivo remineralization after air-rotor stripping. *J Clin Orthod.* 1991, 25(2): 75-8.
80. Enlow DH. A study of the post-natal growth and remodeling of bone. *Am J Anat.* 1962, 110(2): 79-101.
81. Enlow DH. Growth and the problem of the local control mechanism. *Am J Anat.* 1973, 136: 403-5.

82. Enlow DH. Enlow on craniofacial growth. *J Clin Orthod.* 1983, 17(10): 669-79.
83. Enlow DH & Bang S. Growth and remodeling of the human maxilla. *Am J Orthod.* 1965, 51: 446-64.
84. Enlow DH et al. A procedure for the analysis of sutural and remodeling growth in the human face. *Am J Orthod.* 1969, 56: 6-23.
85. Epstein WN. Analysis of changes in molar relationships by means of extraoral anchorage (head-cap) in treatment of malocclusion. *Angle Orthod.* 1948, 18: 63-9.
86. Ericsson I & Lindhe J. Effect of longstanding jiggling on experimental marginal periodontitis in the beagle dog. *J Clin Periodontol.* 1982, 9: 497-503.
87. Farrar WB & McCarty WL. A Clinical *Outline of Temporomandibular Joint Diagnosis and Treatment.* 7th edn. Montgomery: Normandie Study Group for TMJ Disfunction, 1983.
88. Fillion D. *De la Mutilanon à la Sculpture Amélaire Progressive*. Paris: Geol Dec, 1991.
89. Fillion D. Apport de la sculpture amèlaire interproximale à l'orthodontie de l'adulte (premiere partie). *Rev Orthop Dento Faciale.* 1992, 26: 279-93.
90. Fillion D. Appart de la sculpture amélaire interproximale à l'orthodontie de l'adulte (deuxième partie). *Rev Orthop Dento Faciale.* 1993, 27: 189-214.
91. Fournier A et al. Orthodontic considerations in the treatment of maxillary impacted canines. *Am J Orthod.* 1982, 81(3): 236-9.
92. Fontenelle A. Esthétique en orthodonties: les appareillages linguaux. *Acta Odont.* 1988, 164: 743-66.
93. Flander LB. Influence of chronic respiratory allergy on orofacial growth. *Am J Phys Anthrop.* 1982, 57: 188.
94. Franceschi C. Prevenzione delle malposizioni dentali e abitudini viziate nel bambino. *Medico e Paziente.* 1991, 14.
95. Fränkel R. The treatment of Class II, Division 1 malocclusion with functional correctors. *Am J Orthod.* 1969, 55(3): 265-75.
96. Fränkel R. *Technik und Handhabung der Funktionsregler.* Berlin: VEB Verlag Vilk und Gesundheit, 1976.
97. Fränkel R. A functional approach to orofacial orthopedics. *Br J Orthod.* 1980, 7: 41-51.
98. Fujita K. [Development of lingual-bracket technique. (Esthetic and hygienic approach to orthodontic treatment.) (Part 2) Manufacture and treatment.] *Shika Rikogaku Zasshi.* 1978, 19(46): 87-94.
99. Funk AC. Mandibular response to headgear therapy and its clinical significance. *Am J Orthod.* 1967, 53(3): 182-216.
100. Genone B, Olivotto R & Ronmin M. Edgewise della scuola di Tweed: il divenire di una concezione di ortognatodonzia clinica. *Mondo Ortod.* 1983, 1: 39-44.
101. Gianelly AA et al. Condylar position and extraction treatment. *Am J Orthod Dentofacial Orthop.* 1988, 93(3): 201-5.
102. Gianelly AA, Cozzani M & Boffa J. Condylar position and maxillary first premolar extraction. *Am J Orthod Dentofacial Orthop*. 1991, 99(5): 473-6.
103. Gianelly AA. *La Tecnica Bidimensionale.* Orteam, 1994.
104. Gianelly AA. *Considerazioni Sulle Tecniche di Trattamento delle I-II-III Classi*. La Spezia: Collana d' Ortodonzia, Centro Studi di Ortodonzia, 1978.
105. Gianelly AA, Arena SA & Bernstein L. A comparison of Class II treatment changes noted with the light wire, edgewise and Fränkel appliances. *Am J Orthod.* 1984, 86(4): 269-76.
106. Giannì E. *La Nuova Ortognatodonzia*. Padova: Piccin, 1980.

2** Gianelly AA. Rapid palatal expansion in the absence of crossbites: added value?. *Am J Orthod Dentofacial Orthop*. 2003, 124(4): 362-5.

3** Gianelly AA. Distal movement of maxillary molars. *Am J Orthod Dentofacial Orthop.* 1998, 114(1): 66-72.

8*1 Gianelly AA, Cozzani M & Boffa J. Condylar position and upper first premolars extraction. *Am J Orthod Dentofacial Orthop*. 1991, 99(5): 473-6.

107. Goldin B. Labial root torque: effect on the maxilla and incisor root apex. *Am J Orthod Dentofacial Orthop.* 1989, 95(3): 208-19.

108. Gonzáles-Ulloa M & Stevens E. Role of chin correction in profileplasty. *Plast Reconstr Surg*. 1968, 41(5): 477-86.

8**1 Gonzalez YM, Greene CS & Mohl ND. Technological devices in the diagnosis of temporomandibular disorders. *Oral Maxillofac Surg Clin North Am*. 2008, 20(2): 211-20, vi.

109. Greenfield RL. Apparecchiature a pistoni fissa per una correzione rapida della Classe II. *Mondo Ort*. 1996, 2: 161-9.

110. Greenspan RA. Reference charts for controlled extraoral force application to maxillary molars. *Am J Orthod.* 1970, 58(5): 486-91.

111. Gros E. Tractions extrabuccales sur baillon rétro-labial. Vol 37:691Orthod Fr. 1966

112. Gundlach KKH. Der naso-pharinx bei der kieferkompression kraniometrische und rhinologische daten. *Dtsch Zanhartzl.* 1976, 31: 792-9.

113. Haas AJ. Palatal expansion: just the beginning of dentofacial orthopedics. *Am J Orthod*. 1970, 57(3): 219-55.

114. Harry MR & Sims MR. Root resorption in bicuspid intrusion. A scanning electron microscope study. *Angle Orthod.* 1982, 52(3): 235-58.

115. Harvold EP, Chierici G & Vargervik K. Experiments on the development of dental malocclusions. *Am J Orthod*. 1972, 61(1): 38-44.

116. Harvold EP. Neuromuscular and morphological adaptations in experimentally induced oral respiratiom. In: McNamara, JA & Riddens, KA editors. *Nasorespiratory Function and Craniofacial Growth*. Monograph 9, Craniofacial growth series, Centre for human growth and development, University of Michigan, Ann Arbor, 1979, 149-64, Stockholm, Sweden, 1985.

117. Harvold EP. *The Activator in Interceptive Orthodontics*. St Louis: CV Mosby Co, 1974.

118. Heckmann U. The treatment of anterior open bite with removable appliances. *Trans Eur Orthod Soc.* 1974: 173-80.

119. Herbst E. Dreissigjahrige erfahrungen mit dem retentions-schamier. Part 1. *Zahn Rundschr*. 1934, 43: 1515-24.

120. Herren P. The activator's mode of action. *Am J Orthod.* 1959, 45(7): 512-27.

121. Hirose H et al. Cephalometric evaluation on the orthopedic therapy applied to the skeletal open bite patients during the growth periods. *J Japan Ort Soc*. 1981, 40: 365-77.

122. Hixon EH & Oldfather RE. Estimation of the sizes of unerupted and bicuspid teeth. *Angle Orthodont.* 1958, 28: 236-40.

123. Hocevar RA. Begg-edgewise diagnosis-determined totally individualized orthodontic technique: introduction to clinical applications. *Am J Orthod Dentofacial Orthop.* 1987, 92(1): 50-69.

124. Holdaway RA. Soft tissue cephalometric analysis and its use in orthodontic treatment planning. *Am J Orthod.* 1983, Part I: 84(1): 1-28, Part II: 85(4): 279-93.

125. Howard CC. Inherent growth and its influence on malocclusion. *J Am Dent Assoc.* 1932, 19: 642-51.

126. Huggins DG & McBride LJ. The eruption of the lower third molars following the loss of lower second molars: a longitudinal cephalometric study. *Brit J Orthod.* 1978, 5(1): 13-20.
127. Hunter WS, Balbach DH & Lamphiear DE. The heritability of attained growth in the human face. *Am J Orthod.* 1970, 58(2): 126-34. .
128. Jacoby H. The etiology of maxillary canine impactions. *Am J Orthod.* 1983, 84(2): 125-32.
129. Jann W & Engel GA. Treatment of skeletal openbite cases by molar extraction. *Proc Found Orth Res.* 1978, 33-38.
130. Jarabak JR & Fizzel JA. *Technique and treatment with light-wire edgewise appliances.* St. Louis: Mosby Co, 1972.
177. Jensen E et al. Mesiodistal crown diameters of the deciduous and permanent teeth in individuals. *J Dent Res.* 1957, 36(1): 39-47.
131. Jeiroudi MT. Enamel fracture caused by ceramic brackets. *Am J Orthod Dentofacial Orthop.* 1991, 99(2): 97-9.
132. Joho JP, Grobéty D & Pfeiffer JP. [The origin of class II.] *SSO Schwiez Monatsschr Zahnheilkd.* 1978, 88(8): 869-73.
133. Khier SE, Brantley WA & Fournelle RA. Bending properties of superelastic and non-superelastic nickel-titanium orthodontic wires. *Am J Orthod Dentofacial Orthop.* 1991, 99(4): 310-8.
5**1 Katzberg RW et al. Orthodontics and temporomandibular joint internal derangement. *Am J Orthod Dentofacial Orthop.* 1996, 109(5): 515-20.
6**1 Kim MR, Graber TM & Viana MA. Orthodontics and temporomandibular disorder: a meta-analysis. *Am J Orthod Dentofacial Orthop.* 2002, 121(5): 438-46.
134. King EW. Cervical anchorage in Class II division I treatment: a cephalometric appraisal. *Angle Orthod.* 1957, 27: 98-104.
5** Kizinger GSM et al. Efficiency of a pendulum appliance for molar distalization related to the second and third molar eruption stage. *Am J Orthod Dentofacial Orthop.* 2004, 125(1): 8-23.
135. Kloehn SJ. Guiding alveolar growth and eruption of the teeth to reduce treatment time and produce a more balanced denture and face. *Angle Orthod.* 1947, 17(1-2): 10-33.
136. Kloehn SJ. Evaluation of cervical anchorage force in treatment. *Angle Orthod.* 1961, 31(2): 91-104.
137. Kokich V et al. Ankylosed teeth as abutments for maxillary protraction: a case report. *Am J Orthod.* 1985, 88(4): 303-7.
138. Korn M. *Postural Orthodontics.* Boston, Ma, Tuft University. 1985.
139. Koski K. Some aspects of the growth of the cranial base and the upper face. *Odont Tidskr.* 1960, 68: 344-358.
140. Koski K. Growth changes in the relationships between some basicranial planes and the palatal plane. *Suomen Hammaslaak Toim.* 1961, 57: 15-26.
141. Koski K. Growth potential of the mandibular condyle in light of transplantation studies. *Studieweek.* 1965, 35.
142. Koski K. Cranial growth centers: facts or fallacies? *Am J Orthod.* 1968, 54(8): 566-83.
143. Koski K & Odont D. Variability of the craniofacial skeleton. An exercise in roentgen-cephalmoetry. *Am J Orth.* 1973, 64(2): 188-96.
144. Kremenak CR et al. Orthodontics as a risk factor for temporomandibular disorders (TMD). II. *Am J Orthod Dentofacial Orthop.* 1992, 101(1): 21-7.
2**1 Kremenak CR. Orthodontic risk factors for temporomandibular disorders (TMJ). I. *Am J Orthod Dentofacial Orthop.* 1992, 101(1): 13-20.

145. Kristerson L. Autotransplantation of teeth. Influence of different factors on periodontal and pulp healing. Thesis, Kongl Karolinska Medio Chrirurgiska Institutet.
146. Kubein D, Jäger A & Bormann V. [System for distalization of the upper 6-year molar with indirect headgear.] *Forlschr Kieferorthop.* 1984, 45(2): 128-40.
147. Kusy RP. Comparison of nickel-titanium and beta titanium wire sizes to conventional orthodontic arch wire materials. *Am J Orthod.* 1981, 79(6): 625-9.
148. Kusy RP & Whitley JQ. Effects of surface roughness on the coefficients of friction in model orthodontic systems. *J Biomech.* 1990, 23(9): 913-25.
149. Kutin G & Hawes RR. Posterior cross-bites in the deciduous and mixed dentitions. *Am J Orthod.* 1969, 56(5): 491-504.
150. Langlade M. *Thérapeutique Orthodontique*. Paris: Maloine, 1978.
151. Langlade M. *Terapia Ortodontica*. Milan: Scienza e tecnica dentistica, Ed Internazionali, 1982.
152. Langlade M. Contribution à la thérapeutique orthopédique fonctionnelle simplifiée. Soulet-Besombes. *Orthod Fr.* 1966, 37: 487-90.
153. Langlade M. Problema degli eccessi verticali di alto grado. *Communication a la Société Italienne d'Orthodontie*. Sept, 1982.
154. Lawlor J. The effects on the lower third molar of the extraction of the lower second molar. *Brit J Orthod.* 1978, 5(2): 99-103.
155. Leclere JF. Etat de surface de l'émail après remodelage amélaire proximat. *J Edge.* 1992, 25: 25-34.
156. Lehman R. A consideration of the advantages of second molar extractions in orthodontics. *Europ J Orthod.* 1979, 1: 119-24.
157. Linge BO & Linge L. Apical root resorption in upper anterior teeth. *Eur J Orthod.* 1983, 5(3): 173-83.
158. Little R, Riedel RA & Artun J. An evaluation of changes in mandibular anterior alignment from l0 to 20 years post retention. *Am J Orthod Dentofacial Orthop.* 1988, 93(5): 423-8.
159. Little R. Stabilità e recidiva dell'allineamento e della forma dell'arcata dentale. *Ortognatodonzia Italiana*. 1994, 3(2): 179-93.
160. Luecke PE & Johnston LE. The effect of maxillary first premolar extraction and incisor retraction on mandibular position: testing the central dogma of "functional orthodontics". *Am J Orthod Dentofacial Orthop.* 1992, 101(1): 4-12
1** Lundner AS & Warunek SP. Patent nasopalatine after rapid maxillary expansion. *Am J Orthod Dentofacial Orthop*. 2006, 130(1): 96-9.
162. Masotti D. Collaborazione tra logopedia e ortodonzia: la spinta in avanti della lingua. *Logopedia Contemporanea.* 1987, 4: 3.
163. Mclnaney JB, Adams RM & Freeman M. A nonextraction approach to crowded dentitions in young children: early recognition and treatment. *J Am Dent Assoc.* 1980, 101(2): 251-7.
164. McNamara JA. Forma e funzione degli apparecchi funzionali in ortognatodonzia. *Quaderno SIDO*. 1985, 22: 49-59.
165. McNamara JA et al. Cephalometric standards of adults with well-balanced faces. Unpublished data.
166. Melsen B, Agerbaek N & Markenstam G. Intrusion of incisors in adult patients with marginal bone loss. *Am J Orthod Dentofacial Orthop*. 1989, 96(3): 232-41.
167. Melsen B. Treatment problems in adult patients. *Studieweek. Am J Orthod Dentofacial Orthop* 1980, 219-36
168. Melsen B et al. New attachment through periodontal treatment and orthodontic intrusion. *Am J Ort Dentofac Orthop.* 1988, 94(2): 104-16.

169. Merlini C et al. [Retained teeth, impacted teeth: diagnostic, clinical, and therapeutic problems.] *Mondo Ortod*. 1983, 8(4): 9-26.
170. Merrifield LL. The profile line as an aid in critically evaluating facial esthetics. *Am J Orthod*. 1966, 52(11): 804-22.
171. Merrifield LL. *Directional Force Treatment Syllabus*. CH Tweed International Foundation for Orthodontic Research, Ed Tucson, 1985.
7** Mihalik CA, Proffit WR & Philips C. Long-term follow-up of Class II adults treated with orthodontic camouflage: a comparison with orthognatic surgery outcomes. *Am J Orthod Dentofacial Orthop*. 2003, 123(3): 266-78.
172. Miura F et al. The super-elastic property of the Japanese NiTi alloy wire for use in orthodontics. *Am J Orthod Dentofacial.* 1986, 90(1): 1-10.
7**1 Mohl ND. Reliability and validity of diagnostic modalities for temporomandibular disorders. *Adv Dent Res.* 1993, 7(2): 113-9.
173. Moyers RE. *Handbook of Orthodontics*. Ed 3. Chicago: Mosby, Year Book, 1973.
174. Molina M. *Disturbi dell' Articolazione Temporomandibolare*. Milano: Ilic Ed, 1994.
175. Mongini F. Condylar remodeling after occlusal therapy. *J Prosthet Dent*. 1980, 43(5): 568-77.
176. Moore A. Observations on mouthbreathing. *Bull NZ Soc Periodont*. 1972, 33: 9-11.
178. Moss ML. The functional matrix. In: Kraus BS & Riedel RA, editors. *Visitas in Orthodontics*. Philadelphia: Lea & Febiger, 1962.
179. Moss ML. Twenty years of functional cranial analysis. *Am J Orthod*. 1972, 61(5): 479-85.
180. Moss ML. Genetics, epigenetics and causation. *Am J Orthod.* 1981, 80(4): 366-75.
181. Moss ML & Rankow RM. The role of the functional matrix in mandibular growth. *Angle Orthod.* 1968, 38(2): 95-103.
182. Moss JP. Function-fact or fiction? *Am J Orthod.* 1975, 67(6): 625-46.
183. Nance HN. The limitations of orthodontic treatment; mixed dentition diagnosis and treatment. *Arm J Orthod*. 1947, 33(4): 177-223.
184. Nelson BG. What does extraoral anchorage accomplish? *Am J Orthod.* 1952, 38(6): 422-34.
185. Newman WG. Possible etiologic factors in external root resorption. *Am J Orthod.* 1975, 67(5): 522-39.
4** Ngantung V, Nanda RS & Bowman SJ. Post-treatment evaluation of the distal jet appliance. *Am J Orthod Dentofacial Orthop*. 2001, 120(2): 178-85.
186. Nidoli G, Macchi A & Lazzati M. La tecnica degli attacchi linguali. Varese: Forestadental giugno, 1992.
187. Owen AH III. Frontal facial changes with the Fränkel appliance. *Angle Orthod*. 1988, 58(3): 257-87.
188. Pancherz H. *La Terapia delle II Classi Scheletriche con Cerniera di Herbst*. Sillabus SIDO, 1992.
*** Pandis N, Polychronopoulou A, & Eliades T. Self-ligating vs conventional brackets in the treatment of mandibular crowding: a prospective clinical trial of treatment duration and dental effects. *Am J Orthod Dentofacial Orthop*. 2007, 132(2): 208-15.
189. Paradise I & Bluestone CD. Longitudinal study of nasopharyngeal airway obstruction. *J Speech Hear Disord.* 1965, 30: 87-99.
190. Parfitt GI, Mjor IA. A clinical evaluation of local gingival recession in children. *J Dentistry for Children*. 1964, 31: 3.
191. Paskow H. Self-alignment following interproximal stripping. *Am J Orthod*. 1970, 58(3): 240-9.

1*2 Patterson TR, Staja SR & Tuncay OC. Outcomes of an inappropriate orthodontic treatment plan – a case series. *Prog Orthod.* 2000, (1)1: 37-42.
192. Patti Balestrino D & van Venrooy JR. Meccanica di scorrimento nel trattamento ortodontico con arco diritto. *Mondo Ort.* 1990, 15(2): 179-90.
193. Pearson LE. Vertical control in treatment of patients having backward-rotational growth tendencies. *Angle Orthod.* 1978, 48(2): 132-40.
194. Peck H & Peck S. A concept of facial esthetics. *Angle Orthod.* 1970, 40(4): 284-318.
195. Peck H & Peck. S. An index for assessing tooth shape deviations as applied to the mandibular incisors. *Am J Orthod.* 1972, 61(4): 384-401.
196. Petrovic AG, Stutzmann JJ (note di) Deli R. Crescita saggitale della mandibola mediante edgewise ed elastici di II classe. *Ortognatodonzia Italiana.* 1994, III(1): 93-108.
197. Petrovic AG, Stutzmann J & Oudet C. Orthopedic appliances modulate the bone formation in the mandible as a whole. *Swed Dent J Suppl.* 1982, 15: 192-201.
198. Planas P. Equi-plan. *Ort Fr.* 1981, 31.
199. Planchè P. TI nuovo edgewise. *Mondo Ort.* 1992, 1: 63-75.
200. Prattern DH et al. Frictional resistance of ceramic and stainless steel orthodontic brackets. *Am J Orthod Dentofacial Orthop.* 1990, 98(5): 398-403.
201. Proffit WR. *Ortodonzia Moderna.* Masson S.p.A, 1995.
202. Quinn RS & Yoshikawa DK. A reassessment of force magnitude in orthodontics. *Am J Orthod.* 1985, 88(3): 252-60.
203. Ramfjord SP & Ash MM. *Occlusion.* Philadelphia; WB Saunders Ed, 1971.
204. Ranta R. Treatment of unilateral posterior crossbite: comparison of the quad-helix and removable plate. *ASDC J Dent Child.* 1988, 55(2): 102-4.
205. Reitan K. Tissue behavior during orthodontic tooth movement. *Am J Orthod.* 1960, 46(12): 881-900.
7*1 Reynders RM. Orthodontics and temporomandibular disorders: a review of the literature (1966-1988). *Am J Orthod Dentofacial Orthop.* 1990, 97(6): 463-71.
206. Ricketts RM. Mechanisms of mandibular growth: a series of inquires of the growth of the mandible. In: McNamara JA jr, editor. *Determinants of Mandibular Form and Growth.* University of Michigan, Ann Arbor, 1975: 77-100.
207. Ricketts RM et al. Third molar enucleation: diagnosis and technique. *J Calif Dent Assoc.* 1976, 4(4): 52-7.
208. Ricketts RM. Respiratory obstruction syndrome. *Am J Orthod.* 1968, 54(7): 495-507.
209. Ricketts RM et al. *Bioprogressive Therapy.* Denver: Rocky Mountain Orthodontics, 1979.
210. Ricketts RM. Esthetics, environment, and the law of lip relation. *Am J Orthod.* 1968, 54(4): 272-89.
211. Ricketts RM. Perspectives in the clinical application of cephalometrics. *Angle Orthod.* 1981, 51(2): 115-50.
212. Richardson M. [Development of 3rd molar impaction and its prevention.] *Mondo Orthod.* 1988, 13(5): 143-52.
213. Riedel RA. An analysis of dental relationships. *Am J Orthod.* 1957, 43: 103-19.
** Rinchuse DJ & Miles PG. Self ligating brackets: present and future. *Am J Orthod Dentofacial Orthop.* 2007; 132: 216-22.
* Rinchuse DJ, Rinchuse DJ & Kapur-Wadhwa R. Orthodontic appliance design. *Am J Orthod Dentofacial Orthop.* 2007; 131(1): 76-82.
214. Roth RH. Functional occlusion for the orthodontist. *J Clin Orthod.* 1981, 15(1): 32-40, 44-51.
215. Sadowsky C, Theisen TA & Sakols EI. Orthodontic treatment and temporomandibular joint sounds – a longitudinal study. *Am J Orthod.* 1991, 99(5): 441-7.

216. Salagnac JM. [Procedure to follow after postero-anterior traction with Delaire's orthopaedic mask in the treatment of class II lesions.] *Rev Stomatol Chir Maxillofac.* 1987, 88(5): 321-5.
217. Salzmann JA. Elastics. In: *Practice of Orthodontics.* 1983, 745.
218. Sander FG. Biomechanische untersuchungen zur bewegung des unterkiefers bei der Headgear-Aktivator Behandlung. *Fortschr Kieferorthop.* 1979, 40: 61-9.
219. Sassouni V. The face in five dimensions. Philadelphia: Centre for research in child growth, 1960.
220. Sassouni V & Nanda S. Analysis of dentofacial vertical proportions. *Am J Orthod.* 1969. 55: 109-23.
221. Schonherr E. Extraction of the first molar in orthodontic practice. *Trans Eur Orthod Soc.* 1970, 46° Congress, 389-402.
222. Schudy FF. Vertical growth versus anteroposterior growth as related to function and treatment. *Angle Orthod.* 1964, 34: 75-93.
223. Schwartz O, Bergmann P & Klausen B. Autotransplantation of human teeth. A life-table analysis of prognostic factors. *Int J Oral Surg.* 1985, 14(3): 245-58.
224. Schwarz AM. *Gebissregelung mit Platten.* Wien: Urban und Schwarzenberg, 1938.
225. Scott JH. *Dentofacial Development and Growth.* Oxford: Pergamon Press, 1967.
**** Scott P et al. Alignment efficiency of Damon 3 self-ligating and conventional orthodontic brackets systems. *Am J Orthod Dentofacial Orthop.* 2008; 134: 470-1.
226. Sheridan JJ. Air rotor stripping update. *J Clin Orthod.* 1987, 21(11): 781-8.
227. Sheridan JJ & Ledoux PM. Air-rotor stripping and proximal sealants. An SEM evaluation. *J Clin Orthod.* 1989, 23(12): 790-4.
228. Sicher H. *Oral Anatomy.* London: Henry Kimpton, 1952.
229. Slagsvold O & Bjercke B. *Autotransplantation of Premolars.* Göteborgs Tandläkare-Sällskaps Artkelserie. 1967, 351: 45-85.
230. Slagsvold O, Bjercke B. Autotransplantation of premolars in cases of missing anterior teeth. *Rep Congr Eur Orthod Soc.* 1970, 473-85.
231. Smith DI. The eruption of third molars following extraction of second molars. *Brit Soc Orthod Trans.* 1957, 55-7.
232. Spurrier S et al. Riassorbimento apicale radicolare in corso di trattamento ortodontiro in pazienti trattati endooonticamente e con denti vitali. *Am J Orthod,* Ed It. 1990, 4: 290-4.
233. Staggers JA. Vertical changes following first premolar extractions. *Am J Orthod Dentofacial Orthop.* 1994, 105(1): 19-24.
234. Steiner CC. Cephalometric for you and me. *Am J Orthod.* 1953, 39: 729-75.
235. Steward R et al. *Pediatric Dentistry: scientific foundation and clinical practice.* St Louis: Mosby Co, 1982.
236. Stockfisch H. Possibilities and limitations of the Kinetor bimaxillary appliance. *Trans Eur Orthod Soc.* 1971, 317-28.
237. Sugawara J et al. Long term effects on the skeletal profile by using a chin cup for mandibular prognathism. *Am J Orthod Dentofacial Orthop.* 1990, 98(2): 127-33.
238. Tanaka MM & Johnston LE. The prediction of the size of unerupted canines and premolars in contemporary orthodontic population. *J Aro Dent Assoc.* 1974, 88(4): 798-801.
239. Teuscher U. Terapia ortopedica con trazione e attivatore syllabus. *Quaderno SIDO.* 2, 1991.
240. Thilander B. Orthodontic tooth movement in periodontal therapy. In: Lindhe J, editor. *Textbook of Clinical Perodontology.* Copenhagen: Muskgaard, 1984.

241. Thordarson A, Zachrisson BU & Mjör IA. Remodelling of canines to the shape of lateral incisors by grinding: a long-term clinical and radiographic evaluation. *Am J Orthod Dentofacial Orthop.* 1991, 100(2): 123-32.
242. Tuenge RH & Elder JR. Posttreatment changes following extraoral high-pull traction to the maxilla of the Macaca mulatta. *Am J Orthod.* 1974, 66(6): 618-44.
243. Tweed CH. *Clinical Orthodontics.* St Louis: CV Mosby, 1966.
244. Van der Klaauw CJ. Cerebral skull and facial skull. A contribution to the knowledge of skull structure. *Arch Neerl Zoo.* 1946, 9: 16.
245. Van der Klaauw CJ. Size and position of the functional components of the skull. *Arch Neerl Zoo.* 1948, 9: 176.
246. Van der Klaauw CJ. Size and position of the functional components of the skull (continuation). *Arch Neerl Zoo.* 1951, 9: 369.
247. Van der KJaauw CJ. Size and position of the functional components of the skull (continuation). *Arch Neerl Zoo.* 1952, 9: 559.
248. Vanarsdall RL, Musich DR. Adult orthodontics: diagnosis and treatment. In: Graber TM, Swain BF, editors. *Orthodontics Current Principles and Techniques.* The CV Mosby Company, 1984.
249. Vanarsdall RL. Periodontal considerations in corrective orthodontics. In: *Principles of Orthodontic Tooth Movement.* Vol 2, chap 22.
1*4 Vanzin GD et al. Considerações sobre recessão gengival e proclinação excessiva dos incisivos inferiores. *J Bras Ortod Ortop.* 2003, 8: 318-25.
250. Verdon P. *Le Masque Orthopédique Facial.* Soc Franç D'Orthop Dento-Fac Comm. Nov. 1988.
251. Watnick SS. Inheritance of craniofacial morphology. *Angle Ort.* 1947, 17: 97.
1*1 Wennström JL et al. Some peridontal tissue reactions to orthodontic tooth movement in monkeys. *Clin Periodontol.* 1987, 14(3): 121-9.
252. Wieslander L. Intensive treatment of severe Class II malocclusions with a headgear-Herbst appliance in the early mixed dentition. *Am J Orthod.* 1984, 86(1): 1-13.
253. Williams R & Hosila FJ. The effect of different extraction sites upon incisor retraction. *Am J Orthod.* 1976, 69(4): 388-410.
254. Witt E & Komposch G. [Intermaxillary forces of bimaxillary appliances.] *Fortschr Kieferorthop.* 1971, 32(2): 345-52.
255. Wendell PO et al. The effects of chin cup therapy on the mandible: a longitudinal study. *Am J Orthod.* 1985, 87(4): 265-74.
256. Woodside DG, Metaxas A & Altuna G. The influence of functional appliance therapy on glenoid fossa remodeling. *Am J Orthod Dentofacial Orthop.* 1987, 92(3): 181-98.
257. Woodside DG. The Harvold-Woodside activator. In: Graber TM, Neuman B, editors. *Removable Orthodontics.* Ed 2. Philadelphia: WB Saunders Co, 1984.
258. Wright CH. A study of the maxillary sutures. *Dent Cosmos.* 1911, 52: 633.
1*3 Yared KF, Zenobio EG & Pacheco W. Periodontal status of mandibular central incisors after orthodontic proclination in adults. *Am J Orthod Dentofacial Orthop.* 2006, 130(1):6 e 1-8.
259. Zachrisson BU. Improving orthodontic results in cases with maxillary incisors missing. *Am J Orthod.* 1978, 73(3): 274-89.